NEUROLOGY MCQs
for Postgraduate and Superspecialty Medical Entrance Examinations

NEUROLOGY MCQs
for Postgraduate and Superspecialty Medical Entrance Examinations

Based on 20th Edition of Harrison's Prinicples of Internal Medicine

Dr Ajay Mathur
Senior Professor
Department of Medicine
SMS Medical College and Hospital
Jaipur, Rajasthan, India

Foreword
Dr Ramesh Roop Rai

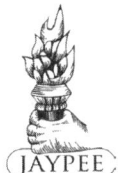

JAYPEE BROTHERS MEDICAL PUBLISHERS
The Health Sciences Publisher
New Delhi | London | Panama

Jaypee Brothers Medical Publishers (P) Ltd.

Headquarters
Jaypee Brothers Medical Publishers (P) Ltd
4838/24, Ansari Road, Daryaganj
New Delhi 110 002, India
Phone: +91-11-43574357
Fax: +91-11-43574314
E-mail: jaypee@jaypeebrothers.com

Overseas Offices

J.P. Medical Ltd
83, Victoria Street, London
SW1H 0HW (UK)
Phone: +44 20 3170 8910
Fax: +44 (0)20 3008 6180
E-mail: info@jpmedpub.com

Jaypee-Highlights Medical Publishers Inc
City of Knowledge, Bld. 235, 2nd Floor, Clayton
Panama City, Panama
Phone: +1 507-301-0496
Fax: +1 507-301-0499
E-mail: cservice@jphmedical.com

Jaypee Brothers Medical Publishers (P) Ltd
Bhotahity, Kathmandu, Nepal
Phone: +977-9741283608
E-mail: kathmandu@jaypeebrothers.com

Website: www.jaypeebrothers.com
Website: www.jaypeedigital.com

© 2019, Jaypee Brothers Medical Publishers

The views and opinions expressed in this book are solely those of the original contributor(s)/author(s) and do not necessarily represent those of editor(s) of the book.

All rights reserved. No part of this publication may be reproduced, stored or transmitted in any form or by any means, electronic, mechanical, photocopying, recording or otherwise, without the prior permission in writing of the publishers.

All brand names and product names used in this book are trade names, service marks, trademarks or registered trademarks of their respective owners. The publisher is not associated with any product or vendor mentioned in this book.

Medical knowledge and practice change constantly. This book is designed to provide accurate, authoritative information about the subject matter in question. However, readers are advised to check the most current information available on procedures included and check information from the manufacturer of each product to be administered, to verify the recommended dose, formula, method and duration of administration, adverse effects and contraindications. It is the responsibility of the practitioner to take all appropriate safety precautions. Neither the publisher nor the author(s)/editor(s) assume any liability for any injury and/or damage to persons or property arising from or related to use of material in this book.

This book is sold on the understanding that the publisher is not engaged in providing professional medical services. If such advice or services are required, the services of a competent medical professional should be sought.

Every effort has been made where necessary to contact holders of copyright to obtain permission to reproduce copyright material. If any have been inadvertently overlooked, the publisher will be pleased to make the necessary arrangements at the first opportunity. The **CD/DVD-ROM** (if any) provided in the sealed envelope with this book is complimentary and free of cost. **Not meant for sale.**

Inquiries for bulk sales may be solicited at: jaypee@jaypeebrothers.com

Neurology MCQs for Postgraduate and Superspecialty Medical Entrance Examinations

First Edition: **2019**

ISBN: 978-93-5270-810-9

Printed at Rajkamal Electric Press, Kundli, Haryana.

Foreword

As a professional who has been practicing medicine for over four decades now, I appreciate the value this book brings to the table in times like today. As we move from a largely descriptive era to the bullet-point generation, this academic initiative appears profoundly relevant.

Dr Mathur is bringing to the students and others, Neurology MCQs in an individual book format. This would be more handy and subject specific. The book has been a reference point for many medical entrance examinations and has left an impact on medical professionals who look for high quality of academic material.

Knowledge is a more processed form of information. Dr Mathur stays true to his pledge by presenting well-digested bytes of knowledge across different fields of medicine. His relying on good old word-of-mouth to make this book a success rather than enthusiastic marketing adds further credibility to his initiative. I recommend this book, without a shadow of doubt, to every medical professional who is looking to continue learning.

Dr Ramesh Roop Rai
Former, Professor and Head
Department of Gastroenterology
SMS Medical College and Hospital, Jaipur
Past President, Indian Society of Gastroenterology (2008)

Preface

Medicine, in all its vastness, needs to be understood in a way that makes most sense to how it is applied today. Memorizing each word is elusive and therefore, testing knowledge of a discipline remains an evergreen challenge.

It is a widely accepted fact that taking a quiz soon after studying helps one retain knowledge better and apply the lessons in practice. Multiple Choice Questions (MCQs) are an effective way of remembering the gist of the matter. This is precisely the reason why most examinations today follow this format. This book is committed to honing your skills to retain knowledge, help diagnose medical conditions, and maximize your impact, as a doctor.

A tremendous volume of questions has been generated over the past ten years. As it stands today, the approach needs to be adjusted according to the knowledge available at hand. This time around, my team has decided that each specialism merits its own edition. This will help you to study existing literature with recent advances in medicine and glean deeper insights into the subject matter. Based on the epic 20th edition of Harrison's Principles of Internal Medicine, published by The McGraw-Hill Companies, Inc., this book is dedicated to the field of Neurology in all its endless scope. This book caters to medical professionals at all levels. Not only can this be used by aspiring doctors to prepare for medical entrance examinations, but also by seasoned physicians to update knowledge long after it has been acquired. The book is sign-posted with references should the reader require elaboration on any given topic.

The book contains 3600 questions and still counting, I continue to keep my promise to continually refine the content of my book and chronicle the advances of medical science.

Dr Ajay Mathur

Contents

1. Neurologic Causes of Weakness and Paralysis 1
2. Numbness, Tingling, and Sensory Loss 5
3. Gait Disorders, Imbalance, and Falls 9
4. Confusion and Delirium 11
5. Dementia 13
6. Aphasia, Memory Loss, Hemispatial Neglect, Frontal Syndromes, and Other Cerebral Disorders 17
7. Disorders of the Eye 26
8. Pathobiology of Neurologic Diseases 37
9. Headache 39
10. Migraine and Other Primary Headache Disorders 42
11. Coma 49
12. Severe Acute Encephalopathies and Critical Care Weakness 60
13. Neuroimaging in Neurologic Disorders 65
14. Seizures and Epilepsy 68
15. Cerebrovascular Diseases 83
16. Ischemic Stroke 91
17. Intracranial Hemorrhage 103
18. Subarachnoid Hemorrhage 109
19. Alzheimer's Disease 114
20. Frontotemporal Dementia 120
21. Vascular Dementia 126
22. Dementia with Lewy Bodies 128
23. Parkinson's Disease 129
24. Tremor, Chorea, and Other Movement Disorders 141
25. Amyotrophic Lateral Sclerosis and Other Motor Neuron Diseases 152
26. Prion Diseases 157
27. Ataxic Disorders 161
28. Disorders of the Autonomic Nervous System 170
29. Trigeminal Neuralgia, Bell's Palsy, and Other Cranial Nerve Disorders 176

30.	Diseases of the Spinal Cord	186
31.	Transverse Myelitis	200
32.	Multiple Sclerosis	202
33.	Neuromyelitis Optica	210
34.	Peripheral Neuropathy	212
35.	Guillain-Barré Syndrome and Other Immune-Mediated Neuropathies	234
36.	Chronic Inflammatory Demyelinating Polyneuropathy	239
37.	Myasthenia Gravis and Other Diseases of the Neuromuscular Junction	241
38.	Muscular Dystrophies and Other Muscle Diseases	252
39.	Chronic Fatigue Syndrome	266
40.	Biology of Psychiatric Disorders	267
41.	Psychiatric Disorders	269
42.	Schizophrenia	283
43.	Primary and Metastatic Tumors of the Nervous System	289
44.	Encephalitis	295
45.	Acute Meningitis: Bacterial Meningitis	299
46.	Viral Meningitis	303
47.	Chronic and Recurrent Meningitis	306
48.	Brain Abscess and Empyema	307
49.	Alcohol and Alcohol Use Disorders	311

NEUROLOGY

Neurologic Causes of Weakness and Paralysis

1. Motor system dysfunction leads to?
Harrison's 20th Ed. Chapter 21, Page 135

A. Weakness or paralysis
B. Ataxia
C. Abnormal movements
D. All of the above

2. Normal motor function involves integrated muscle activity that is modulated by?
Harrison's 20th Ed. Chapter 21, Page 135

A. Red nucleus
B. Brainstem reticular formation
C. Lateral vestibular nucleus
D. All of the above

Normal motor function involves integrated muscle activity that is modulated by activity of cerebral cortex, basal ganglia, cerebellum, red nucleus, brainstem reticular formation, lateral vestibular nucleus and spinal cord.

3. Which of the following statements is false?
Harrison's 20th Ed. Chapter 21, Page 135

A. Myopathic weakness is most marked in proximal muscles
B. UMN lesion cause weakness in extensors and abductors of upper limb
C. UMN lesion cause weakness in flexors of lower limb
D. None of the above

4. Which of the following is related to muscle tone?
Harrison's 20th Ed. Chapter 21, Page 135

A. Spasticity
B. Rigidity
C. Paratonia (or gegenhalten)
D. All of the above

5. Tone is the resistance of a muscle to?
Harrison's 20th Ed. Chapter 21, Page 135

A. Active stretch
B. Passive stretch
C. Gravitational stretch
D. Anti-gravity stretch

Tone is the resistance of a muscle to passive stretch.

6. Increased muscle tone is found in?
Harrison's 20th Ed. Chapter 21, Page 135

A. Spasticity
B. Rigidity
C. Paratonia
D. All of the above

7. Which of the following is false about spasticity?
Harrison's 20th Ed. Chapter 21, Page 135

A. Associated with disease of upper motor neurons
B. Velocity-dependent
C. Affects antigravity muscles
D. None of the above

Tone is the resistance of a muscle to passive stretch. Spasticity is the increase in tone associated with disease of upper motor neurons. It is velocity-dependent, has a sudden release after reaching a maximum ("clasp-knife" phenomenon), and predominantly affects antigravity muscles (upper-limb flexors & lower-limb extensors).

8. Which of the following is false about rigidity?
Harrison's 20th Ed. Chapter 21, Page 135

A. Hypertonia present throughout the range of motion
B. Affects flexors & extensors equally
C. Occurs with certain extrapyramidal disorders
D. None of the above

9. Which of the following about 'Spasticity' is false?
Harrison's 20th Ed. Chapter 21, Page 135

A. Velocity-dependent
B. Sudden release at maximum
C. Affects antigravity muscles
D. None of the above

Spasticity refers to an increase in tone associated with disease of upper motor neurons. Spasticity is velocity-dependent, has a sudden release after reaching a maximum and predominantly affects the antigravity muscles (upper-limb flexors and lower-limb extensors).

10. Which of the following is false about paratonia?
Harrison's 20th Ed. Chapter 21, Page 135

A. Present throughout the range of motion
B. Affects flexors & extensors equally
C. Results from disease of the frontal lobes
D. None of the above

11. Which of the following about 'Paratonia' is false?
Harrison's 20th Ed. Chapter 21, Page 135

A. Also called gegenhalten
B. Increased tone varies irregularly
C. Present throughout range of motion
D. None of the above

12. Which of the following about 'Paratonia' is false?
Harrison's 20th Ed. Chapter 21, Page 135

A. Increased muscle tone
B. Affects flexors & extensors equally
C. Results from disease of frontal lobes
D. None of the above

Paratonia (gegenhalten) is increased tone that varies irregularly related to the degree of relaxation. It is present throughout the range of motion and affects flexors & extensors equally. Results from disease of frontal lobes.

13. Paratonic rigidity or gegenhalten results from disease of?
Harrison's 20th Ed. Chapter 21, Page 135

A. Frontal lobes
B. Temporal lobes
C. Parietal lobes
D. Occipital lobes

Paratonia (or gegenhalten) is increased tone that varies irregularly in a manner that may seem related to the degree of relaxation, is present throughout the range of motion, and affects flexors and extensors equally; it usually results from disease of the frontal lobes.

14. Which of the following about 'flaccidity' is false?
Harrison's 20th Ed. Chapter 21, Page 135

A. Weakness
B. Decreased tone
C. Disorder of motor unit
D. None of the above

Weakness with decreased tone is called flaccidity. It occurs with disorders of motor units which consists of a single lower motor neuron and all of the muscle fibers that are innervated by it.

15. Which of the following is false about fasciculation?
Harrison's 20th Ed. Chapter 21, Page 135

A. Visible twitch
B. Palpable twitch
C. Spontaneous discharge of a motor unit
D. None of the above

Fasciculations are visible or palpable twitch within a muscle due to spontaneous discharge of a motor unit.

16. Which of the following statements is false?
Harrison's 20th Ed. Chapter 21, Page 135

A. Distal weakness is likely to be neuropathic
B. Symmetric proximal weakness is likely to be myopathic
C. Fasciculations indicate that weakness is myopathic
D. Early atrophy indicate that weakness is neuropathic

Fasciculations & early atrophy indicate that weakness is neuropathic.

17. Which of the following is false about UMN lesions?
Harrison's 20th Ed. Chapter 21, Page 136

A. Distal muscle groups are affected more severely
B. Axial movements are spared
C. Rapid repetitive movements are slowed & coarse
D. Normal rhythmicity is disturbed

Rapid repetitive movements are slowed and coarse, however, normal rhythmicity is maintained.

18. Which of the following is false about upper motor neuron weakness?
Harrison's 20th Ed. Chapter 21, Page 136

A. Proximal muscle groups affected more than distal
B. Axial movements spared
C. Affects ability to perform rapid repetitive movements
D. Normal movement rhythmicity is maintained

In UMN lesions, distal muscle groups are affected more severely than proximal ones.

19. With corticobulbar involvement, which of the following is affected?
Harrison's 20th Ed. Chapter 21, Page 136

A. Pharyngeal muscles
B. Jaw muscles
C. Tongue muscles
D. Upper facial muscles

With corticobulbar involvement, weakness occurs in the lower face & tongue. Typically, extraocular, upper facial, pharyngeal & jaw muscles are spared.

20. Pseudobulbar palsy consists of all except?
Harrison's 20th Ed. Chapter 21, Page 136

A. Dysarthria
B. Dysphagia
C. Dystonia
D. Dysphonia

Bilateral corticobulbar lesions produce a pseudobulbar palsy which consists of dysarthria, dysphagia, dysphonia, bilateral facial weakness and a brisk jaw jerk.

21. Upper motor neurons have their cell bodies in which layer of the primary motor cortex?
Harrison's 20th Ed. Chapter 21, Page 136 Figure 21-1

A. 3
B. 4
C. 5
D. 6

Upper motor neurons have their cell bodies in layer V of the primary motor cortex which consists of the precentral gyrus, or Brodmann's area 4 and the premotor & supplemental motor cortex area 6.

22. What percentage of corticospinal axons remain ipsilateral in the anterior spinal cord?
Harrison's 20th Ed. Chapter 21, Page 136 Figure 21-1

A. 2–10%
B. 5–20%
C. 10–30%
D. 20–50%

At cervicomedullary junction, most corticospinal axons decussate into contralateral corticospinal tract of the lateral spinal cord, but 10–30% remain ipsilateral in the anterior spinal cord.

23. What proportion of pyramidal axons do not decussate and remain ipsilateral?
Harrison's 20th Ed. Chapter 21, Page 136 Figure 21-1

A. 2–10%
B. 5–15%
C. 10–30%
D. 20–35%

At cervicomedullary junction, most pyramidal axons decussate into contralateral corticospinal tract of lateral spinal cord, but 10–30% remain ipsilateral in anterior spinal cord.

24. Corticospinal neurons innervate most densely the lower motor neurons of which of the following?
Harrison's 20th Ed. Chapter 21, Page 136 Figure 21-1

A. Tongue
B. Extra-ocular muscles
C. Hand muscles
D. Muscles of facial expression

Corticospinal neurons innervate most densely the lower motor neurons of hand muscles.

25. Which of the following originates predominantly in the red nucleus?
Harrison's 20th Ed. Chapter 21, Page 136 Figure 21-1

A. Ventromedial bulbospinal pathways
B. Ventrolateral bulbospinal pathways
C. Posteromedial bulbospinal pathways
D. Posterolateral bulbospinal pathways

The descending ventromedial bulbospinal pathways consists of tectospinal pathway, vestibulospinal pathway and the reticulospinal pathway. The descending ventrolateral bulbospinal pathways originates predominantly in the red nucleus (rubrospinal pathway).

26. Which of the following facilitates distal limb muscles?
Harrison's 20th Ed. Chapter 21, Page 136 Figure 21-1

A. Tectospinal pathway
B. Vestibulospinal pathway
C. Reticulospinal pathway
D. Rubrospinal pathway

Pathways that influence axial & proximal muscles are tectospinal pathway, vestibulospinal pathway and reticulospinal pathway. Pathway that facilitates distal limb muscles is rubrospinal pathway.

27. Descending ventromedial bulbospinal pathways include?
Harrison's 20th Ed. Chapter 21, Page 136 Figure 21-1

A. Tectospinal pathway
B. Vestibulospinal pathway
C. Reticulospinal pathway
D. All of the above

Descending ventromedial bulbospinal pathways include tectospinal, vestibulospinal, and reticulospinal pathways. These pathways influence axial & proximal muscles and are involved in the maintenance of posture and integrated movements of the limbs and trunk.

28. All of the following are part of descending ventromedial bulbospinal pathways except?
Harrison's 20th Ed. Chapter 21, Page 136 Figure 21-1

A. Tectospinal pathway
B. Vestibulospinal pathway
C. Reticulospinal pathway
D. Rubrospinal pathway

Descending ventrolateral bulbospinal pathways, which originate predominantly in red nucleus (rubrospinal pathway), facilitate distal limb muscles. Bulbospinal system is also called extrapyramidal upper motor neuron system.

29. Which of the following is false about lower motor neuron weakness?
Harrison's 20th Ed. Chapter 21, Page 136 Figure 21-2

A. Due to loss of α neurons
B. Due to loss of γ motor neurons
C. Absent tendon stretch reflex suggests involvement of spindle afferent fibers
D. Fasciculations signify anterior horn cell disease

Loss of γ-motor neurons does not cause weakness but decreases muscle tone and attenuates the stretch reflexes elicited on examination.

30. Which of the following is false about motor neurons?
Harrison's 20th Ed. Chapter 21, Page 136 Figure 21-2

A. α motor neurons innervate extrafusal muscle fibers
B. γ motor neurons innervate intrafusal muscle fibers
C. α motor neuron receives direct excitatory input from corticomotoneurons & primary muscle spindle afferents
D. α motor neurons receive direct excitation from Renshaw cell interneurons

α-motor neurons receive direct inhibition from Renshaw cell interneurons.

31. Motor neurons receive excitatory input from?
Harrison's 20th Ed. Chapter 21, Page 136 Figure 21-2

A. Descending upper motor neuron pathways
B. Segmental sensory inputs
C. Interneurons
D. All of the above

32. Which of the following is false about myopathic weakness?
Harrison's 20th Ed. Chapter 21, Page 137

A. Due to disorders of muscle fibers
B. Due to defect in neuromuscular junctions
C. In EMG, size of each motor unit action potential is reduced
D. Distribution of weakness is distal

Distribution of myopathic weakness is typically proximal. Lower motor neuron weakness is most profound distally.

33. Which of the following about Pronator Drift is false?
N Engl J Med. 2013;369:16 e20

A. Indicates subtle upper motor neuron disorder
B. May be seen in inborn errors of metabolism
C. Performed with outstretched upper limbs with palms facing upward
D. None of the above

In the presence of an upper motor neuron lesion, the supinator muscles in the upper limb are weaker than the pronator muscles, and as a result, the arm drifts downward and the palm turns toward the floor.

34. Fatigable weakness is suggestive of disorders of?
Harrison's 20th Ed. Chapter 21, Page 137

A. Neuromuscular junction weakness
B. Myopathic weakness
C. Psychogenic weakness
D. All of the above

Fatigable weakness indicates towards disorders of neuromuscular junction, which cause functional loss of muscle fibers due to failure of their repeated activation.

35. Most lesions that produce hemiparesis are?
Harrison's 20th Ed. Chapter 21, Page 137

A. Above the foramen magnum
B. In the upper cervical cord
C. In the lower cervical cord
D. Any of the above

Most lesions that produce hemiparesis are above the foramen magnum.

36. In hemiparesis, simultaneous language disorder point to a lesion in?
Harrison's 20th Ed. Chapter 21, Page 137

A. Cerebral cortical lesion
B. Subcortical hemispheric lesion
C. Brainstem lesion
D. Any of the above

In hemiparesis, simultaneous language disorder point to a cortical lesion.

37. A "pure motor" hemiparesis of face, arm & leg is due to a lesion in?
Harrison's 20th Ed. Chapter 21, Page 137

A. Posterior limb of the internal capsule
B. Cerebral peduncle in the midbrain
C. Upper pons
D. Any of the above

38. Hemiparesis due to a cortical lesion is suggested by all except?
Harrison's 20th Ed. Chapter 21, Page 137

A. "Pure motor" hemiparesis
B. Disorders of visual-spatial integration
C. Apraxia
D. Seizures

Language disorders point to a cortical lesion. Homonymous visual field defects are due to either a cortical or a subcortical hemispheric lesion.

39. Chronic hemiparesis that evolves over months is due to?
Harrison's 20th Ed. Chapter 21, Page 137
- A. Sarcoidosis
- B. Primary central nervous system (CNS) lymphoma
- C. Chronic subdural hematoma
- D. All of the above

Chronic hemiparesis that evolves over months is due to a neoplasm/vascular malformation, chronic subdural hematoma, or a degenerative disease.

40. In the workup of a patient with proximal or distal weakness, the first investigation out of the following is?
Harrison's 20th Ed. Chapter 21, Page 137 Figure 21-3
- A. Computed tomography (CT)
- B. Magnetic resonance imaging (MRI)
- C. Electromyography (EMG) & Nerve conduction studies (NCS)
- D. Myelography

41. Disease of cerebral hemispheres that produces acute paraparesis is?
Harrison's 20th Ed. Chapter 21, Page 137
- A. Anterior cerebral artery ischemia
- B. Superior sagittal sinus or cortical venous thrombosis
- C. Acute hydrocephalus
- D. All of the above

42. Diseases of the cerebral hemispheres that produce acute paraparesis include?
Harrison's 20th Ed. Chapter 21, Page 137
- A. Unpaired anterior cerebral artery ischemia
- B. Superior sagittal sinus or cortical venous thrombosis
- C. Acute hydrocephalus
- D. All of the above

If hemispheric signs are present in a patient with subacute or chronic spastic paraparesis, a parasagittal meningioma or chronic hydrocephalus is likely.

43. Paraparesis can arise due to?
Harrison's 20th Ed. Chapter 21, Page 137
- A. Anterior horn cell disorders
- B. Cauda equina syndrome
- C. Peripheral neuropathies
- D. Any of the above

44. Acute paraparesis can be due to which of the following diseases of cerebral hemispheres?
Harrison's 20th Ed. Chapter 21, Page 137
- A. Superior sagittal sinus thrombosis
- B. Cortical venous thrombosis
- C. Acute hydrocephalus
- D. Any of the above

45. Acute monoparesis due to focal cortical ischemia is characterized by?
Harrison's 20th Ed. Chapter 21, Page 138
- A. Weakness is predominantly distal
- B. Weakness affects non-antigravity muscles
- C. Not associated with sensory impairment or pain
- D. All of the above

46. Weakness limited to respiratory muscles is due to?
Harrison's 20th Ed. Chapter 21, Page 138
- A. Motor neuron disease
- B. Myasthenia gravis
- C. Polymyositis/dermatomyositis
- D. All of the above

47. Which of the following is a cause of episodic generalized weakness?
Harrison's 20th Ed. Chapter 21, Page 138
- A. Myasthenia gravis
- B. Lambert-Eaton myasthenic syndrome
- C. Multiple sclerosis
- D. All of the above

48. Which of the following is false about 'Tetany'?
DeJong's The Neurologic Examination, 7th Ed. Page 766
- A. Tingling around mouth
- B. Manifestation of hypocalcemia
- C. Manifestation of respiratory alkalosis
- D. None of the above

49. Muscular rigidity may occur in?
DeJong's The Neurologic Examination, 7th Ed. Page 473
- A. Epilepsy
- B. Tetany
- C. Tetanus
- D. All of the above

Muscular rigidity may also occur in epilepsy, tetany, and tetanus.

50. Which of the following is a sign of tetany?
DeJong's The Neurologic Examination, 7th Ed. Page 767
- A. Chvostek's sign
- B. Trousseau's sign
- C. Hochsinger's sign
- D. All of the above

In Hochsinger's sign, when pressure on inner aspect of biceps muscle is applied, spasm and contraction of hand occurs in tetany. It is a variant of Trousseau sign.

51. Which of the following is a sign of tetany?
DeJong's The Neurologic Examination, 7th Ed. Page 767
- A. Schultze's sign
- B. Kashida's thermic sign
- C. Escherich's sign
- D. All of the above

52. Characteristics of dystonia include all except?
DeJong's The Neurologic Examination, 7th Ed. Page 767
- A. Ill sustained muscle contractions
- B. Repetitive twisting movements
- C. Abnormal posture
- D. Often has a genetic basis

Dystonia is a disorder characterized by sustained muscle contractions, resulting in repetitive twisting movements and abnormal posture. It often has a genetic basis.

53. Which of the following is labeled as the "Fifth vital sign"?
Harrison's 20th Ed. Chapter 9, Page 51
- A. Pain assessment
- B. Skin hue
- C. Cooperation of patient
- D. Colour of nails

Numbness, Tingling, and Sensory Loss

54. Which of the following is not a positive sensory symptom?
Harrison's 20th Ed. Chapter 22, Page 139
- A. Tingling
- B. Numbness
- C. Burning
- D. Pricking

Loss of sensory function (diminished or absent feeling) is termed negative phenomena experienced as numbness and abnormal finding on sensory examination.

55. Hyperesthesia means pain or increased sensitivity in response to?
Harrison's 20th Ed. Chapter 22, Page 139
- A. Touch
- B. Pain
- C. Warm or cold stimuli
- D. All of the above

Hyperesthesia means pain or increased sensitivity in response to touch.

56. Allodynia refers to?
Harrison's 20th Ed. Chapter 22, Page 139
- A. Pain on imagination
- B. Fear of pain
- C. Painful response to nonpainful stimulus
- D. Nonpainful response to painful stimulus

Painful response to nonpainful stimulus is termed allodynia. Like, elicitation of a painful sensation by application of a vibrating tuning fork.

57. Hyperpathia includes which of the following?
Harrison's 20th Ed. Chapter 22, Page 139
- A. Hyperesthesia
- B. Allodynia
- C. Hyperalgesia
- D. All of the above

Hyperpathia, a broad term, encompasses all the phenomena described by hyperesthesia, allodynia, and hyperalgesia. With hyperpathia, the threshold for a sensory stimulus is increased and perception is delayed, but once felt, is unduly painful.

58. Sense of vibration is tested with a tuning fork that vibrates at?
Harrison's 20th Ed. Chapter 22, Page 139
- A. 128 Hz
- B. 256 Hz
- C. 512 Hz
- D. Any of the above

Sense of vibration is tested with a tuning fork that vibrates at 128 Hz.

59. Cortical sensation are tested by?
Harrison's 20th Ed. Chapter 22, Page 139
- A. Two-point discrimination
- B. Bilateral simultaneous stimulation
- C. Graphesthesia
- D. All of the above

Commonly used tests of cortical function are two-point discrimination, touch localization, bilateral simultaneous stimulation & tests for graphesthesia and stereognosis.

60. Normal individuals can distinguish separation of points by what minimum distance in 2-PD test?
Harrison's 20th Ed. Chapter 22, Page 139
- A. 1 mm
- B. 3 mm
- C. 5 mm
- D. 7 mm

Normal individuals can distinguish separation of points by 3 mm distance in two-point discrimination test.

61. Which of the following is false about small-fiber polyneuropathy?
Harrison's 20th Ed. Chapter 22, Page 139
- A. Burning, painful dysesthesias
- B. Sparing of proprioception
- C. Sparing of motor function
- D. Absent tendon reflexes

62. Which of the following is false about large-fiber polyneuropathy?
Harrison's 20th Ed. Chapter 22, Page 139
- A. Vibration & position sense deficits
- B. Imbalance
- C. Absent tendon reflexes
- D. None of the above

Small-fiber polyneuropathies are characterized by burning, painful dysesthesias with reduced pinprick & thermal sensation but sparing of proprioception, motor function & deep tendon reflexes. Large-fiber polyneuropathies are characterized by vibration & position sense deficits, imbalance, absent tendon reflexes & variable motor dysfunction but preservation of most cutaneous sensation.

63. Which of the following is the prototypical positive symptom?
Harrison's 20th Ed. Chapter 22, Page 139
- A. Raw feelings
- B. Burning
- C. Tingling (pins and needles)
- D. Itch

The prototypical positive symptom is tingling (pins & needles). Other positive sensory phenomena include itch & altered sensations that are described as pricking, band like, lightning-like shooting feelings (lancinations), aching, knife like, twisting, drawing, pulling, tightening, burning, searing, electrical, or raw feelings. Positive phenomena represent excessive activity in sensory pathways.

64. Term hyperpathia includes which of the following?
Harrison's 20th Ed. Chapter 22, Page 139
- A. Hyperesthesia
- B. Allodynia
- C. Hyperalgesia
- D. All of the above

Term hyperpathia encompasses all phenomena described by hyperesthesia, allodynia & hyperalgesia.

65. Sensory ataxia includes which of the following?
Harrison's 20th Ed. Chapter 22, Page 139
- A. Imbalance, particularly with eyes closed or in dark
- B. Clumsiness of precision movements
- C. Unsteadiness of gait
- D. All of the above

66. **Continuous involuntary movements of outstretched hands & fingers with eyes closed is called?**
   Harrison's 20th Ed. Chapter 21, Page 139
   A. Alogia
   B. Spooning
   C. Punding
   D. Pseudoathetosis

   Pseudoathetosis refers to continuous involuntary movements of the outstretched hands & fingers, particularly with eyes closed.

67. **Which of the following cutaneous receptor highly developed in the finger pads?**
   DeJong's The Neurologic Examination, 7th Ed. Page 526
   A. Merkel cell endings
   B. Meissner's corpuscles
   C. Pacinian corpuscles
   D. Ruffini endings

68. **Fibers below which level are grouped together in fasciculus gracilis?**
   DeJong's The Neurologic Examination, 7th Ed. Page 528
   A. About C8
   B. About T4
   C. About T8
   D. About T12

   All the fibers below about T8 are grouped together in the fasciculus gracilis. Analogous fibers above T8 form the fasciculus cuneatus.

69. **Sense of vibration is tested with an oscillating tuning fork that vibrates at?**
   Harrison's 20th Ed. Chapter 22, Page 140
   A. 128 Hz
   B. 256 Hz
   C. 512 Hz
   D. Any of the above

   Sense of vibration is tested with an oscillating tuning fork that vibrates at 128 Hz.

70. **Which of the following statements is false?**
   Harrison's 20th Ed. Chapter 22, Page 140
   A. Vibration is tested over bony points, beginning distally
   B. Examiner may serve as control
   C. Interside comparison are important
   D. None of the above

71. **In two-point discrimination test on fingertips, a normal person can distinguish what distance of separation of points?**
   Harrison's 20th Ed. Chapter 22, Page 141, DeJong's The Neurologic Examination, 7th Ed. Page 542
   A. About 2 mm
   B. About 3 mm
   C. About 4 mm
   D. About 5 mm

   In two-point discrimination test on fingertips, a normal individual can distinguish about 3 mm. separation of points. Normal two-point discrimination is about 1 mm on the tip of the tongue, 2 to 3 mm on the lips, 2 to 4 mm on the fingertips, 4 to 6 mm on the dorsum of fingers, 8 to 12 mm on the palm, 20 to 30 mm on the back of the hand, and 30 to 40 mm on the dorsum of the foot.

72. **Which of the following can be used to demonstrate a sensory level on trunk in myelopathy?**
   DeJong's The Neurologic Examination, 7th Ed. Page 542
   A. Stereognosis
   B. Graphesthesia
   C. Two-point discrimination
   D. All of the above

   Two-point discrimination may also be used to demonstrate a sensory level on the trunk in myelopathy.

73. **Which of the following is true about small-fiber polyneuropathies?**
   Harrison's 20th Ed. Chapter 22, Page 142
   A. Reduced proprioception
   B. Reduced thermal sensation
   C. Variable motor dysfunction
   D. Absent deep tendon reflexes

   Small-fiber polyneuropathies are characterized by burning, painful dysesthesias with reduced pinprick and thermal sensation but with sparing of proprioception, motor function, and deep tendon reflexes.

74. **Large-fiber polyneuropathies are characterized by all except?**
   Harrison's 20th Ed. Chapter 22, Page 142
   A. Vibration and position sense deficits
   B. Absent tendon reflexes
   C. Variable motor dysfunction
   D. Cutaneous sensation dysfunction

   Large-fiber polyneuropathies are characterized by vibration & position sense deficits, imbalance, absent tendon reflexes, and variable motor dysfunction but preservation of most cutaneous sensation.

75. **Sensory neuronopathy (or ganglionopathy) is best related to?**
   Harrison's 20th Ed. Chapter 22, Page 142
   A. Leprosy
   B. Sjögren's syndrome
   C. Vitamin B12 deficiency
   D. Isoniazid

   Sensory neuronopathy (or ganglionopathy) is characterized by pain & numbness that progress to sensory ataxia and impairment of all sensory modalities with time. It is usually paraneoplastic or idiopathic in origin or related to an autoimmune disease, particularly Sjögren's syndrome.

76. **In Déjerine-Roussy syndrome, the lesion is in?**
   Harrison's 20th Ed. Chapter 22, Page 142
   A. Spinal cord
   B. Brainstem
   C. Thalamus
   D. Cortex

   Lesions affecting thalamic VPL nucleus or adjacent white matter, produce a syndrome of persistent, unrelenting unilateral thalamic pain, called Déjerine-Roussy syndrome.

77. **In pseudothalamic syndrome, the lesion is in?**
   Harrison's 20th Ed. Chapter 22, Page 142
   A. Spinal cord
   B. Brainstem
   C. Thalamus
   D. Cortex

   Anterior parietal infarction presents as a pseudothalamic syndrome with contralateral loss of primary sensation from head to toe.

78. The principal symptom of focal sensory seizures is?
Harrison's 20th Ed. Chapter 22, Page 142

A. Sense of warmth
B. Tingling
C. A sense of movement without detectable motion
D. Rushing feeling

The principal symptom of focal sensory seizures is tingling.

79. Which of the following nucleus of thalamus is related to sensory pathway?
DeJong's The Neurologic Examination, 7th Ed. Page 524

A. Lateral geniculate nucleus
B. Medial geniculate nucleus
C. Ventral posterolateral nucleus
D. Ventral anterior nucleus

80. Which of the following is a classic sign of tabes dorsalis?
DeJong's The Neurologic Examination, 7th Ed. Page 537

A. Abadie's sign
B. Biernacki's sign
C. Pitres' sign
D. All of the above

Abadie's sign is the absence of pain on squeezing the Achilles tendon. Biernacki's sign is the absence of pain on pressure on the ulnar nerve. Pitres' sign is loss of pain squeezing testicles. All these are classic signs of tabes dorsalis.

81. General visceral afferent fibers are found in all of the following cranial nerves except?
DeJong's The Neurologic Examination, 7th Ed. Page 539

A. V
B. VII
C. IX
D. X

General visceral afferent fibers are found in cranial nerves VII, IX, and X and in the thoracolumbar and sacral autonomic nerves.

82. Finger agnosia occurs most commonly as part of?
DeJong's The Neurologic Examination, 7th Ed. Page 543

A. Gerstmann's syndrome
B. Central cord syndrome
C. Brown-Séquard syndrome
D. Wallenberg's syndrome

Finger agnosia occurs most commonly as part of Gerstmann's syndrome (finger agnosia, agraphia, acalculia, and right-left disorientation).

83. Which of the following is a cause of dissociated sensory loss?
DeJong's The Neurologic Examination, 7th Ed. Page 545

A. Anterior spinal artery stroke
B. Syringomyelia
C. Wallenberg's syndrome
D. All of the above

Patients with Brown-Séquard syndrome have extreme dissociation of modalities, with loss of pain & temperature on one side of body and loss of touch, pressure, position & vibration on the other side of body.

84. Which of the following is false about Brown-Séquard syndrome?
DeJong's The Neurologic Examination, 7th Ed. Page 545

A. Hemisection of the spinal cord
B. Absent pain & temperature sensation contralaterally
C. Loss of proprioceptive sensation & power ipsilaterally
D. None of the above

Hemisection of spinal cord produces Brown-Séquard syndrome, with absent pain & temperature sensation contralaterally & loss of proprioceptive sensation & power ipsilaterally below the lesion.

85. Which of the following does not cause large fiber sensory neuropathy?
DeJong's The Neurologic Examination, 7th Ed. Page 550

A. Uremia
B. Amyloidosis
C. Sjögren's syndrome
D. Vitamin B12 deficiency

86. Which of the following causes small fiber sensory neuropathy?
DeJong's The Neurologic Examination, 7th Ed. Page 550

A. Amyloidosis
B. Hereditary sensory autonomic neuropathy
C. Diabetes mellitus
D. All of the above

Large fiber sensory neuropathies include uremia, Sjögren's syndrome, vitamin B12 deficiency, toxins (pyridoxine, cisplatin, metronidazole) & some cases of diabetes (pseudotabes). Small fiber neuropathies include amyloidosis, hereditary sensory autonomic neuropathy, and some cases of diabetes mellitus (pseudosyringomyelia).

87. In generalized peripheral neuropathies, which of the following is affected first?
DeJong's The Neurologic Examination, 7th Ed. Page 549

A. Pain
B. Vibration
C. Cold
D. Heat

In generalized peripheral neuropathies, vibration is often the first modality affected.

88. During recovery, which of the following sensation returns first?
DeJong's The Neurologic Examination, 7th Ed. Page 552

A. Tactile
B. Pain
C. Pressure
D. Heat

The pattern of sensory return with recovering spinal lesions, pressure sensation returns first and its recovery is usually the most complete, followed, in turn, by tactile, pain, cold, and heat sensibilities.

89. Which of the following sensory loss occurs in syringomyelia?
DeJong's The Neurologic Examination, 7th Ed. Page 552

A. Pinprick & temperature
B. Light touch
C. Position sense
D. Vibration

In syringomyelia there is a dissociated sensory loss with impairment of pinprick & temperature appreciation. Light touch, position sense and vibration appreciation are preserved.

90. Which of the following is related to Lhermitte's sign?
DeJong's The Neurologic Examination, 7th Ed. Page 552

A. Flexion of the neck
B. Electric shock like sensation
C. Radiation down the back & into the legs
D. All of the above

In Lhermitte's sign, flexion of neck leads to an electric shock like sensation that radiates down the back and into the legs. It is seen in patients with a cervical lesion affecting posterior columns like multiple sclerosis, cervical spondylosis or recent irradiation to the cervical region. Vitamin B12 deficiency syndrome & Cisplatin toxicity can also cause it.

91. Pansensory loss contralaterally is produced by a lesion in?
DeJong's The Neurologic Examination, 7th Ed. Page 552

A. Cervical spinal cord
B. Thalamus
C. Tegmentum of pons & midbrain
D. Lateral medulla

A lesion in tegmentum of pons & midbrain, where lemniscal & spinothalamic tracts merge, causes pansensory loss contralaterally.

Gait Disorders, Imbalance, and Falls

92. Sensory information for postural control is primarily generated by?
Harrison's 20th Ed. Chapter 23, Page 143

- A. Visual system
- B. Vestibular system
- C. Proprioceptive receptors in the muscle spindles & joints
- D. All of the above

Loss of two of the above three pathways is sufficient to compromise standing balance.

93. Gait that results from avoidance of pain associated with weight-bearing is called?
Harrison's 20th Ed. Chapter 23, Page 143

- A. Antalgic gait
- B. Steppage gait
- C. Scissoring gait
- D. Functional gait

94. Which of the following is the commonest etiology of gait disorders?
Harrison's 20th Ed. Chapter 23, Page 143 Table 23-1

- A. Parkinsonism
- B. Cerebellar degeneration
- C. Multiple infarcts
- D. Sensory deficits

95. Which of the following is a feature of cautious gait?
Harrison's 20th Ed. Chapter 23, Page 144

- A. Abbreviated stride
- B. Widened base
- C. Lowered center of mass
- D. All of the above

96. Which of the following is a stiff-legged gait?
Harrison's 20th Ed. Chapter 23, Page 144

- A. Dystonia
- B. Stiff-person syndrome
- C. Spastic gait
- D. All of the above

97. Freezing of gait is seen in?
Harrison's 20th Ed. Chapter 23, Page 144

- A. Progressive supranuclear palsy (PSP)
- B. Multiple-system atrophy
- C. Corticobasal degeneration
- D. All of the above

Freezing gait is a feature of Parkinson's disease, progressive supranuclear palsy, multiple system atrophy, corticobasal degeneration, and primary pallidal degeneration.

98. Pill-rolling tremor is a characteristic feature of?
Harrison's 20th Ed. Chapter 23, Page 144

- A. Progressive supranuclear palsy
- B. Multiple system atrophy
- C. Corticobasal degeneration
- D. Parkinson's disease

99. Pill-rolling tremor of Parkinson's disease is seen in?
Harrison's 20th Ed. Chapter 23, Page 144

- A. Progressive supranuclear palsy (PSP)
- B. Multiple-system atrophy
- C. Corticobasal degeneration
- D. None of the above

100. Which of the following about progressive supranuclear palsy (PSP) is false?
Harrison's 20th Ed. Chapter 23, Page 144

- A. Gait more erect compared to stooped posture of Parkinson's
- B. No pill-rolling tremor
- C. Falls within the first year
- D. None of the above

101. Gait with a dancing quality is a feature of?
Harrison's 20th Ed. Chapter 23, Page 144

- A. Tardive dyskinesia
- B. Huntington's disease
- C. Stiff-Person syndrome
- D. Psychogenic cause

In Huntington's disease, unpredictable occurrence of choreic movements gives gait a dancing quality.

102. "Higher level gait disorder" refers to?
Harrison's 20th Ed. Chapter 23, Page 144

- A. Sensory ataxia
- B. Cerebellar ataxia
- C. Frontal gait disorder
- D. All of the above

Frontal gait disorder is also known as higher level gait disorder.

103. Term "gait apraxia" refers to?
Harrison's 20th Ed. Chapter 23, Page 144

- A. Cautious gait
- B. Cerebellar gait ataxia
- C. Frontal gait disorder
- D. Sensory ataxia

104. Which of the following terms is used to describe frontal gait disorders?
Harrison's 20th Ed. Chapter 23, Page 144

- A. "Slipping clutch" syndrome
- B. Gait ignition failure
- C. Lower-body parkinsonism
- D. All of the above

105. The lesion in frontal gait disorder is in?
Harrison's 20th Ed. Chapter 23, Page 144

A. Locus coeruleus
B. Periaqueductal gray
C. Centrum ovale
D. Substantia nigra pars compacta

Vascular small-vessel disease is the most common cause of frontal gait disorder. The lesion is in subcortical region in deep frontal white matter & centrum ovale.

106. Which of the following is a feature of normal pressure (communicating) hydrocephalus?
Harrison's 20th Ed. Chapter 23, Page 144

A. Gait disorder
B. Mental changes
C. Incontinence
D. All of the above

107. Which of the following is an early feature of cerebellar gait ataxia?
Harrison's 20th Ed. Chapter 23, Page 144

A. Lateral instability of the trunk
B. Erratic foot placement
C. Difficulty maintaining balance when turning
D. Wide base of support

Cerebellar gait ataxia is characterized by a wide base of support, lateral instability of trunk, erratic foot placement, decompensation of balance when attempting to walk on a narrow base, difficulty maintaining balance when turning (early feature), and unable to walk tandem heel to toe. Patients with cerebellar ataxia do not complain of dizziness. Neurologic examination reveals cerebellar signs.

108. Which of the following is false about sensory ataxia?
Harrison's 20th Ed. Chapter 23, Page 145 Table 23-2

A. Narrow base, looks down
B. Normal initiation
C. Regular stride with path deviation
D. None of the above

109. Steppage gait best relates to?
Harrison's 20th Ed. Chapter 23, Page 145

A. Neuromuscular disease
B. Cerebellar gait ataxia
C. Sensory ataxia
D. Functional disorders

110. "Astasia-abasia" best relates to?
Harrison's 20th Ed. Chapter 23, Page 145

A. Cautious gait
B. Cerebellar gait ataxia
C. Functional gait disorder
D. Sensory ataxia

Hysterical gait disorders with odd gyrations of posture & wastage of muscular energy (astasia-abasia), extreme slow motion & dramatic fluctuations over time are seen in somatoform disorders & conversion reaction.

111. Gait disorder associated with urinary urgency & incontinence, point towards the diagnosis of?
Harrison's 20th Ed. Chapter 23, Page 145

A. Cerebellar gait ataxia
B. Sensory ataxia
C. Functional disorders
D. Hydrocephalus

Gait disorder may be associated with urinary urgency & incontinence, particularly in patients with cervical spine disease or hydrocephalus.

112. For assessment of a gait disorder, which of the following must be noted?
Harrison's 20th Ed. Chapter 23, Page 145

A. Cadence (steps per minute)
B. Velocity and stride length
C. Watching the patient rise from a chair
D. All of the above

113. Which of the following favour diagnosis of a vestibular disorder?
Harrison's 20th Ed. Chapter 23, Page 145

A. Vertigo
B. Nystagmus
C. Impaired standing balance
D. All of the above

114. Which of the following is the most common risk factor for falls in older persons?
Harrison's 20th Ed. Chapter 23, Page 146 Table 23-3

A. History of falls
B. Visual deficit
C. Cognitive impairment
D. Muscle weakness

115. Which of the following are at high risk for falls?
Harrison's 20th Ed. Chapter 23, Page 146

A. Polypharmacy (use of ≥ 4 prescription medications)
B. Patients with a history of falls
C. Those requiring >12 seconds to complete TUG test
D. All of the above

The Timed Up & Go ("TUG") test involves timing a patient as they stand up from a chair, walk 10 feet, turn, then sit down. Patients with a history of falls, or those requiring >12 seconds to complete the TUG test, are high risk for falls.

116. Which of the following is a cause of drop attacks and collapsing falls?
Harrison's 20th Ed. Chapter 23, Page 146

A. Syncope or orthostatic hypotension
B. Atonic seizures
C. Myoclonus
D. All of the above

117. Thalamic astasia relates best with?
Harrison's 20th Ed. Chapter 23, Page 146

A. Toppling falls
B. Drop attacks and collapsing falls
C. Falls due to gait freezing
D. Falls related to sensory loss

118. Toppling falls relates best with?
Harrison's 20th Ed. Chapter 23, Page 146

A. Syncope
B. Progressive supranuclear palsy (PSP)
C. Parkinson's disease
D. Acute obstructive hydrocephalus

Toppling falls are an early feature of PSP.

Confusion and Delirium

119. In confusion, which of the following is reduced?
Harrison's 20th Ed. Chapter 24, Page 147

A. Comprehension
B. Coherence
C. Capacity to reason
D. All of the above

120. Which of the following terms are used to describe patients with delirium?
Harrison's 20th Ed. Chapter 24, Page 147

A. Encephalopathy
B. Acute brain failure
C. Acute confusional state
D. All of the above

121. Cognitive domain includes which of the following?
Harrison's 20th Ed. Chapter 24, Page 147

A. Memory
B. Executive function
C. Visuospatial tasks
D. All of the above

Cognitive domains include memory, executive function, visuospatial tasks and language.

122. Which of the following about delirium is false?
Harrison's 20th Ed. Chapter 24, Page 147

A. Hallmark of delirium is a deficit of attention
B. Fluctuates over hours or days
C. It is a clinical diagnosis that is made only at bedside
D. None of the above

123. Which of the following is a feature of hyperactive subtype of delirium?
Harrison's 20th Ed. Chapter 24, Page 147

A. Hallucinations
B. Agitation, and hyperarousal
C. Life-threatening autonomic instability
D. All of the above

Severe alcohol withdrawal (delirium tremens) is the classic example of hyperactive subtype of delirium.

124. Most consistently identified risk factor for delirium is?
Harrison's 20th Ed. Chapter 24, Page 147

A. Preexisting hearing & visual impairment
B. Baseline cognitive dysfunction
C. Malnutrition
D. Medication

Two most consistently identified risk factors for delirium are older age & baseline cognitive dysfunction.

125. Patients with which of the following diseases clinically resembles hyperactive delirium?
Harrison's 20th Ed. Chapter 24, Page 148

A. Alzheimer's disease
B. Dementia with Lewy bodies
C. Parkinson's disease dementia
D. All of the above

Dementia with Lewy bodies (DLB) is characterized by a fluctuating course, prominent visual hallucinations, parkinsonism & attentional deficit that clinically resembles hyperactive delirium. They are vulnerable to delirium.

126. Which of the following is a screening tool for identifying patients with delirium?
Harrison's 20th Ed. Chapter 24, Page 147

A. Confusion Assessment Method (CAM)
B. Nursing Delirium Screening Scale (NuDESC)
C. Organic Brain Syndrome Scale
D. All of the above

127. Presence of which of the following helps in diagnosis of delirium?
Harrison's 20th Ed. Chapter 24, Page 147

A. Acute onset of confusion and fluctuating course
B. Inattention accompanied by disorganized thinking
C. Inattention accompanied by altered level of consciousness
D. All of the above

128. Which of the following best relates to delirium?
Harrison's 20th Ed. Chapter 24, Page 148

A. Sundowning
B. Fast-working
C. Mock sun
D. Rainbow

In delirium, fluctuations may occur over hours or days and may worsen at night. This is called sundowning. It is typical but not essential for the diagnosis of delirium.

129. Which of the following is essential in history taking of a delirium patient?
Harrison's 20th Ed. Chapter 24, Page 149

A. Patient's baseline cognitive function
B. Time course of the present illness
C. Current medications
D. All of the above

130. Which of the following is false about "Digit span forward" test?
Harrison's 20th Ed. Chapter 24, Page 149

A. Test of attention
B. Normal capacity is six numbers
C. Asking patient to repeat digits in same order told
D. None of the above

131. Which of the following is false about "Digit span backward" test?
Harrison's 20th Ed. Chapter 24, Page 149

A. Test of working memory
B. Normal capacity is five numbers
C. Asking patient to repeat digits in reverse order
D. None of the above

Most common bedside test of working memory involves asking patients to repeat a series of digits orally, with the clinician gradually increasing the number of to-be-retained digits. Asking the patient to repeat digits in the same order as they were delivered is called digit span forward which is a test of attention. Clinician may also ask the patient to repeat digits in reverse order. This is called digit span backward which is a test of working memory. Capacity for digit span forward is typically six numbers, while normal adults can generally repeat five digits backward.

132. Deficiency of which of the following can cause delirium?
Harrison's 20th Ed. Chapter 24, Page 150 Table 24-2
   A. Vitamin B12
   B. Thiamine
   C. Niacin
   D. All of the above

133. Which of the following can cause delirium?
Harrison's 20th Ed. Chapter 24, Page 150 Table 24-2
   A. Anticholinergic drugs
   B. Narcotics
   C. Benzodiazepines
   D. All of the above

134. Which of the following is a drug of abuse?
Harrison's 20th Ed. Chapter 24, Page 149
   A. γ-hydroxybutyrate (GHB)
   B. Phencyclidine (PCP)
   C. Bath salts
   D. All of the above

135. Which of the following sedatives is less likely to lead to delirium in critically ill patients?
Harrison's 20th Ed. Chapter 24, Page 151
   A. Dexmedetomidine
   B. Propofol
   C. Fentanyl
   D. Midazolam

136. Which of the following drug may be effective for delirium prevention?
Harrison's 20th Ed. Chapter 24, Page 151
   A. Agomelatine
   B. Luzindole
   C. Ramelteon
   D. Prazosin

Melatonin and its agonist ramelteon have shown beneficial results for delirium prevention.

Dementia

137. Which of the following does not appear in the definition of dementia?
Harrison's 20th Ed. Chapter 25, Page 152

A. Acquired
B. Deterioration in cognitive abilities
C. Impairment in activities of daily living
D. Co-morbid diseases

It is defined as an acquired deterioration in cognitive abilities that impairs the successful performance of activities of daily living. The common forms of dementia are progressive.

138. Which of the following is most commonly affected in dementia?
Harrison's 20th Ed. Chapter 25, Page 152

A. Visuospatial ability
B. Calculation
C. Episodic memory
D. Language

Episodic memory is the most common cognitive ability lost with dementia. Other mental faculties like language, visuospatial, praxis, calculation, judgment, and problem-solving abilities are also affected. Neuropsychiatric and social deficits may also develop in dementia syndromes resulting in depression, withdrawal, hallucinations, delusions, agitation, insomnia, and disinhibition.

139. Clinical course of dementia may be static in which of the following?
Harrison's 20th Ed. Chapter 25, Page 152

A. Alzheimer's disease
B. Anoxic encephalopathy
C. Dementia with Lewy bodies
D. Frontotemporal dementia

Clinical course of dementia may be slowly progressive (Alzheimer's disease), static (anoxic encephalopathy) or may fluctuate from day to day or minute to minute (dementia with Lewy bodies).

140. Memory loss is not typically a presenting feature in?
Harrison's 20th Ed. Chapter 25, Page 152

A. Alzheimer's disease
B. Anoxic encephalopathy
C. Dementia with Lewy bodies
D. Frontotemporal dementia

Memory loss is not typically a presenting feature in Frontotemporal dementia (FTD). They are more likely to present with difficulties with judgment, mood, executive control, movement, and behavior.

141. Behavior and mood are modulated by which of the following pathway?
Harrison's 20th Ed. Chapter 25, Page 152

A. Noradrenergic pathway
B. Serotonergic pathway
C. Dopaminergic pathway
D. All of the above

142. Which of the following pathways is critical for attention & memory functions?
Harrison's 20th Ed. Chapter 25, Page 152

A. Noradrenergic pathway
B. Serotonergic pathway
C. Dopaminergic pathway
D. Cholinergic pathway

Behavior and mood are modulated by noradrenergic, serotonergic, and dopaminergic pathways, while cholinergic signaling is critical for attention and memory functions.

143. Pathological process in Alzheimer's disease (AD) begins in?
Harrison's 20th Ed. Chapter 25, Page 152

A. Entorhinal cortex
B. Hippocampus
C. Posterior temporal neocortex
D. Parietal neocortex

AD begins in entorhinal cortex of the medial temporal lobe, then involves hippocampus, posterior temporal & parietal neocortex and eventually causes a relatively diffuse degeneration throughout cerebral cortex.

144. Dorsolateral prefrontal cortex has connections with?
Harrison's 20th Ed. Chapter 25, Page 152

A. Central band of caudate nucleus
B. Ventromedial caudate nucleus
C. Nucleus accumbens
D. All of the above

Dorsolateral prefrontal cortex has connections through frontal-striatal pathways with a central band of caudate nucleus. Lesions here result in executive dysfunction, manifesting as poor organization and planning, decreased cognitive flexibility & impaired working memory. Lateral orbital frontal cortex connects with ventromedial caudate, and lesions cause impulsiveness, distractibility, and disinhibition. Anterior cingulate cortex and adjacent medial prefrontal cortex project to nucleus accumbens and interruption here produces apathy, poverty of speech, emotional blunting, or even akinetic mutism.

145. The striatum comprises of all except?
Harrison's 20th Ed. Chapter 25, Page 152

A. Caudate nucleus
B. Putamen
C. Globus pallidus
D. Nucleus accumbens

The striatum comprises of caudate, putamen and nucleus accumbens.

146. Which of the following is the single strongest risk factor for dementia?
Harrison's 20th Ed. Chapter 25, Page 152

A. Race/ethnicity
B. Geographical location
C. Intoxications
D. Age

The single strongest risk factor for dementia is increasing age.

147. After Alzheimer disease, which of the following is the most common cause of dementia?
Harrison's 20th Ed. Chapter 25, Page 153

A. Vascular dementia
B. Multiple system atrophy
C. Parkinson disease dementia
D. Frontotemporal dementia

Vascular disease is considered the second most frequent cause for dementia after Alzheimer disease.

148. In patients aged <65 years, which of the following is the most common cause of dementia?
Harrison's 20th Ed. Chapter 25, Page 153

A. Vascular dementia
B. Multiple system atrophy
C. Parkinson disease dementia
D. Frontotemporal dementia

In patients aged <65 years, Frontotemporal dementia (FTD) is the most common cause of dementia.

149. Binswanger's syndrome best relates to?
Harrison's 20th Ed. Chapter 25, Page 152 Table 25-1

A. Alcoholism
B. Encephalopathy
C. Head trauma
D. Diffuse white matter disease

150. Pseudodementia is best related to?
Harrison's 20th Ed. Chapter 25, Page 152 Table 25-1

A. Depression
B. Schizophrenia
C. Conversion reaction
D. HIV

Severely depressed or anxious individuals may appear demented, a phenomenon called pseudodementia. Dementia associated with depression (pseudodementia), schizophrenia, and conversion reaction are potentially reversible while that with HIV is not.

151. Which of the following is not a potentially reversible dementia?
Harrison's 20th Ed. Chapter 25, Page 152 Table 25-1

A. Depression
B. Normal-pressure hydrocephalus
C. HIV
D. Alcoholism

The three most common potentially reversible dementias are depression, normal pressure hydrocephalus (NPH), alcohol dependence. Others include subacute combined degeneration, pellagra, adrenal insufficiency and Cushing's syndrome, due to drug, medication, and narcotic poisoning.

152. Which of the following is false about "Benign forgetfulness of the elderly"?
Harrison's 20th Ed. Chapter 25, Page 153, JMAJ 2001;44(6):274-278

A. Not so progressive
B. Does not impair productive daily functioning
C. Revised Hasegawa's Dementia Scale (HDS-R) useful
D. None of the above

"Benign forgetfulness of the elderly" or "benign senescent forgetfulness" or benign senescent amnesia (BSA) implies that changes in memory functions are part of "normal" aging and not associated with central nervous system pathology. Features of BSA include nonprogressive, partial disturbance of episodic memory or word amnesia, with no disorientation, no disturbance of judgement or abstract thinking, aware of memory decline, and mild and not affecting daily life. In contrast, features of AD include progressive, disturbance of memory in general (first-delayed recall), with disorientation (first-temporal disorientation), reduction of all intellectual capabilities, unaware of memory decline, and affecting daily life.

153. Factors that predict progression from MCI to an AD dementia include?
Harrison's 20th Ed. Chapter 25, Page 153

A. Apolipoprotein ε4 (Apo ε4) allele
B. Low cerebrospinal fluid Aβ
C. Elevated tau on PET imaging
D. All of the above

Factors that predict progression from MCI to an AD dementia include a prominent memory deficit, family history of dementia, presence of apolipoprotein ε4 (Apo ε4) allele, small hippocampal volumes, an AD-like signature of cortical atrophy, low cerebrospinal fluid Aβ, & elevated tau or evidence of brain amyloid deposition on positron emission tomography (PET) imaging.

154. Which of the following can predict progression from mild cognitive impairment (MCI) to Alzheimer's disease (AD)?
Harrison's 20th Ed. Chapter 25, Page 153

A. Diffuse white matter disease
B. Ventricular system dilatation
C. Hippocampal atrophy
D. Subdural effusion

In neuroimaging studies, factors that predict progression from MCI to AD include a memory deficit >1.5 SD from normal, family history of dementia, presence of an apolipoprotein ε4 (Apo ε4) and small hippocampal volumes + posterior-predominant cortical atrophy.

155. Major degenerative dementias include?
Harrison's 20th Ed. Chapter 25, Page 153

A. Alzheimer's disease
B. Creutzfeldt-Jakob disease
C. Dementia with Lewy bodies
D. All of the above

Major degenerative dementias include AD, DLB, FTD, HD & prion diseases like CJD.

156. Which of the following specific protein is abnormal aggregated in frontotemporal dementia?
Harrison's 20th Ed. Chapter 25, Page 153 Table 25-2

A. Tau
B. TDP-43
C. FUS
D. All of the above

157. FUS refers to?
Harrison's 20th Ed. Chapter 25, Page 153

A. Fused in sarcoplasm
B. Fused in synuclein
C. Fused in sarcoma
D. Fused in specimen

158. Which of the following specific protein is abnormal aggregated in Alzheimer's disease?
Harrison's 20th Ed. Chapter 25, Page 153 Table 25-2

A. Aβ
B. α-Synuclein
C. PrP^{sc}
D. All of the above

159. α-Synuclein best relates to?
Harrison's 20th Ed. Chapter 25, Page 153 Table 25-2

A. Alzheimer's disease
B. Creutzfeldt-Jakob disease
C. Dementia with Lewy bodies
D. Frontotemporal dementia

Lewy bodies are α-Synuclein neuronal inclusions, found in Dementia with Lewy bodies (DLB).

160. The major degenerative dementias can be distinguished by?
Harrison's 20th Ed. Chapter 25, Page 153

A. Initial or first symptoms
B. Neuroimaging features
C. Neurologic findings
D. All of the above

The major degenerative dementias can be distinguished by the initial symptoms, neuropsychological, neuropsychiatric, neurologic findings and neuroimaging features.

161. Which of the following suggests FTD and not AD?
Harrison's 20th Ed. Chapter 25, Page 153

A. Personality change
B. Disinhibition
C. Weight gain or compulsive eating
D. All of the above

Personality change, disinhibition & weight gain or compulsive eating suggest FTD and not AD. FTD is also suggested by prominent apathy, compulsivity, loss of empathy for others, or progressive loss of speech fluency or single word comprehension and by a relative sparing of memory & visuo-spatial abilities.

162. The diagnosis of DLB is suggested by?
Harrison's 20th Ed. Chapter 25, Page 153

A. Early visual hallucinations
B. Parkinsonism
C. Capgras syndrome
D. All of the above

Diagnosis of DLB is suggested by early visual hallucinations, parkinsonism, proneness to delirium or sensitivity to psychoactive medications, rapid eye movement (REM) behavior disorder (RBD) or Capgras syndrome, the delusion that a familiar person has been replaced by an impostor.

163. Rapid progression of dementia with motor rigidity & myoclonus suggests?
Harrison's 20th Ed. Chapter 25, Page 153

A. Alzheimer's disease
B. Frontotemporal dementia
C. Cortical basal degeneration
D. Creutzfeldt-Jakob disease

Rapid progression of dementia in association with diffuse motor rigidity, akinetic-mute state & startle-sensitive myoclonus suggests CJD.

164. Rapid progression of the dementia with motor rigidity & myoclonus suggests which of the following?
Harrison's 20th Ed. Chapter 25, Page 153

A. Alzheimer's disease
B. Prion disease
C. Frontotemporal dementia
D. Parkinson's disease

Rapid progression of dementia with motor rigidity & myoclonus suggests a prion disease.

165. Gait disturbance is common in?
Harrison's 20th Ed. Chapter 25, Page 153

A. Vascular dementia
B. PD/DLB
C. NPH
D. Any of the above

Gait disturbance is common in vascular dementia, PD/DLB, or NPH.

166. Dementia in a patient with a history of recurrent head trauma suggests?
Harrison's 20th Ed. Chapter 25, Page 153

A. Chronic subdural hematoma
B. Chronic traumatic encephalopathy
C. NPH
D. Any of the above

Dementia in a patient with a history of recurrent head trauma suggests chronic subdural hematoma, chronic traumatic encephalopathy, intracranial hypotension, or NPH.

167. Which of the following statements is false?
Harrison's 20th Ed. Chapter 25, Page 154

A. Typical AD spares motor systems until later in the course
B. FTD patients may mimic amyotrophic lateral sclerosis (ALS)
C. DLB often starts with visual hallucinations or dementia
D. None of the above

168. Which of the following is a feature of Corticobasal syndrome (CBS)?
Harrison's 20th Ed. Chapter 25, Page 154

A. Dystonia
B. Myoclonus
C. Alien limb phenomena
D. All of the above

Features of Corticobasal syndrome (CBS) include asymmetric akinesia & rigidity, dystonia, myoclonus, alien limb phenomena, pyramidal signs, prefrontal deficits (nonfluent aphasia with or without motor speech impairment), executive dysfunction, apraxia, or a behavioral disorder.

169. Unexplained falls is a feature of?
Harrison's 20th Ed. Chapter 25, Page 154

A. Alzheimer's disease
B. Frontotemporal dementia
C. Cortical basal degeneration
D. Progressive supranuclear palsy

Progressive supranuclear palsy (PSP) is associated with unexplained falls, axial rigidity, dysphagia, and vertical gaze deficits.

170. CJD is suggested by the presence of?
Harrison's 20th Ed. Chapter 25, Page 154

A. Diffuse rigidity
B. Akinetic-mute state
C. Startle-sensitive myoclonus
D. All of the above

CJD is suggested by the presence of diffuse rigidity, akinetic-mute state & prominent startle-sensitive myoclonus.

171. Dementia with peripheral neuropathy suggests?
Harrison's 20th Ed. Chapter 25, Page 154

A. Vitamin B12 deficiency
B. Thyroid dysfunction
C. Lyme disease
D. All of the above

Dementia with a peripheral neuropathy suggests vitamin B12 deficiency, heavy metal intoxication, thyroid dysfunction, Lyme disease, or vasculitis.

172. Brief screening tools used to detect dementia & follow progression include?
Harrison's 20th Ed. Chapter 25, Page 155

- A. Mini-Mental State Examination (MMSE)
- B. Montreal Cognitive Assessment (MOCA)
- C. Cognistat
- D. All of the above

Brief screening tools that can be used to identify dementia and follow its progression include Mini-Mental State Examination (MMSE), the Montreal Cognitive Assessment (MOCA), and Cognistat.

173. In Mini-Mental Status Examination (MMSE), scoring is done out of?
Harrison's 20th Ed. Chapter 25, Page 155

- A. 20
- B. 30
- C. 40
- D. 50

Mini-mental status examination (MMSE) is a brief screening tool to confirm the presence of cognitive impairment & to follow progression of dementia. It is a 30-point test of cognitive function.

174. MMSE contains tests for?
Harrison's 20th Ed. Chapter 25, Page 155

- A. Orientation
- B. Working memory
- C. Episodic memory
- D. All of the above

MMSE contains tests of orientation, working memory (spell world backwards), episodic memory (orientation & 3-word recall), language comprehension, naming, and figure copying.

175. MMSE is named after?
Harrison's 20th Ed. Chapter 25, Page 155

- A. Samuels
- B. Blumenthal
- C. Campbell
- D. Folstein

Folstein mini-mental status examination (MMSE) is an easy, standardized screening examination of cognitive function especially working and episodic memory. The test is 85% sensitive and 85% specific for the diagnosis of dementia.

176. Mini-Mental Status Examination (MMSE) provides information regarding?
Harrison's 20th Ed. Chapter 25, Page 155

- A. Orientation
- B. Language
- C. Visuospatial skills
- D. All of the above

Mini-Mental Status Examination (MMSE) can provide information regarding orientation, language, and visuospatial skills.

177. Capgras syndrome is best related to?
Harrison's 20th Ed. Chapter 25, Page 154 Table 25-4

- A. Alzheimer's disease
- B. Cortical basal degeneration
- C. Creutzfeldt-Jakob disease
- D. Dementia with Lewy bodies

178. Posterior parietal atrophy on imaging is seen in?
Harrison's 20th Ed. Chapter 25, Page 154 Table 25-4

- A. Alzheimer's disease
- B. Cortical basal degeneration
- C. Creutzfeldt-Jakob disease
- D. Dementia with Lewy bodies

179. Cortical ribboning and basal ganglia or thalamus hyperintensity on imaging is seen in?
Harrison's 20th Ed. Chapter 25, Page 154 Table 25-4

- A. Alzheimer's disease
- B. Cortical basal degeneration
- C. Creutzfeldt-Jakob disease
- D. Dementia with Lewy bodies

180. Which of the following is a cholinesterase inhibitor?
Harrison's 20th Ed. Chapter 25, Page 157

- A. Ropinirole
- B. Galantamine
- C. Clomipramine
- D. Doxylamine

181. Which of the following is not a cholinesterase inhibitor?
Harrison's 20th Ed. Chapter 25, Page 157

- A. Donepezil
- B. Rivastigmine
- C. Galantamine
- D. All of the above

Clomipramine is a tricyclic antidepressant, pramipexole and ropinirole are agonists of dopamine D2/3 receptors while doxylamine is an antihistaminic.

182. Which of the following drugs is useful in moderate to severe Alzheimer's disease?
Harrison's 20th Ed. Chapter 25, Page 157

- A. Memantine
- B. Amifostine
- C. Trientine
- D. All of the above

Memantine acts by blocking overexcited N-methyl-D-aspartate (NMDA) glutamate receptors.

Aphasia, Memory Loss, Hemispatial Neglect, Frontal Syndromes, and Other Cerebral Disorders

183. Cerebral cortex of human brain contains approximately how many neurons?
    Harrison's 20th Ed. Chapter 26, Page 157
    A. 5 billion
    B. 10 billion
    C. 20 billion
    D. 50 billion

184. Cerebral cortex of human brain has an area of?
    Harrison's 20th Ed. Chapter 26, Page 157
    A. $0.5 m^2$
    B. $1.5 m^2$
    C. $2.5 m^2$
    D. $3.5 m^2$

    Human cerebral cortex contains ~20 billion neurons spread over an area of $2.5 m^2$.

185. Primary sensory & motor areas constitute what percentage of cerebral cortex?
    Harrison's 20th Ed. Chapter 26, Page 157
    A. 10%
    B. 15%
    C. 20%
    D. 25%

    Primary sensory & motor areas constitute 10% of the cerebral cortex.

186. Which of the following is part of association cortex?
    Harrison's 20th Ed. Chapter 26, Page 157
    A. Heteromodal area
    B. Paralimbic area
    C. Limbic area
    D. All of the above

    Modality-selective, heteromodal, paralimbic, and limbic areas collectively known as the association cortex.

187. In the brain, there are no centers for?
    Harrison's 20th Ed. Chapter 26, Page 157
    A. Hearing words
    B. Perceiving space
    C. Storing memories
    D. All of the above

    In the brain, there are no centers for "hearing words," "perceiving space," or "storing memories."

188. Which of the following large-scale neural network is meant for face & object recognition?
    Harrison's 20th Ed. Chapter 26, Page 157
    A. Perisylvian network
    B. Parietofrontal network
    C. Occipitotemporal network
    D. Prefrontal network

    Five anatomically defined large scale networks perform cognitive and behavioral functions in human brain. They are a left-dominant perisylvian network for language, a right-dominant parietofrontal network for spatial orientation, occipitotemporal network for face and object recognition, limbic network for retentive memory and prefrontal network for the executive control of cognition and compartment.

189. Which of the following Brodmann area corresponds to the primary auditory cortex?
    Harrison's 20th Ed. Chapter 26, Page 158 Figure 26-1
    A. 33–34
    B. 36–37
    C. 39–40
    D. 41–42

190. Which of the following Brodmann area corresponds to primary motor cortex?
    Harrison's 20th Ed. Chapter 26, Page 158 Figure 26-1
    A. 1
    B. 2
    C. 3
    D. 4

191. Which of the following Brodmann area corresponds to primary somatosensory cortex?
    Harrison's 20th Ed. Chapter 26, Page 158 Figure 26-1
    A. 1–3
    B. 2–4
    C. 3–5
    D. 4–6

192. Which of the following Brodmann area corresponds to primary visual cortex?
    Harrison's 20th Ed. Chapter 26, Page 158 Figure 26-1
    A. 11
    B. 13
    C. 17
    D. 21

193. Wernicke's area is located in?
    Harrison's 20th Ed. Chapter 26, Page 158
    A. Anterior temporal lobe
    B. Parietotemporal junction
    C. Inferior frontal gyrus
    D. Superior frontal gyrus

    Broca's area is situated in the inferior frontal gyrus. Wernicke's area is located at the parietotemporal junction.

194. 'Recovery from aphasia will be best for the language most used' refers to?
    DeJong's The Neurologic Examination, 7th Ed. Page 98
    A. Pitres' law
    B. Hering's law
    C. Alexander's law
    D. Brodmann law

    Pitres' law states that recovery from aphasia will be best for the language most used.

195. Which of the following is the single most common finding in aphasic patients?
Harrison's 20th Ed. Chapter 26, Page 158

A. Anomia
B. Apraxia
C. Aphemia
D. Alexia

A deficit of naming, called anomia, is the single most common finding in aphasic patients.

196. Anomia refers to?
Harrison's 20th Ed. Chapter 26, Page 158

A. Naming with the wrong word
B. Deficit of naming
C. Naming a different object
D. Any of the above

Deficit of naming or anomia is the single most common finding in aphasic patients. Naming with the wrong word is called paraphasia that can be semantic or phonemic.

197. Inability to read aloud or comprehend single words and simple sentences is called?
Harrison's 20th Ed. Chapter 26, Page 158

A. Alexia
B. Agraphia
C. Anomia
D. Paraphasia

Alexia means an inability to read aloud or comprehend written words & sentences. Agraphia (or dysgraphia) means an acquired deficit in spelling or grammar of written language.

198. Which of the following is impaired in Wernicke's aphasia?
Harrison's 20th Ed. Chapter 26, Page 158 Table 26-1

A. Comprehension
B. Repetition of spoken language
C. Naming
D. All of the above

Comprehension, repetition of spoken language and naming are impaired in Wernicke's aphasia. Fluency is preserved or increased.

199. Which of the following is preserved in Broca's aphasia?
Harrison's 20th Ed. Chapter 26, Page 158 Table 26-1

A. Comprehension
B. Repetition of spoken language
C. Naming
D. Fluency

200. Which of the following is considered as "minimal dysfunction" syndrome of the language network?
Harrison's 20th Ed. Chapter 26, Page 160

A. Anomic aphasia
B. Isolation aphasia
C. Wernicke's aphasia
D. Conduction aphasia

201. Anomic aphasia is the single most common language disturbance seen in?
Harrison's 20th Ed. Chapter 26, Page 160

A. Head trauma
B. Metabolic encephalopathy
C. Alzheimer's disease
D. All of the above

Anomic aphasia is the single most common language disturbance seen in head trauma, metabolic encephalopathy, and Alzheimer's disease.

202. Which of the following results when superior temporal gyrus is damaged?
Harrison's 20th Ed. Chapter 26, Page 160

A. Isolation aphasia
B. Anomic aphasia
C. Pure word deafness
D. Pure alexia without agraphia

203. Fluency is severely impaired in?
Harrison's 20th Ed. Chapter 26, Page 160

A. Aphemia
B. Alexia
C. Anomia
D. Wernicke's aphasia

Aphemia is an acute onset of severely impaired fluency.

204. Apraxia refers to?
Harrison's 20th Ed. Chapter 26, Page 160

A. Repetition of spoken language
B. Disorder of initiating skilled/learned movement
C. Impaired comprehension
D. No purposeful speech

205. In apraxia, complex motor deficit is attributed to?
Harrison's 20th Ed. Chapter 26, Page 160

A. Pyramidal dysfunction
B. Extrapyramidal dysfunction
C. Cerebellar dysfunction
D. None of the above

Apraxia refers to a complex motor deficit that cannot be attributed to pyramidal, extrapyramidal, cerebellar, or sensory dysfunction. It is a disorder of planning & initiating a skilled or learned movement unrelated to a significant motor or sensory deficit.

206. Alien hand syndrome best relates to?
Harrison's 20th Ed. Chapter 26, Page 160

A. Sympathetic dyspraxia
B. Ideational apraxia
C. Ideomotor apraxia
D. Limb-kinetic apraxia

207. Gerstmann's Syndrome includes all except?
Harrison's 20th Ed. Chapter 26, Page 160

A. Acalculia
B. Aphasia
C. Right-left confusion
D. Finger anomia

Gerstmann tetrad comprises of acalculia, alexia, finger anomia and right-left confusion. Pure Gerstmann syndrome is without aphasia.

208. In isolated Gerstmann's syndrome, the damage is in?
Harrison's 20th Ed. Chapter 26, Page 160

A. Superior parietal lobule in dominant hemisphere
B. Inferior parietal lobule in dominant hemisphere
C. Superior parietal lobule in non-dominant hemisphere
D. Inferior parietal lobule in non-dominant hemisphere

Isolated Gerstmann's syndrome results from damage to inferior parietal lobule (angular gyrus) in the left hemisphere.

209. Statements uttered in a monotone are termed?
Harrison's 20th Ed. Chapter 26, Page 160

A. Primary progressive aphasia (PPA)
B. Anomic aphasia
C. Aprosodia
D. Prosopagnosia

210. Which of the following is a subtype of primary progressive aphasia (PPA)?
Harrison's 20th Ed. Chapter 26, Page 161

A. Agrammatic
B. Semantic
C. Logopenic
D. All of the above

211. Which of the following PPAs is not seen with CVAs?
Harrison's 20th Ed. Chapter 26, Page 161

A. Agrammatic
B. Semantic
C. Logopenic
D. All of the above

212. Which symptom can occur in Bálint's syndrome?
Harrison's 20th Ed. Chapter 26, Page 162

A. Optic ataxia
B. Oculomotor apaxia
C. Simultagnosia
D. All of the above

Bálint's syndrome is a state of severe spatial disorientation involving deficits in orderly visuomotor scanning of the environment (oculomotor apraxia) and in accurate manual reaching toward visual targets (optic ataxia) and simultanagnosia and reflects an inability to integrate visual information in the center of gaze with more peripheral information.

213. Bálint's syndrome may result from?
Harrison's 20th Ed. Chapter 26, Page 162

A. Hypoglycemia
B. Sagittal sinus thrombosis
C. Atypical forms of Alzheimer's disease
D. All of the above

214. Face recognition deficit is termed as?
Harrison's 20th Ed. Chapter 26, Page 162

A. Primary progressive aphasia (PPA)
B. Apperceptive agnosia
C. Aprosodia
D. Prosopagnosia

Face & object recognition deficits are known as prosopagnosia & visual object agnosia. Lesions in prosopagnosia & visual object agnosia consist of bilateral infarctions in the territory of posterior cerebral arteries.

215. Which of the following artery is involved in lesions in prosopagnosia?
Harrison's 20th Ed. Chapter 26, Page 163

A. Anterior cerebral artery
B. Middle cerebral artery
C. Posterior cerebral artery
D. Internal carotid artery

The characteristic lesions in prosopagnosia & visual object agnosia of acute onset consist of bilateral infarctions in the territory of posterior cerebral arteries that involve fusiform gyrus.

216. Combination of progressive associative agnosia & fluent aphasia with word comprehension impairment is known as?
Harrison's 20th Ed. Chapter 26, Page 163

A. Amnestic dementia
B. Behavioral variant of frontotemporal dementia (bvFTD)
C. Semantic dementia
D. Semantic PPA

217. Which of the following is not included in paralimbic area?
Harrison's 20th Ed. Chapter 26, Page 164

A. Hippocampus
B. Hypothalamus
C. Amygdala
D. Entorhinal cortex

Limbic system is a distributed network consisting of limbic & paralimbic areas (hippocampus, amygdala & entorhinal cortex), anterior & medial nuclei of thalamus, medial & basal parts of striatum, and hypothalamus.

218. Which of the following functions is related to limbic system?
Harrison's 20th Ed. Chapter 26, Page 164

A. Coordination of emotion
B. Autonomic tone
C. Endocrine function
D. All of the above

Functions related to limbic system include coordination of emotion, motivation, autonomic tone, endocrine function and declarative (explicit) memory for recent episodes & experiences.

219. Cause of transient global amnesia is?
Harrison's 20th Ed. Chapter 26, Page 165

A. Migraine
B. Temporal lobe seizures
C. TIA in the posterior cerebral territory
D. All of the above

220. Which of the following is best related to visuospatial disorientation?
N Engl J Med. 2005;352:692-9

A. Optic ataxia
B. Ocular apraxia
C. Simultanagnosia
D. All of the above

Bilateral parietal lesions produce Bálint's syndrome, which is characterized by impaired eye-hand coordination (optic ataxia), difficulty initiating voluntary eye movements (ocular apraxia), and visuospatial disorientation (simultanagnosia).

221. Which of the following is not a major type of memory?

- A. Working
- B. Sequential
- C. Episodic
- D. Remote

Memory is divided into three major types - working, episodic, and remote.

222. Working memory lasts for what duration?

- A. < 5 seconds
- B. < 10 seconds
- C. < 20 seconds
- D. < 30 seconds

Working memory lasts for <30 seconds.

223. Which of the following types of memory is tested by asking the patient to recall digits backwards?

- A. Working
- B. Episodic
- C. Remote
- D. All of the above

Working memory is highly vulnerable to distraction, requiring attention and vigilance for its maintenance. It is tested by asking the patient to recall digits backwards.

224. Which of the following types of memory is tested by asking the patient to recall three words after 3 to 5 minutes?

- A. Working
- B. Episodic
- C. Remote
- D. All of the above

Episodic memory is tested by asking a patient to recall three words after 3 to 5 minutes.

225. Hippocampal complex is critical for which of the following types of memory?

- A. Working
- B. Episodic
- C. Remote
- D. All of the above

Hippocampal complex is critical for episodic memory, and physiologic changes in synapses in this brain region accompany new episodic memories.

226. More permanent stores of words, dates, historic facts or names require which of the following?

- A. Hippocampal complex
- B. Left anterior temporal cortex
- C. Prefrontal lobe
- D. Parietal lobe

More permanent stores of words, dates, facts or names require left anterior temporal cortex.

227. Most common cognitive deficits that follow seizures, hypoglycemia, hypoxia is?

- A. Working memory deficits
- B. Episodic memory deficits
- C. Remote memory deficits
- D. None of the above

Hippocampal complex is vulnerable to metabolic insults such as seizures, hypoglycemia, hypoxia, and neurodegenerative processes, which explains why episodic memory deficits are the most common cognitive deficits that follow these disorders.

228. The process of memory retrieval requires which of the following cerebral lobes?

- A. Frontal lobe
- B. Temporal lobe
- C. Parietal lobe
- D. All of the above

The process of memory encoding is dependent upon frontal lobes and hippocampal complex, while the process of retrieval requires frontal lobes.

229. Memory function includes which of the following?

- A. Registration (encoding or acquisition)
- B. Retention (storage or consolidation)
- C. Retrieval (decoding or recall)
- D. All of the above

Memory function includes registration (encoding or acquisition), retention (storage or consolidation), stabilization (consolidation), and retrieval (decoding or recall).

230. The basal ganglia, cerebellum, and supplementary motor area are critical for?

- A. Episodic memory
- B. Semantic memory
- C. Procedural memory
- D. Working memory

Procedural (implicit) memory involves centers outside the hippocampus such as amygdala, basal ganglia, cerebellum, and sensory cortex.

231. The medial temporal lobes, including the hippocampus and parahippocampus, are critical for?

- A. Episodic memory
- B. Semantic memory
- C. Procedural memory
- D. Working memory

Episodic memory requires dorsomedial nucleus of thalamus and medial temporal lobes.

232. Which of the following is damaged in Korsakoff's syndrome due to thiamine deficiency?

- A. Dorsomedial nucleus of thalamus
- B. Medial temporal lobes
- C. Amygdala
- D. Basal ganglia

Dorsomedial nucleus of thalamus is damaged in Korsakoff's syndrome due to thiamine deficiency resulting in loss of episodic memory.

233. **Inferolateral temporal lobes are critical for?**
   N Engl J Med. 2005;352:692-9
   A. Episodic memory
   B. Semantic memory
   C. Procedural memory
   D. Working memory

234. **Prefrontal cortex, Broca's area, Wernicke's area are critical for?**
   N Engl J Med. 2005;352:692-9
   A. Episodic memory
   B. Semantic memory
   C. Procedural memory
   D. Phonologic working memory

235. **Prefrontal cortex, visual-association areas are critical for?**
   N Engl J Med. 2005;352:692-9
   A. Episodic memory
   B. Semantic memory
   C. Procedural memory
   D. Spatial working memory

236. **Which memory is involved in remembering unchanging facts, principles & rules (number of days in a week)?**
   N Engl J Med. 2005;352:692-9
   A. Semantic memory
   B. Declarative (explicit) memory
   C. Procedural (implicit) memory
   D. All of the above

   Semantic memory contains unchanging facts, principles, associations, and rules (number of days in a week). Injury to anterior temporal neocortex leads to loss of semantic memory.

237. **Which kind of memory is involved in remembering facts about the world and past personal events?**
   N Engl J Med. 2005;352:692-9
   A. Semantic memory
   B. Declarative (explicit) memory
   C. Procedural (implicit) memory
   D. All of the above

   Declarative (explicit) memory refers to facts about world & past personal events that must be consciously retrieved to be remembered. Episodic is prototypical declarative explicit memory.

238. **Which kind of memory is involved in learning and retaining a skill or procedure like riding a bicycle, getting dressed, or driving a car?**
   N Engl J Med. 2005;352:692-9
   A. Semantic memory
   B. Declarative (explicit) memory
   C. Procedural (implicit) memory
   D. All of the above

   Procedural (implicit) memory is involved in learning and retaining a skill or procedure such as riding a bicycle, getting dressed, or driving a car. Abilities stored in procedural memory become automatic and do not require conscious implementation.

239. **Executive memory function is highly dependent upon which of the following?**
   N Engl J Med. 2005;352:692-9
   A. Working
   B. Episodic
   C. Remote
   D. All of the above

   Executive function refers to mental activity involved in planning, initiating, and regulating behavior. It is highly dependent upon working memory.

240. **Which of the following is not a part of the components of medial temporal lobe memory system?**
   Harrison's 20th Ed. Chapter 423 Page 3109
   A. Hippocampus
   B. Amgdala
   C. Entorhinal region
   D. Perirhinal region

   Components of medial temporal lobe memory system include hippocampus and adjacent cortex, including the entorhinal, perirhinal, and parahippocampal regions.

241. **In AD, the early deficits involve which class of memory?**
   Harrison's 20th Ed. Chapter 25 Page 155
   A. Working memory
   B. Episodic memory
   C. Executive function
   D. Language

   In AD the early deficits involve verbal or visual episodic memory, category generation ("name as many animals as you can in one minute"), and visuoconstructive ability. Tasks requiring patient to recall a long list of words or a series of pictures after a predetermined delay will demonstrate deficits.

242. **An autosomal dominant family history of dementia can be found in which of the following?**
   Harrison's 20th Ed. Chapter 25 Page 154
   A. Huntington's disease
   B. Alzheimer's disease
   C. Frontotemporal dementia
   D. All of the above

   An autosomal dominant family history is found in HD and in familial forms of AD, FTD, DLB, or prion disorders.

243. **Early presence of visual hallucinations is a feature of which of the following dementias?**
   Harrison's 20th Ed. Chapter 426 Page 3119
   A. Creutzfeldt-Jakob disease
   B. Schizophrenia
   C. Frontotemporal dementia
   D. Dementia with Lewy bodies

   Diagnosis of DLB is suggested by early presence of visual hallucinations, parkinsonism, delirium, rapid-eye-movement (REM) sleep disorder or Capgras syndrome (delusion that a familiar person has been replaced by an impostor).

244. **Capgras syndrome is an early feature in which of the following degenerative diseases?**
   Harrison's 20th Ed. Chapter 25 Page 153
   A. Alzheimer's disease
   B. Creutzfeldt-Jakob disease
   C. Frontotemporal dementia
   D. Dementia with Lewy bodies

   Capgras syndrome—delusion that a familiar person has been replaced by an impostor, is an early feature of Dementia with Lewy bodies.

245. Early prominent gait disturbance is a feature of?
Harrison's 20th Ed. Chapter 423 Page 3109

A. Alzheimer's disease
B. Dementia with Lewy bodies
C. Creutzfeldt-Jakob disease
D. Vascular dementia

Early prominent gait disturbance with only mild memory loss suggests vascular dementia. Gait disturbance is common in vascular dementia, PD/DLB, or normal-pressure hydrocephalus (NPH).

246. On neuroimaging studies, extensive white matter abnormalities correlate best with?
Harrison's 20th Ed. Chapter 425 Page 3118

A. Alzheimer's disease
B. Frontotemporal dementia
C. Vascular etiology
D. Creutzfeldt-Jakob disease

On neuroimaging studies, extensive white matter abnormalities correlate best with a vascular etiology for dementia.

247. In amyloid imaging of brain for diagnosis of Alzheimer's disease (AD), which of the following is used?
Harrison's 20th Ed. Chapter 25 Page 156

A. Pittsburgh Compound-A
B. Pittsburgh Compound-B
C. Pittsburgh Compound-C
D. Pittsburgh Compound-D

Amyloid imaging with radioligands like Pittsburgh Compound-B (PiB), 18F-AV-45 and tau PET tracers, such as 18F-T807 and T808 help in detecting brain amyloid associated with amyloid angiopathy or neuritic plaques of AD.

248. EEG is helpful in the diagnosis of which of the following?
Harrison's 20th Ed. Chapter 25 Page 156

A. Alzheimer's disease
B. Frontotemporal dementia
C. Cortical basal degeneration
D. Creutzfeldt-Jakob disease

Electroencephalogram (EEG) is rarely helpful except in CJD (repetitive bursts of diffuse high-amplitude sharp waves, or "periodic complexes").

249. Which of the following is the major source of cholinergic input to the cerebral cortex?
Harrison's 20th Ed. Chapter 423 Page 3109

A. Globus pallidus
B. Thalamus
C. Nucleus accumbens
D. Nucleus basalis of Meynert

Nucleus basalis of Meynert is the major source of cholinergic input to the cerebral cortex.

250. Agents useful for reducing the signs of dementia include?
N Engl J Med. 2004;351:56-67

A. Donepezil
B. Rivastigmine
C. Galantamine
D. All of the above

251. Which of the following drugs used in management of dementia is not a cholinesterase inhibitor?
N Engl J Med. 2004;351:56-67

A. Donepezil
B. Rivastigmine
C. Galantamine
D. Memantine

252. Which of the following drugs used in the management of dementia is a NMDA-receptor antagonist?
N Engl J Med. 2004;351:56-67

A. Donepezil
B. Rivastigmine
C. Galantamine
D. Memantine

253. Ribot's law states that?
N Engl J Med. 2005;352:692-9

A. Events just before ictus are most vulnerable to dissolution
B. Remote memories are most resistant
C. A+B
D. None of the above

254. The most common clinical disorder disrupting semantic memory is?
N Engl J Med. 2005;352:692-9

A. Alzheimer's disease
B. Parkinsons's disease
C. Multiple sclerosis
D. Progressive supranuclear palsy

255. Disorders affecting procedural memory include all except?
N Engl J Med. 2005;352:692-9

A. Alzheimer's disease
B. Parkinsons's disease
C. Huntington's disease
D. Olivopontocerebellar degeneration

256. After Alzheimer disease, which of the following is the most common cause of dementia?
Cleveland Clinic Journal of Medicine 2014;81(4):243

A. Vascular dementia
B. Multiple system atrophy
C. Parkinson disease dementia
D. Frontotemporal dementia

After Alzheimer disease, vascular dementia is the most common dementia, accounting for ~ 20%–30% of cases.

257. Which of the following is used as a bedside tool to differentiate Alzheimer dementia from vascular dementia?
Cleveland Clinic Journal of Medicine 2014;81(4):243

A. Trail making test
B. Folstein mini-mental state examination
C. Hachinski ischemic score
D. Montreal cognitive assessment

The Hachinski ischemic score is a good bedside tool to help differentiate Alzheimer dementia from vascular dementia.

258. Executive dysfunction may be identified by which of the following?
Cleveland Clinic Journal of Medicine 2014;81(4):243

A. St. Louis University mental status examination
B. Folstein mini-mental state examination
C. Montreal cognitive assessment
D. All of the above

Executive dysfunction may be identified using the Trail making test or Executive Interview (EXIT25). Office-based tools like Folstein mini-mental state examination, Montreal cognitive assessment, or St. Louis University mental status examination may also uncover these deficits.

259. Out of the following, which is the most common neurodegenerative dementia in the elderly?
Cleveland Clinic Journal of Medicine 2014;81(4):243

A. Progressive supranuclear palsy
B. Frontotemporal dementia
C. Corticobasal degeneration
D. Dementia with Lewy bodies

After Alzheimer disease and Vascular dementias, Dementia with Lewy bodies is the next most common neurodegenerative dementia in the elderly.

260. Which of the following is a less common feature of Dementia with Lewy bodies?
Cleveland Clinic Journal of Medicine 2014;81(4):243

A. Progressive loss of cognitive function
B. Prominent visual hallucinations
C. Autonomic failure
D. Parkinsonism

Progressive loss of cognitive function, prominent visual hallucinations and parkinsonism (bradykinesia, masked facies & rigidity. Resting tremor is less common. Dementia occurs before or concurrently with parkinsonism) are characteristic features of Dementia with Lewy bodies, progression of which usually occurs over years but can be more rapid than in Alzheimer disease.

261. McKeith consensus criteria is the gold standard for diagnosing which of the following?
Cleveland Clinic Journal of Medicine 2014;81(4):243

A. Progressive supranuclear palsy
B. Frontotemporal dementia
C. Corticobasal degeneration
D. Dementia with Lewy bodies

McKeith criteria is the gold standard for diagnosing probable Lewy body dementia, based on clinical and imaging features.

262. Which of the following about progressive supranuclear palsy is false?
Cleveland Clinic Journal of Medicine 2014;81(4):243

A. Sporadic atypical parkinsonian disorder
B. Onset between age 50 and 70
C. Accumulation of tau protein aggregates in basal ganglia
D. None of the above

Progressive supranuclear palsy is a sporadic atypical parkinsonian disorder with onset between age 50 and 70 and gradual progression. Familial cases are infrequent. Histologically, PSP is characterized by accumulation of tau protein aggregates in basal ganglia, brainstem, and cerebral cortex.

263. Degenerative process in progressive supranuclear palsy involves which of the following neurons?
Cleveland Clinic Journal of Medicine 2014;81(4):243

A. Dopaminergic neurons
B. Cholinergic neurons
C. Gamma-aminobutyric acid (GABA) neurons
D. All of the above

Degenerative process in progressive supranuclear palsy involves dopaminergic, cholinergic, and gamma-aminobutyric acid (GABA)-ergic neurons.

264. Which of the following is not a feature of progressive supranuclear palsy?
Cleveland Clinic Journal of Medicine 2014;81(4):243

A. Vertical gaze palsy
B. Gait and balance impairment
C. Limb rigidity is more prominent than axial rigidity
D. Cognitive impairment

The hallmark of progressive supranuclear palsy is vertical gaze palsy. Earliest symptom is gait & balance impairment (falls usually backward). Axial (especially neck) rigidity is more prominent than limb rigidity. Retrocollis (the head is drawn back) occurs in <25% of patients.

265. Which of the following signs is related to progressive supranuclear palsy?
DeJong's The Neurologic Examination, 7th Ed. Page 253

A. Negro's sign
B. Myerson's sign
C. Omega sign
D. Hanes sign

In progressive supranuclear palsy, omega sign refers to a characteristic facial dystonia with knitting of the brows and widening of the palpebral fissures.

266. "Leonine facies" is a feature of which of the following?
Cleveland Clinic Journal of Medicine 2014;81(4):243

A. Progressive supranuclear palsy
B. Frontotemporal dementia
C. Corticobasal degeneration
D. Dementia with Lewy bodies

In PSP, gaze abnormality combined with rare blinking & facial dystonia form the classic facial expression of astonishment called "leonine facies." The face is stiff and deeply furrowed, with a look of surprise.

267. 'Hummingbird sign' and "morning glory flower" on MRI is a feature of which of the following?
Cleveland Clinic Journal of Medicine 2014;81(4):243

A. Progressive supranuclear palsy
B. Frontotemporal dementia
C. Corticobasal degeneration
D. Dementia with Lewy bodies

In PSP, brain MRI shows atrophy of brainstem, particularly midbrain. Thinning of superior part of midbrain & dilation of third ventricle ("hummingbird sign" on sagittal sections or "morning glory flower" on axial sections) support the diagnosis and differentiate it from Parkinson disease and other atypical parkinsonian disorders.

268. 'Hot cross bun' sign on MRI is a feature of which of the following?
Cleveland Clinic Journal of Medicine 2014;81(4):243

A. Multiple system atrophy
B. Frontotemporal dementia
C. Corticobasal degeneration
D. Dementia with Lewy bodies

In MSA, Brain MRI shows atrophy of putamen (hypointensity of putamen with a hyperintense rim). Pons atrophy may also be present, revealing a "hot cross bun" sign in axial images.

269. Rapid-eye-movement sleep behavior disorders are infrequent in which of the following?
Cleveland Clinic Journal of Medicine 2014;81(4):243

A. Parkinson disease
B. Multiple system atrophy
C. Progressive supranuclear palsy
D. Lewy body dementia

Rapid-eye-movement sleep behavior disorders are infrequent in PSP, unlike in Parkinson disease, multiple system atrophy, and Lewy body dementia.

270. Which of the following clinical features is least common in corticobasal degeneration?
Cleveland Clinic Journal of Medicine 2014;81(4):243

A. Dementia
B. Parkinsonism
C. Higher cortical dysfunction
D. Gait disorder

In corticobasal degeneration, the frequency of clinical features is : parkinsonism (100%), higher cortical dysfunction (93%), dyspraxia (82%), gait disorder (80%), unilateral limb dystonia (71%), tremor (55%), and dementia (25%).

271. MRI of which of the following diseases may show asymmetric cortical atrophy especially in posterior frontal and parietal lobes?
Cleveland Clinic Journal of Medicine 2014;81(4):243

A. Progressive supranuclear palsy
B. Frontotemporal dementia
C. Corticobasal degeneration
D. Dementia with Lewy bodies

In CBD, MRI may be normal initially. As the disease progresses, asymmetric cortical atrophy may be seen, especially in the posterior frontal and parietal lobes.

272. Which of the following is not a prominent feature of Multiple system atrophy (MSA)?
Cleveland Clinic Journal of Medicine 2014;81(4):243

A. Psychiatric symptoms
B. Parkinsonism
C. Cerebellar signs
D. Pyramidal tract dysfunction

Multiple system atrophy is characterized by sporadic parkinsonism, cerebellar signs (involving balance and coordination), pyramidal tract dysfunction, and autonomic insufficiency in varying combinations. In contrast to dementia with Lewy bodies, psychiatric symptoms are not a major feature, except possibly depression.

273. In Parkinson disease dementia, volume of which of the following is reduced?
Cleveland Clinic Journal of Medicine 2014;81(4):243

A. Temporal
B. Occipital
C. Subcortical areas
D. All of the above

In Parkinson disease dementia, reduced volume extends to temporal, occipital, and subcortical areas.

274. In patients with Parkinson disease dementia, which of the following drugs is effective?
Cleveland Clinic Journal of Medicine 2014;81(4):243

A. Selective serotonin reuptake inhibitors
B. Midodrine
C. Memantine
D. Rivastigmine

Acetylcholinesterase inhibitor rivastigmine (FDA-approved) has a positive impact on global assessment, cognitive function, behavioral disturbance, and activities of daily living rating scales in patients with Parkinson disease dementia.

275. Behavioral & language changes accompany which of the following forms of dementia?
Cleveland Clinic Journal of Medicine 2014;81(4):243

A. Alzheimer disease
B. Vascular dementia
C. Primary progressive aphasia
D. All of the above

Behavioral & language changes accompany Alzheimer disease, vascular dementia, primary progressive aphasia.

276. Which of the following is not a feature of the classic triad of normal-pressure hydrocephalus?
Cleveland Clinic Journal of Medicine 2014;81(4):243

A. Gait impairment
B. Cognitive impairment
C. Progressive aphasia
D. Urinary frequency or incontinence

Normal-pressure hydrocephalus is characterized by the classic triad of gait impairment, cognitive impairment, and urinary frequency or incontinence.

277. Degree of enlargement of cerebral ventricles is calculated by?
Cleveland Clinic Journal of Medicine 2014;81(4):243

A. Armstrong ratio
B. Litvan ratio
C. Evans ratio
D. Cooper ratio

In 1942, William Evans calculated degree of enlargement of cerebral ventricles and defined its normal limits. He defined & computed a ratio of transverse diameter of the anterior horns to the greatest internal diameter of the skull in the sagittal direction. This index was for children and the normal range was 0.20 to 0.25, and that a ratio of 0.25 to 0.30 represents early ventricular enlargement while values above 0.30 define ventricular enlargement.

278. Which of the following is a rapidly progressive dementia?
Cleveland Clinic Journal of Medicine 2014;81(4):243

A. Hashimoto encephalopathy
B. Paraneoplastic limbic encephalitis
C. Creutzfeldt-Jakob disease
D. All of the above

279. Which of the following is true for Creutzfeldt-Jakob disease?
Cleveland Clinic Journal of Medicine 2014;81(4):243

A. EEG positive for periodic sharp-wave complexes
B. CSF with a positive 14-3-3 protein assay
C. MRI with high signal abnormalities in caudate nucleus & putamen
D. All of the above

For the diagnosis of Creutzfeldt-Jakob disease, two of the following must be present : Myoclonus (muscle twitching), Pyramidal or extrapyramidal findings, Visual or cerebellar deficits and Akinetic mutism (patient appears alert but is unresponsive). In addition, one of the above three tests must be positive.

280. **Progression of which of the following neurodegenerative dementias is sudden, stepwise?**
   Cleveland Clinic Journal of Medicine 2014;81(4):243
   A. Vascular dementia
   B. Multiple system atrophy
   C. Parkinson disease dementia
   D. Frontotemporal dementia

281. **Progression of which of the following neurodegenerative dementias is gradual with fluctuation in cognition?**
   Cleveland Clinic Journal of Medicine 2014;81(4):243
   A. Vascular dementia
   B. Multiple system atrophy
   C. Parkinson disease dementia
   D. Dementia with Lewy bodies

282. **Visual hallucinations is a typical feature of which of the following neurodegenerative dementias?**
   Cleveland Clinic Journal of Medicine 2014;81(4):243
   A. Vascular dementia
   B. Multiple system atrophy
   C. Parkinson disease dementia
   D. Dementia with Lewy bodies

Disorders of the Eye

283. About how many rods are present in human retina?
Harrison's 20th Ed. Chapter 28, Page 177

- A. 10 million
- B. 50 million
- C. 75 million
- D. 100 million

284. About how many cones are present in human retina?
Harrison's 20th Ed. Chapter 28, Page 177

- A. 1 million
- B. 3 million
- C. 5 million
- D. 10 million

285. Which of the following statements about vision is false?
Harrison's 20th Ed. Chapter 28, Page 177

- A. Rods operate in dim (scotopic) illumination
- B. Cones function under daylight (photopic) conditions
- C. Rods specialized for color perception
- D. Fovea is packed exclusively with cones

The cone system is specialized for color perception and high spatial resolution.

286. Which of the following statements is false?
Harrison's 20th Ed. Chapter 28, Page 28, 177

- A. Rods operate in scotopic illumination
- B. Cones function under photopic conditions
- C. Cone system is specialized for color perception
- D. Rod system is specialized for high spatial resolution

Rods operate in dim (scotopic) illumination. Cones function under daylight (photopic) conditions. Cone system is specialized for color perception & high spatial resolution.

287. How many fibers are present in each optic nerve?
Harrison's 20th Ed. Chapter 28, Page, 177

- A. 1 million
- B. 2 million
- C. 3 million
- D. 4 million

288. How many ganglion cells are present in each retina?
Harrison's 20th Ed. Chapter 28, Page, 177

- A. One million
- B. Five million
- C. Ten million
- D. Twenty million

After processing of photoreceptor responses, the flow of sensory information converges on a final common pathway, i.e. ganglion cells. There are a million ganglion cells in each retina and hence a million fibers in each optic nerve.

289. The majority of cones are within?
Harrison's 20th Ed. Chapter 28, Page 177

- A. Macula
- B. Optic disc
- C. Peripheral retina
- D. Evenly distributed all over retina

Majority of cones are within macula which is that portion of retina that serves the central 10° of vision. Fovea is In the middle of macula and is packed exclusively with cones.

290. Which cell in the inner nuclear layer of retina is activated when photoreceptors hyperpolarize in response to light?
Harrison's 20th Ed. Chapter 28, Page 177

- A. Bipolar cells
- B. Amacrine cells
- C. Horizontal cells
- D. All of the above

Photoreceptors hyperpolarize in response to light, activating bipolar, amacrine & horizontal cells in the inner nuclear layer of retina.

291. Majority of ganglion cell axons synapse on cells in?
Harrison's 20th Ed. Chapter 28, Page 177

- A. Medical geniculate body
- B. Lateral geniculate body
- C. Edinger-Westphal nuclei
- D. Primary visual cortex

Majority of ganglion cell axons synapse on cells in the lateral geniculate body, a thalamic relay station. Cells in lateral geniculate body project in turn to the primary visual cortex.

292. Melanopsin is best related to?
Harrison's 20th Ed. Chapter 28, Page 177

- A. Pupillary constriction
- B. Visual orientation
- C. Eye movements
- D. Gaze stabilization

Ganglion cells that mediate pupillary constriction and circadian rhythms are light sensitive owing to a novel visual pigment, melanopsin.

293. Pupil responses are mediated by input to?
Harrison's 20th Ed. Chapter 28, Page 177

- A. Superior colliculus
- B. Pretectal olivary nuclei
- C. Suprachiasmatic nucleus
- D. All of the above

Pupil responses are mediated by input to pretectal olivary nuclei in the midbrain which send their output to the Edinger-Westphal nuclei, which in turn provide parasympathetic innervation to the iris sphincter via an interneuron in the ciliary ganglion.

294. Circadian rhythms are timed by a retinal projection to?
Harrison's 20th Ed. Chapter 28, Page 177

- A. Superior colliculus
- B. Pretectal olivary nuclei
- C. Suprachiasmatic nucleus
- D. All of the above

Circadian rhythms are timed by a retinal projection to the suprachiasmatic nucleus.

295. Visual orientation & eye movements are served by retinal input to?
Harrison's 20th Ed. Chapter 28, Page 177

A. Superior colliculus
B. Pretectal olivary nuclei
C. Suprachiasmatic nucleus
D. All of the above

Visual orientation & eye movements are served by retinal input to superior colliculus.

296. Brainstem accessory optic system is best related to?
Harrison's 20th Ed. Chapter 28, Page 177

A. Pupillary constriction
B. Visual orientation
C. Eye movements
D. Gaze stabilization and optokinetic reflexes

Gaze stabilization & optokinetic reflexes are governed by a group of small retinal targets known collectively as brainstem accessory optic system.

297. Phenomenon by which eyes maintain targets of visual interest on the fovea is called?
Harrison's 20th Ed. Chapter 28, Page 177

A. Acculization
B. Focussation
C. Foveation
D. Maculization

Eyes maintain targets of visual interest on fovea. This activity is called foveation.

298. Each eye is moved by how many extraocular muscles?
Harrison's 20th Ed. Chapter 28, Page 177

A. 4
B. 5
C. 6
D. 8

299. Which of the following control brainstem eye movement centers?
Harrison's 20th Ed. Chapter 28, Page 177

A. Frontal cortex
B. Temporal cortex
C. Cingulate gyrus
D. Limbic system

Large regions of frontal and parietooccipital cortex control brainstem ocular motor nuclei eye movement centers by providing descending supranuclear input.

300. Bell's reflex refers to?
Harrison's 19th Ed. 2647

A. Elevation & adduction of eyes on attempted lid closure
B. Elevation & abduction of eyes on attempted lid closure
C. Depression & adduction of eyes on attempted lid closure
D. Depression & abduction of eyes on attempted lid closure

Bell's reflex, also called palpebral oculogyric reflex, refers to elevation & abduction of eyes on attempted lid closure.

301. Term used to describe parallel rays from infinity focused perfectly on the retina is?
Harrison's 20th Ed. Chapter 28, Page 178

A. Emmetropia
B. Immetropia
C. Ammetropia
D. Smmetropia

In emmetropia, parallel rays from infinity are focused perfectly on retina.

302. To test acuity, Rosenbaum card is held at what distance from the patient?
Harrison's 20th Ed. Chapter 28, Page 178

A. 9 inches
B. 12 inches
C. 14 inches
D. 18 inches

The Snellen chart is used to test acuity at a distance of 6 meters (20 feet). A scale version of Snellen chart called Rosenbaum card is held at 36 cm or 14 inches from the patient.

303. Legal blindness is defined as a best corrected acuity of?
Harrison's 20th Ed. Chapter 28, Page 178

A. 6/20
B. 6/30
C. 6/40
D. 6/60

Legal blindness is defined by Internal Revenue Service as a best corrected acuity of 6/60 (20/200) or less in the better eye or a binocular visual field subtending 20° or less.

304. Patients with which of the following disorders should avoid driving?
Harrison's 20th Ed. Chapter 28, Page 178

A. Bitemporal hemianopia
B. Homonymous hemianopia
C. Junctional scotoma
D. All of the above

Patients with a homonymous hemianopia should not drive.

305. In abbreviation PERRLA, "A" stands for?
Harrison's 20th Ed. Chapter 28, Page 178

A. Absent
B. Asymmetric
C. Accommodation
D. Alignment

Abbreviation PERRLA stands for pupils equal, round, and reactive to light and accommodation.

306. Light-near dissociation occurs with?
Harrison's 20th Ed. Chapter 28, Page 178

A. Neurosyphilis
B. Parinaud's syndrome
C. Adie's tonic pupil
D. All of the above

Light-near dissociation occurs with neurosyphilis (Argyll Robertson pupil), with lesions of dorsal midbrain (Parinaud's syndrome), and after aberrant regeneration (oculomotor nerve palsy, Adie's tonic pupil).

307. Marcus Gunn pupil is best related to?
Harrison's 20th Ed. Chapter 28, Page 178

A. Neurosyphilis
B. Cataract
C. Oculomotor nerve palsy
D. Retrobulbar optic neuritis

Direct pupillary response is weaker than the consensual pupillary response evoked by shining a light into the other eye. This relative afferent pupillary defect is called Marcus Gunn pupil elicited with the swinging flashlight test. It is an extremely useful sign in retrobulbar optic neuritis and other optic nerve diseases.

308. Tonic pupils is associated with?
Harrison's 20th Ed. Chapter 28, Page 178

A. Shy-Drager syndrome
B. Diabetes mellitus
C. Amyloidosis
D. All of the above

309. Marcus Gunn pupil indicates?
Harrison's 20th Ed. Chapter 28, Page 178

A. Retrobulbar optic neuritis
B. Herpes zoster infection
C. Diabetes mellitus
D. All of the above

An eye with no light perception has no pupillary response to direct light stimulation. If the retina or optic nerve is only partially injured, direct pupillary response will be weaker than consensual pupillary response evoked by shining a light into other eye. This relative afferent pupillary defect (Marcus Gunn pupil) can be elicited with the swinging flashlight test. It is an extremely useful sign in retrobulbar optic neuritis & optic nerve diseases.

310. Which of the following is not a feature of Horner's syndrome?
Harrison's 20th Ed. Chapter 28, Page 178

A. Miosis
B. Ipsilateral ptosis
C. Anisocoria
D. Anhidrosis

Horner's syndrome is a triad of miosis, ipsilateral ptosis & anhidrosis. Anhidrosis is an inconstant feature. Brainstem stroke, carotid dissection & neoplasm impinging on the sympathetic chain cause of Horner's syndrome, but most cases are idiopathic.

311. Which of the following feature of Horner's syndrome is inconstant?
Harrison's 20th Ed. Chapter 28, Page 192

A. Miosis
B. Ipsilateral ptosis
C. Anhidrosis
D. All of the above

312. In Adie's syndrome, a tonic pupil occurs in conjunction with?
Harrison's 20th Ed. Chapter 28, Page 178

A. Weak or absent tendon reflexes in lower extremities
B. Weak or absent tendon reflexes in upper extremities
C. Xerophthalmia
D. Strabismus

Adie's syndrome is a benign disorder in which tonic pupil occurs in conjunction with weak or absent tendon reflexes in lower extremities. It is assumed to represent a mild dysautonomia mostly seen in healthy young women.

313. Tonic pupils are associated with?
Harrison's 20th Ed. Chapter 28, Page 178

A. Shy-Drager syndrome
B. Diabetes
C. Amyloidosis
D. All of the above

Tonic pupils are associated with Shy-Drager syndrome, segmental hypohidrosis, diabetes, amyloidosis or incidentally in an otherwise completely normal, asymptomatic individual.

314. Gardener's pupil best relates to?
Harrison's 20th Ed. Chapter 28, Page 179

A. Narcotic use
B. Exposure to tropane alkaloids contained in plants
C. Perforating injury of eye
D. Adhesions (synechia)

Gardener's pupil refers to mydriasis induced by exposure to tropane alkaloids, contained in plants like deadly nightshade, jimsonweed, or angel's trumpet.

315. Retina does not contain cones for which of the following colour?
Harrison's 20th Ed. Chapter 28, Page 179

A. Red
B. Yellow
C. Green
D. Blue

For colour vision, retina contains three classes of cones, with visual pigments of differing peak spectral sensitivity. Red (560 nm), green (530 nm), and blue (430 nm).

316. In retina, which of the following is not a class of cones?
Harrison's 20th Ed. Chapter 28, Page 179

A. Red
B. Green
C. Yellow
D. Blue

317. Which of the following is false about colour vision?
Harrison's 20th Ed. Chapter 28, Page 179

A. Red & green cone pigments are encoded on X chromosome
B. Blue cone pigment is encoded on chromosome 7
C. Mutations of blue cone pigment are common
D. Ishihara color plates is used to detect red-green color blindness

318. Blue cone pigment is encoded on chromosome?
Harrison's 20th Ed. Chapter 28, Page 179

A. 5
B. 6
C. 7
D. 8

Red & green cone pigments are encoded on X chromosome, while blue cone pigment is on chromosome 7. Mutations of the blue cone pigment are exceedingly rare.

319. Ishihara color plates are used to detect?
Harrison's 20th Ed. Chapter 28, Page 179

A. Red color blindness
B. Green color blindness
C. Blue color blindness
D. Red-green color blindness

Ishihara color plates can be used to detect red-green color blindness.

320. Which of the following statements about colour blindness is false?
Harrison's 20th Ed. Chapter 28, Page 179
- A. Mutations of blue cone pigment are exceedingly rare
- B. Mutations of red & green pigments cause congenital X-linked color blindness
- C. Only male children must be screened
- D. None of the above

321. Acquired defects in color vision can result from?
Harrison's 20th Ed. Chapter 28, Page 179
- A. Disease of macula
- B. Disease of optic nerve
- C. Bilateral strokes involving occipital lobe
- D. All of the above

322. Vision can be impaired by all except?
Harrison's 20th Ed. Chapter 28, Page 179
- A. Colour blindness
- B. Damage to Optic chiasma
- C. Damage to Optic tract
- D. Damage to Occipital lobes

Vision can be impaired by damage to the visual system anywhere from the eyes to the occipital lobes. Anomalous trichromats and dichromats have 6/6 (20/20) visual acuity. Also, a unilateral postchiasmal lesion leaves the visual acuity in each eye unaffected.

323. Dimension of central binocular field is?
Harrison's 20th Ed. Chapter 28, Page 180 Figure 28-3
- A. 40°
- B. 80°
- C. 120°
- D. 160°

Visual fields overlap partially, creating 120° of central binocular field flanked by a 40° monocular crescent on either side.

324. Arcuate scotomas shaped like a Turkish scimitar result from?
Harrison's 20th Ed. Chapter 28, Page 181
- A. Ischemic optic neuropathy
- B. Glaucoma
- C. Optic disc drusen
- D. All of the above

Glaucoma selectively destroys axons that enter superotemporal or inferotemporal poles of optic disc, resulting in arcuate scotomas shaped like a Turkish scimitar, which emanate from the blind spot & curve around fixation to end flat against the horizontal meridian. Arcuate or nerve fiber layer scotomas also result from optic neuritis, ischemic optic neuropathy, optic disc drusen, and branch retinal artery or vein occlusion.

325. In visual field analysis, which of the following indicates that lesion anterior to the optic chiasm?
Harrison's 20th Ed. Chapter 28, Page 181
- A. Scotoma is confined to one eye
- B. Cecocentral scotoma
- C. Arcuate or nerve fiber layer scotomas
- D. All of the above

326. Homonymous hemianopia is produced by a postchiasmal lesion in?
Harrison's 20th Ed. Chapter 28, Page 181
- A. Optic tract
- B. Lateral geniculate body
- C. Optic radiations
- D. Any of the above

A postchiasmal lesion anywhere in the optic tract, lateral geniculate body, optic radiations, or visual cortex can produce a homonymous hemianopia (temporal hemifield defect in contralateral eye and a matching nasal hemifield defect in ipsilateral eye).

327. Damage to the optic radiations in the temporal lobe (Meyer's loop) produces?
Harrison's 20th Ed. Chapter 28, Page 181
- A. Bitemporal hemianopia
- B. Superior quadrantic homonymous hemianopia
- C. Inferior quadrantic homonymous hemianopia
- D. Total homonymous hemianopia

Symmetric compression of optic chiasm by a pituitary adenoma, meningioma, craniopharyngioma, glioma, or aneurysm results in a bitemporal hemianopia. Damage to the optic radiations in the temporal lobe (Meyer's loop) produces a superior quadrantic homonymous hemianopia, whereas injury to the optic radiations in the parietal lobe results in an inferior quadrantic homonymous hemianopia. Occlusion of posterior cerebral artery supplying occipital lobe causes total homonymous hemianopia.

328. Cortical blindness is distinguished from bilateral prechiasmal visual loss by?
Harrison's 20th Ed. Chapter 28, Page 181
- A. Normal visual acuity
- B. Normal color vision
- C. Normal pupillary responses
- D. All of the above

Cortical blindness is distinguished from bilateral prechiasmal visual loss by normal pupillary responses and normal optic fundi.

329. Hutchinson's sign is best related to?
Harrison's 20th Ed. Chapter 28, Page 182
- A. Herpes simplex
- B. Herpes zoster
- C. Sarcoidosis
- D. Sjögren's syndrome

Hutchinson's sign refers to vesicles forming on tip of the nose, reflecting nasociliary (V1) nerve involvement due to Herpes Zoster. Vesicles may precede the development of sight-threatening ophthalmic herpes zoster.

330. Hutchinson pupil best relates to?
DeJong's The Neurologic Examination, 7th Ed. Page 750
- A. Mastication muscles
- B. Macula lutea
- C. Uncal herniation
- D. Seizures

Hutchinson pupil refers to third nerve palsy due to uncal herniation presenting as unilaterally dilated pupil, unreactive to light, in the setting of coma.

331. Law of equal innervation is known by the name of?
DeJong's The Neurologic Examination, 7th Ed. Page 204
- A. Pitres' law
- B. Hering's law
- C. Alexander's law
- D. Brodmann law

Hering's law, or the law of equal innervation, states that the same amount of innervation goes to an extraocular muscle and to its yoked fellow.

332. Which of the following is a cause of scleritis?
Harrison's 20th Ed. Chapter 28, Page 182

A. Rheumatoid arthritis
B. Lupus erythematosus
C. Polyarteritis nodosa
D. All of the above

Scleritis is associated with connective tissue diseases like rheumatoid arthritis, lupus erythematosus, polyarteritis nodosa, granulomatosis with polyangiitis, or relapsing polychondritis.

333. Which of the following can cause panuveitis?
Harrison's 20th Ed. Chapter 28, Page 182

A. Sarcoidosis
B. Behçet's disease
C. Inflammatory bowel disease
D. All of the above

334. Chronic inflammation occurs in which of the following structures in intermediate uveitis?
Harrison's 20th Ed. Chapter 28, Page 182

A. Anterior vitreous
B. Ciliary body
C. Peripheral retina
D. All of the above

Term "intermediate uveitis" describes inflammation of anterior vitreous, ciliary body & peripheral retina, which may or may not be associated with infection or systemic disease. Term "pars planitis" refers to a subset of intermediate uveitis associated with snowbank & snowball formation in the absence of an infectious or systemic disease.

335. Which of the following is a cause of Roth's spots?
Harrison's 20th Ed. Chapter 28, Page 183

A. Subacute bacterial endocarditis
B. Leukemia
C. Diabetes
D. All of the above

Roth's spots are white-centered retinal hemorrhages. They are pathognomonic for subacute bacterial endocarditis (SABE), but they also appear in leukemia, diabetes.

336. Amaurosis in Greek language means?
Neurology. 1989;39(12):1622-4

A. Fake
B. Dangerous
C. Dark
D. Slow

Amaurosis in Greek means darkening, dark, or obscure.

337. Fugax in Latin language means?
Neurology. 1989;39(12):1622-4

A. Below the ground
B. Water
C. Fleeting
D. Sleep

Latin meaning of fugax is fleeting.

338. Amaurosis Fugax is best related to?
Harrison's 20th Ed. Chapter 28, Page 183

A. Multiple sclerosis
B. Schizophrenia
C. Transient ischemic attack of retina
D. All of the above

Amaurosis Fugax or refers to a transient ischemic attack of the retina. Interruption of blood flow to retina for more than a few seconds, mostly by an embolus, results in transient monocular blindness. Emboli are composed of cholesterol (Hollenhorst plaque), calcium, or platelet-fibrin debris mostly coming from an atherosclerotic plaque in carotid artery or aorta.

339. Retinal arterial occlusion occurs in which of the following?
Harrison's 20th Ed. Chapter 28, Page 183

A. Retinal migraine
B. Pregnancy
C. Blood dyscrasias
D. All of the above

340. Susac's syndrome consists of?
American Journal of Neuroradiology. 2004;25(3):351-352

A. Encephalopathy
B. Branch retinal artery occlusions
C. Hearing loss
D. All of the above

Susac's syndrome refers to clinical triad of encephalopathy, branch retinal artery occlusions & hearing loss.

341. Cotton-wool spots in optic fundus refer to?
Harrison's 20th Ed. Chapter 28, Page 184

A. Sclerosis of retinal arterioles
B. Splinter hemorrhages
C. Focal infarcts of the nerve fiber layer of retina
D. Leakage of lipid & fluid into the macula

342. Hard exudate in optic fundus refer to?
Harrison's 20th Ed. Chapter 28, Page 184

A. Sclerosis of retinal arterioles
B. Splinter hemorrhages
C. Focal infarcts of the nerve fiber layer of retina
D. Leakage of lipid & fluid into the macula

Marked systemic hypertension causes sclerosis of retinal arterioles, splinter hemorrhages, focal infarcts of the nerve fiber layer of retina (cotton-wool spots), & leakage of lipid and fluid (hard exudate) into the macula.

343. "Blood and thunder" appearance in optical fundus is best related to?
Harrison's 20th Ed. Chapter 28, Page 184

A. Marked systemic hypertension
B. Retinal arterial occlusion
C. Central retinal vein occlusion
D. Optic neuritis

In central retinal vein occlusion due to frank obstruction may result in extensive retinal bleeding ("blood and thunder" appearance of optical fundus), infarction, and visual loss.

344. Which of the following is false about anterior ischemic optic neuropathy (AION)?
Harrison's 20th Ed. Chapter 28, Page 184

A. Decreased blood flow through posterior ciliary arteries
B. Causes painless & sudden monocular visual loss
C. Consists of two forms: arteritic and nonarteritic
D. None of the above

345. Risk factor for nonarteritic form of AION is?
Harrison's 20th Ed. Chapter 28, Page 184

A. Diabetes
B. Renal failure
C. Hypertension
D. All of the above

Erectile dysfunction drugs may cause AION. AION in one eye increases the likelihood of AION in the other eye. Glucocorticoids should not be prescribed in nonarteritic AION.

346. Which of the following occurs in conjunction with giant cell (temporal) arteritis?
Harrison's 20th Ed. Chapter 28, Page 184

A. Anterior ischemic optic neuropathy (AION)
B. Posterior ischemic optic neuropathy
C. Optic neuritis
D. Toxic optic neuropathy

~5% of patients, especially those >age 60, develop the arteritic form of AION in conjunction with giant cell (temporal) arteritis that causes insufficient blood flow through the posterior ciliary arteries that supply the optic disc. High doses of glucocorticoids or Tocilizumab is useful.

347. Acute visual loss, induced by the combination of severe anemia and hypotension is best related to?
Harrison's 20th Ed. Chapter 28, Page 185

A. Anterior ischemic optic neuropathy (AION)
B. Posterior ischemic optic neuropathy
C. Optic Neuritis
D. Leber's hereditary optic neuropathy

Posterior ischemic optic neuropathy causes acute visual loss, induced by the combination of severe anemia and hypotension.

348. Phrase "the doctor sees nothing, and the patient sees nothing" is best related to?
Harrison's 20th Ed. Chapter 28, Page 185 Figure 28-10

A. Anterior ischemic optic neuropathy (AION)
B. Posterior ischemic optic neuropathy
C. Retrobulbar optic neuritis
D. Leber's hereditary optic neuropathy

349. Which of the following is false about Optic Neuritis?
Harrison's 20th Ed. Chapter 28, Page 185

A. Ocular pain with eye movements
B. Female preponderance
C. Gradual recovery of vision after a single episode
D. None of the above

Virtually all patients experience a gradual recovery of vision after a single episode of optic neuritis, even without treatment.

350. Clinically definite multiple sclerosis develops after optic neuritis in?
Harrison's 20th Ed. Chapter 28, Page 185

A. 25%
B. 50%
C. 75%
D. 100%

Clinically definite multiple sclerosis develops after optic neuritis in 50% cases.

351. Leber's optic neuropathy is caused by a point mutation at codon?
Harrison's 20th Ed. Chapter 28, Page 185

A. 11776
B. 11777
C. 11778
D. 11779

Leber's Hereditary Optic Neuropathy is caused by a point mutation at codon 11778 in the mitochondrial gene encoding nicotinamide adenine dinucleotide dehydrogenase (NADH) subunit 4. These mitochondrial mutations are inherited from the mother by all her children, but usually only sons develop symptoms.

352. Toxic Optic Neuropathy results from exposure to?
Harrison's 20th Ed. Chapter 28, Page 185

A. Ethambutol
B. Methyl alcohol
C. Carbon monoxide
D. All of the above

Toxic Optic Neuropathy results in acute visual loss with bilateral optic disc swelling and central or cecocentral scotomas due to exposure to ethambutol, methyl alcohol (moonshine), ethylene glycol (antifreeze), or carbon monoxide. Other potential offending drugs or toxins are disulfiram, etchlorvynol, chloramphenicol, amiodarone, monoclonal anti-CD3 antibody, ciprofloxacin, digitalis, streptomycin, lead, arsenic, thallium, d-penicillamine, isoniazid, emetine, and sulfonamides. Deficiency states induced by starvation, malabsorption, or alcoholism can lead to insidious visual loss.

353. Optic atrophy refers to?
Harrison's 20th Ed. Chapter 28, Page 185 Figure 28-11

A. Optic disc pallor
B. Arteriolar narrowing
C. Nerve fiber layer destruction
D. All of the above

Optic atrophy is not a specific diagnosis but refers to the combination of optic disc pallor, arteriolar narrowing & nerve fiber layer destruction produced by various eye diseases, especially optic neuropathies.

354. Which of the following is false about papilledema?
Harrison's 20th Ed. Chapter 28, Page 185

A. Optic disc edema
B. Optic disc swelling
C. Due to raised intracranial pressure
D. Visual acuity is not affected

Papilledema refers to bilateral optic disc swelling due to raised intracranial pressure. Other forms of optic disc swelling like optic neuritis or ischemic optic neuropathy are called "optic disc edema."

355. Which of the following is false regarding 'Papilledema'?
Harrison's 20th Ed. Chapter 28, Page 185

A. Bilateral optic disc swelling
B. Due to raised intracranial pressure
C. Transient visual obscuration
D. Visual acuity is generally affected by papilledema

356. Which of the following is a classic symptom of papilledema?
Harrison's 20th Ed. Chapter 28, Page 185

A. Central or cecocentral scotoma
B. Transient visual obscurations
C. Loss of color perception
D. All of the above

Transient visual obscurations are a classic symptom of papilledema. Obscurations follow abrupt shifts in posture or happen spontaneously.

357. Papilledema is a feature of?
Harrison's 20th Ed. Chapter 28, Page 185
- A. High-altitude cerebral edema (HACE)
- B. Brain leukostasis
- C. POEMS syndrome
- D. All of the above

358. Papilledema is a feature of?
Harrison's 20th Ed. Chapter 28, Page 185
- A. Cat-scratch disease
- B. Hypoparathyroidism
- C. Acute toxicity of vitamin A
- D. All of the above

359. Papilledema is a feature of?
Harrison's 20th Ed. Chapter 28, Page 185
- A. Cerebral malaria
- B. Malignant hypertension
- C. Chronic hypocalcemia
- D. All of the above

360. In papilledema, the earliest change is?
DeJong's The Neurologic Examination, 7th Ed. Page 170
- A. Pallor of the temporal portion of the disc
- B. Loss of previously observed spontaneous venous pulsations
- C. Disc margins stand out distinctly
- D. All of the above

In papilledema, the earliest change is loss of previously observed spontaneous venous pulsations (SVPs). It is an old saying that when the patient sees (normal vision) and the doctor sees (observes disc abnormalities), it is papilledema; when patient doesn't see (impaired vision) and the doctor sees (observes disc abnormalities), it is papillitis; when the patient doesn't see (has impaired vision) and the doctor doesn't see (observes no disc abnormality), it is retrobulbar neuritis.

361. "Champagne cork" disc best relates to?
DeJong's The Neurologic Examination, 7th Ed. Page 170
- A. Anterior ischemic optic neuropathy (AION)
- B. Optic neuritis
- C. Papilledema
- D. Optic disc drusen

In chronic papilledema, hemorrhages & exudates resolve. What is left is a markedly swollen "champagne cork" disc bulging up from the plane of retina.

362. Which of the following best relates to optic disc drusen?
Harrison's 20th Ed. Chapter 28, Page 186 Figure 28-13
- A. Refractile deposits within the substance of optic nerve head
- B. Fulminant papilledema
- C. Optic nerve fiber layer destruction
- D. Optic pallor

Optic disc drusen are refractile calcified, mulberry-like deposits of unknown etiology within the optic disc, giving rise to "pseudopapilledema."

363. Which of the following is false about optic disc drusen?
Harrison's 20th Ed. Chapter 28, Page 186
- A. Innocuous in nature
- B. Unrelated to drusen of the retina
- C. B-ultrasound is the most sensitive way to detect them
- D. None of the above

364. Fragile neovascular vessels that proliferate on surface of retina are seen in?
Harrison's 20th Ed. Chapter 28, Page 186
- A. Diabetes
- B. Sickle cell anemia
- C. Ischemic ocular diseases
- D. All of the above

Fragile neovascular vessels that proliferate on the surface of the retina in diabetes, sickle cell anemia, and other ischemic ocular diseases.

365. Retinal detachment can produce which of the following symptoms?
Harrison's 20th Ed. Chapter 28, Page 186
- A. Floaters
- B. Flashing lights
- C. Scotoma in peripheral visual field corresponding to detachment
- D. All of the above

366. In most eyes, retinal detachment starts with a?
Harrison's 20th Ed. Chapter 28, Page 186
- A. Hole in the peripheral retina
- B. Flap in the peripheral retina
- C. Tear in the peripheral retina
- D. Any of the above

In most eyes, retinal detachment starts with a hole, flap, or tear in the peripheral retina (rhegmatogenous retinal detachment). Patients with peripheral retinal thinning (lattice degeneration) are vulnerable to this process.

367. Which of the following is false about scintillating scotomas of migraine?
Harrison's 20th Ed. Chapter 28, Page 187
- A. Remain visible in the dark
- B. Remain visible with the eyes closed
- C. Headache develops afer visual symptoms recede
- D. None of the above

368. Which of the following is a sign of brainstem ischemia?
Harrison's 20th Ed. Chapter 28, Page 187
- A. Diplopia
- B. Vertigo
- C. Dysarthria
- D. All of the above

Signs of brainstem ischemia are diplopia, vertigo, numbness, weakness, and dysarthria.

369. Which of the following is a cause of hemianopic cortical visual loss?
Harrison's 20th Ed. Chapter 28, Page 187
- A. Occipital lobe stroke
- B. Lobar hemorrhage
- C. Arteriovenous malformation
- D. All of the above

In a case of occipital lobe stroke due to thrombotic occlusion of vertebrobasilar system, embolus, or dissection, the only finding on examination is a homonymous visual field defect that stops abruptly at the "vertical meridian". Lobar hemorrhage, tumor, abscess, and arteriovenous malformation are other common causes of hemianopic cortical visual loss.

370. Formation of cataract occurs more rapidly in patients with a history of?
Harrison's 20th Ed. Chapter 28, Page 187

- A. Uveitis
- B. Diabetes mellitus
- C. Vitrectomy
- D. All of the above

371. Genetic disease leading to the formation of cataract is?
Harrison's 20th Ed. Chapter 28, Page 187

- A. Myotonic dystrophy
- B. Neurofibromatosis type 2
- C. Galactosemia
- D. All of the above

372. In glaucoma, axons entering which of the following aspects of optic disc are damaged first?
Harrison's 20th Ed. Chapter 28, Page 187

- A. Inferotemporal
- B. Inferonasal
- C. Superonasal
- D. Any of the above

In glaucoma, axons entering inferotemporal and superotemporal aspects of optic disc are damaged first, producing typical nerve fiber bundle or arcuate scotomas on perimetric testing.

373. Which of the following condition is caused due to variants in the gene for complement factor H?
Harrison's 20th Ed. Chapter 28, Page 188

- A. Retinal detachment
- B. Cataract
- C. Glaucoma
- D. Macular degeneration

Susceptibility to macular degeneration is associated with variants in the gene for complement factor H, an inhibitor of alternative complement pathway.

374. Which of the following is useful in macular degeneration?
Harrison's 20th Ed. Chapter 28, Page 188

- A. Bevacizumab
- B. Ranibizumab
- C. Aflibercept
- D. All of the above

Exudative macular degeneration can be treated with intraocular injection of antagonists to vascular endothelial growth factor. Bevacizumab, ranibizumab, or aflibercept is administered by direct injection into the vitreous cavity. These antibodies cause the regression of neovascular membranes by blocking the action of vascular endothelial growth factor.

375. Bone spicules in the peripheral retina best relate to?
Harrison's 20th Ed. Chapter 28, Page 188

- A. Central serous chorioretinopathy
- B. Diabetic retinopathy
- C. Melanoma of the choroid
- D. Retinitis pigmentosa

In retinitis pigmentosa, irregular black deposits of clumped pigment are seen in the peripheral retina. These are called bone spicules because of their resemblance to the spicules of cancellous bone.

376. Retinitis pigmentosa is due to a mutation in the gene for?
Harrison's 20th Ed. Chapter 28, Page 188

- A. Peripherin
- B. Tyrosinase (TYR)
- C. Gene for transcription factor C/EBPα
- D. Gene for Gsα subunit

Retinitis pigmentosa is due to a mutation in the gene for rhodopsin or in the gene for peripherin.

377. Which of the following is false about retinitis pigmentosa?
Harrison's 20th Ed. Chapter 28, Page 188

- A. Progressive night blindness
- B. Visual field constriction with a ring scotoma
- C. Abnormal electroretinogram (ERG)
- D. None of the above

378. Treatment with which of the following drugs causes retinopathy that resembles that of retinitis pigmentosa?
Harrison's 20th Ed. Chapter 28, Page 188

- A. Chloroquine
- B. Hydroxychloroquine
- C. Thioridazine
- D. All of the above

379. Retinitis pigmentosa occur in association with?
Harrison's 20th Ed. Chapter 28, Page 188

- A. Bassen-Kornzweig disease
- B. Kearns-Sayre syndrome
- C. Refsum's disease
- D. All of the above

380. Which is the most common primary tumor of the eye?
Harrison's 20th Ed. Chapter 28, Page 189

- A. Retinoblastoma
- B. Melanoma
- C. Hemangioblastoma
- D. Astrocytic hamartoma

381. Which of the following is not a cause of enophthalmos?
Harrison's 20th Ed. Chapter 28, Page 189

- A. Horner's syndrome
- B. Fracture of the orbital floor
- C. Space-occupying lesion in the orbit
- D. All of the above

382. Protrusion of the globe in orbital inflammation is due particularly to engorgement of which extraocular muscle?
Harrison's 20th Ed. Chapter 28, Page 189

- A. Medial rectus
- B. Lateral rectus
- C. Superior rectus
- D. All of the above

Orbital inflammation & engorgement of extraocular muscles, particularly medial rectus and inferior rectus, account for the protrusion of the globe.

383. Which of the following is a cause of myogenic ptosis?
Harrison's 20th Ed. Chapter 28, Page 190

A. Myasthenia gravis
B. Kearns-Sayre syndrome
C. Myotonic dystrophy
D. All of the above

384. Which of the following is not a feature of Kearns-Sayre syndrome?
Harrison's 20th Ed. Chapter 28, Page 190

A. Frontal balding
B. Retinal pigmentary changes
C. Abnormalities of cardiac conduction
D. "Ragged-red fibers" on peripheral muscle biopsy

In Kearns-Sayre syndrome, retinal pigmentary changes and abnormalities of cardiac conduction develop along with characteristic "ragged-red fibers" on peripheral muscle biopsy. In autosomal dominant myotonic dystrophy, ptosis, ophthalmoparesis, cataract, pigmentary retinopathy, muscle wasting, myotonia, frontal balding, and cardiac abnormalities are seen.

385. Which of the following in not a feature of myasthenia gravis?
Harrison's 20th Ed. Chapter 28, Page 190

A. Muscle wasting
B. Diplopia
C. Pupils are always normal
D. Fluctuating ptosis

Fluctuating ptosis that worsens late in the day is typical of myasthenia gravis.

386. Which of the following is not innervated by oculomotor nerve?
Harrison's 20th Ed. Chapter 28, Page 191

A. Levator palpebrae superioris
B. Inferior oblique
C. Superior oblique
D. Iris sphincter

Third cranial nerve innervates medial, inferior, and superior recti; inferior oblique; levator palpebrae superioris; and iris sphincter. Lateral rectus and superior oblique muscles are not supplied by third cranial nerve. Abducens or the sixth cranial nerve innervates lateral rectus muscle. Trochlear or the fourth cranial nerve innervates the contralateral superior oblique.

387. Total palsy of the oculomotor nerve causes all except?
Harrison's 20th Ed. Chapter 28, Page 191

A. Ptosis
B. Dilated pupil
C. Eye is "down and out"
D. Eye is "down and in"

Total palsy of oculomotor nerve causes ptosis, dilated pupil, and leaves the eye "down and out" because of the unopposed action of lateral rectus and superior oblique muscles.

388. Total palsy of oculomotor nerve leaves the eye?
Harrison's 20th Ed. Chapter 28, Page 191

A. Down and in
B. Down and out
C. Up and in
D. Up and out

389. Which of the following is false about III nerve palsy?
Harrison's 20th Ed. Chapter 28, Page 191

A. Nothnagel's syndrome is ipsilateral III palsy and contralateral cerebellar ataxia
B. Benedikt's syndrome is ipsilateral III nerve palsy and contralateral tremor, chorea, and athetosis
C. Weber's syndrome is ipsilateral III nerve palsy with contralateral hemiparesis
D. None of the above

Nothnagel's syndrome is also called ophthalmoplegia-ataxia syndrome. It is a variant of Parinaud's syndrome, with uni- or bilateral III nerve palsy & ataxia accompanied by vertical gaze deficits & other neurologic signs.

390. Which of the following is not a midbrain syndrome?
DeJong's The Neurologic Examination, 7th Ed. Page 337

A. Millard-Gubler syndrome
B. Weber's syndrome
C. Claude's syndrome
D. Benedikt's syndrome

Millard-Gubler syndrome, Foville syndrome & Raymond's syndrome are pontine syndromes. The three midbrain syndromes are Weber's syndrome, Claude's syndrome & Benedikt's syndrome. Benedikt's is essentially Weber's + Claude's. Parinaud's and Nothnagel's syndrome are also due to lesion in the midbrain.

391. Which of the following is a syndrome of the medulla?
DeJong's The Neurologic Examination, 7th Ed. Page 337

A. Avellis's syndrome
B. Jackson's syndrome
C. Schmidt's syndrome
D. All of the above

The two primary medullary syndromes are the lateral medullary syndrome (Wallenberg) and the medial medullary syndrome (Dejerine). Other syndromes of the medulla include Avellis's, Jackson's, Schmidt's, Céstan-Chenais, and Babinski-Nageotte.

392. Which of the following is called hemimedullary syndrome?
DeJong's The Neurologic Examination, 7th Ed. Page 340

A. Babinski-Nageotte syndrome
B. Céstan-Chenais syndrome
C. Dejerine's syndrome
D. Schmidt's syndrome

393. Injury to the red nucleus causes which of the following?
Harrison's 20th Ed. Chapter 28, Page 191

A. Nothnagel's syndrome
B. Benedikt's syndrome
C. Weber's syndrome
D. All of the above

394. Injury to the superior cerebellar peduncle causes which of the following?
Harrison's 20th Ed. Chapter 28, Page 191

A. Nothnagel's syndrome
B. Benedikt's syndrome
C. Weber's syndrome
D. All of the above

395. Injury to the superior cerebral peduncle causes which of the following?
Harrison's 20th Ed. Chapter 28, Page 191

A. Nothnagel's syndrome
B. Benedikt's syndrome
C. Weber's syndrome
D. All of the above

396. **Ipsilateral oculomotor palsy is a feature of?**
Harrison's 20th Ed. Chapter 28, Page 191

   A. Nothnagel's syndrome
   B. Benedikt's syndrome
   C. Weber's syndrome
   D. All of the above

397. **Contralateral tremor, chorea, and athetosis is a feature of?**
Harrison's 20th Ed. Chapter 28, Page 191

   A. Nothnagel's syndrome
   B. Benedikt's syndrome
   C. Weber's syndrome
   D. All of the above

In Nothnagel's syndrome, injury to the superior cerebellar peduncle causes ipsilateral oculomotor palsy and contralateral cerebellar ataxia. In Benedikt's syndrome, injury to the red nucleus results in ipsilateral oculomotor palsy and contralateral tremor, chorea, and athetosis. Claude's syndrome incorporates features of both of these syndromes, by injury to both the red nucleus and the superior cerebellar peduncle. In Weber's syndrome, injury to the cerebral peduncle causes ipsilateral oculomotor palsy with contralateral hemiparesis.

398. **Which of the following cranial nerves has "head tilt test" as a cardinal diagnostic feature?**
Harrison's 20th Ed. Chapter 28, Page 191

   A. Oculomotor nerve
   B. Trochlear nerve
   C. Abducens nerve
   D. All of the above

Trochlear nerve or fourth cranial nerve originates in midbrain and innervates the contralateral superior oblique. Its action is to depress and intort the eyeball. Its palsy results in hypertropia & excyclotorsion with patients complaining of vertical diplopia, especially upon reading or looking down which is exacerbated by tilting head toward the side with the muscle palsy & alleviated by tilting it away. This "head tilt test" is a cardinal diagnostic feature of trochlear nerve palsy.

399. **Isolated trochlear nerve palsy results from all of the following causes except?**
Harrison's 20th Ed. Chapter 28, Page 191

   A. Aneurysm
   B. Meningitis
   C. Tumor
   D. Infarction

Isolated trochlear nerve palsy does not result from aneurysm.

400. **Which of the following is false about Trochlear Nerve?**
Harrison's 20th Ed. Chapter 28, Page 191

   A. Palsy results in hypertropia
   B. Palsy results in excyclotorsion
   C. Head tilt test is diagnostic
   D. None of the above

401. **Isolated trochlear nerve palsy occurs due to all except?**
Harrison's 20th Ed. Chapter 28, Page 191

   A. Infarction
   B. Herniation
   C. Aneurysm
   D. Tumour

402. **Foville's syndrome includes all except?**
Harrison's 20th Ed. Chapter 28, Page 191

   A. Lateral gaze palsy
   B. Ipsilateral facial palsy
   C. Contralateral hemiparesis
   D. Contralateral hemianesthesia

403. **Which of the following is false about Millard-Gubler syndrome?**
Harrison's 20th Ed. Chapter 28, Page 191

   A. Due to ventral pontine injury
   B. Lateral gaze palsy
   C. Ipsilateral facial palsy
   D. Contralateral hemiparesis

404. **Which of the following is false about Gradenigo's syndrome?**
Harrison's 20th Ed. Chapter 28, Page 191

   A. Mastoiditis
   B. Deafness
   C. Ipsilateral abducens palsy
   D. None of the above

405. **Which of the following can produce ophthalmoplegia?**
Harrison's 20th Ed. Chapter 28, Page 191

   A. Lambert-Eaton myasthenic syndrome
   B. Giant cell (temporal) arteritis
   C. Miller Fisher syndrome
   D. All of the above

406. **Most common cause of internuclear ophthalmoplegia is?**
Harrison's 20th Ed. Chapter 28, Page 191

   A. Multiple sclerosis
   B. Intracranial tumor
   C. Stroke
   D. Concussion trauma

407. **Which of the following is false for Parinaud's syndrome?**
Harrison's 20th Ed. Chapter 28, Page 191

   A. Also known as dorsal midbrain syndrome
   B. Supranuclear vertical gaze disorder
   C. Hydrocephalus from aqueductal stenosis
   D. None of the above

408. **Which of the following has no relation with Parinaud's syndrome?**
Harrison's 20th Ed. Chapter 28, Page 191

   A. Pineal region tumors
   B. Beevor's sign
   C. Setting sun sign
   D. Collier's sign

409. Lateral gaze palsy, ipsilateral facial palsy, and contralateral hemiparesis are features of?
Harrison's 20th Ed. Chapter 28, Page 191

A. Foville's syndrome
B. Millard-Gubler syndrome
C. Gradenigo's syndrome
D. Tolosa-Hunt syndrome

Foville's syndrome occurs as a result of dorsal pontine injury damaging abducens nucleus. It includes lateral gaze palsy, ipsilateral facial palsy, and contralateral hemiparesis incurred by damage to descending corticospinal fibers. Abducens nucleus contains interneurons that project via medial longitudinal fasciculus to the medial rectus subnucleus of the contralateral oculomotor complex. Therefore, abducens nuclear lesion produces a complete lateral gaze palsy from weakness of both the ipsilateral lateral rectus and the contralateral medial rectus.

410. Injury to which of the following leads to Millard-Gubler syndrome?
Harrison's 20th Ed. Chapter 28, Page 191

A. Dorsal pons
B. Ventral pons
C. Medial longitudinal fasciculus
D. Paramedian pontine reticular formation

Millard-Gubler syndrome consists of lateral rectus weakness only, instead of gaze palsy as abducens fascicle is injured rather than the nucleus from ventral pontine injury.

411. Gradenigo's syndrome relates best with which of the following?
Harrison's 20th Ed. Chapter 28, Page 191

A. Subacute sclerosing panencephalitis (SSPE)
B. Progressive multifocal leukoencephalopathy
C. Transverse sinus thrombosis
D. Pituitary adenoma

Headache and earache are the most frequent symptoms of transverse sinus thrombosis. A transverse sinus thrombosis may also present with otitis media, sixth nerve palsy, and retroorbital or facial pain (Gradenigo's syndrome). Sigmoid sinus and internal jugular vein thrombosis may present with neck pain.

412. Which of the following is a cause of abducens palsy?
Harrison's 20th Ed. Chapter 28, Page 191

A. Raised intracranial pressure
B. After lumbar puncture
C. Spontaneous dural cerebrospinal fluid leak
D. All of the above

Unilateral or bilateral abducens palsy is a classic sign of raised intracranial pressure, probably related to rostral-caudal displacement of brainstem. Low intracranial pressure after lumbar puncture, spinal anesthesia, or spontaneous dural cerebrospinal fluid leak may also cause abducens palsy.

413. Which of the intracranial locations can produce multiple ocular motor nerve palsies?
Harrison's 20th Ed. Chapter 28, Page 192

A. Cavernous sinus
B. Superior orbital fissure
C. Orbital apex
D. All of the above

Lesions at cavernous sinus, superior orbital fissure, and orbital apex can produce multiple ocular motor nerve palsies as all three ocular motor nerves are in close proximity.

414. Name of the law that states "jerk nystagmus increases with gaze in the direction of the fast phase" is?
DeJong's The Neurologic Examination, 7th Ed. Page 221

A. Pitres' law
B. Hering's law
C. Alexander's law
D. Brodmann law

Hering's law, or the law of equal innervation, states that the same amount of innervation goes to an extraocular muscle and to its yoked fellow.

415. Nystagmus occurs due to?
Harrison's 20th Ed. Chapter 28, Page 192

A. Vestibular stimulation
B. Optokinetic stimulation
C. Congenital sensory nystagmus
D. All of the above

416. Congenital sensory nystagmus may be due to?
Harrison's 20th Ed. Chapter 28, Page 192

A. Albinism
B. Leber's congenital amaurosis
C. Bilateral cataract
D. All of the above

417. Vestibular nystagmus results from dysfunction of?
Harrison's 20th Ed. Chapter 28, Page 192

A. Labyrinth
B. Vestibular nerve
C. Vestibular nucleus in the brainstem
D. All of the above

418. Downbeat nystagmus results from all except?
Harrison's 20th Ed. Chapter 28, Page 192

A. Chiari malformation
B. Lithium or anticonvulsant intoxication
C. Damage to the pontine tegmentum
D. Alcoholism

Downbeat nystagmus results from lesions near the craniocervical junction, brainstem or cerebellar stroke, lithium or anticonvulsant intoxication, alcoholism & multiple sclerosis. Upbeat nystagmus is associated with damage to pontine tegmentum from stroke, demyelination, or tumor.

419. Saccadomania or dancing eyes best relate to?
Harrison's 20th Ed. Chapter 28, Page 193

A. Opsoclonus
B. Rebound nystagmus
C. Seesaw nystagmus
D. Ocular bobbing

Ocular flutter & opsoclonus are types of saccadic intrusions, spontaneous saccades away from fixation. They may be confused with nystagmus.

420. Which of the following best relates to positional nystagmus?
DeJong's The Neurologic Examination, 7th Ed. Page 294

A. Wartenberg pendulum test
B. Hoover's test
C. Wada test
D. Dix-Hallpike test

421. Who was the inventor of the ophthalmoscope?
DeJong's The Neurologic Examination, 7th Ed. Page 208

A. Helmholtz
B. Welch
C. Allyn
D. Purkinje

Helmholtz was the inventor of ophthalmoscope.

Pathobiology of Neurologic Diseases

422. Neuropil consists of?
Harrison's 20th Ed. Chapter 443, Page 3260

- A. Axons
- B. Dendrites
- C. Glial cell processes
- D. All of the above

423. What proportion of 23,000 genes encoded in human genome are expressed in human nervous system?
Harrison's 20th Ed. Chapter 417 Page 3039

- A. ~ one-fourth
- B. ~ one-third
- C. ~ one-half
- D. ~ three-fourth

Over one-third of 23,000 genes encoded in human genome are expressed in human nervous system.

424. Each mature brain is composed of how many neurons?
Harrison's 20th Ed. Chapter 417 Page 3039

- A. 10 million
- B. 100 million
- C. 10 billion
- D. 100 billion

425. Each mature brain is composed of how many synapses?
Harrison's 20th Ed. Chapter 417 Page 3039

- A. ~ 10^{10}
- B. ~ 10^{15}
- C. ~ 10^{20}
- D. ~ 10^{25}

Each mature brain is composed of 100 billion neurons, several million miles of axons and dendrites, and >10^{15} synapses.

426. Which of the following is false about myelin?
Harrison's 20th Ed. Chapter 416, Page 3030

- A. It speeds impulse conduction
- B. Single oligodendrocyte ensheaths multiple CNS axons
- C. Each Schwann cell myelinates a single PNS axon
- D. It is a protein-rich material

Myelin is a lipid-rich material formed by a spiraling process of the membrane of myelinating cell around the axon.

427. Which of the following about myelin is false?
Harrison's 20th Ed. Chapter 417 Page 3039

- A. Lipid-rich insulating substance that surrounds axons
- B. Speeds impulse conduction
- C. Single oligodendrocyte ensheaths multiple axons in CNS
- D. None of the above

428. Which of the following about oligodendrocyte precursor cells (OPCs) is false?
Harrison's 20th Ed. Chapter 417 Page 3039

- A. Highly motile cells
- B. Migrate along inner surface of endothelial cells
- C. Migration regulated by Wnt pathway signaling
- D. None of the above

429. Which of the following regulate oligodendrocyte differentiation and myelination?
Harrison's 20th Ed. Chapter 417 Page 3039

- A. LINGO-1
- B. PSA-NCAM
- C. Chrm1
- D. All of the above

Oligodendrocyte differentiation & myelination is inhibited by LINGO-1, PSA-NCAM, hyaluronan, Nogo-A, Wnt pathway, notch signaling, and M1 muscarinic receptor Chrm1. Retinoic acid receptor RXRγ have an excitatory influence.

430. Which of the following is a remyelinating agent?
Harrison's 20th Ed. Chapter 417 Page 3039

- A. Prilocaine
- B. Polidocanol
- C. Clemastine
- D. Chlorprothixene

Antihistamine clemastine, that works via binding to Chrm1 muscarinic receptor, has shown efficacy as a remyelinating agent in patients with chronic optic neuropathy due to MS.

431. Brain microglia secrete which of the following?
Harrison's 20th Ed. Chapter 417 Page 3040

- A. Glial-derived neurotrophic factor (GDNF)
- B. Brain derived neurotrophic factor (BDNF)
- C. Ciliary neurotrophic factor
- D. All of the above

432. Which of the function of microglial cell?
Harrison's 20th Ed. Chapter 417 Page 3040

- A. Synaptic pruning
- B. Clearing cellular debris & protein
- C. Promotion of learning and memory
- D. All of the above

433. Which of the following about microglia is false?
Harrison's 20th Ed. Chapter 417 Page 3040

- A. Located throughout the brain parenchyma
- B. Downregulate inflammatory responses & promote tissue repair
- C. Activated microglia promote formation of β-amyloid
- D. None of the above

434. Astrocytes secrete which of the following?
Harrison's 20th Ed. Chapter 417 Page 3041

- A. Apolipoprotein E
- B. Thrombospondins
- C. Glypicans
- D. All of the above

Astrocytes influence synapses by secreting factors (apolipoprotein E, thrombospondins & glypicans) that regulate development, maintenance, and pruning of presynaptic & postsynaptic structures.

435. Which of the following is secreted by activated microglia?
Harrison's 20th Ed. Chapter 417 Page 3041

A. IL-1a
B. TNF
C. C1q
D. All of the above

Activated microglia secrete IL-1a, TNF, and C1q, that induces astrocytes to transform to A1 type which actively participate in the injury process.

436. Glymphatic system best relates to?
Harrison's 20th Ed. Chapter 417 Page 3042

A. Aquaporin-4 water channels
B. Sleep
C. Cervical lymph nodes
D. All of the above

437. Which of the following is a protein involved in protection from oxidative stress?
Harrison's 20th Ed. Chapter 417 Page 3043

A. α-synuclein
B. Parkin
C. PINK1
D. DJ-1

PINK1 is a mitochondrial kinase. DJ-1 is a protein involved in protection from oxidative stress. Parkin is a ubiquitin ligase.

438. Superoxide dismutase mutations are associated with?
Harrison's 20th Ed. Chapter 417 Page 3043

A. Huntington's disease (HD)
B. Familial amyotrophic lateral sclerosis (ALS)
C. Frontotemporal dementia (FTD)
D. Progressive supranuclear palsy (PSP)

439. TAR DNA binding protein 43 (TDP-43) is associated with?
Harrison's 20th Ed. Chapter 417 Page 3043

A. Huntington's disease (HD)
B. Familial amyotrophic lateral sclerosis (ALS)
C. Frontotemporal dementia (FTD)
D. Progressive supranuclear palsy (PSP)

440. Mitochondrial dysfunction is strongly linked to the pathogenesis of?
Harrison's 20th Ed. Chapter 417 Page 3043

A. Gerstmann-Sträussler-Scheinker disease (GSS)
B. Huntington's disease (HD)
C. Creutzfeldt-Jakob disease (CJD)
D. Friedreich's ataxia

441. Autophagy is impaired in?
Harrison's 20th Ed. Chapter 417 Page 3043

A. AD
B. PD
C. HD
D. All of the above

442. Which of the following induces autophagy?
Harrison's 20th Ed. Chapter 417 Page 3043

A. Rapamycin
B. Sorafenib
C. Piaglitazone
D. Metformin

Rapamycin is a selective inhibitor of TORC1 (target of rapamycin complex 1). Resveratrol, rapamycin, spermidine, and metformin have been shown to delay aging in experimental animal models.

Headache

443. Which cranial structure is pain-insensitive?
Harrison's 20th Ed. Chapter 13, Page 85
A. Scalp
B. Choroid plexus
C. Dural sinuses
D. Falx cerebri

444. Which cranial structure is pain-sensitive?
Harrison's 20th Ed. Chapter 13, Page 85
A. Ventricular ependyma
B. Choroid plexus
C. Pial veins
D. Falx cerebri

Pain-producing cranial structures include scalp, middle meningeal artery, dural sinuses, falx cerebri and proximal segments of large pial arteries. Ventricular ependyma, choroid plexus, pial veins, and much of the brain parenchyma are not pain-producing.

445. Which of the following is a type of primary headache?
Harrison's 20th Ed. Chapter 13, Page 85 Table 13-1
A. Migraine
B. Tension-type
C. Cluster
D. All of the above

446. Which of the following is not a type of primary headache?
Harrison's 20th Ed. Chapter 13, Page 85 Table 13-1
A. Idiopathic stabbing
B. Exertional
C. Systemic infection
D. Tension-type

Primary headaches are those in which headache and its associated features are the disorder in itself, whereas secondary headaches are those caused by exogenous disorders. Examples of primary headache are migraine, tension-type, cluster, idiopathic stabbing & exertional. Examples of secondary headache are systemic infection, head injury, vascular disorders, subarachnoid hemorrhage & brain tumor.

447. Of the following cause of primary headache, which one is the most common?
Harrison's 20th Ed. Chapter 13, Page 85 Table 13-1
A. Migraine
B. Tension-type
C. Cluster
D. Exertional

Relative frequency of various types of primary headache is migraine 16%, tension-type 69%, cluster 0.1%, idiopathic stabbing 2% and exertional 1%.

448. Of the following cause of secondary headache, which one is the most common?
Harrison's 20th Ed. Chapter 13, Page 85 Table 13-1
A. Systemic infection
B. Vascular disorders
C. Subarachnoid hemorrhage
D. Brain tumor

Relative frequency of various types of secondary headache is systemic infection 63%, head injury 4%, vascular disorders 1%, subarachnoid hemorrhage <1% and brain tumor 0.1%.

449. Which of the following is a part of the trigeminocervical complex?
Harrison's 20th Ed. Chapter 13, Page 85
A. Trigeminal nucleus caudalis
B. Dorsal horns of C1
C. Dorsal horns of C2
D. All of the above

Caudal portion of trigeminal nucleus along with first & second cervical nerve roots is called the trigeminocervical complex.

450. Which of the following is a cranial autonomic symptom?
Harrison's 20th Ed. Chapter 13, Page 85
A. Lacrimation
B. Rhinorrhea
C. Ptosis
D. All of the above

Cranial autonomic symptoms include lacrimation, conjunctival injection, nasal congestion, rhinorrhea, periorbital swelling, aural fullness, and ptosis. These are prominent in trigeminal autonomic cephalalgias (TACs), including cluster headache and paroxysmal hemicrania, and may be seen in migraine.

451. Which of the following symptoms suggest that the headache has a serious underlying disorder?
Harrison's 20th Ed. Chapter 13, Page 86 Table 13-2
A. Pain induced by bending, lifting, cough
B. Pain that disturbs sleep or presents upon awakening
C. Vomiting that precedes headache
D. All of the above

Features that suggest headache has a serious underlying disorder include sudden-onset headache, first severe headache, "worst" headache ever, vomiting that precedes headache, subacute worsening over days or weeks, pain induced by bending, lifting or cough, pain that disturbs sleep or presents immediately upon awakening, known systemic illness, onset after age 55 years, fever or unexplained systemic signs, abnormal neurologic examination and pain associated with local tenderness (region of temporal artery).

452. Which of the following is not a vascular headache?
Harrison's 20th Ed. Chapter 13, Page 85
A. Migraine
B. Cluster headache
C. Tension-type headache
D. All of the above

Migraine & other primary headache types are not vascular headaches. Migraine is a brain disorder.

453. Acute, severe headache with stiff neck but without fever suggests?
Harrison's 20th Ed. Chapter 13, Page 86
A. Cerebral metastases
B. Carcinomatous meningitis
C. Subarachnoid hemorrhage
D. Posterior fossa mass

Acute, severe headache (maximal in <5 minutes, lasting >5 minutes) with stiff neck but without fever suggests subarachnoid hemorrhage.

454. Vomiting that precedes the appearance of headache by weeks is highly characteristic of?
Harrison's 20th Ed. Chapter 13, Page 86

A. Meningitis
B. Subarachnoid hemorrhage
C. Posterior fossa brain tumors
D. Temporal arteritis

Vomiting that precedes appearance of headache by weeks is highly characteristic of posterior fossa brain tumors.

455. Head pain appearing abruptly after bending, lifting or coughing can be due to?
Harrison's 20th Ed. Chapter 13, Page 86

A. Posterior fossa mass
B. Chiari malformation
C. Low cerebrospinal fluid (CSF) volume
D. All of the above

Head pain appearing abruptly after bending, lifting or coughing can be due to posterior fossa mass, Chiari malformation or low cerebrospinal fluid (CSF) volume.

456. Jaw claudication is a feature of?
Harrison's 20th Ed. Chapter 13, Page 86, 676, 3072

A. Vinca alkaloid use
B. Temporal (giant cell) arteritis
C. Occlusion of common carotid artery
D. All of the above

457. Giant cell arteritis is closely associated with?
Harrison's 20th Ed. Chapter 356, Page 2583

A. Granulomatosis with polyangiitis (Wegener's)
B. Eosinophilic granulomatosis with polyangiitis (Churg-Strauss)
C. Polymyalgia rheumatica
D. Polyarteritis nodosa

Giant cell arteritis is closely associated with polymyalgia rheumatica (40–50%).

458. Which of the following is a feature of temporal arteritis?
Harrison's 20th Ed. Chapter 13, Page 86

A. Head pain is infrequently throbbing
B. Scalp tenderness is present
C. Head pain is worse at night & aggravated by exposure to cold
D. All of the above

459. Chronic daily headache (CDH) means headache for how many days per month?
Harrison's 20th Ed. Chapter 13, Page 87

A. 3 days per month
B. 7 days per month
C. 10 days per month
D. 15 days per month

Chronic daily headache (CDH) or near-daily headache could be suspected when a patient experiences headache on 15 days or more per month. It affects ~4% of adults & encompasses different headache syndromes, both primary and secondary.

460. Which of the following is a secondary cause of Daily or Near-Daily Headache?
Harrison's 20th Ed. Chapter 13, Page 87 Table 13-3

A. Giant cell arteritis
B. Sarcoidosis
C. Behçet's syndrome
D. All of the above

461. In "Coat-hanger headache", the pain is in?
Harrison's 20th Ed. Chapter 18, Page 126

A. Suboccipital region
B. Posterior cervical region
C. Shoulder region
D. All of the above

462. Which of the following is the cause of "coat-hanger headache"?
Harrison's 20th Ed. Chapter 18, Page 126

A. Neck muscle spasm
B. Neck muscle tear
C. Neck muscle ischemia
D. Neck muscle inflammation

"Coat-hanger headache" is most likely due to neck muscle ischemia in a patient of orthostatic hypotension.

463. Which of the following is a feature of new daily persistent headache (NDPH)?
Harrison's 20th Ed. Chapter 422, Page 3107

A. Headache on most if not all days
B. Ipsilateral conjunctival injection and lacrimation
C. Very frequent short-lasting attacks
D. Periodicity

464. Which of the following is false about post-lumbar puncture headache?
Harrison's 20th Ed. Chapter 13, Page 88

A. Usually begins within 48 hours
B. Incidence is between 10 and 30%
C. Is dramatically positional
D. Aggravated by abdominal compression

465. Which of the following is false about lumbar puncture headache?
Harrison's 20th Ed. Chapter 13, Page 88

A. Worsened by head shaking
B. Worsened by jugular vein compression
C. Location is bitemporal
D. Epidural blood patch is an effective treatment

466. Which of the following is not a feature of lumbar puncture headache?
Harrison's 20th Ed. Chapter 13, Page 88

A. Dramatically positional
B. Begins when the patient sits or stands upright
C. Relief by abdominal compression
D. Relief by jugular vein compression

Low CSF volume headache is positional (recumbency improves headache within minutes), occipitofrontal, begins within 48 hours following lumbar puncture, but may be delayed for up to 12 days (incidence 10–30%) & caffeine, abdominal binder & oral theophylline provide temporary relief. Symptoms result from low CSF volume rather than low CSF pressure.

467. Headache on rising in the morning or nocturnal headache is characteristic of?
Harrison's 20th Ed. Chapter 13, Page 88

   A. Obstructive sleep apnea
   B. Poorly controlled hypertension
   C. Raised CSF pressure headache
   D. All of the above

468. Sleep disruption and early morning headaches that improve during the day are characteristics of?
Harrison's 20th Ed. Chapter 13, Page 88

   A. Migraine
   B. Cluster headache
   C. Brain tumors
   D. Unruptured aneurysms

469. Headaches that build up over hours, maintained for several hours to days, relieved by sleep are sugestive of?
Harrison's 20th Ed. Chapter 13, Page 88

   A. Migraine
   B. Cluster headache
   C. Brain tumors
   D. Unruptured aneurysms

470. Headache in the absence of any exogenous cause is a feature of?
Harrison's 20th Ed. Chapter 13, Page 88

   A. Migraine
   B. Tension-type headache
   C. Trigeminal autonomic cephalalgias
   D. All of the above

Migraine and Other Primary Headache Disorders

471. Prevalence of migraine increases steeply at?
N Engl J Med. 2017;377:553-61

A. 10 to 14 years of age
B. 20 to 24 years of age
C. 30 to 34 years of age
D. 40 to 44 years of age

Although migraine may begin early in childhood, but its prevalence increases steeply at 10 to 14 years of age. Prevalence continues to increase until 35 to 39 years of age, after which it gradually decreases, particularly among women after menopause.

472. Migraine is associated with an increased risk of?
N Engl J Med. 2017;377:553-61

A. Asthma
B. Stroke
C. Anxiety and depression
D. All of the above

Migraine is associated with increased risks of asthma, stroke, anxiety & depression, & other pain disorders. Although, it is exceedingly rare for cerebral ischemia or infarction to occur during a migraine attack.

473. Which of the following is a common premonitory symptom in migraine?
N Engl J Med. 2017;377:553-61

A. Eye lid twitching
B. Itching
C. Sneezing
D. Yawning

Yawning, mood change, light sensitivity, neck pain, and fatigue are common premonitory symptoms typical of a migraine attack.

474. Which of the following is an infrequent phase in a migraine attack?
Harrison's 20th Ed. Chapter 422, Page 3096, N Engl J Med. 2017;377:553-61

A. Aura
B. Premonitory (prodrome)
C. Headache phase
D. Postdrome

A migraine attack has three phases—premonitory (prodrome), headache phase and postdrome. ~20–25% of migraine patients have a fourth, aura phase. Aura symptoms may include visual disturbances (wavy lines or bright or dark spots), or sensory changes (numbness or tingling), language dysfunction, and vertigo.

475. Which of the following is a paroxysmal disorder?
DeJong's The Neurologic Examination, 7th Ed. Page 791

A. Migraine
B. Periodic paralysis
C. Narcolepsy
D. All of the above

Some disorders occur episodically in patients who are otherwise well and have no abnormalities on neurologic examination between attacks (paroxysmal disorders). They include migraine, seizures, episodic ataxias, certain movement disorders, narcolepsy, and periodic paralysis.

476. Which of the following is not a category of migraine?
DeJong's The Neurologic Examination, 7th Ed. Page 792

A. Classic migraine
B. Contemporary migraine
C. Common migraine
D. Complicated migraine

Migraine is a very common cause of recurrent headaches. It is divided into two large categories: with aura (classic migraine) and without aura (common migraine). When the neurologic dysfunction (with or without headache) is unusually severe or prolonged, becoming the most prominent part of migraine episode, the condition is called complicated migraine.

477. What percentage of patients have migraine without aura?
DeJong's The Neurologic Examination, 7th Ed. Page 792

A. 25%
B. 55%
C. 75%
D. 85%

~ 85% of patients have migraine without aura.

478. Which of the following is not a feature of prodromal phase of a migraine attack?
Harrison's 20th Ed. Chapter 422, Page 3096

A. Cutaneous allodynia
B. Polyuria
C. Yawning
D. Cognitive dysfunction

Cutaneous allodynia refers to the experience of normal touch as uncomfortable.

479. Which of the following is not a feature of headache phase of a migraine attack?
Harrison's 20th Ed. Chapter 422, Page 3096

A. Photophobia
B. Phonophobia
C. Palinopsia
D. Allodynia

Features of the premonitory (prodromal) phase of migraine include yawning, tiredness, cognitive dysfunction, mood change, neck discomfort, polyuria, and food cravings. Headache phase follows with features like nausea, photophobia, phonophobia and allodynia. During postdrome phase, the patient feels tired/weary, has problems concentrating, and has mild neck discomfort.

480. Which of the following can be a cause of hyperosmia?
DeJong's The Neurologic Examination, 7th Ed. Page 142

A. Functional
B. Substance abuse
C. Migraine
D. All of the above

Hyperosmia is usually functional, but it can occur with certain types of substance abuse and in migraine.

481. To be called as suffering from chronic migraine, episodes of migraine on how many days per month must a patient have?
Harrison's 20th Ed. Chapter 422, Page 3096

A. Two or more days per month
B. Four or more days per month
C. Six or more days per month
D. Eight or more days per month

Patients with episodes of migraine on eight or more days per month and with at least 15 total days of headache per month are considered to have chronic migraine.

482. Status migrainosus refers to a migraine attack that lasts longer than?
DeJong's The Neurologic Examination, 7th Ed. Page 793

A. 12 hours
B. 24 hours
C. 48 hours
D. 72 hours

Status migrainosus refers to a migraine attack that lasts longer than 72 hours despite treatment.

483. Which of the following is not included in the simplified diagnostic criteria for migraine?
Harrison's 20th Ed. Chapter 422, Page 3100 Table 422-3

A. Photophobia
B. Phonophobia
C. Allodynia
D. Throbbing, unilateral headache

Although migraine headache is characteristically severe, unilateral, and throbbing, it may also be moderate, bilateral, and constant in quality. The features of migraine other than headache, particularly sensitivity to light and sound, nausea, and interference with the ability to function, may be more useful in diagnosis than the character of the headache.

484. Out of the following, which is the commonest symptom accompanying severe migraine?
Harrison's 20th Ed. Chapter 422, Page 3098 Table 422-2

A. Photophobia
B. Scalp tenderness
C. Vomiting
D. Vertigo

485. Out of the following, which of the following is the most frequent symptoms accompanying severe migraine?
Harrison's 20th Ed. Chapter 422, Page 3098 Table 422-2

A. Photophobia
B. Vomiting
C. Fortification spectra
D. Light headedness

486. In which patient of headache should we apply the simplified diagnostic criteria for migraine?
Harrison's 20th Ed. Chapter 422, Page 3100 Table 422-3

A. Repeated attacks of headache lasting 4–72 hours
B. Patients of headache with a normal physical examination
C. In whom there is no other reasonable cause for headache
D. All of the above

International Headache Society Classification.

487. Which of the following is a type of complicated migraine?
DeJong's The Neurologic Examination, 7th Ed. Page 792

A. Hemiplegic migraine
B. Ophthalmoplegic migraine
C. Basilar artery migraine
D. All of the above

488. Which of the following episodic syndromes may be associated with migraine?
Harrison's 20th Ed. Chapter 422, Page 3097 Table 422-1

A. Cyclical vomiting syndrome
B. Abdominal migraine
C. Benign paroxysmal vertigo
D. All of the above

Primary Headache Disorders, Modified from International Classification of Headache Disorders-III-Beta (Headache Classification Committee of the International Headache Society, 2018).

489. Which of the following is a feature of visual snow syndrome?
Harrison's 20th Ed. Chapter 422, Page 3096, Brain 2014;137(5): 1419–1428

A. Palinopsia
B. Nyctalopia
C. Entoptic phenomena
D. All of the above

Diagnosis of visual snow syndrome (continuous perception of tiny flickering dots in the entire field of vision) can be confirmed if the symptoms have lasted longer than three months & person has two of the following additional symptoms: sensitivity to light (photophobia), seeing image of an object after it has moved (palinopsia), impaired night vision (nyctalopia) or seeing small floating objects (entoptic phenomena). Most people with visual snow syndrome have normal vision tests and normal brain images. Differential diagnosis includes migraine visual aura.

490. In acephalgic migraine, which of the following is least prominent?
Harrison's 20th Ed. Chapter 422, Page 3096

A. Recurrent neurologic symptoms
B. Nausea or vomiting
C. Headache
D. Vertigo

Patients with acephalgic migraine ((typical aura without headache) have recurrent neurologic symptoms, with nausea or vomiting, but with little or no headache. Vertigo may be prominent.

491. Migraine activators (triggers) include all except?
Harrison's 20th Ed. Chapter 422, Page 3096

A. Red wine
B. Menstruation
C. Pregnancy
D. Lack of sleep

492. Migraine deactivators include all except?
Harrison's 20th Ed. Chapter 422, Page 3096

A. Sleep
B. Pregnancy
C. Exhiliration
D. Hunger

Triggers include glare, bright lights, sounds, or other afferent stimulation; hunger, excess stress, physical exertion, stormy weather or barometric pressure changes, hormonal fluctuations during menses, lack of or excess sleep & alcohol or other chemical stimulation such as with nitrates.

493. Which of the following medication can exacerbate migraine?
N Engl J Med. 2017;377:553-61

A. Nasal decongestants
B. Selective serotonin-reuptake inhibitor antidepressants
C. Proton-pump inhibitors
D. All of the above

Multiple medications can exacerbate migraine, including oral contraceptives, postmenopausal hormone therapy, nasal decongestants, selective serotonin-reuptake inhibitor antidepressants, and proton-pump inhibitors.

494. Sensory sensitivity in migraine is due to dysfunction of monoaminergic sensory control systems located in?
Harrison's 20th Ed. Chapter 422, Page 3096

A. Hypothalamus
B. Thalamus
C. Putamen
D. Globus pallidus

Sensory sensitivity, characteristic of migraine, is probably due to dysfunction of monoaminergic sensory control systems located in brainstem & hypothalamus.

495. Key pain input in migraine is from?
Harrison's 20th Ed. Chapter 422, Page 3098 Figure 422-1

A. Meningeal vessels
B. Pia mater
C. Arachnoid mater
D. All of the above

496. Neurons of trigeminocervical complex (TCC) synapse on neurons in thalamus through which tract?
Harrison's 20th Ed. Chapter 422, Page 3098 Figure 422-1

A. Thalamocapsular tract
B. Thalamogeniculate tract
C. Quintothalamic tract
D. All of the above

497. Modulation of trigeminovascular nociceptive input come from?
Harrison's 20th Ed. Chapter 422, Page 3098 Figure 422-1

A. Dorsal raphe nucleus
B. Locus coeruleus
C. Nucleus raphe magnus
D. All of the above

Key pathway for pain in migraine is trigeminovascular input from meningeal vessels. It then passes through trigeminal ganglion & synapses on second-order neurons in trigeminocervical complex (TCC). These neurons in turn project in quintothalamic tract and, after decussating in brainstem, synapse on neurons in thalamus. Important modulation of trigeminovascular nociceptive input comes from dorsal raphe nucleus, locus coeruleus and nucleus raphe magnus.

498. Which of the following is related to migraine?
Harrison's 20th Ed. Chapter 422, Page 3096

A. Gepants
B. Ditans
C. Triptans
D. All of the above

Activation of cells in the trigeminal nucleus results in the release of vasoactive neuropeptides particularly calcitonin gene-related peptide (CGRP) at vascular terminations of the trigeminal nerve and within the trigeminal nucleus. CGRP receptor antagonists called gepants are effective in the acute treatment of migraine as are monoclonal antibodies to CGRP. Exclusive agonists of 5-HT1F receptor are called ditans.

499. Migraine is associated with the release of?
N Engl J Med. 2017;377:553-61

A. Neurotensin
B. Substance P
C. Calcitonin gene-related peptide (CGRP)
D. Cholecystokinin

Migraine is associated with the release of neurotransmitters & neuromodulators, including neuropeptides calcitonin gene-related peptide (CGRP) & pituitary adenylate cyclase-activating peptide (PACAP).

500. MIDAS stands for?
Harrison's 20th Ed. Chapter 422, Page 3098

A. Migraine Disease Assessment Score
B. Migraine Disability Assessment Score
C. Migraine Drug Assessment Score
D. Migraine Diagnosis Assessment Score

MIDAS stands for Migraine Disability Assessment Score meant to assess the extent of a patient's disease and disability.

501. MIDAS questionnaire assesses migraine disability based on how many questions?
Harrison's 20th Ed. Chapter 422, Page 3100 Figure 422-4

A. 5
B. 8
C. 10
D. 12

502. Severe migraine disability is labeled when MIDAS score is?
Harrison's 20th Ed. Chapter 422, Page 3100 Figure 422-4

A. > 5
B. > 10
C. > 15
D. > 20

For questions 1–5, add the total number of days to arrive at the score. If MIDAS Score is 6 or more, consultation with doctor is needed.

503. MIDAS questionnaire asks about events that happened during last how many months?
Harrison's 20th Ed. Chapter 422, Page 3100 Figure 422-4

A. 1 month
B. 3 months
C. 6 months
D. 12 months

504. Drugs used for prophylactic treatment of migraine include all except?
Harrison's 20th Ed. Chapter 422, Page 3103

A. Amitriptyline
B. Sodium valproate
C. Metoclopramide
D. Cyproheptadine

Drugs that have been approved by the FDA for the prophylactic treatment of migraine include propranolol, timolol, sodium valproate, topiramate, methysergide, amitriptyline, nortriptyline, flunarizine, phenelzine, gabapentin and cyproheptadine.

505. Drugs effective in treatment of migraine are?
Harrison's 20th Ed. Chapter 422, Page 3101 Table 422-4

A. Nonsteroidal anti-inflammatory agents
B. 5-HT$_{1B/1D}$ receptor agonists
C. Dopamine receptor antagonists
D. All of the above

Drugs effective in the treatment of migraine are nonsteroidal anti-inflammatory agents, 5HT$_{1B/1D}$ receptor agonists and dopamine receptor antagonists.

506. Triptans are least potent agonist of which of the following?
Harrison's 20th Ed. Chapter 422, Page 3096

A. 5-HT$_{1A}$ receptor
B. 5-HT$_{1B}$ receptor
C. 5-HT$_{1D}$ receptor
D. 5-HT$_{1F}$ receptor

Triptans are potent agonists of 5-HT$_{1B}$, 5-HT$_{1D}$, and 5-HT$_{1F}$ receptors and are less potent at the 5-HT$_{1A}$ receptor.

507. Antimigraine efficacy of the triptans is due to their ability to stimulate?
Harrison's 20th Ed. Chapter 422, Page 3096

A. 5-HT$_{1A}$ receptors
B. 5-HT$_{1B}$ receptors
C. 5-HT$_{1C}$ receptors
D. 5-HT$_{1E}$ receptors

Antimigraine efficacy of triptans relates to their ability to stimulate 5-HT$_{1B/1D}$ receptors, which are located on both blood vessels and nerve terminals.

508. Which of the following about triptans is false?
Harrison's 20th Ed. Chapter 422, Page 3096

A. Potent agonists of 5-HT$_{1B}$ & 5-HT$_{1D}$ receptors
B. Arrest nerve signaling in nociceptive pathways of trigeminovascular system
C. Promote cranial vasoconstriction
D. None of the above

509. Which of the following about ditans is false?
Harrison's 20th Ed. Chapter 422, Page 3096

A. Exclusive agonists of 5-HT$_{1F}$ receptor
B. Act only at neural & not vascular targets
C. Effective in acute migraine
D. None of the above

510. Which of the following about migraineurs is false?
Harrison's 20th Ed. Chapter 422, Page 3096, 131

A. Dopamine receptor hypersensitivity
B. Sensitive to environmental & sensory stimuli
C. Experience more prolonged periods of disequilibrium
D. None of the above

511. Which of the following gene has been incriminated in the causation of Familial hemiplegic migraine (FHM)?
Harrison's 20th Ed. Chapter 422, Page 3096

A. tRNAL$^{eu(UUR)}$
B. CACNA1A
C. DRD2
D. All of the above

Mutations involving the Cav2.1 (P/Q) type voltage-gated calcium channel CACNA1A gene cause familial hemiplegic migraine 1 (FHM 1). Mutations in Na$^+$-K$^+$ATPase ATP1A2 gene causes FHM 2. Mutations in neuronal voltage-gated sodium channel SCN1A cause FHM 3.

512. In PET examination in migraine patients, activation of which of the following area is fundamental to expression of migraine?
Harrison's 20th Ed. Chapter 422, Page 3099 Figure 422-2

A. Hypothalamic
B. Dorsal midbrain
C. Dorsolateral pontine
D. Thalamus

When seen in Positron emission tomography (PET) imaging in migraine patients, activation of dorsolateral pontine area, which includes noradrenergic locus coeruleus, is fundamental to the expression of migraine.

513. Which of the following is a 5-HT$_{1F}$ receptor agonist?
Harrison's 20th Ed. Chapter 422, Page 3100

A. Rimegepant
B. Ubrogepant
C. Lasmiditan
D. All of the above

Two new classes of therapeutic agents for migraine treatment, CGRP receptor antagonists (rimegepant & ubrogepant), and 5-HT$_{1F}$ receptor agonist (lasmiditan), should soon be available.

514. Which of the following is most efficacious amongst triptans?
Harrison's 20th Ed. Chapter 422, Page 3100

A. Frovatriptan
B. Naratriptan
C. Almotriptan
D. Rizatriptan

Rizatriptan & eletriptan are the most efficacious of the triptans.

515. Which of the following about 5HT$_{1B/1D}$ receptor agonists is false?
Harrison's 20th Ed. Chapter 422, Page 3101

A. Not effective in migraine with aura
B. Contraindicated in patients with a h/o cardiovascular & cerebrovascular disease
C. Recurrence of headache common
D. None of the above

516. Which of the following triptan is documented porphyrinogenic and unsafe in porphyria?
Harrison's 20th Ed. Chapter 422, Page 2991 Table 409-4

A. Rizatriptan
B. Sumatriptan
C. Zolmitriptan
D. All of the above

Triptans available for treatment of migraine include sumatriptan, almotriptan, eletriptan, frovatriptan, naratriptan, rizatriptan, and zolmitriptan.

517. Which of the following drugs for treatment of acute migraine can be administered by nasal route?
Harrison's 20th Ed. Chapter 422, Page 3101 Table 422-4

A. Dihydroergotamine
B. Sumatriptan
C. Zolmitriptan
D. All of the above

518. Route of administration of sumatriptan is?
Harrison's 20th Ed. Chapter 422, Page 3101 Table 422-4

A. Oral
B. Nasal
C. Subcuteneous
D. All of the above

519. In migraine, use of which of the following may decrease the likelihood of a response to triptans in future?
Harrison's 20th Ed. Chapter 422, Page 3102

A. Isometheptene
B. Meperidine
C. Prochlorperazine
D. Dihydroergotamine

There is evidence that use of opioids may decrease the likelihood of a response to triptans in future.

520. Methysergide may cause retroperitoneal or cardiac valvular fibrosis when used for more than?
Harrison's 20th Ed. Chapter 422, Page 3103

A. 3 months
B. 6 months
C. 9 months
D. 12 months

Methysergide may cause retroperitoneal or cardiac valvular fibrosis when it is used for > 6 months. Risk of fibrosis is about 1:1500 and is likely to reverse after drug is stopped.

521. For instituting prophylactic treatment of migraine, what should be the frequency of attacks?
Harrison's 20th Ed. Chapter 422, Page 3103

A. At least three attacks per day
B. At least three attacks per week
C. At least three attacks per month
D. At least three attacks per year

522. Drugs used for prophylactic treatment of migraine include all except?
Harrison's 20th Ed. Chapter 422, Page 3103

A. Timolol
B. Sodium valproate
C. Methysergide
D. Sumatriptan

Antihypertensive agents (betaadrenergic blockers & candesartan), anticonvulsant agents (topiramate & divalproex sodium), and tricyclic antidepressants (amitriptyline & nortriptyline) are standard preventive therapies for migraine.

523. Which of the following is useful for prevention of chronic migraine?
N Engl J Med. 2017;377:553-61

A. Coenzyme Q10
B. Melatonin
C. Petasites
D. OnabotulinumtoxinA

OnabotulinumtoxinA is a Food and Drug Administration (FDA) approved therapy for prevention of chronic migraine, defined as headache occurring on more than 15 days per month, with migraine features on at least 8 of those days.

524. Which of the following drug is useful in patients of migraine who are obese?
N Engl J Med. 2017;377:553-61

A. Divalproex sodium
B. Topiramate
C. Candesartan
D. Nortriptyline

525. Electrical stimulation of which part of brain results in migraine-like headache?
Harrison's 20th Ed. Chapter 422, Page 3103

A. Temporal lobe
B. Midbrain in the region of dorsal raphe
C. Putamen
D. Globus pallidum

526. Which of the following is a monoclonal antibody to CGRP receptor?
Harrison's 20th Ed. Chapter 422, Page 3103

A. Erenumab
B. Eptinezumab
C. Fremanezumab
D. Galcanezumab

Monoclonal antibodies to the CGRP receptor (erenumab) or to the peptide (eptinezumab, fremanezumab & galcanezumab) are effective and well tolerated in migraine. They can be used as preventive agents.

527. Chronic head-pain syndrome best relates to?
Harrison's 20th Ed. Chapter 422, Page 3103

A. Migraine
B. Tension-type headache (TTH)
C. Cluster headache
D. All of the above

Term tension-type headache (TTH) is commonly used to describe a chronic head-pain syndrome characterized by bilateral tight, band like discomfort.

528. Which of the following is an accompanying feature of tension-type headache?
Harrison's 20th Ed. Chapter 422, Page 3103

A. Nausea, vomiting
B. Photophobia, phonophobia
C. Aggravation with movement
D. None of the above

TTH patients have headaches without accompanying features like nausea, vomiting, photophobia, phonophobia, osmophobia, throbbing & aggravation with movement.

529. For chronic TTH, which is the only proven treatment?
Harrison's 20th Ed. Chapter 422, Page 3104

A. Amitriptyline
B. Selective serotonin reuptake inhibitors
C. Benzodiazepines
D. Acupuncture

For chronic TTH, amitriptyline is the only proven treatment.

530. Trigeminal autonomic cephalalgias include all except?
Harrison's 20th Ed. Chapter 422, Page 3104

A. Cluster headache
B. Migraine
C. Paroxysmal hemicrania
D. SUNCT

Trigeminal autonomic cephalalgias (TACs) includes cluster headache, paroxysmal hemicrania & SUNCT (short-lasting unilateral neuralgiform headache attacks with conjunctival injection & tearing). TAC features are short-lasting attacks of head pain with cranial autonomic symptoms (lacrimation, conjunctival injection, or nasal congestion).

531. Short-lasting headaches without prominent cranial autonomic syndromes include?
Harrison's 20th Ed. Chapter 422, Page 3104

A. Trigeminal neuralgia
B. Primary stabbing headache
C. Hypnic headache
D. All of the above

Short-lasting headaches without prominent cranial autonomic syndromes are trigeminal neuralgia, primary stabbing headache & hypnic headache.

532. Which of the following is false about cluster headache?
Harrison's 20th Ed. Chapter 422, Page 3104

A. Men are affected more than women
B. Ipsilateral autonomic features
C. Propranolol and amitriptyline are ineffective
D. Lithium is not beneficial

533. Which of the following is false about cluster headache?
Harrison's 20th Ed. Chapter 422, Page 3104

A. Pain is strictly unilateral
B. Pain affects the same side in subsequent episodes
C. Certain foods or emotional factors precipitate pain
D. On-off vulnerability to alcohol

534. Which of the following is false about cluster headache?
Lancet 2005; 366: 843–55

A. Circadian rhythmicity of painful attacks
B. Autonomic symptoms
C. Severe unilateral pain
D. Hypothalamic dysfunction has no role in acute attacks

535. Which of the following is most useful during acute attack of cluster headache?
Lancet 2005; 366: 843–55

A. 100% oxygen inhalation
B. Valsalva manuevre
C. Hyperventilation
D. All of the above

536. Which of the following is a feature of cluster headache?
Harrison's 20th Ed. Chapter 422, Page 3104

A. Periodicity
B. Unilateral pain
C. A pain-free interval
D. All of the above

537. Drugs used for preventive treatment of cluster headache include all except?
Harrison's 20th Ed. Chapter 422, Page 3105

A. Prednisone
B. Lithium
C. Cyproheptadine
D. Methysergide

Oral glucocorticoids, methysergide, lithium are useful for chronic form of cluster headache.

538. Which of the following is a feature of paroxysmal hemicrania?
Harrison's 20th Ed. Chapter 422, Page 3105

A. Very frequent short-lasting attacks
B. Equal male: female ratio
C. Excellent response to indomethacin
D. All of the above

539. Which of the following is a feature of SUNCT?
Harrison's 20th Ed. Chapter 422, Page 3106

A. Ipsilateral conjunctival injection and lacrimation
B. Lack of refractory period to triggering
C. Lack of response to indomethacin
D. All of the above

540. Secondary SUNCT is seen in?
Harrison's 20th Ed. Chapter 422, Page 3106

A. Anterior communicating artery aneurysm
B. Post head injury
C. Posterior fossa or pituitary lesions
D. Hypertension

SUNCT (short-lasting unilateral neuralgiform headache attacks with conjunctival injection and tearing) can be seen with posterior fossa or pituitary lesions.

541. Most effective treatment for prevention of SUNCT is?
Harrison's 20th Ed. Chapter 422, Page 3106

A. Prednisone
B. Lamotrigine
C. Cyproheptadine
D. Lithium

Most effective treatment for prevention of SUNCT is lamotrigine. Topiramate, gabapentin and carbamazepine offer modest benefit.

542. "Fortification spectrum" is characteristic of?
Harrison's 20th Ed. Chapter 422, Page 187

A. Cluster headache
B. Migraine
C. Pseudotumour cerebri
D. Giant cell arteritis

In classic Migraine a visual aura lasting about 20 minutes occurs in both eyes (open or closed) with a small central disturbance in the field of vision marching toward the periphery leaving a transient scotoma. The expanding border of migraine scotoma has a scintillating, dancing or zigzag edge resembling the bastions of a fortified city, hence the term fortification spectra. It can be confused with amaurosis fugax (briefer and occurs in only one eye).

543. Which of the following best relates to migraine?
DeJong's The Neurologic Examination, 7th Ed. Page 164

A. Quadrantopsia
B. Teichopsias
C. Achromatopsia
D. Metamorphopsia

Scintillating scotomas of migraine are called teichopsias.

544. Which of the following is false about Bickerstaff migraine?
Lancet 1961a;1:15-7

A. Episodes begin with total blindness
B. Symptoms (vertigo, ataxia) persist for 20–30 minutes
C. Occurs only in males
D. Full recovery after the episode is the rule

Basilar-type migraine, basilar migraine, basilar artery migraine, and Bickerstaff migraine is now referred to as migraine with brainstem aura. According to the ICHD-3 beta, there must be at least 2 of the following non-ischemic "brainstem" symptoms present: dysarthria, vertigo, tinnitus, impaired hearing, double vision, ataxia, and decreased level consciousness.

545. Lower-half headache or facial migraine is called?
American Journal of Neuroradiology. 2000;21(4):766-769

A. Basilar migraine
B. Carotidynia
C. Raeder's syndrome
D. Ophthalmoplegic migraine

546. Common precipitant of carotidynia attacks is?
American Journal of Neuroradiology. 2000;21(4):766-769

A. Cervical spondylosis
B. Dental trauma
C. Hypertension
D. All of the above

Carotidynia or Fay syndrome was described by Fay in 1927 as an atypical neuralgia in neck & face. It was classified by the International Headache Society in 1988 as an idiopathic neck pain syndrome associated with tenderness over the carotid bifurcation without structural abnormality. Carotydinia was removed as a pathological entity from the second International Headache Society classification in 2004.

Coma

547. Which of the following is a feature of coma?
Harrison's 20th Ed. Chapter 300, Page 2068

A. Deep sleep like state
B. Eyes closed
C. Patient cannot be aroused
D. All of the above

Coma is defined as a deep sleep like state, with eyes closed and the patient cannot be aroused. Stupor refers to a state where in patient can be transiently awakened by vigorous stimuli, accompanied by motor behavior of avoidance or withdrawal from uncomfortable or aggravating stimuli. Drowsiness simulates light sleep & is characterized by easy arousal and persistence of alertness for brief periods. Stupor and drowsiness are usually accompanied by some degree of confusion.

548. At bedside, which of the following term is not ambiguous and is preferred?
Harrison's 20th Ed. Chapter 300, Page 2068

A. Lethargy
B. Drowsiness
C. Semicoma
D. Obtundation

At bedside, stupor, drowsiness and coma are precise narrative descriptions of the level of arousal and of the type of responses evoked by various stimuli and are preferable to ambiguous terms such as lethargy, semicoma, or obtundation.

549. Which of the following is false about vegetative state?
Harrison's 20th Ed. Chapter 300, Page 2068

A. Awake-appearing but nonresponsive state
B. Respiratory and autonomic functions are retained
C. Yawning, swallowing, limb & head movements persist
D. None of the above

A vegetative state signifies an awake-appearing but nonresponsive state often in a patient who has come out of coma. The eyelids may open periodically, giving the appearance of wakefulness. Respiratory & autonomic functions are retained. Yawning, coughing, swallowing, and limb & head movements persist, often meaningless.

550. Which of the following is false about minimally conscious state?
Harrison's 20th Ed. Chapter 300, Page 2068

A. Patient displays rudimentary vocal or motor behaviors
B. Patient displays response to touch, visual stimuli, or command
C. Cerebral hypoperfusion & head trauma are common causes
D. None of the above

551. Persistent vegetative state is the term used when prognosis for regaining mental faculties is almost nil after being in a vegetative state for?
Harrison's 20th Ed. Chapter 300, Page 2068

A. Three months
B. Six months
C. Nine months
D. One year

Patients in the minimally conscious state carry a better prognosis for some recovery compared to those in a persistent vegetative state.

552. Which of the following is false about akinetic mutism?
Harrison's 20th Ed. Chapter 300, Page 2069

A. Partially or fully awake state
B. Patient is able to form impressions and think
C. Patient remains virtually immobile and mute
D. None of the above

Akinetic mutism refers to a partially or fully awake state wherein the patient is able to form impressions & think, as demonstrated by later recounting of events, but remains virtually immobile & mute.

553. Akinetic mutism results from damage in?
Harrison's 20th Ed. Chapter 300, Page 2069

A. Ventral pons
B. Medial thalamic nuclei
C. Temporal lobe
D. Any of the above

Akinetic mutism results from damage in regions of medial thalamic nuclei or frontal lobes (particularly orbitofrontal surfaces) or from extreme hydrocephalus.

554. Abulia describes a milder form of?
Harrison's 20th Ed. Chapter 300, Page 2069

A. Parkinsonism
B. Akinetic mutism
C. Catatonia
D. Locked-in state

Abulia is a milder form of akinetic mutism characterized by mental & physical slowness with diminished ability to initiate activity. It is usually the result of damage to frontal lobes and its connections.

555. Which of the following occurs as part of a major psychosis?
Harrison's 20th Ed. Chapter 300, Page 2069

A. Akinetic mutism
B. Abulia
C. Catatonia
D. Locked-in state

Catatonia occurs as part of a major psychosis (schizophrenia or major depression).

556. Catatonia is differentiated from akinetic mutism by?
Harrison's 20th Ed. Chapter 300, Page 2069

A. Level of awakening
B. Babinski signs
C. Blinking
D. Mobility

Catatonia is differentiated from akinetic mutism by clinical evidence of cerebral damage such as Babinski signs and hypertonicity of the limbs present in akinetic mutism.

557. "Waxy flexibility" is a feature of which of the following?
Harrison's 20th Ed. Chapter 300, Page 2069

A. Abulia
B. Akinetic mutism
C. Catatonia
D. Locked-in state

In catatonia, the patient retains the posture in which they have been placed by the examiner ("waxy flexibility," or catalepsy).

558. "Locked-in state" results from damage in?
Harrison's 20th Ed. Chapter 300, Page 2069

A. Ventral pons
B. Medial thalamic nuclei
C. Temporal lobe
D. Any of the above

"Locked-in state" results from an infarction or hemorrhage of ventral pons that transects all descending motor (corticospinal and corticobulbar) pathways.

559. "Locked-in state" like condition may be seen in?
Harrison's 20th Ed. Chapter 300, Page 2069

A. Guillain-Barré syndrome
B. Critical illness neuropathy
C. Pharmacologic neuromuscular blockade
D. Any of the above

These are awake but de-efferented states.

560. The principal cause of coma is?
Harrison's 20th Ed. Chapter 300, Page 2069

A. Lesions that damage substantial portion of RAS
B. Destruction of large portions of both cerebral hemispheres
C. Suppression of thalamocerebral function by drugs, toxins, hypoglycemia, anoxia, azotemia, or hepatic failure
D. All of the above

Principal causes of coma are lesions that damage the reticular activating system (RAS) or its projections, destruction of large portions of both cerebral hemispheres and suppression of reticulo-cerebral function by drugs, toxins, or metabolic derangements such as hypoglycemia, anoxia, azotemia, or hepatic failure.

561. Metabolic derangement that can lead to suppression of reticulocerebral function is?
Harrison's 20th Ed. Chapter 300, Page 2069

A. Hypoglycemia
B. Uremia
C. Hepatic failure
D. All of the above

Metabolic derangements that can lead to suppression of reticulocerebral function are hypoglycemia, anoxia, uremia, and hepatic failure.

562. Which of the following is false about brain herniation?
Harrison's 20th Ed. Chapter 300, Page 2069

A. Displacement of brain tissue into a contiguous compartment
B. Displacement of brain tissue by an overlying or adjacent mass
C. "False localizing" signs
D. None of the above

563. Brain herniation can be?
Harrison's 20th Ed. Chapter 300, Page 2069 Figure 300-1

A. Transfalcial
B. Uncal
C. Foraminal
D. All of the above

Brain herniations can be of the following types : uncal, central, transfalcial and foraminal.

564. Which is the most common form of brain herniation?
Harrison's 20th Ed. Chapter 300, Page 2069

A. Transfalcial
B. Foraminal herniation
C. Transtentorial herniation
D. Any of the above

The most common form of herniation is transtentorial herniation, in which brain tissue is displaced from supratentorial to infratentorial compartment through tentorial opening.

565. Uncus refers to which of the following?
Harrison's 20th Ed. Chapter 300, Page 2069

A. Lingual gyrus
B. Cingulate gyrus
C. Anterior medial temporal gyrus
D. Parahippocampal gyrus

Uncus refers to anterior medial temporal gyrus.

566. Kernohan-Woltman sign best relates to?
Harrison's 20th Ed. Chapter 300, Page 2069

A. Hypoglycemia
B. Central fever
C. Transtentorial herniation
D. Epileptic coma

Transtentorial herniation refers to part of brain being displaced from supratentorial to infratentorial compartment through the tentorial opening. Consequent lateral displacement of midbrain may compress the opposite cerebral peduncle against the tentorial edge, thus eliciting Kernohan-Woltman sign.

567. Kernohan-Woltman sign refers to?
Harrison's 20th Ed. Chapter 300, Page 2069

A. Contralateral pupillary dilatation in brain mass lesion
B. Waxing and waning levels of consciousness
C. Hemiparesis contralateral to original hemiparesis
D. Bilateral nystagmus

Kernohan-Woltman sign refers to a Babinski response and hemiparesis contralateral to the original hemiparesis due to compression of the opposite cerebral peduncle.

568. Brain herniation can cause which of the following?
Harrison's 20th Ed. Chapter 300, Page 2069

A. Cranial nerve palsy
B. Compression of anterior and posterior cerebral arteries
C. Hydrocephalus
D. All of the above

569. Coma results due to damage in reticular activating system (RAS) at the level of?
Harrison's 20th Ed. Chapter 300, Page 2069

A. Medulla oblongata
B. Pons
C. Lower midbrain
D. Upper midbrain

Coma results due to damage in reticular activating system (RAS) at the level of upper midbrain or its projections.

570. Which of the following finding suggests that the lesion is in the upper brainstem?
Harrison's 20th Ed. Chapter 300, Page 2069

A. Pupillary enlargement
B. Loss of light reaction
C. Loss of vertical and adduction movements of eyes
D. All of the above

Pupillary enlargement with loss of light reaction and loss of vertical and adduction movements of the eyes suggests that the lesion is in the upper brainstem. On the other hand, if pupillary light reaction and eye movements are intact, the lesion is more widespread or the cause of coma is metabolic suppression of the cerebral hemispheres.

571. The term 'coma dépassé' means?
N Engl J Med. 2001;344:1215

A. Hysteria
B. Irreversible coma
C. Coma during pregnancy
D. Coma in children

In 1959, Mollaret & Goulon introduced the term coma dépassé (irreversible coma) in 23 comatose patients who lost consciousness, brainstem reflexes & respiration & whose EEGs were flat.

572. As brain death occurs, which is the last part of brain to cease to function?
N Engl J Med. 2001;344:1216

A. Cerebral cortex
B. Midbrain
C. Pons
D. Medulla oblongata

As brain death occurs, patients lose their reflexes in a rostral-to-caudal direction, and medulla oblongata is the last part of brain to cease to function.

573. Misdiagnosis of brain death is possible in?
N Engl J Med. 2001;344:1215

A. Locked-in syndrome
B. Hypothermia
C. Drug intoxication
D. All of the above

Misdiagnosis of brain death is possible in locked-in syndrome, hypothermia or drug intoxication.

574. In the tests to confirm brain death, "hollow-skull sign" is a finding in which of the following?
N Engl J Med. 2001;344:1215

A. EEG
B. Dynamic radionuclide brain scan
C. Cerebral angiography
D. Transcranial Doppler measurements

When brain death has occurred, a dynamic radionuclide brain scan shows no intracranial filling - the so called hollow-skull sign.

575. Which part of brain is damaged in "locked-in syndrome"?
N Engl J Med. 2001;344:1215

A. Medulla oblongata
B. Pons
C. Midbrain
D. Thalamus

The locked-in syndrome (pseudocoma) is a consequence of destruction of base of pons mostly caused by acute embolus to basilar artery. Patient cannot move limbs, grimace, or swallow (damaged corticospinal & corticobulbar tracts), but upper rostral mesencephalic structures involved in voluntary blinking and vertical eye movements remain intact. Consciousness persists because tegmentum, with the reticular formation, is not affected.

576. Cingulate gyrus is likely to be involved in which of the following brain herniations?
Harrison's 20th Ed. Chapter 300, Page 2070

A. Temporal transtentorial herniation
B. Central transtentorial herniation
C. Transfalcial herniation
D. Foraminal herniation

In transfalcial herniation, the cingulate gyrus is displaced under the falx and across the midline.

577. Cerebellar tonsils are likely to be involved in which of the following brain herniations?
Harrison's 20th Ed. Chapter 300, Page 2070

A. Temporal transtentorial herniation
B. Central transtentorial herniation
C. Transfalcial herniation
D. Foraminal herniation

In foraminal herniation, cerebellar tonsils move downward into foramen magnum, causing compression of medulla that may result in respiratory arrest and death.

578. Drowsiness occurs when horizontal displacement of the pineal calcification occurs by?
Harrison's 20th Ed. Chapter 300, Page 2070

A. 1 to 3 mm
B. 3 to 5 mm
C. 6 to 8 mm
D. > 9 mm

579. Stupor occurs when horizontal displacement of the pineal calcification occurs by?
Harrison's 20th Ed. Chapter 300, Page 2070

A. 1 to 3 mm
B. 3 to 5 mm
C. 6 to 8 mm
D. > 9 mm

580. Coma occurs when horizontal displacement of the pineal calcification occurs by?
Harrison's 20th Ed. Chapter 300, Page 2070

A. 1 to 3 mm
B. 3 to 5 mm
C. 6 to 8 mm
D. > 9 mm

On CT/MRI, horizontal displacement of pineal calcification of 3 to 5 mm is associated with drowsiness, 6 to 8 mm with stupor, and >9 mm with coma, in acutely appearing masses.

581. Cerebral blood flow is principally influenced by all except?
Harrison's 20th Ed. Chapter 300, Page 2070

A. Systemic blood pressure
B. pH
C. PCO_2
D. PO_2

CBF is strongly influenced by systemic blood pressure, pH and PCO_2. CBF increases with hypercapnia and acidosis and decreases with hypocapnia and alkalosis.

582. In adults, volume of CSF within ventricles and surrounding the brain and spinal cord is about?
Harrison's 20th Ed. Chapter 300, Page 2075

A. 50 mL
B. 100 mL
C. 150 mL
D. 200 mL

583. Brain volume is normally about?
DeJong's The Neurologic Examination, 7th Ed. Page 740

A. 1000 mL
B. 1200 mL
C. 1400 mL
D. 1600 mL

Brain volume is normally approximately 1400 mL.

584. Monro-Kellie hypothesis best relates to?
DeJong's The Neurologic Examination, 7th Ed. Page 741

A. Intracranial pressure
B. Intracranial volume
C. Intraocular pressure
D. Intraocular volume

Monro-Kellie hypothesis refers to the fact that because cranium cannot expand, and brain cannot be significantly compressed, when volume of one of the compartments increases (blood, brain & CSF), volume in the other compartments must undergo a compensatory decrease.

585. Cerebral blood volume is about?
Harrison's 20th Ed. Chapter 300, Page 2075

A. 50 mL
B. 100 mL
C. 150 mL
D. 200 mL

About 150 mL of CSF is present within the ventricles and surrounding the brain and spinal cord. Cerebral blood volume is also ~150 mL.

586. Cerebral blood flow (CBF) in gray matter is about?
Harrison's 20th Ed. Chapter 300, Page 2070

A. 25 mL per 100 gram/minute
B. 50 mL per 100 gram/minute
C. 75 mL per 100 gram/minute
D. 100 mL per 100 gram/minute

587. Cerebral blood flow (CBF) in white matter is about?
Harrison's 20th Ed. Chapter 300, Page 2070

A. 10 mL per 100 gram/minute
B. 20 mL per 100 gram/minute
C. 30 mL per 100 gram/minute
D. 40 mL per 100 gram/minute

588. Mean cerebral blood flow (CBF) is about?
Harrison's 20th Ed. Chapter 300, Page 2070

A. 25 mL per 100 gram/minute
B. 35 mL per 100 gram/minute
C. 45 mL per 100 gram/minute
D. 55 mL per 100 gram/minute

589. Oxygen consumption of brain tissue is?
Harrison's 20th Ed. Chapter 300, Page 2070

A. 1.5 mL per 100 gram/minute
B. 2.5 mL per 100 gram/minute
C. 3.5 mL per 100 gram/minute
D. 4.5 mL per 100 gram/minute

590. Glucose utilization of brain tissue is?
Harrison's 20th Ed. Chapter 300, Page 2070

A. 1 mg per 100 gram/minute
B. 3 mg per 100 gram/minute
C. 5 mg per 100 gram/minute
D. 7 mg per 100 gram/minute

591. After the cessation of blood flow, brain stores of glucose provide energy for approximately?
Harrison's 20th Ed. Chapter 300, Page 2070

A. 1 minute
B. 2 minutes
C. 3 minutes
D. 4 minutes

592. After the cessation of cerebral blood flow, oxygen stores last for approximately?
Harrison's 20th Ed. Chapter 300, Page 2070

A. 3 to 5 seconds
B. 8 to 10 seconds
C. 12 to 15 seconds
D. 20 to 30 seconds

Cerebral neurons are fully dependent on cerebral blood flow (CBF) and the related delivery of oxygen and glucose. CBF approximates 75 mL per 100 gram/minute in gray matter and 30 mL per 100 gram/minute in white matter (mean of 55 mL per 100 gram/minute). Oxygen consumption is 3.5 mL per 100 gram/minute, and glucose utilization is 5 mg per 100 gram/minute. Brain stores of glucose provide energy for ~2 minutes after blood flow is interrupted, and oxygen stores last 8 to 10 seconds after cessation of blood flow.

593. Normal CSF pressure is?
Harrison's 20th Ed. Chapter 300, Page 2075

A. 20–70 mm H_2O
B. 80–120 mm H_2O
C. 50–180 mm H_2O
D. 120–280 mm H_2O

594. Normal CSF osmolarity is?
Harrison's 20th Ed. Chapter 300, Page 2075

A. 280–285 mOsm/L
B. 285–292 mOsm/L
C. 292–297 mOsm/L
D. 298–302 mOsm/L

595. Normal CSF pH is?
Harrison's 20th Ed. Chapter 300, Page 2075

A. 7.31–7.34
B. 7.34–7.37
C. 7.37–7.40
D. 7.40–7.44

596. Which receptor for PGE2 in brain is essential for fever?
Harrison's 20th Ed. 103

A. EP-1
B. EP-2
C. EP-3
D. EP-4

Elevation of PGE2 in brain starts the process of raising hypothalamic set point for core temperature. Out of the 4 receptors for PGE2, EP-3 is essential for fever.

597. In metabolic disorders, most neuronal damage is caused by which of the following?
Harrison's 20th Ed. Chapter 300, Page 2070

A. Hypoglycemia
B. Hyponatremia
C. Hypoxia-ischemia
D. All of the above

Hypoxia-ischemia causes most neuronal destruction. Other metabolic disorders like hypoglycemia, hyponatremia, hyperosmolarity, hypercapnia, hypercalcemia, and hepatic and renal failure cause only minor neuropathologic changes.

598. Which of the following changes occur in hepatic encephalopathy (HE)?
Harrison's 20th Ed. Chapter 300, Page 2070

A. Increased synthesis of glutamine in astrocytes
B. Increases in inhibitory neurotransmitter GABA
C. Synthesis of putative "false" neurotransmitters
D. All of the above

In hepatic encephalopathy (HE), high ammonia concentrations lead to increased synthesis of glutamine in astrocytes with osmotic swelling, mitochondrial energy failure, production of reactive nitrogen & oxygen species, increases in inhibitory neurotransmitter GABA, and synthesis of putative "false" neurotransmitters.

599. Which of the following is typical of chronic hepatic encephalopathy (HE)?
Harrison's 20th Ed. Chapter 300, Page 2070

A. Development of diffuse astrocytosis
B. Depletion of catecholamines
C. Increases in brain calcium
D. All of the above

Over a period of time, development of a diffuse astrocytosis is typical of chronic HE.

600. Which of the following does not contribute to the development of uremic encephalopathy?
Harrison's 20th Ed. Chapter 300, Page 2070

A. Urea
B. Creatinine
C. Guanidine
D. Calcium

601. Which of the following occur in uremic encephalopathy?
Harrison's 20th Ed. Chapter 300, Page 2070

A. Accumulation of creatinine and guanidine
B. Depletion of catecholamines
C. Increases in brain calcium
D. All of the above

Contributors to uremic encephalopathy include accumulation of neurotoxic substances (creatinine, guanidine), depletion of catecholamines, altered glutamate & GABA tone, increases in brain calcium, inflammation with disruption of blood brain barrier.

602. Sodium below what level is associated with coma and convulsions?
Harrison's 20th Ed. Chapter 300, Page 2070

A. 125 mmol/L
B. 121 mmol/L
C. 119 mmol/L
D. 115 mmol/L

Sodium levels <125 mmol/L induce confusion & <119 mmol/L are associated with coma & convulsions.

603. In hyperosmolar coma, the serum osmolarity is generally more than?
Harrison's 20th Ed. Chapter 300, Page 2070

A. >280 mOsmol/L
B. >300 mOsmol/L
C. >320 mOsmol/L
D. >350 mOsmol/L

In hyperosmolar coma, the serum osmolarity is generally >350 moSmol/L.

604. Disorder that occlude small blood vessels throughout the brain causing bihemispheral damage is?
Harrison's 20th Ed. Chapter 300, Page 2070

A. Cerebral malaria
B. Thrombotic thrombocytopenic purpura
C. Hyperviscosity
D. All of the above

Disorders that occlude small blood vessels throughout the brain causing bihemispheral damage are cerebral malaria, thrombotic thrombocytopenic purpura, and hyperviscosity.

605. In coma, which of the following is not included initially in determining severity and nature of coma?
Harrison's 20th Ed. Chapter 300, Page 2070

A. Vital signs
B. Funduscopy
C. Nuchal rigidity
D. Respiratory patterns

606. Which of the following is the least likely cause of fever in coma?
Harrison's 20th Ed. Chapter 300, Page 2071

A. Heat stroke
B. Neuroleptic malignant syndrome
C. Central fever
D. Anticholinergic drug intoxication

607. Hypothermia in coma is observed in?
Harrison's 20th Ed. Chapter 300, Page 2071

A. Phenothiazine intoxication
B. Hypoglycemia
C. Extreme hypothyroidism
D. All of the above

Hypothermia in coma is observed with alcohol, barbiturate, sedative, or phenothiazine intoxication; hypoglycemia; peripheral circulatory failure; or extreme hypothyroidism.

608. Hypothermia itself causes coma only when the temperature is?
Harrison's 20th Ed. Chapter 300, Page 2071

A. <34°C
B. <33°C
C. <32°C
D. <31°C

Hypothermia itself causes coma only when the temperature is <31°C (87.8°F), regardless of the underlying etiology.

609. Marked hypertension in coma suggests?
Harrison's 20th Ed. Chapter 300, Page 2071

A. Cerebral hemorrhage
B. Large cerebral infarction
C. Head injury
D. All of the above

Marked hypertension suggests hypertensive encephalopathy, cerebral hemorrhage, large cerebral infarction, or head injury.

610. Cushing response best relates to?
Harrison's 20th Ed. Chapter 300, Page 2071

A. Hypertension
B. Cyanosis
C. Convulsion
D. Hypothermia

Cushing response refers to marked hypertension in a case of coma that may be secondary to a rapid rise in intracranial pressure (ICP), most often after cerebral hemorrhage or head injury.

611. Hypotension is characteristic of coma due to?
Harrison's 20th Ed. Chapter 300, Page 2071

A. Profound hypothyroidism
B. Sepsis
C. Alcohol intoxication
D. All of the above

Hypotension is characteristic of coma from alcohol or barbiturate intoxication, internal hemorrhage, myocardial infarction, sepsis, profound hypothyroidism, or Addisonian crisis.

612. On funduscopic examination, subhyaloid hemorrhage suggests?
Harrison's 20th Ed. Chapter 300, Page 2071

A. Meningococcemia
B. Subarachnoid hemorrhage
C. Bleeding diathesis
D. All of the above

Subhyaloid hemorrhages on funduscopic examination indicate subarachnoid hemorrhage.

613. Cutaneous petechiae in coma suggest?
Harrison's 20th Ed. Chapter 300, Page 2071

A. Thrombotic thrombocytopenic purpura
B. Meningococcemia
C. Bleeding diathesis associated with an ICH
D. All of the above

Cutaneous petechiae suggest thrombotic thrombocytopenic purpura, meningococcemia, or a bleeding diathesis associated with an intracerebral hemorrhage.

614. Multifocal myoclonus indicates which of the following?
Harrison's 20th Ed. Chapter 300, Page 2071

A. Uremia
B. Haloperidol intoxication
C. Prion disease
D. Any of the above

Multifocal myoclonus almost always indicates a metabolic disorder (uremia, anoxia), drug intoxication (lithium or haloperidol), or a prion disease.

615. In a drowsy and confused patient, bilateral asterixis is a certain sign of?
Harrison's 20th Ed. Chapter 300, Page 2071

A. Drug intoxication
B. Cerebral malaria
C. Septicemia
D. Head injury

In a drowsy and confused patient, bilateral asterixis is a certain sign of metabolic encephalopathy or drug intoxication.

616. Bilateral damage rostral to the midbrain produces which of the following?
Harrison's 20th Ed. Chapter 300, Page 2071

A. Extension of elbows and wrists with pronation of arm
B. Flexion of elbows and wrists with supination of arm
C. Arm extension with leg flexion
D. Arm extension with flaccid legs

617. Bilateral damage to motor tracts in midbrain or caudal diencephalon produces which of the following?
Harrison's 20th Ed. Chapter 300, Page 2071

A. Extension of elbows and wrists with pronation of arm
B. Flexion of elbows and wrists with supination of arm
C. Arm extension with leg flexion
D. Arm extension with flaccid legs

Flexion of elbows and wrists and supination of arm (decortication) suggests bilateral damage rostral to the midbrain, whereas extension of elbows and wrists with pronation (decerebration) indicates damage to motor tracts in midbrain or caudal diencephalon.

618. Combination of arm extension with leg flexion or flaccid legs is associated with lesions in?
Harrison's 20th Ed. Chapter 300, Page 2071

A. Basal ganglia
B. Midbrain
C. Pons
D. Medulla oblongata

Combination of arm extension with leg flexion or flaccid legs is associated with lesions in pons.

619. Which of the following stimuli is useful in eliciting abduction withdrawal movements of limbs?
Harrison's 20th Ed. Chapter 300, Page 2071

A. Tickling the nostrils with a cotton wisp
B. Pressure on the knuckles or bony prominences
C. Pinprick stimulation
D. Pinching the skin

Abduction-avoidance movement of a limb is usually purposeful and denotes an intact corticospinal system. Posturing in response to noxious stimuli indicates severe damage to corticospinal system.

620. Which of the following is not a brainstem reflex?
Harrison's 20th Ed. Chapter 300, Page 2071

A. Pupillary responses to light
B. Spontaneous and elicited eye movements
C. Corneal responses
D. Jaw jerk

Brainstem reflexes include pupillary responses to light, spontaneous and elicited eye movements, corneal responses, and respiratory pattern. As a rule, if these brainstem activities, particularly pupillary reactions and eye movements, are preserved, coma is due to bilateral hemispheral disease.

621. Normally reactive and round pupils of midsize excludes?
Harrison's 20th Ed. Chapter 300, Page 2072

A. Midbrain damage
B. Pontine damage
C. Temporal lobe damage
D. Occipital lobe damage

In coma, normally reactive & round pupils of midsize (2.5–5 mm) essentially excludes midbrain damage, either primary or secondary to compression.

622. Reaction to light is difficult to appreciate in pupils?
Harrison's 20th Ed. Chapter 300, Page 2072

A. < 2 mm in diameter
B. < 3 mm in diameter
C. < 4 mm in diameter
D. < 5 mm in diameter

Reaction to light is often difficult to appreciate in pupils <2 mm in diameter.

623. A transitional sign that accompanies early midbrain–third nerve compression is?
Harrison's 20th Ed. Chapter 300, Page 2072

A. Pupil > 6 mm is diameter
B. Oval and slightly eccentric pupil
C. Unilateral miosis
D. Reactive and bilaterally small

In coma, an oval & slightly eccentric pupil is a transitional sign that accompanies early midbrain–third nerve compression.

624. Bilaterally dilated and unreactive pupils indicate?
Harrison's 20th Ed. Chapter 300, Page 2072

A. Severe cortical damage
B. Severe thalamic damage
C. Severe midbrain damage
D. Severe pontine damage

In coma, bilaterally dilated & unreactive pupils, indicates severe midbrain damage, usually from compression by a supratentorial mass.

625. Which of the following causes fixed pupils in drug induced coma?
DeJong's The Neurologic Examination, 7th Ed. Page 199

A. Digoxin
B. Glutethimide
C. Piperidine
D. Methyprylon

Glutethimide intoxication causes fixed pupils in drug induced coma, has fortunately become rare.

626. Reactive pupils are smaller in size in which of the following?
Harrison's 20th Ed. Chapter 300, Page 2072

A. Metabolic encephalopathies
B. Hydrocephalus
C. Thalamic hemorrhage
D. All of the above

627. Reactive pupils are smaller in size in which of the following?
Harrison's 20th Ed. Chapter 300, Page 2072

A. Narcotic overdose
B. Barbiturate overdose
C. Pontine hemorrhage
D. All of the above

628. Cause of misleading pupillary enlargement is?
Harrison's 20th Ed. Chapter 300, Page 2072

A. Nebulizer treatments
B. Direct ocular trauma
C. Use of drugs with anticholinergic activity
D. All of the above

Ingestion of drugs with anticholinergic activity, use of mydriatic eye drops, nebulizer treatments, and direct ocular trauma can cause misleading pupillary enlargement. Horizontal divergence of eyes at rest is normal in drowsiness.

629. Unilateral miosis in coma is due to lesion in?
Harrison's 20th Ed. Chapter 300, Page 2072

A. Lower brainstem (medulla)
B. Sympathetic efferents originating in posterior hypothalamus
C. Medial longitudinal fasciculus (MLF)
D. Any of the above

630. Eyes turn down & inward with which of the following lesion?
Harrison's 20th Ed. Chapter 300, Page 2072

A. Frontal lobe lesions
B. Thalamic lesions
C. Pontine lesions
D. Medullary lesions

Eyes turn down & inward with thalamic hemorrhage & upper midbrain lesions.

631. Which of the following statements about eyes in a state of coma is correct?
Harrison's 20th Ed. Chapter 300, Page 2072

A. Eyes look toward hemispheral lesion & away from brainstem lesion
B. Eyes look away from hemispheral lesion & toward a brainstem lesion
C. Eyes look away from hemispheral or a brainstem lesion
D. Eyes look towards hemispheral or a brainstem lesion

Conjugate horizontal ocular deviation to one side indicates damage to pons on the opposite side or to frontal lobe on the same side. The rule therefore is "eyes look toward a hemispheral lesion and away from a brainstem lesion". "Wrong-way eyes" refers to eyes that may on a rare occasion turn paradoxically away from the side of a deep hemispheral lesion.

632. "Ocular bobbing" is diagnostic of?
Harrison's 20th Ed. Chapter 300, Page 2072

A. Bilateral occipital infarct
B. Bilateral pontine damage
C. Bilateral temporal lobe infarct
D. Cerebellar damage

"Ocular bobbing" describes a brisk downward and slow upward movement of the eyes associated with loss of horizontal eye movements and is diagnostic of bilateral pontine damage, usually from thrombosis of the basilar artery.

633. "Ocular dipping" is diagnostic of?
Harrison's 20th Ed. Chapter 300, Page 2072

A. Diffuse cortical anoxic damage
B. ICSOL
C. SAH
D. Tubercular meningitis

"Ocular dipping" is a slower, arrhythmic downward movement followed by a faster upward movement in patients with normal reflex horizontal gaze indicating diffuse cortical anoxic damage.

634. "Doll's eye" oculocephalic reflex is indicative of which of the following?
Harrison's 20th Ed. Chapter 300, Page 2072

A. Reduced cortical influence on brainstem & damaged brainstem pathways
B. Reduced cortical influence on brainstem & intact brainstem pathways
C. Normal cortical influence on brainstem & damaged brainstem pathways
D. Normal cortical influence on brainstem & intact brainstem pathways

The oculocephalic reflexes, elicited by moving the head from side to side or vertically and observing eye movements in the direction opposite to the head movement, depend on the integrity of the ocular motor nuclei and their interconnecting tracts that extend from the midbrain to the pons and medulla. The movements, called somewhat inappropriately "doll's eyes" (which refers more accurately to the reflex elevation of the eyelids with flexion of the neck), are normally suppressed in the awake patient. The ability to elicit them therefore indicates both reduced cortical influence on the brainstem and intact brainstem pathways, indicating that coma is caused by a lesion or dysfunction in the cerebral hemispheres. Oculovestibular & oculocephalic reflexes provide essentially the same information.

635. Midbrain and third nerve function are tested by?
Harrison's 20th Ed. Chapter 300, Page 2071, Figure 300-3

A. Pupillary reaction to light
B. Spontaneous and reflex eye movements
C. Corneal responses
D. Respiratory & pharyngeal responses

636. Pontine function is tested by?
Harrison's 20th Ed. Chapter 300, Page 2071, Figure 300-3

A. Pupillary reaction to light
B. Spontaneous and reflex eye movements
C. Respiratory responses
D. Pharyngeal responses

637. Pontine function is tested by?
Harrison's 20th Ed. Chapter 300, Page 2071, Figure 300-3

A. Spontaneous eye movements
B. Reflex eye movements
C. Corneal responses
D. All of the above

638. Medullary function is tested by?
Harrison's 20th Ed. Chapter 300, Page 2071, Figure 300-3

A. Pupillary reaction to light
B. Spontaneous and reflex eye movements
C. Corneal responses
D. Respiratory & pharyngeal responses

In coma, midbrain & third nerve function are tested by pupillary reaction to light, pontine function by spontaneous & reflex eye movements & corneal responses, and medullary function by respiratory and pharyngeal responses.

639. Reflex conjugate, horizontal eye movements are dependent on?
Harrison's 20th Ed. Chapter 300, Page 2071, Figure 300-3

A. Medial longitudinal fasciculus (MLF)
B. Superior colliculus
C. Cerebellum
D. Temporal radiation

Reflex conjugate, horizontal eye movements are dependent on medial longitudinal fasciculus (MLF) that interconnects sixth & contralateral third nerve nuclei.

640. Acronym "COWS" that refers to "cold water opposite, warm water same" is for which of the following?
Harrison's 20th Ed. Chapter 300, Page 2072

A. Tonic deviation of head
B. Tonic deviation of both eyes
C. Direction of nystagmus
D. All of the above

Head rotation (oculocephalic reflex) or caloric stimulation of the labyrinths (oculovestibular reflex) elicits contraversive eye movements. Oculovestibular test is performed by irrigating the external auditory canal with cool water in order to induce convection currents in labyrinths. After a brief latency, result is tonic deviation of both eyes to the side of cool-water irrigation and nystagmus in the opposite direction. (Acronym "COWS" refers to direction of nystagmus - "cold water opposite, warm water same.") Loss of induced conjugate ocular movements indicates brainstem damage.

641. Presence of corrective nystagmus indicates which of the following?
Harrison's 20th Ed. Chapter 300, Page 2072

A. Frontal lobes are functioning
B. Frontal lobes are connected to the brainstem
C. Functional or hysterical coma is likely
D. All of the above

Presence of corrective nystagmus indicates that the frontal lobes are functioning and connected to the brainstem; thus functional or hysterical coma is likely.

642. Corneal reflex depends on the integrity of pontine pathways between?
Harrison's 20th Ed. Chapter 300, Page 2072

A. Fifth and same sided seventh cranial nerve
B. Fifth and opposite sided seventh cranial nerve
C. Fifth and both seventh cranial nerves
D. Any of the above

Corneal reflex depends on the integrity of pontine pathways between fifth (afferent) & both seventh (efferent) cranial nerves.

643. Corneal reflex in conjunction with reflex eye movements is a useful test of?
Harrison's 20th Ed. Chapter 300, Page 2072

A. Midbrain function
B. Pontine function
C. Medullary function
D. All of the above

Corneal reflex in conjunction with reflex eye movements is a useful test of pontine function.

644. When CNS-depressant drugs are given, which of these is the first to disappear?
Harrison's 20th Ed. Chapter 300, Page 2072

A. Corneal responses
B. Reflex eye movements
C. Non-reactivity of pupils to light
D. Any of the above

CNS-depressant drugs diminish or eliminate the corneal responses soon after reflex eye movements are paralyzed but before the pupils become unreactive to light.

645. Agonal gasps are the result of damage to?
Harrison's 20th Ed. Chapter 300, Page 2072

A. Cortex
B. Midbrain
C. Pons
D. Medulla

Agonal gasps are the result of lower brainstem (medullary) damage and are recognized as the terminal respiratory pattern of severe brain damage.

646. Which of the following abnormalities of respiration may be seen in coma?
DeJong's The Neurologic Examination, 7th Ed. Page 38

A. Cheyne - Stokes breathing
B. Biot breathing
C. Kussmaul breathing
D. All of the above

Abnormalities of respiration, such as Cheyne-Stokes, Biot, or Kussmaul breathing may be seen in coma and other neurologic disorders.

647. Which of the following respiratory pattern is seen in ponto-mesencephalic lesions?
Harrison's 20th Ed. Chapter 300, Page 2072

A. Shallow, slow, regular
B. Cheyne-Stokes respiration
C. Kussmaul breathing
D. Tachypnea

Kussmaul or rapid, deep breathing is usually seen in metabolic acidosis but may also occur with pontomesencephalic lesions.

648. Cheyne-Stokes respiration in its classic cyclic form is seen in which of the following conditions?
Harrison's 20th Ed. Chapter 300, Page 2072

A. Light coma
B. Deep coma
C. Sleep
D. Awake state

Cheyne-Stokes respiration in its classic cyclic form signifies bihemispheral damage or metabolic suppression and commonly accompanies light coma.

649. Tachypnea occurs in which of the following conditions?
Harrison's 20th Ed. Chapter 300, Page 2072

A. Tuberculosis of CNS
B. Lymphoma of CNS
C. Fungal infection of CNS
D. All of the above

Tachypnea occurs with lymphoma of the CNS.

650. In nonhabituated patients, what level of ethanol causes impaired mental activity?
Harrison's 20th Ed. Chapter 300, Page 2072

A. 0.2 gram/dL
B. 0.3 gram/dL
C. 0.4 gram/dL
D. 0.5 gram/dL

651. In nonhabituated patients, what level of ethanol is associated with stupor?
Harrison's 20th Ed. Chapter 300, Page 2072

A. 0.2 gram/dL
B. 0.3 gram/dL
C. 0.4 gram/dL
D. 0.5 gram/dL

In nonhabituated patients, generally an ethanol level of 43 mmol/L (0.2 gram/dL) causes impaired mental activity and a level of >65 mmol/L (0.3 gram/dL) is associated with stupor.

652. Most cases of coma (and confusion) are due to?
Harrison's 20th Ed. Chapter 300, Page 2072, DeJong's The Neurologic Examination, 7th Ed. Page 748

A. Hemorrhage
B. Tumor
C. Metabolic or toxic origin
D. Hydrocephalus

Most cases of coma (and confusion) are metabolic or toxic in origin. With rare exception, metabolic encephalopathies are characterized by reactive pupils and a symmetric neurologic examination. Any asymmetry in motor or sensory responses and any pupillary or eye movement abnormality should prompt an immediate, vigorous search for structural disease.

653. Which of the score is used to assess level of coma?
DeJong's The Neurologic Examination, 7th Ed. Page 749

A. FOUR score
B. ACDU
C. AVPU
D. All of the above

The FOUR (Full Outline of UnResponsiveness) score has four components (eye, motor, brainstem, and respiration). Other coma scales are the Innsbruck, Glasgow-Liege, reaction level, coma recovery, ACDU (Alert, Confused, Drowsy, Unresponsive), and AVPU (Alert, responds to Voice, responds to Pain, Unresponsive).

654. Coma must be distinguished from?
DeJong's The Neurologic Examination, 7th Ed. Page 749

A. Persistent vegetative state (PVS)
B. Locked-in syndrome
C. Mutism
D. All of the above

655. Which of the following reflex is related to brain death?
DeJong's The Neurologic Examination, 7th Ed. Page 759

A. Lazarus reflex
B. Galant reflex
C. Churchill Cope reflex
D. Bezold-Jarisch reflex

The Lazarus reflex is a reflex movement in brain-dead. Patient briefly raise their arms & drop them crossed on their chests. The phenomenon is named after the Biblical figure Lazarus of Bethany, whom Jesus raised from the dead in the Gospel of John.

656. In a case of coma, which of the following may not be detected by CT scan?
Harrison's 20th Ed. Chapter 300, Page 2072

A. Acute brainstem infarction
B. Sagittal sinus thrombosis
C. Encephalitis
D. All of the above

Bilateral hemisphere infarction, acute brainstem infarction, encephalitis, meningitis, mechanical shearing of axons (closed head trauma), sagittal sinus thrombosis, and subdural hematoma isodense to adjacent brain may not be detected.

657. In coma, EEG is useful in which of the following conditions?
Harrison's 20th Ed. Chapter 300, Page 2072

A. Clinically unrecognized seizure
B. Herpesvirus encephalitis
C. Prion (Creutzfeldt-Jakob) disease
D. All of the above

The EEG is useful in metabolic or drug-induced states and is diagnostic when coma is due to clinically unrecognized seizure, to herpesvirus encephalitis, or to prion (Creutzfeldt-Jakob) disease.

658. Which of the following is typical of metabolic coma?
Harrison's 20th Ed. Chapter 300, Page 2073

A. Delta or triphasic waves in the frontal regions
B. Widespread fast beta activity
C. Widespread variable 8- to 12-Hz activity
D. Normal alpha activity

Predominant high-voltage slowing (delta or triphasic waves) in the frontal regions is typical of metabolic coma.

659. Which of the following is typical of coma due to sedative drugs (diazepines, barbiturates)?
Harrison's 20th Ed. Chapter 300, Page 2073

A. Delta or triphasic waves in the frontal regions
B. Widespread fast beta activity
C. Widespread variable 8- to 12-Hz activity
D. Normal alpha activity

Widespread fast beta activity implies sedative drugs (diazepines, barbiturates) as a cause of coma.

660. Alpha coma results from?
Harrison's 20th Ed. Chapter 300, Page 2073

A. Hyperventilation
B. Hypoglycemia
C. Pontine damage
D. Subdural hematoma

Alpha coma results from pontine or diffuse cortical damage and is associated with a poor prognosis.

661. Which of the following is typical of locked-in syndrome?
Harrison's 20th Ed. Chapter 300, Page 2073

A. Delta or triphasic waves in the frontal regions
B. Widespread fast beta activity
C. Widespread variable 8- to 12-Hz activity
D. Normal alpha activity

Normal alpha activity on EEG is found in locked-in syndrome, hysteria or catatonia.

662. Which of the following condition causes sudden coma?
Harrison's 20th Ed. Chapter 300, Page 2073

A. Acute hydrocephalus
B. Basilar artery embolism
C. Cerebral infarction
D. Encephalitis

Conditions that cause sudden coma include drug ingestion, cerebral hemorrhage, trauma, cardiac arrest, epilepsy, or basilar artery embolism.

663. Gaze paresis is a feature of which cerebrovascular disease?
Harrison's 20th Ed. Chapter 300, Page 2073

A. Thalamic hemorrhage
B. Pontine hemorrhage
C. Cerebellar hemorrhage
D. Subarachnoid hemorrhage

Occipital headache, vomiting, gaze paresis, and inability to stand are features of cerebellar hemorrhage.

664. Asymmetric limb paresis is a feature of which cerebrovascular disease?
Harrison's 20th Ed. Chapter 300, Page 2073

A. Basilar artery thrombosis
B. Infarction in middle cerebral artery territory
C. Acute hydrocephalus
D. Subarachnoid hemorrhage

665. Neurologic prodrome or warning spells are a feature of which of the following?
Harrison's 20th Ed. Chapter 300, Page 2073

A. Basilar artery thrombosis
B. Infarction in middle cerebral artery territory
C. Acute hydrocephalus
D. Subarachnoid hemorrhage

Neurologic prodrome or warning spells, diplopia, dysarthria, vomiting, eye movement and corneal response abnormalities, and asymmetric limb paresis are features of basilar artery thrombosis.

666. Hyperventilation and excessive sweating are a feature of which cerebrovascular disease?
Harrison's 20th Ed. Chapter 300, Page 2073

A. Thalamic hemorrhage
B. Pontine hemorrhage
C. Cerebellar hemorrhage
D. Subarachnoid hemorrhage

Sudden onset, pinpoint pupils, loss of reflex eye movements and corneal responses, ocular bobbing, posturing, hyperventilation, and excessive sweating are features of pontine hemorrhage.

667. Vomiting is a feature of which of the following?
Harrison's 20th Ed. Chapter 300, Page 2073

A. Thalamic hemorrhage
B. Cerebellar hemorrhage
C. Subarachnoid hemorrhage
D. All of the above

668. Precipitous coma after headache and vomiting is a feature of which of the following?
Harrison's 20th Ed. Chapter 300, Page 2073

- A. Thalamic hemorrhage
- B. Pontine hemorrhage
- C. Cerebellar hemorrhage
- D. Subarachnoid hemorrhage

Precipitous coma after headache and vomiting is a feature of subarachnoid hemorrhage.

669. Acute hydrocephalus accompanies particularly which of the following?
Harrison's 20th Ed. Chapter 300, Page 2073

- A. Thalamic hemorrhage
- B. Pontine hemorrhage
- C. Cerebellar hemorrhage
- D. Subarachnoid hemorrhage

The syndrome of acute hydrocephalus accompanies particularly subarachnoid hemorrhage.

670. Which of the following diseases cause meningeal irritation?
Harrison's 20th Ed. Chapter 300, Page 2073, Table 300-1

- A. Fat embolism
- B. Cholesterol embolism
- C. Carcinomatous meningitis
- D. All of the above

Fat embolism, cholesterol embolism, carcinomatous and lymphomatous meningitis cause meningeal irritation with or without fever, and with an excess of WBCs or RBCs in CSF, usually without focal or lateralizing cerebral or brainstem signs. CT or MRI shows no mass lesion.

671. Which of the following diseases cause focal brainstem or lateralizing cerebral signs?
Harrison's 20th Ed. Chapter 300, Page 2073, Table 300-1

- A. Herpes simplex encephalitis
- B. Thrombotic thrombocytopenic purpura
- C. Pituitary apoplexy
- D. All of the above

672. Cellular content of the CSF is not normal in which of the following?
Harrison's 20th Ed. Chapter 300, Page 2073, Table 300-1

- A. Malaria
- B. Fat embolism
- C. Typhoid fever
- D. Eclampsia

673. Which of the following is a feature of brain death?
Harrison's 20th Ed. Chapter 300, Page 2073

- A. Heart rate unresponsive to atropine
- B. Diabetes insipidus
- C. Absent Babinski signs
- D. All of the above

674. In a valid apnea testing, PCO_2 should be at least?
Harrison's 20th Ed. Chapter 300, Page 2073

- A. 30–40 mm Hg
- B. 40–50 mm Hg
- C. 50–60 mm Hg
- D. 60–70 mm Hg

To confirm brain death, apnea is confirmed if no respiratory effort is observed in the presence of a sufficiently elevated PCO_2, i.e. 50-60 mm Hg.

675. A "coma cocktail," consists of all except?
DeJong's The Neurologic Examination, 7th Ed. Page 746

- A. Dextrose
- B. Flumazenil
- C. Cobalamin
- D. Naloxone

A "coma cocktail," consisting of dextrose, flumazenil, naloxone, and thiamine, is sometimes used in the initial management of the comatose patient.

Severe Acute Encephalopathies and Critical Care Weakness

676. Encephalopathy is a general term describing brain dysfunction that is?
Harrison's 20th Ed. Chapter 301, Page 2074

- A. Diffuse
- B. Global
- C. Multi-focal
- D. Any of the above

677. Which of the following is false about vasogenic brain edema?
Harrison's 20th Ed. Chapter 301, Page 2074

- A. Abnormal permeability of blood-brain barrier (BBB)
- B. Influx of fluid & solutes into brain
- C. Caused by ischemia, trauma, infection & metabolic derangements
- D. None of the above

678. Which of the following is false about cytotoxic brain edema?
Harrison's 20th Ed. Chapter 301, Page 2074

- A. Due to cellular swelling & membrane breakdown
- B. Caused by head trauma & stroke
- C. Leads to necrotic cell death & tissue infarction
- D. None of the above

679. Release of which of the following leads to influx of calcium & sodium ions?
Harrison's 20th Ed. Chapter 301, Page 2074

- A. Dopamine
- B. Serotonin
- C. Histamine
- D. Glutamate

Ischemic cascade is initiated when delivery of substrates like oxygen & glucose is inadequate to sustain brain cellular functions. Release of excitatory amino acids like glutamate leads to influx of calcium & sodium ions, which disrupt cellular homeostasis.

680. Which of the following is related to ischemic cascade?
Harrison's 20th Ed. Chapter 301, Page 2074

- A. Increased intracellular calcium concentration
- B. Activation of proteases & lipases
- C. Lipid peroxidation & free radical–mediated cell membrane injury
- D. All of the above

681. Events that can cause "secondary brain insults" include all except?
Harrison's 20th Ed. Chapter 301, Page 2075

- A. Systemic hypertension
- B. Hypoxia
- C. Seizures
- D. Hyperglycemia

Systemic hypotension & hypoxia reduce substrate delivery to vulnerable brain tissue (penumbra). Fever, seizures & hyperglycemia can increase cellular metabolism. Clinically these events are known as secondary brain insults because they lead to exacerbation of the primary brain injury.

682. Which of the following about penumbra is false?
Harrison's 20th Ed. Chapter 301, Page 2075

- A. Ischemic but reversibly dysfunctional tissue surrounding a core area of infarction
- B. Can be imaged by perfusion imaging using MRI or CT
- C. Immediate goal of treatment is to optimize cerebral perfusion in ischemic penumbra
- D. None of the above

683. In MRI, which of the following provides an estimate of ischemic penumbra?
Harrison's 20th Ed. Chapter 301, Page 2075

- A. Perfusion defect
- B. Diffusion deficit
- C. Diffusion-perfusion mismatch
- D. All of the above

The discrepancy between the region of poor perfusion and diffusion deficit is called diffusion-perfusion mismatch and is a measure of ischemic penumbra.

684. Which of the following about apoptosis is false?
Harrison's 20th Ed. Chapter 301, Page 2075

- A. Programmed cell death
- B. Occurs without cerebral edema
- C. Not seen on brain imaging
- D. None of the above

685. Cerebral perfusion pressure (CPP) is defined as?
Harrison's 20th Ed. Chapter 301, Page 2075

- A. Systolic blood pressure – intracranial pressure
- B. Diastolic blood pressure – intracranial pressure
- C. Mean arterial pressure – intracranial pressure
- D. Mean arterial pressure (MAP) + intracranial pressure

Cerebral perfusion pressure (CPP) is defined as the mean systemic arterial pressure (MAP) minus the intracranial pressure (ICP).

686. Which of the following is responsible for autoregulation of cerebral blood flow?
Harrison's 20th Ed. Chapter 301, Page 2075

- A. Stems of ACA, MCA, PCA
- B. Circle of Willis
- C. Microcirculation
- D. All of the above

Cerebral blood flow (CBF) remains relatively constant over a wide range of blood pressures due to physiologic autoregulation that occur in microcirculation or by vessels below the resolution of those seen on angiography.

687. Cerebral blood flow is principally influenced by all except?
Harrison's 20th Ed. Chapter 301, Page 2075

- A. Systemic blood pressure
- B. pH
- C. PCO_2
- D. PO_2

CBF is strongly influenced by systemic blood pressure, pH and PCO_2. CBF increases with hypercapnia and acidosis and decreases with hypocapnia and alkalosis.

688. Which of the following statements is false?
Harrison's 20th Ed. Chapter 301, Page 2075
A. CBF increases with hypercapnia & acidosis
B. CBF decreases with hypocapnia and alkalosis
C. CBF becoming pressure-dependent is ominous
D. None of the above

689. Volume of CSF within ventricles and surrounding the brain and spinal cord is about?
Harrison's 20th Ed. Chapter 301, Page 2075
A. 50 mL
B. 100 mL
C. 150 mL
D. 200 mL

690. Cerebral blood volume is about?
Harrison's 20th Ed. Chapter 301, Page 2075
A. 50 mL
B. 100 mL
C. 150 mL
D. 200 mL

About 150 mL of CSF is present within the ventricles and surrounding the brain and spinal cord. Cerebral blood volume is also ~150 mL.

691. To avoid secondary ischemic brain injury, intracranial pressure should be maintained at?
Harrison's 20th Ed. Chapter 301, Page 2077
A. < 5 mm Hg
B. < 10 mm Hg
C. < 15 mm Hg
D. < 20 mm Hg

In general, ICP should be maintained at <20 mm Hg.

692. To avoid secondary ischemic brain injury, cerebral perfusion pressure (CPP) should be maintained at?
Harrison's 20th Ed. Chapter 301, Page 2077
A. ≥ 40 mm Hg
B. ≥ 50 mm Hg
C. ≥ 60 mm Hg
D. ≥ 70 mm Hg

In treatment of SAH, cerebral perfusion pressure should be maintained at ≥ 60 mm Hg.

693. Which of the following is an early sign of elevated ICP?
Harrison's 20th Ed. Chapter 301, Page 2077
A. Drowsiness and a diminished level of consciousness
B. Unilateral pupillary changes
C. Coma
D. All of the above

Early signs of elevated ICP include drowsiness and a diminished level of consciousness while coma and unilateral pupillary changes are late signs.

694. Which of the following has been shown to improve outcome in patients with elevated ICP?
Harrison's 20th Ed. Chapter 301, Page 2078
A. Intubation and hyperventilation to $PaCO_2$ 30–35 mm Hg
B. High dose barbiturates ("pentobarb coma")
C. Decompressive hemicraniectomy
D. Hypothermia to 33°C

695. "Histotoxic hypoxia" is produced by?
Harrison's 20th Ed. Chapter 301, Page 2078
A. Shock
B. Asphyxiation
C. Carbon monoxide poisoning
D. Any of the above

Carbon monoxide & cyanide poisoning are termed histotoxic hypoxia because they cause a direct impairment of the respiratory chain.

696. Which of the following reflexes pertain to brainstem function?
Harrison's 20th Ed. Chapter 301, Page 2078
A. Oculocephalic (doll's eyes) reflex
B. Oculovestibular (caloric) reflex
C. Corneal reflex
D. All of the above

697. Selective persistent memory deficits after brief cardiac arrest is due to injury to?
Harrison's 20th Ed. Chapter 301, Page 2078
A. Cerebral cortex
B. Basal ganglia
C. Hippocampus
D. Hypothalamus

Selective persistent memory deficits after brief cardiac arrest is due to injury to hippocampal CA1 neurons which are vulnerable to even brief episodes of hypoxia-ischemia.

698. Which of the following convey a poor prognosis after a severe hypoxic-ischemic insult?
Harrison's 20th Ed. Chapter 301, Page 2078
A. Myoclonic status epilepticus
B. Absence of pupillary light reflex day 3 after injury
C. Bilateral absence of N20 somatosensory evoked response
D. All of the above

Absence of pupillary light reflex or absence of a motor response to pain on day 3 following injury, bilateral absence of early cortical somatosensory evoked response (SSEPs) and myoclonic status epilepticus within 24 hours after a primary circulatory arrest convey a poor prognosis.

699. Neuron-specific enolase (NSE) has relevance in which of the following conditions?
Harrison's 20th Ed. Chapter 301, Page 2078
A. Creutzfeldt-Jakob disease (CJD)
B. Small-cell cancer of the lung
C. Gastrointestinal neuroendocrine tumors (Carcinoids)
D. All of the above

Elevations of CSF neuron-specific enolase & tau occur in CJD but lack specificity for diagnosis. Plasma NSE levels are also used as a marker of GI-NETs (carcinoids). A very elevated serum level (>33 μg/L) of biochemical marker neuron-specific enolase (NSE) within first 3 days is indicative of brain damage after resuscitation from cardiac arrest & predicts a poor outcome.

700. Which of the following about watershed distribution of brain is false?
Harrison's 20th Ed. Chapter 301, Page 2078
A. Most metastases develop at watershed areas of brain
B. Balint's syndrome results from infarctions in watershed areas between distal PCA & MCA territories
C. Watershed infarcts occurs at distal territories between major cerebral arteries in low flow states
D. None of the above

701. **Which of the following CNS injuries may occur following open heart or coronary artery bypass grafting (CABG) surgery?**
Harrison's 20th Ed. Chapter 301, Page 2079
   A. Acute encephalopathy
   B. Stroke
   C. Chronic syndrome of cognitive impairment
   D. All of the above

702. **Which of the following is preferred to reduce delirium & shorten the duration of mechanical ventilation in critically ill patients requiring sedation?**
Harrison's 20th Ed. Chapter 301, Page 2079
   A. Haloperidol
   B. Lorazepam
   C. Midazolam
   D. Dexmedetomidine

In critically ill patients requiring sedation, use of the centrally acting α2 agonist dexmedetomidine reduces delirium & shortens the duration of mechanical ventilation.

703. **Biomarkers of blood brain barrier (BBB) dysfunction include?**
Harrison's 20th Ed. Chapter 301, Page 2080
   A. S-100β
   B. Plasma-soluble prion protein (PrPc)
   C. Ubiquitin carboxyl-terminal hydrolase isoenzyme L1 (UCHL1)
   D. All of the above

704. **Which of the following about osmotic demyelination syndrome is false?**
Harrison's 20th Ed. Chapter 301, Page 2080
   A. Demyelination without inflammation in base of pons
   B. Relative sparing of axons & nerve cells
   C. Presents as quadriplegia & pseudobulbar palsy
   D. None of the above

Previously called central pontine myelinolysis.

705. **Which of the following is a feature of acute Wernicke's disease?**
Harrison's 20th Ed. Chapter 301, Page 2080
   A. Global confusion
   B. Impairment of eye movements
   C. Gait ataxia
   D. All of the above

Characteristic clinical triad of acute Wernicke's disease is ophthalmoplegia, ataxia & global confusion.

706. **Ocular motor abnormalities in acute Wernicke's disease include?**
Harrison's 20th Ed. Chapter 301, Page 2080
   A. Horizontal nystagmus on lateral gaze
   B. Lateral rectus palsy
   C. Conjugate gaze palsies
   D. All of the above

Ocular motor abnormalities in acute Wernicke's disease include horizontal nystagmus on lateral gaze, usually bilateral lateral rectus palsy, conjugate gaze palsies, and rarely ptosis. Pupils are usually spared. Horizontal nystagmus may persist even after treatment.

707. **Gait ataxia in acute Wernicke's disease results from?**
Harrison's 20th Ed. Chapter 301, Page 2080
   A. Polyneuropathy
   B. Cerebellar involvement
   C. Vestibular paresis
   D. All of the above

Gait ataxia results from a combination of polyneuropathy, cerebellar involvement & vestibular paresis.

708. **Feature of amnestic syndrome (Korsakoff's syndrome) is?**
Harrison's 20th Ed. Chapter 301, Page 2081
   A. Gaps in memory
   B. Confabulation
   C. Disordered temporal sequencing
   D. All of the above

Damage to medial thalamic nuclei & mammillary bodies occur in Korsakoff's syndrome. Mammillary body atrophy may be visible on MRI in the chronic phase. Amnestic defect is related to lesions in dorsal medial nuclei of thalamus.

709. **Thiamine is a cofactor of which of the following enzymes?**
Harrison's 20th Ed. Chapter 301, Page 2081
   A. Transketolase
   B. Pyruvate dehydrogenase
   C. α-ketoglutarate dehydrogenase
   D. All of the above

Thiamine is a cofactor of transketolase, pyruvate dehydrogenase, and α-ketoglutarate dehydrogenase and others. Thiamine deficiency leads to glutamate accumulation due to impairment of α-ketoglutarate dehydrogenase activity resulting in excitotoxic cell damage. Glucose infusions may precipitate Wernicke's Zdisease.

710. **Which of the following about posterior reversible encephalopathy syndrome (PRES) is false?**
Harrison's 20th Ed. Chapter 301, Page 2081
   A. Pathogenesis of hyperperfusion due to endothelial dysfunction
   B. Vasogenic edema
   C. Affects posterior rather than anterior portions of brain
   D. None of the above

711. **Which of the following can lead to posterior reversible encephalopathy syndrome (PRES)?**
Harrison's 20th Ed. Chapter 301, Page 2082 Table 301-3
   A. Cyclosporine
   B. Tacrolimus
   C. Methotrexate
   D. All of the above

712. **Which of the following can lead to posterior reversible encephalopathy syndrome (PRES)?**
Harrison's 20th Ed. Chapter 301, Page 2082 Table 301-3
   A. HELLP syndrome
   B. Hemolytic-uremic syndrome (HUS)
   C. Cocaine use
   D. All of the above

713. **Clinical presentation of posterior reversible encephalopathy syndrome include?**
Harrison's 20th Ed. Chapter 301, Page 2081
   A. Prominent headaches
   B. Seizures
   C. Focal neurologic deficits
   D. All of the above

714. Typical focal deficit in hyperperfusion states is?
Harrison's 20th Ed. Chapter 301, Page 2081

A. Glaucoma
B. Cortical visual loss
C. Posterior Uveitis
D. Amaurosis Fugax

Typical focal deficit in hyperperfusion states is cortical visual loss, given the tendency of the process to involve the occipital lobes. Increased capillary pressure or endothelial dysfunction play a role in its pathophysiology. The rapidity of rise, rather than absolute value of pressure, is the most important risk factor.

715. Most common peripheral nervous system (PNS) complication related to critical illness is?
Harrison's 20th Ed. Chapter 301, Page 2083

A. Critical illness polyneuropathy
B. Critical illness myopathy
C. Guillain-Barré syndrome
D. Myasthenia gravis

716. Medication that impairs neuromuscular transmission is?
Harrison's 20th Ed. Chapter 301, Page 2083

A. Aminoglycosides
B. Beta-blocking agents
C. Cisatracurium
D. All of the above

717. Risk factors for prolonged action of neuromuscular blocking agents include?
Harrison's 20th Ed. Chapter 301, Page 2083

A. Female sex
B. Metabolic acidosis
C. Renal failure
D. All of the above

718. Which of the following about cachectic myopathy is false?
Harrison's 20th Ed. Chapter 301, Page 2083

A. Serum creatine kinase levels normal
B. Electromyography (EMG) normal
C. Muscle biopsy shows type II fiber atrophy
D. None of the above

719. Which of the following about acute necrotizing intensive care myopathy is false?
Harrison's 20th Ed. Chapter 301, Page 2083

A. Elevations in serum creatine kinase
B. Elevations in urine myoglobin
C. Both EMG & muscle biopsy may be normal initially
D. None of the above

720. Which of the following about thick-filament myopathy is false?
Harrison's 20th Ed. Chapter 301, Page 2083

A. Occurs in the setting of glucocorticoid & nd-NMBA use
B. Actual myopathy with muscle damage
C. Invariably improves & most patients return to normal
D. None of the above

721. Amaurosis Fugax is best related to?
Harrison's 20th Ed. Chapter 28, Page 183

A. Cluster headache
B. Transient ischemic attack of retina
C. Hysterical conversion reaction
D. All of the above

Amaurosis fugax or a transient ischemic attack of the retina or transient monocular blindness, occurs from emboli to central retinal artery of one eye indicating carotid stenosis or local ophthalmic artery disease as the cause.

722. Amaurosis Fugax is the result of?
Harrison's 20th Ed. Chapter 28, Page 183

A. Trauma
B. Emboli
C. Vascular spasm
D. Any of the above

Amaurosis fugax usually results from an embolus stuck in a retinal arteriole. Complete occlusion of the central retinal artery produces arrest of blood flow and a milky retina with a cherry-red fovea.

723. Emboli causing amaurosis fugax are composed of?
Harrison's 20th Ed. Chapter 28, Page 183

A. Cholesterol
B. Calcium
C. Platelet-fibrin debris
D. Any of the above

Emboli causing amaurosis fugax are composed of cholesterol (Hollenhorst plaque), calcium, or platelet-fibrin debris. Most common source is atherosclerotic plaque in carotid artery or aorta.

724. Which of the following statements about amaurosis fugax is false?
Harrison's 20th Ed. Chapter 28, Page 183, 187

A. Briefer duration than migraine
B. Occurs in both eyes
C. Not followed by headache
D. Associated with antiphospholipid antibody syndrome

Amaurosis fugax refers to a transient ischemic attack of retina and occurs in only one eye (painless monocular loss of vision). It can be a part of high-altitude neurologic events.

725. Which of the following is false about Charcot-Bouchard miliary aneurysm?
Angiology. 2018;69(1):17-30

A. Aneurysms of brain blood vessels of <300 μm diameter
B. Located in brainstem
C. Associated with chronic hypertension
D. None of the above

Charcot-Bouchard miliary aneurysms (French physicians Jean-Martin Charcot and Charles-Joseph Bouchard) are aneurysms of brain small blood vessels (<300 μm diameter). While, saccular aneurysms (berry aneurysms) occur in larger-sized blood vessels. Charcot-Bouchard aneurysms are most often located in the brainstem and are associated with chronic hypertension.

726. Hypothesis of homunculus organization of fibers in internal capsule means?
Brain. 2017;140:3055-3061

A. Sensory & motor fibers have same orientation
B. Sensory & motor fibers have different orientation
C. Adjacent regions on cortex correspond on adjacent areas on body surface
D. None of the above

Homunculus means 'little man' in Latin, first described by Penfield and Boldrey, 1937. Functional mapping & lesion studies have shown that primary motor & somatosensory cortices are so arranged that adjacent regions on cortex correspond on adjacent areas on body surface. In somatotropic representations, arms are always medial to legs except in primary sensiromotor cortex & in posterior columns.

727. Which of the following tracts is not present in the posterior limb of internal capsule?

DeJong's The Neurologic Examination, 7th Ed. Page 59

A. Cortico-pontine
B. Superior thalamic radiation
C. Anterior thalamic radiation
D. Corticospinal tract

Anterior thalamic radiation is part of anterior limb of internal capsule.

728. Genu of the internal capsule is at the level of?

DeJong's The Neurologic Examination, 7th Ed. Page 59

A. Foremen of Lushka
B. Foramen of Magendie
C. Foramen of Monro
D. Foramen magnum

729. Hippocampus-fornix-anterior thalamus-cingulate gyrus-cingulum bundle-perihippocampal cortex-hippocampus - this circuit is called?

DeJong's The Neurologic Examination, 7th Ed. Page 51

A. Papez's circuit
B. Hafez's circuit
C. Parkinson's circuit
D. Peter's circuit

Structures of limbic lobe are connected in Papez circuit (cigulate gyrus → parahippocampal gyrus → hippocampus → fornix → mammillary body → anterior nucleus of thalamus → cingulate gyrus).

Neuroimaging in Neurologic Disorders

730. Which of the following investigation is recommended in meningeal disease?
Harrison's 20th Ed. Chapter 416, Page 3030 Table 416-1

A. CT (noncontrast)
B. CT contrast
C. MRI
D. MRI with contrast

731. Which of the following investigation is recommended in myelopathy?
Harrison's 20th Ed. Chapter 416, Page 3030 Table 416-1

A. CT (noncontrast)
B. CT contrast
C. MRI
D. MRI with contrast

732. MRI + contrast is the investigation of choice for all of the following except?
Harrison's 20th Ed. Chapter 416, Page 3030 Table 416-1

A. Neoplasm (primary or metastatic)
B. White matter disorders
C. Infection/abscess
D. Immunosuppressed with focal findings

733. Which of the following is the most sensitive technique for detecting acute ischemic stroke of brain?
Harrison's 20th Ed. Chapter 416, Page 3030

A. CT angiography (CTA)
B. Perfusion CT (pCT)
C. MR angiography (MRA)
D. Diffusion MR

Diffusion MR is the most sensitive technique for detecting acute ischemic stroke of brain or spinal cord, encephalitis, abscesses and prion diseases.

734. In normal CNS, which of the following structure lacks blood-brain barrier (BBB)?
Harrison's 20th Ed. Chapter 416, Page 3031

A. Pituitary gland
B. Choroid plexus
C. Dura
D. All of the above

In normal CNS, the pituitary gland, choroid plexus, and dura lack blood-brain barrier (BBB) and enhance after contrast administration.

735. In a routine brain CT study, radiation dose is normally about?
Harrison's 20th Ed. Chapter 416, Page 3031

A. 0.2 to 1 mSv
B. 2 to 5 mSv
C. 6 to 12 mSv
D. 22 to 50 mSv

In a routine brain CT study, radiation dose is normally between 2 and 5 mSv (millisievert).

736. Rise in serum creatinine of at least 1 mg/dL within how many hours of contrast administration defines contrast nephropathy?
Harrison's 20th Ed. Chapter 416, Page 3031

A. 6 hours
B. 12 hours
C. 24 hours
D. 48 hours

737. Risk factors for contrast nephropathy include all except?
Harrison's 20th Ed. Chapter 416, Page 3031

A. Solitary kidney
B. Diabetes mellitus
C. Hypertension
D. Advanced age (>80 years)

Risk factors for contrast nephropathy include advanced age (>80 years), preexisting renal disease (serum creatinine exceeding 2 mg/dL), solitary kidney, diabetes mellitus, dehydration, paraproteinemia, concurrent use of nephrotoxic medication or chemotherapeutic agents, and high contrast dose.

738. What is the eGFR threshold below which iodinated contrast should not be given?
Harrison's 20th Ed. Chapter 416, Page 3033

A. 90 mL/min/1.73 meter^2
B. 75 mL/min/1.73 meter^2
C. 60 mL/min/1.73 meter^2
D. 30 mL/min/1.73 meter^2

The American College of Radiology suggests using an estimated glomerular filtration rate (eGFR) of 30 mL/min/1.73 meter^2 as a threshold below which iodinated contrast should not be given without serious consideration of the potential for contrast nephropathy.

739. Use of which of the following may reduce the incidence of contrast nephropathy?
Harrison's 20th Ed. Chapter 416, Page 3033

A. Acetylcysteine
B. Oxygen inhalation
C. Osmolar diuretics
D. Loop diuretics

Apart from hydration and reduction in dose of contrast media, use of bicarbonate & acetylcysteine may reduce the incidence of contrast nephropathy.

740. Severe allergic reactions occur in what proportion of patients receiving nonionic media?
Harrison's 20th Ed. Chapter 416, Page 3033

A. 0.04%
B. 0.12%
C. 0.18%
D. 0.24%

Severe allergic reactions occur in 0.04% of patients receiving nonionic media, sixfold lower than with ionic media.

741. Which of the following is not related to magnetic resonance imaging (MRI)?
Harrison's 20th Ed. Chapter 416, Page 3033

A. Hydrogen protons in biologic tissues
B. Dynamic magnetic field
C. Static magnetic field
D. Radiofrequency (Rf) waves

MRI is a complex interaction between hydrogen protons in biologic tissues, a static magnetic field (the magnet), and energy (echo) in the form of radiofrequency (Rf) waves of a specific frequency.

742. T2W images are more sensitive than T1W images to all of the following except?
Harrison's 20th Ed. Chapter 416, Page 3034

A. Edema
B. Fat-containing structures
C. Demyelination
D. Infarction

T2-weighted (T2W) images are more sensitive than T1-weighted (T1W) images to edema, demyelination, infarction, and chronic hemorrhage, while T1W Imaging is more sensitive to subacute hemorrhage and fat-containing structures.

743. MRI involves imaging of?
N Engl J Med. 1993; 328:708-716

A. Electron
B. Proton
C. Neutron
D. All of the above

MRI involves imaging of the proton which is the positively charged spinning nucleus of hydrogen atoms found in abundance in tissues containing water, proteins, lipids & other macromolecules. Protons align with or against the direction of the magnetic field.

744. Which of the following is related to MRI?
N Engl J Med. 1993; 328:708-716

A. Larmor or resonance frequency
B. Body coil
C. Pulse sequence
D. All of the above

745. Which of the following is an MRI image?
N Engl J Med. 1993; 328:708-716

A. T1-weighted
B. T2-weighted
C. Proton-density-weighted
D. All of the above

746. In MRI, the degree of weighting depends on?
N Engl J Med. 1993; 328:708-716

A. Pulse sequence
B. Repetition time
C. Echo time
D. All of the above

747. Which of the following statements is false?
N Engl J Med. 1993; 328:708-716

A. Fluids appear dark in T1-weighted images
B. Fluids appear bright in proton-density-weighted images
C. Fluids appear bright in T2-weighted images
D. None of the above

748. Which of the following statements about gadolinium is false?
Harrison's 20th Ed. Chapter 416, Page 3034

A. Heavy-metal element
B. Paramagnetic substance
C. Chelated to DTPA
D. Approximate dose 2 mL/kg IV

Approximate dose of gadolinium is 0.2 mL/kg body weight administered intravenously. Gadolinium has the greatest ability to capture thermal neutrons.

749. Gadolinium is produced from which of the following minerals?
N Engl J Med. 2007;357:720-722

A. Ilmenite
B. Zircon
C. Monazite
D. Sillimanite

Gadolinium is produced both from monazite and bastnäsite.

750. Which of the following countries has deposits of monazite sands?
N Engl J Med. 2007;357:720-722

A. India
B. Brazil
C. South Africa
D. All of the above

751. Symbol of Gadolinium is?
N Engl J Med. 2007;357:720-722

A. Ga
B. Gd
C. Gl
D. Gm

Symbol of Gadolinium is Gd with atomic number 64 and atomic weight of 157.25.

752. Which of the following is best related to gadolinium contrast agents?
Harrison's 20th Ed. Chapter 416, Page 3035

A. Nephrogenic diabetes insipidus (NDI)
B. Nephrogenic Syndrome of Inappropriate Antidiuresis
C. Nephrogenic systemic fibrosis (NSF)
D. Nephrotic syndrome

Patients with renal insufficiency exposed to gadolinium contrast agents may develop a rare complication - nephrogenic systemic fibrosis (NSF) between 5 and 75 days following exposure.

753. Nephrogenic systemic fibrosis (NSF) involves which of the following parts of the body most?
Cleveland Clinic Journal of Medicine 2008;75(2):95-111

A. Upper extremities
B. Between ankles and thighs
C. Trunk
D. Face

754. Nephrogenic systemic fibrosis (NSF) involves which of the following parts of the body least?
Cleveland Clinic Journal of Medicine 2008;75(2):95-111

A. Upper extremities
B. Between ankles and thighs
C. Trunk
D. Face

NSF typically presents between ankles and the thighs (symmetric, progresses to involve the entire lower extremities). Upper extremity involvement occurs frequently, but usually with lower extremity disease. Trunk is involved less commonly than legs and arms. The face is typically spared.

755. Which of the following is a laboratory biomarker for NSF?
Cleveland Clinic Journal of Medicine 2008;75(2):95-111

A. Anti nuclear antibodies
B. Rheumatoid factor
C. Anti-SCL70 antibodies
D. None of the above

There is no laboratory biomarker for NSF.

756. Which of the following is characteristic and pathognomonic of NSF?
Cleveland Clinic Journal of Medicine 2008;75(2):95-111

A. Proliferation of dermal spindle cells
B. Thick collagen bundles with surrounding clefts
C. Immunohistochemically CD34 reactivity in fibroblast-like cells
D. Absence of mucin and elastic fibers

A characteristic and almost pathognomonic staining profile is the immunohistochemical identification of CD34 reactivity in the fibroblast-like cells. Cells expressing CD34 are normally found in the umbilical cord, the bone marrow (as pluripotential hematopoietic stem cells), and in the vascular endothelium.

757. Disorder that causes thickening & hardening of skin of extremities & trunk is?
Cleveland Clinic Journal of Medicine 2008;75(2):95-111

A. Systemic sclerosis
B. Scleromyxedema
C. Eosinophilic fasciitis
D. All of the above

Besides NSF, other disorders that can cause thickening & hardening of skin of extremities & trunk include systemic sclerosis or scleroderma, scleromyxedema, and eosinophilic fasciitis.

758. Most frequently used radionuclide moiety in Positron Emission Tomography (PET) is?
Harrison's 20th Ed. Chapter 416, Page 3037

A. 2-[^{16}F]fluoro-2-deoxy-d-glucose
B. 2-[^{17}F]fluoro-2-deoxy-d-glucose
C. 2-[^{18}F]fluoro-2-deoxy-d-glucose
D. 2-[^{19}F]fluoro-2-deoxy-d-glucose

In Positron Emission Tomography (PET), the most frequently used moiety is 2-[^{18}F]fluoro-2-deoxy-d-glucose (FDG), an analogue of glucose. It is taken up by cells competitively with 2-deoxyglucose.

Seizures and Epilepsy

759. Seizure is derived from a Latin word "sacire" that means?
Harrison's 20th Ed. Chapter 418, Page 3050

A. "to invade"
B. "to destroy"
C. "to silence"
D. "to take possession of"

Seizure is derived from Latin word "sacire" meaning "to take possession of".

760. What percentage of population will have at least one seizure in lifetime?
Harrison's 20th Ed. Chapter 418, Page 3050

A. ~1–3%
B. ~3–5%
C. ~5–10%
D. ~10–15%

761. Highest incidence of seizure is in which of the following age groups?
Harrison's 20th Ed. Chapter 418, Page 3050

A. Infancy
B. Early childhood & late adulthood
C. Middle age
D. Old age

~5–10% percentage of population will have at least one seizure in lifetime and the highest incidence is in early childhood and late adulthood.

762. Which of the following is false about epilepsy?
Harrison's 20th Ed. Chapter 418, Page 3050

A. Single seizure
B. Acute
C. No correctable or avoidable circumstance
D. All of the above

Epilepsy is a clinical phenomenon & is said to be present when a person has recurrent seizures due to a chronic, underlying process. A person with a single seizure or recurrent seizures due to correctable or avoidable circumstances, does not have epilepsy. By definition, epilepsy is two or more unprovoked seizures.

763. What is the prevalence of epilepsy?
Harrison's 20th Ed. Chapter 418, Page 3050

A. 2 – 6 persons per 1000
B. 3 – 9 persons per 1000
C. 4 – 20 persons per 1000
D. 5 – 30 persons per 1000

The prevalence of epilepsy is estimated at 5 - 30 persons per 1000.

764. In which year did the International League Against Epilepsy (ILAE) classify seizure disorders?
Harrison's 20th Ed. Chapter 418, Page 3050, Harrison's 19th Ed. 2542

A. 1965
B. 1978
C. 1981
D. 1995

In 1981, the International League against Epilepsy (ILAE) classification is based on clinical features of seizures and associated EEG findings. Etiology or cellular substrate are not considered. ILAE (2005-2009) has updated approach to classify seizures. ILAE Commission on Classification and Terminology provided an updated approach to classification of seizures in 2017.

765. Which of the following term is no longer used in classification of seizures?
Harrison's 20th Ed. Chapter 418, Page 3050

A. Partial seizures
B. Focal onset seizures
C. Generalized onset seizures
D. Unknown Onset seizures

In the new classification system (International League against Epilepsy (ILAE) Commission on Classification and Terminology, 2017), term partial seizures is no longer used and subcategories of "simple focal seizures" and "complex focal seizures" have been eliminated.

766. Focal seizures are associated with?
Harrison's 20th Ed. Chapter 418, Page 3051

A. Structural abnormalities of brain
B. Cellular abnormalities
C. Biochemical abnormalities
D. All of the above

Focal seizures are associated with structural abnormalities of brain, there are exception though.

767. Generalized seizures are associated with?
Harrison's 20th Ed. Chapter 418, Page 3051

A. Cellular abnormality
B. Biochemical abnormality
C. Structural abnormality
D. Any of the above

Generalized seizures may result from cellular, biochemical, or structural abnormalities.

768. Main difference between simple partial and complex partial seizure is?
Harrison's 20th Ed. Chapter 418, Page 3051

A. Unilateral or bilateral
B. Focal or generalized
C. Consciousness or unconsciousness
D. Absence or presence of aura

If consciousness is fully preserved during seizure, it was termed simple partial seizure. If consciousness is impaired, the seizure was termed complex partial seizure.

769. Motor manifestations of focal seizures can be all except?
Harrison's 20th Ed. Chapter 418, Page 3051

A. Tonic
B. Clonic
C. Myoclonic
D. Atonic

770. Nonmotor manifestations of focal seizures can be?
Harrison's 20th Ed. Chapter 418, Page 3051

A. Sensory
B. Autonomic
C. Emotional
D. All of the above

Focal seizures can have motor manifestations (tonic, clonic, or myoclonic movements) or nonmotor manifestations (sensory, autonomic, or emotional symptoms).

771. Which of the following is a feature of focal motor seizure?
Harrison's 20th Ed. Chapter 418, Page 3051

A. Jacksonian march
B. Todd's paralysis
C. Epilepsia partialis continua
D. All of the above

In focal motor seizures, after initiation from a restricted region, abnormal discharges may spread to other wider areas. This is called a "Jacksonian march". Following focal motor seizure, patient may have localized paresis in the involved region for minutes to many hours (Todd's paralysis). Focal motor seizure may continue for hours or days (epilepsia partialis continua).

772. Which of the following is often refractory to medical therapy?
Harrison's 20th Ed. Chapter 418, Page 3051

A. Jacksonian march
B. Todd's paralysis
C. Epilepsia partialis continua
D. All of the above

Focal motor seizure may continue for hours or days. Epilepsia partialis continua is the term applied to this condition. It is often refractory to medical therapy.

773. Which of the following is false about auras?
Harrison's 20th Ed. Chapter 418, Page 3051

A. Subjective
B. "Internal" events
C. Not directly observable by someone else
D. None of the above

Subjective, "internal" events that are not directly observable by someone else are referred to as auras.

774. Which of the following about focal seizures with dyscognitive features is false?
Harrison's 20th Ed. Chapter 418, Page 3051

A. Begins with an aura
B. Behavioral arrest denotes beginning of ictal phase
C. Reterograde amnesia
D. Automatisms

Focal seizures with dyscognitive features are characterized by focal seizure activity with transient unconsciousness, beginning with an aura which are subjective, internal events that are not directly observable by others. Behavioral arrest or motionless stare denotes beginning of ictal phase which marks the onset of the period of amnesia & automatisms. Following seizure anterograde amnesia, confusion or postictal aphasia may be present. Automatisms are involuntary, automatic behaviors that have a wide range of manifestations.

775. In seizure, retrograde component of amnesia may dominate in?
Harrison's 20th Ed. Chapter 418, Page 164

A. Absence seizure
B. Temporal lobe epilepsy
C. Myoclonic seizure
D. Febrile seizure

Occasionally associated with temporal lobe epilepsy or herpes simplex encephalitis, the retrograde component of amnesia may dominate.

776. Which of the following is false about seizures that may occur exclusively during sleep?
Harrison's 20th Ed. Chapter 418, Page 170

A. Mimic a primary sleep disorder
B. Typically occur during episodes of NREM sleep
C. May occur as generalized tonic-clonic movements
D. None of the above

777. A focal seizure that evolves into a generalized seizure frequently arise from?
Harrison's 20th Ed. Chapter 418, Page 3051

A. Frontal lobe
B. Temporal lobe
C. Parietal lobe
D. Occipital lobe

A focal seizure that evolves into a generalized seizure frequently arises from a region in frontal lobe. But, may happen with focal seizures occurring elsewhere in the brain.

778. Which of the following is false about typical absence seizures?
Harrison's 20th Ed. Chapter 418, Page 3051

A. Sudden, brief loss of consciousness with loss of postural control
B. Typically lasts for only seconds
C. Consciousness returns as suddenly as it was lost
D. No postictal confusion

Absence seizures are characterized by sudden, brief lapses of consciousness "without" loss of postural control. Patients stare & cease normal activity for a few seconds, return immediately to normal & have no memory of the event or no postictal confusion.

779. Which of the following occurs as bilateral motor sign in typical absence seizures?
Harrison's 20th Ed. Chapter 418, Page 3051

A. Small-amplitude, clonic movements of hands
B. Large-amplitude, clonic movements of hands
C. Small-amplitude, tonic movements of hands
D. Large-amplitude, tonic movements of hands

Absence seizures are usually accompanied by subtle, bilateral motor signs such as rapid blinking of eyelids, chewing movements, or small-amplitude, clonic movements of hands.

780. Which of the following is false about typical absence seizures?
Harrison's 20th Ed. Chapter 418, Page 3052

A. Usually begin in childhood (4 to 8 yrs)
B. EEG shows generalized, symmetric, 3-Hz spike-&-wave
C. EEG discharge begin & end suddenly on an abnormal background
D. Hyperventilation provokes EEG discharges & seizures

The EEG hallmark of typical absence seizures is a generalized, symmetric, 3-Hz spike-and-wave discharge that begins and ends suddenly, superimposed on a "normal" EEG background. Hyperventilation provokes these EEG discharges.

781. Which of the following will trigger a seizure in most patients with untreated typical absence seizures?
Harrison's 20th Ed. Chapter 418, Page 3052

A. Exercise
B. Hyperventilation
C. Breath holding
D. Lack of sleep

Hyperventilation for 3 minutes will trigger a seizure in most patients with untreated absence seizures.

782. Absence seizures were also called?
Epilepsy Currents, 2013;13(3):135–140

A. Narcolepsy
B. Cataplexy
C. Pyknolepsy
D. All of the above

The term "absence" was first used to describe seizures in 1705 and was reported as pyknolepsy ("heaped up, closely packed, aggregated attacks") in the early 20th century. Childhood absence epilepsy (CAE), also known as pyknolepsy, is an idiopathic generalized epilepsy which occurs in otherwise normal children.

783. What percentage of patients of typical absence seizures will have a spontaneous remission during adolescence?
Harrison's 17th Ed. 2499

A. ~ 10–20%
B. ~ 30–40%
C. ~ 50–60%
D. ~ 60–70%

~ 60-70% patients of absence seizures have a spontaneous remission during adolescence.

784. In atypical absence seizures, EEG finding of generalized, spike-and-wave pattern has a frequency of?
Harrison's 20th Ed. Chapter 418, Page 3052

A. <= 4.0 per second
B. <= 3.5 per second
C. <= 3.0 per second
D. <= 2.5 per second

EEG in atypical absence seizures shows a generalized, slow spike-and-wave pattern with a frequency of <= 2.5 per second, as well as other abnormal EEG activity.

785. When compared to typical absence seizures, patients with atypical absence seizures have?
Harrison's 20th Ed. Chapter 418, Page 3052

A. Lapse of consciousness of longer duration
B. Less abrupt onset and cessation
C. Less responsive to anticonvulsants
D. All of the above

786. The most common seizure type resulting from metabolic derangements is?
Harrison's 20th Ed. Chapter 418, Page 3052

A. Absence seizures
B. Myoclonic seizures
C. Grand Mal seizures
D. Atonic seizures

Grand Mal seizures are the main seizure type in ~10% of all persons with epilepsy. They are also the most common seizure type resulting from metabolic derangements.

787. "Ictal cry" is related to tonic contraction of which of the following?
Harrison's 20th Ed. Chapter 418, Page 3052

A. Muscles of inspiration and larynx
B. Muscles of expiration and larynx
C. Muscles of inspiration and pharynx
D. Muscles of expiration and pharynx

Tonic contraction of muscles of expiration and larynx at the onset will produce a loud moan or "Ictal cry".

788. Ictal cry is observed in which phase of Grand Mal seizure?
Harrison's 20th Ed. Chapter 418, Page 3052

A. Preictal phase
B. Ictal phase
C. Postictal phase
D. Any of the above

Initial phase of Grand Mal seizure is tonic contraction of muscles throughout the body. Tonic contraction of muscles of expiration and larynx at the onset produces a loud moan or "ictal cry".

789. During tonic phase of Grand Mal seizure, which of the following does not occur?
Harrison's 20th Ed. Chapter 418, Page 3052

A. Increase in heart rate
B. Increase in blood pressure
C. Impaired respiration
D. Constriction of pupils

A marked enhancement of sympathetic tone during ictal phase of Grand Mal seizure leads to increases in heart rate, blood pressure, and pupillary size. Respiration is impaired.

790. In Grand Mal seizure, initial tonic phase evolves into clonic phase after?
Harrison's 20th Ed. Chapter 418, Page 3052

A. 10–20 seconds
B. 30–60 seconds
C. 60–120 seconds
D. 120–180 seconds

In Grand Mal seizure, initial tonic phase evolves into clonic phase after 10 - 20 seconds. Ictal phase usually lasts no more than 1 minute.

791. Postictal phase in Grand Mal seizures is characterized by all except?
Harrison's 20th Ed. Chapter 418, Page 3052

A. Irritability
B. Bladder or bowel incontinence
C. Muscular flaccidity
D. Excessive salivation

Postictal phase in Grand Mal seizures is characterized by unresponsiveness, muscular flaccidity, excessive salivation and bladder or bowel incontinence.

792. Which of the following is typical of EEG of clonic phase of Grand Mal seizure?
Harrison's 20th Ed. Chapter 418, Page 3052

A. High-amplitude activity interrupted by slow waves
B. High-amplitude activity interrupted by fast waves
C. Low-amplitude activity interrupted by slow waves
D. Low-amplitude activity interrupted by fast waves

EEG during the tonic phase of Grand Mal seizure shows a progressive increase in generalized low-voltage fast activity, followed by generalized high-amplitude, polyspike discharges. In clonic phase, high-amplitude activity is typically interrupted by slow waves to create a spike-and-slow-wave pattern.

793. Which of the following is false about atonic seizures?
Harrison's 20th Ed. Chapter 418, Page 3052

A. Sudden loss of postural muscle tone
B. Consciousness is briefly impaired
C. Significant postictal confusion
D. Seen in association with known epilepsy syndromes

Atonic seizures are characterized by sudden loss of postural muscle tone lasting 1-2 seconds. Consciousness is briefly impaired, but there is usually no postictal confusion. Atonic seizures are usually seen in association with known epilepsy syndromes.

794. Myoclonic seizure is a type of?
Harrison's 20th Ed. Chapter 418, Page 3052

A. Focal seizure
B. Generalized seizure
C. Focal, generalised or unclear seizure
D. Any of the above

795. Pathologic myoclonus is mostly seen in association with?
Harrison's 20th Ed. Chapter 418, Page 3052

A. Metabolic disorders
B. Degenerative CNS diseases
C. Anoxic brain injury
D. All of the above

Pathologic myoclonus is commonly seen with metabolic disorders, degenerative CNS diseases or anoxic brain injury.

796. Myoclonic seizures are caused by?
Harrison's 20th Ed. Chapter 418, Page 3052

A. Cortical dysfunction
B. Subcortical dysfunction
C. Spinal dysfunction
D. Any of the above

Myoclonic seizures are considered to be true epileptic events becacuse they are caused by cortical (versus subcortical or spinal) dysfunction.

797. Which of the following is false about myoclonic jerks associated with syncope?
Harrison's 20th Ed. Chapter 418, Page 128

A. May be multifocal or generalized
B. Typically arrhythmic
C. Short duration (<30 seconds)
D. None of the above

Whereas tonic-clonic movements are the hallmark of a generalized seizure, myoclonic & other movements may occur in ~90% of syncopal episodes. Myoclonic jerks associated with syncope may be multifocal or generalized. They are typically arrhythmic and of short duration (<30 seconds).

798. Which of the following is false about autonomic epilepsy?
Harrison's 20th Ed. Chapter 418, Page 128

A. Cardiovascular
B. Gastrointestinal
C. Pulmonary
D. All of the above

Autonomic manifestations of seizures (autonomic epilepsy or seizures have cardiovascular, gastrointestinal, pulmonary, urogenital, pupillary, and cutaneous manifestations that are similar to the premonitory features of syncope.

799. Which of the following differentiates seizure from syncope?
Harrison's 20th Ed. Chapter 418, Page 128

A. Seizures are rarely provoked by emotions or pain
B. Loss of consciousness in seizure is longer with postictal drowsiness & disorientation
C. Fecal incontinence occurs very rarely with syncope
D. All of the above

Loss of consciousness in seizure usually lasts >5 minutes and has postictal drowsiness & disorientation, whereas reorientation occurs almost immediately after a syncopal event. Muscle aches last longer and are more severe following a seizure. Seizures, unlike syncope, are rarely provoked by emotions or pain. Incontinence of urine may occur with seizures & syncope, but fecal incontinence occurs very rarely with syncope.

800. Tornado epilepsy best relates to?
DeJong's The Neurologic Examination, 7th Ed. Page 73

A. Sleep
B. Vertigo
C. Vision
D. Hearing

Tornado epilepsy refers to vertigo due to involvement of the vestibular cortex in a seizure discharge.

801. Giant slow waves relate best with which of the following?
Harrison's 20th Ed. Chapter 418, Page 3052

A. Atonic seizures
B. Myoclonic seizure
C. Epileptic spasms
D. Atypical absence seizures

EEG in epileptic spasms which if an unclassifiable seizure disorder shows hypsarrhythmias (diffuse, giant slow waves with a chaotic background of irregular, multifocal spikes and sharp waves).

802. "Electrodecremental response" in EEG is a feature of?
Harrison's 20th Ed. Chapter 418, Page 3052

A. Atonic seizures
B. Myoclonic seizure
C. Epileptic spasms
D. Atypical absence seizures

"Electrodecremental response" or a marked suppression of EEG background is a feature of epileptic spasms.

803. Rhomboid pattern seen in electromyogram is a feature of?
Harrison's 20th Ed. Chapter 418, Page 3052

A. Atonic seizures
B. Myoclonic seizure
C. Epileptic spasms
D. Atypical absence seizures

804. Which of the following is an epilepsy syndrome?
Harrison's 20th Ed. Chapter 418, Page 3052

A. Juvenile myoclonic epilepsy (JME)
B. Lennox-Gastaut syndrome
C. Mesial temporal lobe epilepsy (MTLE)
D. All of the above

805. Which of the following gene for various epilepsy syndromes is associated with severe mental retardation?
Harrison's 20th Ed. Chapter 418, Page 3053 Table 418-2

A. CHRNA4
B. KCNQ2
C. SCN1B
D. Doublecortin

Doublecortin (Xq21-24), expressed primarily in frontal lobes directly regulates microtubule polymerization and bundling. X-linked dominant classic lissencephaly is associated with severe mental retardation and seizures in males, subcortical band heterotopia with more subtle findings in females.

806. Gene associated with autosomal dominant nocturnal frontal lobe epilepsy (ADNFLE) is?
Harrison's 20th Ed. Chapter 418, Page 3053 Table 418-2

A. CHRNA4
B. KCNQ2
C. SCN1A
D. LGI1

807. **Gene associated with autosomal dominant partial epilepsy with auditory features (ADPEAF) is?**
Harrison's 20th Ed. Chapter 418, Page 3053 Table 418-2
   A. CHRNA4
   B. KCNQ2
   C. SCN1A
   D. LGI1

808. **Gene associated with benign familial neonatal seizures is?**
Harrison's 20th Ed. Chapter 418, Page 3053 Table 418-2
   A. CHRNA4
   B. KCNQ2
   C. SCN1A
   D. LGI1

809. **Gene associated with benign familial neonatal seizures is?**
Harrison's 20th Ed. Chapter 418, Page 3053 Table 418-2
   A. CHRNA4
   B. KCNQ2
   C. SCN1A
   D. LGI1

810. **Gene associated with autosomal dominant familial focal epilepsy with variable foci (FFEVF) is?**
Harrison's 20th Ed. Chapter 418, Page 3053 Table 418-2
   A. CSTB
   B. DEPDC5
   C. EPM2A
   D. LGI1

811. **Gene associated with Unverricht-Lundborg disease is?**
Harrison's 20th Ed. Chapter 418, Page 3053 Table 418-2
   A. CSTB
   B. DEPDC5
   C. EPM2A
   D. LGI1

812. **Seizures in Juvenile myoclonic epilepsy (JME) are most frequent in?**
Harrison's 20th Ed. Chapter 418, Page 3052, N Engl J Med. 1999;340:1565
   A. Morning
   B. Afternoon
   C. Evening
   D. Night

Syndrome of JME, also known as Janz syndrome, accounts for ~7% of all cases of epilepsy. It is characterized by onset of myoclonic seizures, generalized tonic-clonic seizures, & absence seizures in adolescents (12 - 18 years) who have normal intellectual function, with EEG findings of rapid, generalized spike-wave & polyspike-wave discharges. They are most frequent in morning after awakening and can be provoked by sleep deprivation. Consciousness is preserved.

813. **Which of the following statements about Lennox-Gastaut syndrome is true?**
Harrison's 20th Ed. Chapter 418, Page 3052
   A. Multiple seizure types
   B. EEG shows slow (<3 Hz) spike-&-wave discharges
   C. Impaired cognitive function
   D. All of the above

Triad of Lennox-Gastaut syndrome includes multiple seizure types, slow (<3 Hz) spike-and-wave discharges on EEG and impaired cognitive function.

814. **Seizure types in Lennox-Gastaut syndrome include all except?**
Harrison's 20th Ed. Chapter 418, Page 3052
   A. Generalized tonic-clonic
   B. Atonic
   C. Myoclonic
   D. Atypical absence seizures

In children with Lennox-Gastaut syndrome, multiple seizure types include generalized tonic-clonic, atonic and atypical absence seizures.

815. **Which of the following is a feature of epilepsia partialis continua?**
N Engl J Med. 2014;371:1737-46
   A. Continuous muscular clonic twitching affecting limited part of body
   B. Consciousness is preserved
   C. Involves the face, arms, or both
   D. All of the above

Epilepsia partialis continua is defined as almost continuous (at least 1 hour) regular or irregular muscular clonic twitching affecting a limited part of the body. Consciousness is typically preserved, and the twitching most commonly involves the face, arms, or both occurring at least once every 10 seconds, typically in isolation or in clusters of 1 to 2 Hz.

816. **Epilepsia Partialis Continua is seen in?**
N Engl J Med. 2014;371:1737-46
   A. Rasmussen's encephalitis
   B. Cerebral venous sinus thrombosis
   C. Hyponatremia
   D. All of the above

Differential Diagnosis of Epilepsia Partialis Continua include nonprogressive causes (Vascular causes (stroke, cerebral venous sinus thrombosis), Metabolic causes (hyperosmolar hyperglycemic nonketotic syndrome, hyponatremia), Neoplasm (central nervous system neoplasm or hematologic neoplasm), Infectious or immunologic causes (human immunodeficiency virus, encephalitis), Cortical dysplasia, Mitochondrial causes or inborn error of metabolism, Perinatal central nervous system injury, Cryptogenic causes. Progressive cause include Rasmussen's encephalitis.

817. **Which of the following about Rasmussen's encephalitis is false?**
N Engl J Med. 2014;371:1737-46
   A. Epilepsia partialis continua
   B. Hemiparesis
   C. Seizures are typically refractory to medication
   D. None of the above

Rasmussen's encephalitis, which was first described in 1958 by Dr. Theodore Rasmussen, is a progressive neurologic disease of unknown cause. Patients typically present in childhood with focal-onset seizures, which then progress over a period of months to refractory epilepsy with progressive hemiparesis. Epilepsia partialis continua develops in approximately 50 to 90% of persons with Rasmussen's encephalitis, and fixed hemiparesis typically occurs within 2 to 3 years after the onset of seizures. Seizures are typically refractory to medication, as was the case with this patient, but glucocorticoids and intravenous immune globulin can be effective in controlling seizures. Various other immunosuppressive medications have been tried, but the most effective therapy remains hemispherectomy.

818. **Most common syndrome associated with focal seizures with dyscognitive features is?**
Harrison's 20th Ed. Chapter 418, Page 3053
   A. Mesial temporal lobe epilepsy (MTLE)
   B. Lennox-Gastaut syndrome
   C. Juvenile myoclonic epilepsy (JME)
   D. All of the above

Mesial temporal lobe epilepsy (MTLE) is the most common syndrome associated with focal seizures with dyscognitive features. Formerly it was known as "psychomotor epilepsy" (Gibbs et al, 1940).

819. In mesial temporal lobe epilepsy (MTLE), the characteristic MRI finding is?
Harrison's 20th Ed. Chapter 418, Page 3053

A. Hippocampal calcification
B. Hippocampal sclerosis
C. Increased signal intensity in fronto-temporal region
D. Normal MRI

On high-resolution MRI, characteristic & essential finding of MTLE is hippocampal sclerosis.

820. In mesial temporal lobe epilepsy (MTLE), the MRI finding in-include all except?
Harrison's 20th Ed. Chapter 418, Page 3054 Table 418-3

A. Small hippocampus
B. Small temporal lobe
C. Small temporal horn
D. Hippocampal sclerosis

MRI findings in Mesial Temporal Lobe Epilepsy Syndrome include small hippocampus, small temporal lobe, enlarged temporal horn and hippocampal sclerosis.

821. Which of the following is an MRI finding of hippocampal sclerosis?
Harrison's 20th Ed. Chapter 418, Page 3054 Table 418-1

A. Abnormal high signal intensity
B. Blurring of internal laminar architecture
C. Reduced size of hippocampus
D. All of the above

This triad of imaging findings is consistent with hippocampal sclerosis includes abnormal high signal intensity, blurring of internal laminar architecture and reduced size of hippocampus.

822. Word Hippocampus best relates to?
American Journal of Roentgenology. 1998;171:1139-46

A. Hippopotamus
B. Seahorse
C. Hippocrates
D. Snail

Hippocampus means "Seahorse".

823. Which of the following is a part of hippocampus?
American Journal of Roentgenology. 1998;171:1139-46

A. Subiculum
B. Ammon's horn
C. Dentate gyrus
D. All of the above

824. Which of the following is a part of Ammon's horn?
American Journal of Roentgenology. 1998;171:1139-46

A. CA1
B. CA2
C. CA3
D. All of the above

Hippocampus consists of 3 major regions: subiculum, hippocampus proper (Ammon's horn) & dentate gyrus. Hippocampus & dentate gyrus have a three layered cortex. Subiculum is the transition zone from the three to six layered cortex. Important regions of hippocampus proper include CA1, CA2, CA3.

825. Intracranial amobarbital or Wada test is performed for?
Harrison's 20th Ed. Chapter 418, Page 3054 Table 418-3

A. Circulation adequacy of cerebral hemispheres
B. IQ level
C. Cerebral functions are localized to which hemisphere
D. Sleep pattern

Named after Canadian neurologist Juhn A. Wada (University of British Columbia), this test is used to establish which cerebral functions are localized to which hemisphere. It is also known as the "intracarotid sodium amobarbital procedure" (ISAP) and is performed prior to ablative surgery for epilepsy and prior to tumor resection. The aim is to determine which side of the brain is responsible for certain vital cognitive functions, namely speech and memory. Sodium amobarbital is injected into one cerebral hemisphere at a time. Material-specific memory deficits on intracranial amobarbital (Wada) test is a feature of MTLE.

826. Which of the following is an idiopathic epilepsy associated with identified gene mutations?
Harrison's 20th Ed. Chapter 418, Page 3054 Table 418-2

A. Generalized epilepsy with febrile seizures plus (GEFS+)
B. Benign familial neonatal convulsions (BFNC)
C. Autosomal dominant partial epilepsy with auditory features
D. All of the above

ADNFLE, BFNC, GEFS+, ADPEAF and FFEVF are idiopathic epilepsies associated with identified gene mutations.

827. Which of the following about Generalized epilepsy with febrile seizures plus (GEFS+) is false?
Harrison's 20th Ed. Chapter 418, Page 3054 Table 418-2

A. Autosomal dominant inheritance
B. Presents with febrile seizures
C. May have variable seizure types not associated with fever
D. Autosomal recessive inheritance

"Generalized epilepsy with febrile seizures plus" is a genetic syndrome consisting of febrile seizures plus at least one other type of seizure (absence, myoclonic, atonic, or afebrile generalized tonic–clonic seizures). It has autosomal dominant inheritance.

828. Dravet's syndrome best relates to which of the following?
Harrison's 20th Ed. Chapter 418, Page 3054 Table 418-2

A. Myoclonic epilepsies due to storage diseases
B. Severe myoclonic epilepsy in infancy
C. Febrile convulsions
D. Early cryptogenic focal epilepsy

829. Which of the following gene is associated with Generalized epilepsy with febrile seizures plus (GEFS+)?
Harrison's 20th Ed. Chapter 418, Page 3054 Table 418-2

A. CHRNA4
B. SCN1A
C. KCNQ2
D. LGI1

In Generalized epilepsy with febrile seizures plus (GEFS+), mutation occurs in the SCN1A gene for the voltage-gated sodium channel which modifies gating and inactivation properties of the channel. Mutations in other sodium channel subunits (SCN2A) and GABAA receptor subunit (GABRG2 and GABRA1) have been reported.

830. Which of the following about benign familial neonatal convulsions (BFNC) is false?
Harrison's 20th Ed. Chapter 418, Page 3054 Table 418-2

A. Autosomal dominant inheritance
B. Onset in first week of life
C. Mutations in KCNQ2 (20q13.3)
D. None of the above

BFNC has autosomal dominant inheritance with onset in 1st week of life. Infants are normal with no neurologic or metabolic abnormality. Mutations have been identified in KCNQ2, gene for potassium channels on chromosomes 20q.

831. Gene responsible for progressive myoclonus epilepsy (PME) or Unverricht-Lundborg disease is?
Harrison's 20th Ed. Chapter 418, Page 3054 Table 418-2

A. LGI1
B. EPM2A
C. CSTB
D. SCN1B

Progressive myoclonus epilepsy (PME) (Unverricht-Lundborg disease) has autosomal recessive inheritance with age of onset between 6-15 years presenting as myoclonic seizures, ataxia and progressive cognitive decline. CSTB mutation causes PME.

832. Gene responsible for Autosomal dominant familial focal epilepsy with variable foci (FFEVF) is?
Harrison's 20th Ed. Chapter 418, Page 3054 Table 418-2

A. LGI1
B. EPM2A
C. CSTB
D. DEPDC5

833. Which of the following is false about progressive myoclonus epilepsy (Lafora's disease)?
Harrison's 20th Ed. Chapter 418, Page 3054 Table 418-2

A. Autosomal recessive inheritance
B. Age of onset - 6 to 19 years
C. Polyglucosan intracellular inclusion bodies
D. Gene mution in SCN1B

Gene mution occurs in EPM2A (6q24). The protein tyrosine phosphatase (PTP) - Laforin influences glycogen metabolism.

834. Gene responsible for autosomal dominant nocturnal frontal lobe epilepsy (ADNFLE) is?
Harrison's 20th Ed. Chapter 418, Page 3054 Table 418-2

A. CHRNA4
B. EPM2A
C. CSTB
D. SCN1B

Autosomal dominant nocturnal frontal lobe epilepsy (ADNFLE) occurs during childhood & presents as brief, nighttime seizures with prominent motor movements. Gene responsible is CHRNA4 (20q13.2).

835. Which of the following about autosomal dominant partial epilepsy with auditory features (ADPEAF) is false?
Harrison's 20th Ed. Chapter 418, Page 3054 Table 418-2

A. Type of idiopathic lateral temporal lobe epilepsy
B. Age of onset usually between 10 and 25 years
C. Gene mutation in LGI1 (10q24)
D. None of the above

836. Episodic dyscontrol syndrome is also called?
Archives of Disease in Childhood 2010;95:841-842

A. Rage attacks
B. Time attacks
C. Ground attacks
D. Wall attacks

837. West syndrome includes?
DeJong's The Neurologic Examination, 7th Ed. Page 504, Lancet 1841;1:724-725

A. Infantile spasms
B. Mental retardation
C. Hypsarrhythmic EEG
D. All of the above

West syndrome is a triad of infantile spasms, mental retardation & hypsarrhythmic EEG pattern (electroclinical epileptic syndrome). The syndrome is called 'West syndrome' after Dr. West, who first described the condition in his 4-month-old son in 1841. This type of epilepsy occurs in about one in 2,500-3,000 children.

838. Characteristics of Landau-Kleffner syndrome include?
Neurology 1957;7:523-530

A. Auditory agnosia or "word deafness"
B. Normal hearing
C. Abnormal electrical brain activity
D. All of the above

A childhood disorder, in LKS there occurs gradual or sudden loss of ability to understand and use spoken language (auditory agnosia or "word deafness"). All children with LKS have abnormal EEG and may have epileptic seizures usually at night. Hearing tests show normal hearing.

839. Which of the following factor is important in the genesis of seizures and epilepsy?
Harrison's 20th Ed. Chapter 418, Page 3054

A. Endogenous factors
B. Epileptogenic factors
C. Precipitating factors
D. All of the above

Seizures & epilepsy result from a dynamic interplay between endogenous factors, epileptogenic factors and precipitating factors.

840. Which of the following schistosomes causes Jacksonian epilepsy?
Harrison's 20th Ed. Chapter 216, Page 1639

A. S. japonicum
B. S. mansoni
C. S. haematobium
D. S. mekongi

S. japonicum is associated with granulomatous lesions in brain, causing epileptic seizures, encephalopathy with headache, visual impairment, motor deficit & ataxia.

841. Which of the following schistosomes is associated with transverse myelitis?
Harrison's 20th Ed. Chapter 216, Page 1552

A. S. japonicum
B. S. intercalatum
C. S. haematobium
D. S. mekongi

842. Which of the following schistosomes is associated with transverse myelitis?
Harrison's 20th Ed. Chapter 216, Page 1552

A. S. japonicum
B. S. mansoni
C. S. intercalatum
D. S. mekongi

843. Which of the following schistosomes presents with urinary manifestations?
Harrison's 20th Ed. Chapter 216, Page 1552

A. S. japonicum
B. S. haematobium
C. S. intercalatum
D. S. mekongi

CNS schistosomiasis presents as Jacksonian epilepsy due to S. japonicum infection. S. mansoni & S. haematobium infections have been associated with transverse myelitis. S. haematobium infection leads to dysuria, frequency and hematuria.

844. Which of the following is false about seizures due to inborn errors of metabolism?
Harrison's 20th Ed. Chapter 418, Page 3054

A. Occur once regular feeding begins
B. Occur typically 2 - 3 days after birth
C. Idiosyncratic side effect to Valproic acid common
D. None of the above

Seizures due to inborn errors of metabolism usually present once regular feeding begins, typically 2-3 days after birth.

845. Pyridoxine deficiency causes seizures during?
Harrison's 20th Ed. Chapter 418, Page 3054

A. Neonatal period (<1 month)
B. Infants and children (>1 month and <12 years)
C. Adolescents (12–18 years)
D. Young adults (18–35 years)

Pyridoxine (vitamin B6) deficiency is an important cause of neonatal seizures.

846. Febrile seizures have a peak incidence between?
Harrison's 20th Ed. Chapter 418, Page 3054

A. 1 and 3 months
B. 3 and 9 months
C. 9 and 18 months
D. 18 and 24 months

Febrile seizures usually occur between 3 months and 5 years of age and have a peak incidence between 18 and 24 months.

847. Febrile seizure is likely to occur during?
Harrison's 20th Ed. Chapter 418, Page 3054

A. Rising phase of temperature curve
B. Peak of temperature curve
C. Declining phase of temperature curve
D. Any of the above

Febrile seizure is likely to occur during rising phase of the temperature curve i.e. during 1st day.

848. Which of the following is false about simple febrile seizure?
Harrison's 20th Ed. Chapter 418, Page 3054

A. Single, isolated event
B. Brief in duration
C. Symmetric in appearance
D. None of the above

A simple febrile seizure is a single, isolated event, brief in duration and symmetric in appearance. Simple febrile seizures are not associated with an increase in risk of developing epilepsy subsequently.

849. Which of the following is false about complex febrile seizures?
Harrison's 20th Ed. Chapter 418, Page 3054

A. Duration > 15 minutes
B. Repeated seizure activity
C. Not associated with increased risk of developing epilepsy
D. Focal features

Complex febrile seizures are characterized by repeated seizure activity, duration >15 minutes, or by focal features. Recurrences are more likely when febrile seizure occurs in first year of life. Complex febrile seizures have a risk of 2–5% of developing epilepsy subsequently.

850. Mild head injury is defined as a concussion with amnesia or loss of consciousness of?
Harrison's 20th Ed. Chapter 418, Page 3055

A. < 30 minutes
B. < 45 minutes
C. < 60 minutes
D. < 90 minutes

Mild head injury is defined as a concussion with amnesia or loss of consciousness of <30 minutes.

851. Primary epilepsy syndromes present during which of the following age groups?
Harrison's 20th Ed. Chapter 418, Page 3055 Table 418-4

A. Neonatal period (<1 month)
B. Infants and children (>1 month and <12 years)
C. Adolescents (12–18 years)
D. Young adults (18–35 years)

852. Seizure disorder due to brain tumor is seen in which of the following age groups?
Harrison's 20th Ed. Chapter 418, Page 3055 Table 418-4

A. Adolescents (12–18 years)
B. Young adults (18–35 years)
C. Older adults (> 35 years)
D. All of the above

853. Hypocalcemia or hypomagnesemia are a cause of seizure disorder in which of the following age groups?
Harrison's 20th Ed. Chapter 418, Page 3055 Table 418-4

A. Neonatal period (<1 month)
B. Infants and children (>1 month and <12 years)
C. Adolescents (12–18 years)
D. Young adults (18–35 years)

854. Which of the following anti-tubercular drug cause epilepsy?
Harrison's 20th Ed. Chapter 418, Page 3056 Table 418-5

A. Isoniazid
B. Rifampin
C. Pyrazinamide
D. Ethambutol

855. Which of the following analgesics can cause epilepsy?
Harrison's 20th Ed. Chapter 418, Page 3056 Table 418-5

A. Aspirin
B. Diclofenac sodium
C. Tramadol
D. Nimusilide

856. Which of the following antimicrobial/antiviral can cause epilepsy?
Harrison's 20th Ed. Chapter 418, Page 3056 Table 418-5

A. Quinolones
B. Acyclovir
C. Ganciclovir
D. All of the above

857. Which of the following antimalarials can cause seizure?
Harrison's 20th Ed. Chapter 418, Page 3056 Table 418-5

A. Mefloquine
B. Quinine
C. Artemether
D. Halofantrine

Antimalarials - chloroquine and mefloquine can cause seizure.

858. Acute seizure in older adults is mostly due to?
Harrison's 20th Ed. Chapter 418, Page 3055

A. Embolic stroke
B. Hemorrhagic stroke
C. Thrombotic stroke
D. All of the above

Acute seizures occurring at the time of stroke are seen more often with embolic rather than hemorrhagic or thrombotic stroke. Chronic seizures are associated with all forms of stroke.

859. Diseases due to ion-channel mutations "channelopathies" include?
N Engl J Med. 2003;349:1257-66

A. Episodic ataxia
B. Familial hemiplegic migraine
C. Long-QT syndrome
D. All of the above

Ion-channel mutations "channelopathies" are characterized by paroxysmal episodes of neurologic or cardiac dysfunction, include episodic ataxia, periodic paralysis, familial hemiplegic migraine, and the long-QT syndrome.

860. The initial bursting activity in seizure is caused by?
Harrison's 20th Ed. Chapter 418, Page 3055

A. Influx of extracellular calcium (Ca^{2+})
B. Opening of voltage-dependent sodium (Na^+) channels
C. Gamma-aminobutyric acid (GABA) receptors
D. All of the above

861. Hyperpolarizing after potential during seizure is mediated by?
Harrison's 20th Ed. Chapter 418, Page 3055

A. Influx of extracellular calcium (Ca^{2+})
B. Opening of voltage-dependent sodium (Na^+) channels
C. Gamma-aminobutyric acid (GABA) receptors
D. All of the above

The initiation phase of focal seizure activity is characterized by two concurrent events in an aggregate of neurons: (1) high-frequency bursts of action potentials and (2) hypersynchronization. The bursting activity is caused by a relatively long-lasting depolarization of the neuronal membrane due to influx of extracellular calcium (Ca^{2+}), which leads to the opening of voltage-dependent sodium (Na^+) channels, influx of Na^+, and generation of repetitive action potentials. This is followed by a hyperpolarizing after potential mediated by gamma-aminobutyric acid (GABA) receptors or potassium (K^+) channels, depending on cell type.

862. Which of the following is a co-agonist of glutamate at the NMDA receptor?
Harrison's 20th Ed. Chapter 418, Page 3055

A. Tyrosine
B. Glycine
C. L-tryptophan
D. Arginine

Glycine is a co-agonist of glutamate at the (N-methyl D-aspartate) NMDA receptor. NMDA glutaminergic receptors are excitatory.

863. Which of the following is an analogue of glutamate?
Harrison's 20th Ed. Chapter 418, Page 3056

A. Glunamic acid
B. Tranaxemic acid
C. Tritoin acid
D. Domoic acid

Domoic acid is an analogue of glutamate (principal excitatory neurotransmitter in brain), causes profound seizures via direct activation of excitatory amino acid receptors throughout CNS.

864. Which of the following about gamma-aminobutyric acid (GABA) is false?
Harrison's 20th Ed. Chapter 418, Page 3056

A. GABA is an inhibitory neurotransmitter in adult CNS
B. $GABA_A$ receptors are located postsynaptically
C. $GABA_B$ receptors are located presynaptically
D. None of the above

865. Which of the following is a precipitant of epilepsy?
Harrison's 20th Ed. Chapter 418, Page 3056

A. Psychological or physical stress
B. Sleep deprivation
C. Hormonal changes with menstrual cycle
D. All of the above

Precipitating factors of epilepsy include sleep deprivation, fever, hypoxia, systemic diseases, electrolyte or metabolic derangements, acute infection, drugs that lower the seizure threshold, or alcohol or illicit drug use/withdrawal.

866. Pronator drift is an indicator of?
Harrison's 20th Ed. Chapter 418, Page 3027

A. Lower motor neuron weakness
B. Upper motor neuron weakness
C. Muscle wasting
D. Sensory neuropathy

Pronator drift is a pathologic sign and indicates UMN type weakness. Person is asked to extend arms by 90 degrees, supinate forearms, close eyes and hold the position. If a forearm pronates then the person is said to have pronator drift on that side.

867. Antiepileptic drug that acts by potentiation of GABA receptor function is?
Harrison's 20th Ed. Chapter 418, Page 3057

A. Phenytoin
B. Lamotrigine
C. Benzodiazepine
D. Valproic acid

868. Antiepileptic drug that acts by increasing the availability of GABA is?
Harrison's 20th Ed. Chapter 418, Page 3057

A. Phenytoin
B. Lamotrigine
C. Benzodiazepine
D. Valproic acid

869. Antiepileptic drug that acts by increasing the availability of GABA is?
Harrison's 20th Ed. Chapter 418, Page 3057

A. Tiagabine
B. Valproic acid
C. Gabapentin
D. All of the above

870. Antiepileptic drug that acts by decreasing glutamate release is?
Harrison's 20th Ed. Chapter 418, Page 3057

A. Phenytoin
B. Lamotrigine
C. Benzodiazepine
D. Valproic acid

871. Antiepileptic drug that acts by inhibiting voltage-gated Ca++ channels is?
Harrison's 20th Ed. Chapter 418, Page 3057

A. Phenytoin
B. Lamotrigine
C. Benzodiazepine
D. Valproic acid

Antiepileptic drugs that act by inhibiting Na+ dependent action potentials are phenytoin, carbamazepine, lamotrigine, topiramate, zonisamide, lacosamide & rufinamide. One that acts by inhibiting voltage-gated Ca++ channels are phenytoin, gabapentin & pregabalin while lamotrigine, topiramate & felbamate act by decreasing glutamate release. Ezogabine acts by facilitating opening of potassium channels. Benzodiazepines & barbiturates potentiate GABA receptor function, while valproic acid, gabapentin & tiagabine increase availability of GABA. Ethosuximide & valproic acid act by inhibiting T-type Ca++ channels in thalamic neurons.

872. Which of the following is a glutamate receptor?
Front. Mol. Neurosci. 2018;11:217

A. AMPA
B. Kainate (Ka)
C. NMDA
D. All of the above

Major excitatory neurotransmitter is amino acid glutamate. Glutamate receptors are postsynaptic. Ionotropic subclasses are alpha-amino-2,3-dihydro-5-methyl-3-oxo-4-isoxazolepropanoic acid (AMPA), kainate receptors (Ka) & N-methyl-D-aspartate (NMDA). These allow ion influx upon activation by glutamate.

873. Antagonists to which of the following glutamate receptor suppresses seizure activity?
Front. Mol. Neurosci. 2018;11:217

A. AMPA
B. Kainate (Ka)
C. NMDA
D. All of the above

NMDA, AMPA & kainate agonists induce seizure activity, whereas their antagonists suppress seizure activity.

874. Which of the following is a $GABA_B$ agonist?
Front. Mol. Neurosci. 2018;11:217

A. Baclofen
B. Barbiturate
C. Benzodiazepine
D. All of the above

$GABA_A$ receptor agonists are barbiturates and benzodiazepines. They suppress seizure activity. $GABA_B$ receptors agonist is baclofen and exacerbates hyperexcitability and seizures.

875. In an individual known to have epilepsy, initial routine interictal EEG may be normal up to what percentage of time?
Harrison's 20th Ed. Chapter 418, Page 3059

A. 10%
B. 30%
C. 60%
D. 75%

In an individual known to have epilepsy, the initial routine interictal EEG may be normal up to 60% of the time.

876. Which of the following investigation can be useful to localize potential seizure foci?
Harrison's 20th Ed. Chapter 418, Page 3059

A. EEG
B. Magnetoencephalography (MEG)
C. Magnetic source image (MSI)
D. MRI

Magnetic source image (MSI) can be useful to localize potential seizure foci.

877. Which of the following about EEG is false?
Harrison's 20th Ed. Chapter 418, Page 3059

A. Presence of epileptiform activity is not specific for epilepsy
B. In epileptic, initial interictal EEG is normal in ~ 60%
C. A normal EEG implies a better prognosis
D. None of the above

878. Which of the following is useful in the evaluation of a patient with epilepsy?
Harrison's 20th Ed. Chapter 418, Page 3059

A. FLAIR
B. SPECT
C. PET
D. All of the above

FLAIR has increased sensitivity for detection of abnormalities of cortical architecture. Positron emission tomography (PET) & single photon emission computed tomography (SPECT) are used to evaluate patients with medically refractory seizures.

879. FLAIR stands for?
Harrison's 20th Ed. Chapter 418, Page 3059

A. Fluid-attenuated inversion radiation
B. Fluid-augmented inversion radiography
C. Fluid-attenuated inversion radiography
D. Fluid-attenuated inversion recovery

880. Estimation of which of the following helps to distinguish between organic and psychogenic seizures?
Harrison's 20th Ed. Chapter 418, Page 3061

A. Serum insulin levels
B. Serum growth hormone levels
C. Serum prolactin levels
D. Serum vasopressin levels

Most generalized seizures and some focal seizures are accompanied by rises in serum prolactin during the immediate 30 minute postictal period, whereas psychogenic seizures are not. Peripheral WBC count also increase significantly after a generalized seizure.

881. "Reflex epilepsy" best relates to?
Harrison's 20th Ed. Chapter 418, Page 3061

A. Alcohol intake
B. Sleep deprivation
C. Specific music or an individual's voice
D. Physical exertion

Seizures that are induced by highly specific stimuli such as a video game monitor, music, or an individual's voice are categorized as "reflex epilepsy".

882. Risk factors associated with recurrent seizures include?
Harrison's 20th Ed. Chapter 418, Page 3061

A. Abnormal neurologic examination
B. Seizures presenting as status epilepticus
C. Abnormal EEG
D. All of the above

Risk factors associated with recurrent seizures include an abnormal neurologic examination, seizures presenting as status epilepticus, postictal Todd's paralysis, strong family history of seizures, an abnormal EEG.

883. In EEG, rhythmic activity of vertically oriented pyramidal cells of cerebral cortex normally recorded represents?
Harrison's 20th Ed. Chapter 418, Page 3057

A. Presynaptic potentials
B. Postsynaptic potentials
C. Difference of Pre- and Postsynaptic potentials
D. None of the above

The rhythmic activity normally recorded represents the postsynaptic potentials of vertically oriented pyramidal cells of the cerebral cortex and is characterized by its frequency..

884. In EEG, which of the following rhythm is faster than alpha rhythm?
Harrison's 20th Ed. Chapter 418, Page 3057

A. Beta
B. Theta
C. Delta
D. All of the above

EEG waveforms are divided into four major frequency bands: delta (0–3⁺ Hz), theta (4–7⁺ Hz), alpha (8–13 Hz), and beta (>14 Hz). They are named in Greek order of historical discovery rather than low to high frequency numbers Muscle artifact is high amplitude irregular activity, usually in the frequency range of about 20–50 Hz.

885. Out of the following, which is the slowest frequency in EEG?
Harrison's 20th Ed. Chapter 418, Page 3057

A. Alpha
B. Beta
C. Theta
D. Delta

886. "Posterior dominant rhythm" is also called?
Harrison's 20th Ed. Chapter 418, Page 3057

A. Alpha rhythm
B. Beta rhythm
C. Theta rhythm
D. Delta rhythm

A symmetrical rhythm is observed over the posterior head regions during relaxed wakefulness with eyes closed, that undergoes amplitude attenuation with eye opening or mental alerting activities. It is called the posterior dominant rhythm or alpha rhythm, as in adults it has a frequency of 8–13 Hz. Alpha rhythm is also called Berger rhythm.

887. Which rhythm produces an underlying undulation of EEG?
Harrison's 20th Ed. Chapter 418, Page 3057

A. Alpha rhythm
B. Beta rhythm
C. Theta rhythm
D. Delta rhythm

Delta activity produces an underlying undulation of EEG. Riding on top of delta activity may be frequencies in the other bands, such as components of alpha & high frequency "jittery" activity in the beta range.

888. In EEG, calibration marker shows what level of voltage as standard?
Britton JW. American Epilepsy Society; 2016

A. 1 microvolt
B. 10 microvolt
C. 100 microvolt
D. 1000 microvolt

Each EEG channel is a record of voltage over time. The calibration marker shows one second and 100-microvolt standards.

889. Normal EEG background voltages are in the range of?
Britton JW. American Epilepsy Society; 2016

A. 10–20 microvolts
B. 20–50 microvolts
C. 30–100 microvolts
D. 40–150 microvolts

Normal EEG background voltages are in the range of 30–100 microvolts.

890. Which of the following about alpha rhythm is false?
Britton JW. American Epilepsy Society; 2016

A. Most prominent when subject is quietly relaxed with eyes closed, but not asleep
B. Waxing and waning
C. Higher on right side of the brain
D. None of the above

Alpha rhythm is 8 and 12 Hz, waxing and waning, with a posterior maximum, (parieto-occipital). It can spread into any electrodes of 10–20 system except Fp1 & Fp2. It is most prominent when subject is quietly relaxed with eyes closed, but not asleep. Alpha rhythm usually is higher on right side of brain.

891. Which of the following medication increase β activity in EEG?
Britton JW. American Epilepsy Society; 2016

A. Barbiturates
B. Benzodiazepines
C. Chloral hydrate
D. All of the above

Beta activity is a fast rhythm of 13 per second and greater, is visualized on the EEG as a "jitteriness" of the trace. Barbiturates, benzodiazepines and chloral hydrate increase beta activity.

892. In EEG, which of the following signifies an encephalopathy?
Britton JW. American Epilepsy Society; 2016

A. Localized slow frequency
B. Localized fast frequency
C. Diffuse slow frequency
D. Diffuse fast frequency

Alterations of brain function results in abnormal slow frequency activity in EEG. Diffuse slow activity signifies an encephalopathy.

893. In EEG, which of the following suggest epileptiform activity?
Britton JW. American Epilepsy Society; 2016

A. Spikes
B. Sharp waves
C. Spike-wave complexes
D. Any of the above

Epileptiform activity characteristic of epilepsy includes spikes, sharp waves and spike-wave complexes.

894. Each EEG electrode can detect synchronous activity generated by how much area of surface cerebral cortex?
Britton JW. American Epilepsy Society; 2016

A. ~ 3 sq. cm.
B. ~ 6 sq. cm.
C. ~ 9 sq. cm.
D. ~ 12 sq. cm.

Each EEG electrode can detect synchronous activity generated by ~ 6 sq. cm. of cortex.

895. Usually, EEG is performed after how many hours after a seizure episode?
N Engl J Med. 2001;344:1146

A. 6 hours
B. 12 hours
C. 24 hours
D. 48 hours

896. EEG should include recordings during?
N Engl J Med. 2001;344:1146

A. Sleep
B. Photic stimulation
C. Hyperventilation
D. All of the above

It is customary to perform EEG 48 hours or more after a suspected seizure, because EEG shortly after a seizure may give misleading findings. To provoke abnormalities, EEG should be recorded during sleep, sleep deprivation, photic stimulation, and hyperventilation (Activating procedures).

897. Electrocerebral silence is observed in?
Britton JW. American Epilepsy Society; 2016

A. Irreversible brain damage
B. Hypothermia
C. Drug overdose
D. All of the above

In electrocerebral silence, there is a reduction in amplitude of EEG until activity cannot be detected. It happens in irreversible brain damage, hypothermic patients or with drug overdose.

898. In visual evoked potentials (VEPs), the component of major clinical importance is?
J Neurol Neurosurg Psychiatry 2005;76(Suppl II):ii16–ii22

A. P100 response
B. P200 response
C. P300 response
D. P400 response

Visual evoked potentials (VEPs) are elicited by monocular stimulation with a reversing checkerboard pattern and are recorded from the occipital region in the midline and on either side of scalp. The component of major clinical importance is P100 response, a positive peak having a latency of approximately 100 ms.

899. VEPs are most useful in detecting dysfunction of visual pathways at the level?
J Neurol Neurosurg Psychiatry 2005;76(Suppl II):ii16–ii22

A. Anterior to optic chiasm
B. Optic chiasm
C. Optic radiation
D. Visual cortex

VEPs are most useful in detecting dysfunction of the visual pathways anterior to the optic chiasm. In acute severe optic neuritis, P100 is frequently lost or grossly attenuated and as clinical recovery occurs and visual acuity improves, P100 is restored. VEP findings are helpful in indicating previous or subclinical optic neuritis. In cortical blindness, VEPs may be normal. Multifocal VEP is likely to be more sensitive than routine VEP.

900. Which of the following statements is false about EEG?
Britton JW. American Epilepsy Society; 2016

A. Normal EEG shows posteriorly situated 8-13 Hz a rhythm
B. Alpha rhythm attenuates with eye opening
C. Right-sided placements are indicated by even numbers, left-sided placements by odd numbers
D. Midline placements are indicated by M

Right-sided electrode placements are indicated by even numbers, left-sided placements by odd numbers, and midline placements by Z.

901. Delta activity in EEG is seen in which stage of Hepatic Encephalopathy?
Harrison's 20th Ed. Chapter 300, Page 2073

A. Stage I
B. Stage II
C. Stage III
D. Stage IV

Hepatic encephalopathy is associated with triphasic or δ waves.

902. In EEG, periodic lateralized epileptiform discharges (PLEDs) is typical of?
Britton JW. American Epilepsy Society; 2016

A. Subacute sclerosing panencephalitis (SSPE)
B. Herpes simplex encephalitis
C. Jakob-Creutzfeldt disease
D. Hepatic encephalopathy

In EEG, periodic lateralized epileptiform discharges (PLEDs) is typical of herpes simplex encephalitis.

903. The specific order of electrode pairs is called?
Britton JW. American Epilepsy Society; 2016

A. Montage
B. Prelage
C. Consure
D. Primark

The specific order of electrode pairs is called a montage.

904. Which of the following statements about therapeutic range of antiepileptic drugs is false?
Harrison's 20th Ed. Chapter 418, Page 3061 Table 418-8

A. Carbamazepine   15 - 20 µg/ml
B. Valproic acid   50 - 100 µg/ml
C. Phenytoin   10 - 20 µg/ml
D. Phenobarbital   15 - 40 µg/ml

Therapeutic range of Carbamazepine is 4–10 µg/ml. Ethosuximide 40–100 µg/ml, Primidone 5–12 µg/ml, Lamotrigine 3–14 µg/ml, Levetiracetam 5–30 µg/ml, Gabapentin 2–20 µg/ml.

905. Which of the following is the first-line medication in focal seizures?
Harrison's 20th Ed. Chapter 418, Page 3061 Table 418-8

A. Valproic acid
B. Lamotrigine
C. Topiramate
D. Ethosuximide

906. **Which of the following is the first-line medication in typical absence seizures?**
   Harrison's 20th Ed. Chapter 418, Page 3061 Table 418-8
   A. Valproic acid
   B. Levetiracetam
   C. Carbamazepine
   D. Phenytoin

907. **Which of the following is the first-line medication in atypical absence seizures?**
   Harrison's 20th Ed. Chapter 418, Page 3061 Table 418-8
   A. Valproic acid
   B. Phenytoin
   C. Carbamazepine
   D. Ethosuximide

908. **Which of the following is the first-line medication in myoclonic seizures?**
   Harrison's 20th Ed. Chapter 418, Page 3061 Table 418-8
   A. Valproic acid
   B. Phenytoin
   C. Carbamazepine
   D. Ethosuximide

909. **Which of the following is not a first-line medication in seizures?**
   Harrison's 20th Ed. Chapter 418, Page 3061 Table 418-8
   A. Valproic acid
   B. Lamotrigine
   C. Carbamazepine
   D. Gabapentin

910. **Which of the following anti-epileptic drugs is preferred in Lennox-Gastaut syndrome?**
   Harrison's 20th Ed. Chapter 418, Page 3062 Table 418-9
   A. Phenobarbital
   B. Valproic acid
   C. Gabapentin
   D. Lamotrigine

Anti-epileptic drugs useful in Lennox-Gastaut syndrome include Lamotrigine, Topiramate, Felbamate, Rufinamide. Corpus callosotomy has been shown to be effective for disabling tonic or atonic seizures, usually when they are part of a mixed-seizure syndrome (e.g., Lennox-Gastaut syndrome).

911. **Which of the following anti-epileptic drugs does not have significant drug interactions?**
   Harrison's 20th Ed. Chapter 418, Page 3062 Table 418-9
   A. Phenobarbital
   B. Valproic acid
   C. Gabapentin
   D. Lamotrigine

912. **Which of the following anti-epileptic medications have enzyme-inducing effects?**
   Harrison's 20th Ed. Chapter 418, Page 3062 Table 418-9
   A. Phenytoin
   B. Phenobarbital
   C. Primidone
   D. All of the above

Enzyme-inducing anti-epileptic drugs (phenytoin, carbamazepine, oxcarbazepine, topiramate, phenobarbital, and primidone) cause a transient and reversible deficiency of vitamin K–dependent clotting factors in about 50% of newborn infants.

913. **Carbamazepine and phenytoin are contraindicated in which of the following epilepsies?**
   N Engl J Med. 1999;340:1565
   A. Juvenile myoclonic epilepsy (JME)
   B. Absence seizures
   C. Myoclonic seizures
   D. All of the above

Carbamazepine, oxcarbazepine, and phenytoin can worsen certain types of generalized seizures, including absence, myoclonic, tonic, and atonic seizures.

914. **Which of the following is an adverse effect of carbamazepine?**
   Harrison's 20th Ed. Chapter 418, Page 3062 Table 418-9
   A. Leukopenia
   B. Aplastic anemia
   C. Hepatotoxicity
   D. All of the above

Carbamazepine can cause leukopenia, aplastic anemia, or hepatotoxicity

915. **Treatment of choice for juvenile myoclonic epilepsy is?**
   N Engl J Med. 1999;340:1565
   A. Valproic acid
   B. Lamotrigine
   C. Acetazolamide
   D. Topiramate

Valproic acid is the treatment of choice for juvenile myoclonic epilepsy, but lamotrigine, clonazepam, acetazolamide, primidone & topiramate are useful.

916. **Which of the following anti-epileptic medications rarely cause skin rashes?**
   Harrison's 20th Ed. Chapter 418, Page 3062 Table 418-9
   A. Gabapentin
   B. Divalproex sodium
   C. Levetiracetam
   D. All of the above

917. **Which of the following anti-epileptic drug causes skin rashes?**
   Harrison's 20th Ed. Chapter 418, Page 3062 Table 418-9
   A. Gabapentin
   B. Divalproex sodium
   C. Levetiracetam
   D. Lamotrigine

Lamotrigine causes skin rash during initiation of therapy. This can be extremely severe and lead to Stevens-Johnson syndrome if unrecognized and if the medication is not discontinued immediately.

918. **What percentage of patients with epilepsy do not respond to treatment with a single antiepileptic drug?**
   Harrison's 20th Ed. Chapter 418, Page 3065
   A. ~ one-fourth
   B. ~ one-third
   C. ~ one-half
   D. ~ two-third

About one-third of epileptic patients do not respond to treatment with a single antiepileptic drug.

919. Most recurrences of epilepsy occur how many months after discontinuing therapy?
Harrison's 20th Ed. Chapter 418, Page 3065

A. 3 months
B. 4 months
C. 5 months
D. 6 months

Most recurrences occur in the first 3 months after discontinuing therapy.

920. Most common surgical procedure for patients with temporal lobe epilepsy involves resection of?
Harrison's 20th Ed. Chapter 418, Page 3065

A. Anteromedial temporal lobe
B. Anterolateral temporal lobe
C. Posteromedial temporal lobe
D. Posterolateral temporal lobe

Most common surgical procedure for temporal lobe epilepsy is resection of anteromedial temporal lobe.

921. One of the most specific signs of a metabolic encephalopathy is?
Harrison's 20th Ed. Chapter 300, Page 2071

A. Bilateral asterixis
B. Confusion
C. Seizure
D. Vomiting

Bilateral asterixis, a negative myoclonus, is a certain sign of metabolic encephalopathy or drug intoxication.

922. Asterixis can be found in?
Harrison's 20th Ed. Chapter 300, Page 2071

A. Any tonically held posture
B. Tonically held tongue
C. Voluntary limb motion
D. All of the above

923. In an awake patient of uremic encephalopathy, the typical movement abnormality is?
Harrison's 20th Ed. Chapter 300, Page 2071

A. Myoclonic jerking and tremor
B. Partial seizure
C. Primary generalized seizure
D. Absence seizure

924. Which of the following statements about status epilepticus is false?
Harrison's 20th Ed. Chapter 418, Page 3066

A. Continuous seizures
B. Repetitive, discrete seizures
C. Impaired consciousness in the interictal period
D. May be nonconvulsive

Status epilepticus refers to continuous seizures or repetitive, discrete seizures with impaired consciousness in the interictal period. Its subtypes include generalized convulsive status epilepticus (GCSE) and nonconvulsive status epilepticus (persistent absence seizures or focal seizures).

925. In generalized convulsive status epilepticus (GCSE), which of the following leads to irreversible neuronal injury?
Harrison's 20th Ed. Chapter 418, Page 3066

A. Cardiorespiratory dysfunction
B. Hyperthermia
C. Metabolic derangements
D. All of the above

926. Which of the following is the first medicine that is recommended for generalized tonic-clonic status epilepticus in adults?
Harrison's 20th Ed. Chapter 418, Page 3067 Figure 418-5

A. Lorazepam
B. Fosphenytoin
C. Valproate
D. Phenobarbital

Lorazepam is recommended for generalized tonic-clonic status epilepticus in adults in doses of 0.1 - 0.15 mg/kg IV over 1 - 2 minutes to be repeated once if no response is obtained after 5 minutes.

927. Which of the following drugs should be given concomitantly with lorazepam in management of status epilepticus?
Harrison's 20th Ed. Chapter 418, Page 3066

A. Carbamazepine
B. Fosphenytoin
C. Valproate
D. Phenobarbital

Lorazepam is the most effective benzodiazepine for treating status epilepticus. Phenytoin or fosphenytoin should be given concomitantly since Lorazepam has a short half-life. Other drugs, like gabapentin, carbamazepine and phenobarbital should be reserved for patients with contraindications to phenytoin (allergy or pregnancy) or ongoing seizures despite phenytoin.

928. Nonconvulsive status epilepticus best relates to?
Harrison's 20th Ed. Chapter 418, Page 3066

A. Hysterical conversion reaction
B. Epileptic coma
C. Sleep
D. Excessive exercise

Epileptic coma refers to generalized electrical seizures are associated with coma, even in the absence of motor convulsions (nonconvulsive status epilepticus).

929. Which of the following is false about "Sudden unexpected death in epileptic patients (SUDEP)?
Harrison's 20th Ed. Chapter 418, Page 3066

A. Affects young people with convulsive seizures
B. Tends to occur at night
C. May result from brainstem-mediated effects of seizures on cardiac rhythms or pulmonary function
D. None of the above

Sudden unexpected death in epileptic patients (SUDEP) affects young people with convulsive seizures and tends to occur at night. It may result from brainstem-mediated effects of seizures on cardiac rhythms or pulmonary function.

930. Which of the following drug is effective as adjunctive therapy in catamenial epilepsy?
Harrison's 20th Ed. Chapter 418, Page 3067

A. Prednisolone
B. Beta blockers
C. Medroxyprogesterone
D. Diuretics

There may be an increase in seizure frequency around menses due to effects of estrogen or progesterone on neuronal excitability or changes in antiepileptic drug levels due to altered protein binding. Natural progestins or intramuscular medroxyprogesterone may be of benefit to a subset of women.

931. During pregnancy, seizure frequency decreases in what percentage of women?

Harrison's 20th Ed. Chapter 418, Page 3067

A. 10%
B. 20%
C. 30%
D. 40%

During pregnancy, seizure frequency will remain unchanged in ~50% of women, increase in 30%, and decrease in 20%.

932. Which of the following anti-epileptic medications can significantly antagonize effects of oral contraceptives?

Harrison's 20th Ed. Chapter 418, Page 3068

A. Carbamazepine
B. Phenytoin
C. Topiramate
D. All of the above

Carbamazepine, phenytoin, phenobarbital, and topiramate can significantly antagonize the effects of oral contraceptives via enzyme induction.

933. Ratio of drug concentration in breast milk relative to serum is maximum with which of the following antiepileptic drug?

Harrison's 20th Ed. Chapter 418, Page 3068

A. Levetiracetam
B. Phenobarbital
C. Carbamazepine
D. Phenytoin

934. Ratio of drug concentration in breast milk relative to serum is minimum with which of the following antiepileptic drug?

Harrison's 20th Ed. Chapter 418, Page 3068

A. Valproic acid
B. Phenobarbital
C. Carbamazepine
D. Phenytoin

Ratio of drug concentration in breast milk relative to serum is 300% for levetiracetam, ~80% for ethosuximide, 40–60% for phenobarbital, 40% for carbamazepine, 15% for phenytoin, and 5% for valproic acid.

935. Neonatal unconjugated hyperbilirubinemia & resultant clinical jaundice affect what percentage of newborns?

N Engl J Med. 2013;369:2021-30

A. Approximately 35%
B. Approximately 55%
C. Approximately 70%
D. Approximately 85%

Neonatal unconjugated hyperbilirubinemia & resultant clinical jaundice affect up to approximately 85% of newborns.

936. Which out of the following best relates to kernicterus?

N Engl J Med. 2013;369:2021-30

A. Acute bilirubin encephalopathy
B. Chronic bilirubin encephalopathy
C. Hyperoxic brain injury
D. None of the above

937. Which of the following is a feature of Kernicterus?

N Engl J Med. 2013;369:2021-30

A. Extrapyramidal movement disorders
B. Auditory neuropathy spectrum disorders
C. Oculomotor pareses
D. All of the above

938. In Kernicterus, bilirubin-induced neuropathology is seen in which of the following?

N Engl J Med. 2013;369:2021-30

A. Globus pallidus
B. Hippocampal CA2 neurons
C. Cerebellar Purkinje's cells
D. All of the above

Kernicterus or chronic bilirubin encephalopathy is a permanent disabling neurologic condition that is classically characterized by the extrapyramidal movement disorders of dystonia, choreoathetosis, or both; hearing loss due to auditory neuropathy spectrum disorders; and oculomotor pareses. These central nervous system (CNS) sequelae reflect the regional CNS topography of bilirubin-induced neuropathology, which involves the globus pallidus, subthalamic nucleus, brainstem nuclei, hippocampal CA2 neurons, and cerebellar Purkinje's cells.

939. Medical condition that increases risk of severe hyperbilirubinemia or bilirubin neurotoxicity is?

N Engl J Med. 2013;369:2021-30

A. Glucose-6-phosphate dehydrogenase deficiency
B. Rh isoimmunization
C. Sepsis
D. All of the above

Medical conditions that increase the risk of severe hyperbilirubinemia or bilirubin neurotoxicity, such as glucose-6-phosphate dehydrogenase deficiency, Rh isoimmunization, and sepsis.

940. Phenobarbital increases bilirubin clearance by activating the phenobarbital enhancer module in promoter sequence of?

N Engl J Med. 2013;369:2021-30

A. MRP2
B. UGT1A1
C. FIC1
D. BSEP

Phenobarbital increases bilirubin clearance by activating the phenobarbital enhancer module in the promoter sequence of bilirubin-UDP-glucuronosyltransferase (UGT1A1), which enhances bilirubin conjugation.

941. Which of the following has protective effect against bilirubin-induced neuromotor dysfunction?

N Engl J Med. 2013;369:2021-30

A. Ciprofloxacin
B. Rifampin
C. Minocycline
D. Atorvastatin

Minocycline has protective effect against bilirubin-induced neuromotor dysfunction, cerebellar hypoplasia & auditory-pathway abnormalities in Gunn rat pups.

Cerebrovascular Diseases

942. By definition, neurologic signs and symptoms of transient ischemic attack (TIA) last for less than?
Harrison's 20th Ed. Chapter 419, Page 3068

- A. < 1 hour
- B. < 6 hours
- C. < 12 hours
- D. < 24 hours

Typically the neurologic signs and symptoms of a TIA last for 5 to 15 minutes but, by definition, must last for <24 hours, without evidence of brain infarction on brain imaging.

943. A generalized reduction in cerebral blood flow due to systemic hypotension produces?
Harrison's 20th Ed. Chapter 419, Page 3068

- A. Syncope
- B. Transient ischemic attack
- C. Hypoxic-ischemic encephalopathy
- D. Any of the above

A generalized reduction in cerebral blood flow due to systemic hypotension (cardiac arrhythmia, myocardial infarction or hemorrhagic shock) usually produces syncope.

944. Focal brain ischemia or infarction is usually caused by?
Harrison's 20th Ed. Chapter 419, Page 3068

- A. Thrombosis of cerebral vessels
- B. Emboli from a proximal arterial source
- C. Emboli from the heart
- D. All of the above

Focal brain ischemia or infarction is caused by thrombosis of cerebral vessels or by emboli from a proximal arterial source or heart.

945. Neurologic symptoms in intracranial hemorrhage is caused by?
Harrison's 20th Ed. Chapter 419, Page 3068

- A. Mass effect on neural structures
- B. From the toxic effects of blood itself
- C. By increasing intracranial pressure
- D. All of the above

Intracranial hemorrhage is caused by bleeding directly into or around the brain. It leads to neurologic symptoms by producing a mass effect on neural structures, from the toxic effects of blood itself, or by increasing intracranial pressure.

946. Acute stroke may begins as which of the following?
Harrison's 20th Ed. Chapter 419, Page 3068

- A. Sudden severe headache
- B. Change in vision
- C. Change in gait
- D. Any of the above

947. What percentage of ischemic stroke patients have hemiparesis?
Harrison's 20th Ed. Chapter 419, Page 3068

- A. 30%
- B. 50%
- C. 85%
- D. 100%

Acute stroke has a sudden onset of loss of sensory and/or motor function on one side of the body (nearly 85% of ischemic stroke patients have hemiparesis), change in vision, gait or ability to speak or understand; or a sudden severe headache.

948. In the acronym FAST, "S" stands for?
Harrison's 20th Ed. Chapter 419, Page 3068

- A. Stroke
- B. Sensory deficit
- C. Speech abnormality
- D. Sleep

In the acronym FAST about common physical symptoms of stroke & its treatment, F stands for Facial weakness, A for Arm weakness, S for Speech abnormality and T for Time.

949. Conditions that may mimic stroke include?
Harrison's 20th Ed. Chapter 419, Page 3069, N Engl J Med. 2000;343:710

- A. Seizure
- B. Metabolic encephalopathy
- C. Migraine
- D. All of the above

Causes of sudden-onset neurologic symptoms that may mimic stroke include hypoglycemia, seizure, intracranial tumor, (acephalgic) migraine, hypertensive encephalopathy and metabolic encephalopathy.

950. Intracranial tumor may present with acute neurologic symptoms due to?
Harrison's 20th Ed. Chapter 419, Page 3069

- A. Hemorrhage
- B. Seizure
- C. Hydrocephalus
- D. Any of the above

Intracranial tumor may present with acute neurologic symptoms due to hemorrhage, seizure or hydrocephalus.

951. Which of the following is a stroke syndrome?
Harrison's 20th Ed. Chapter 419, Page 3069

- A. Large-vessel stroke within the anterior circulation
- B. Large-vessel stroke within the posterior circulation
- C. Small-vessel disease of anterior/posterior circulation
- D. All of the above

Stroke syndromes are divided into large vessel stroke within anterior circulation, large-vessel stroke within posterior circulation and small-vessel disease of either vascular bed. Internal carotid artery & its branches comprise the anterior circulation of brain.

952. Occlusion of proximal MCA is most often due to?
Harrison's 20th Ed. Chapter 419, Page 3069

- A. Embolus
- B. Intracranial atherothrombosis
- C. Vasospasm
- D. None of the above

Occlusion of proximal MCA or one of its major branches is mostly due to embolus (artery-to-artery, cardiac, or of unknown source) rather than intracranial atherothrombosis.

953. Collateral formation via which of the following prevents MCA stenosis from becoming symptomatic?
Harrison's 20th Ed. Chapter 419, Page 3069

A. Deep penetrating arterioles
B. Venous sinuses
C. Leptomeningeal vessels
D. All of the above

Collateral formation via leptomeningeal vessels prevents MCA stenosis from becoming symptomatic.

954. Cortical branches of MCA supply which of the following?
Harrison's 20th Ed. Chapter 419, Page 3069

A. Frontal pole
B. Lower temporal pole convolution
C. Occipital pole convolution
D. None of the above

Cortical branches of MCA supply the lateral surface of hemisphere except for frontal pole and a strip along the superomedial border of frontal and parietal lobes (supplied by ACA), and lower temporal and occipital pole convolutions (supplied by PCA).

955. Lenticulostriate arteries from proximal MCA (M1 segment) supply all except?
Harrison's 20th Ed. Chapter 419, Page 3069

A. Putamen
B. Outer globus pallidus
C. Anterior limb of internal capsule
D. Body of caudate nucleus

Proximal MCA (M1 segment) gives rise to penetrating lenticulostriate arteries that supply putamen, outer globus pallidus, posterior limb of internal capsule, adjacent corona radiata & most of caudate nucleus.

956. Temporal cortex is supplied by?
Harrison's 20th Ed. Chapter 419, Page 3069

A. Inferior division of MCA
B. Superior division of MCA
C. ACA
D. PCA

MCA divides into superior & inferior divisions (M2 branches) in sylvian fissure. Branches of the inferior division supply inferior parietal and temporal cortex, and superior division supply the frontal and superior parietal cortex.

957. In a right handed person, occlusion of right MCA leads to all except?
Harrison's 20th Ed. Chapter 419, Page 3069

A. Global aphasia
B. Anosognosia
C. Constructional apraxia
D. Dysarthria

Global aphasia occurs when the dominant hemisphere is involved. When nondominant hemisphere is affected, anosognosia, constructional apraxia, and neglect are found. Contralateral hemiplegia, hemianesthesia, homonymous hemianopia occur in both instances. Dysarthria is common because of facial weakness.

958. Which of the following is a partial syndrome?
Harrison's 20th Ed. Chapter 419, Page 3071

A. Brachial syndrome
B. Broca aphasia
C. Frontal opercular syndrome
D. All of the above

959. Which of the following artery supplying dominant hemisphere is occluded in Wernicke's aphasia without weakness?
Harrison's 20th Ed. Chapter 419, Page 3071

A. Stem of MCA
B. Penetrating lenticulostriate arteries of MCA
C. Proximal superior division of MCA
D. Inferior division of MCA

If a fluent (Wernicke's) aphasia occurs without weakness, inferior division of MCA supplying posterior part (temporal cortex) of dominant hemisphere is probably involved.

960. Which of the following artery supplying the nondominant hemisphere is occluded in a case of hemineglect or spatial agnosia without weakness?
Harrison's 20th Ed. Chapter 419, Page 3071

A. Stem of MCA
B. Penetrating lenticulostriate arteries of MCA
C. Proximal superior division of MCA
D. Inferior division of MCA

Hemineglect or spatial agnosia without weakness indicates that the inferior division of MCA in the nondominant hemisphere is occluded.

961. Which of the following artery is occluded in a case of pure motor stroke contralateral to the lesion?
Harrison's 20th Ed. Chapter 419, Page 3071

A. Stem of MCA
B. Penetrating lenticulostriate arteries of MCA
C. Proximal superior division of MCA
D. Inferior division of MCA

Occlusion of a lenticulostriate vessel of MCA produces lacunar stroke within the internal capsule producing pure motor stroke or sensory-motor stroke contralateral to the lesion.

962. Lacunar infarction affecting which of the following areas produces very few clinical signs?
Harrison's 20th Ed. Chapter 419, Page 3071

A. Genu of internal capsule
B. Posterior limb of internal capsule
C. Globus pallidus and putamen
D. All of the above

Lacunar infarction affecting the globus pallidus and putamen often produce few clinical signs, but parkinsonism and hemiballismus occur.

963. Anterior cerebral artery (ACA) arises from the Internal carotid artery at the level of?
Journal of Neurosurgery 2000;93(6): 1084-1088, JMS 2018;1(1):5-9

A. Anterior clinoid process
B. Optic chiasma
C. Optic nerve
D. Olfactory trigone

Term Heubner's artery was first used in 1909 by Aitken, after Heubner's classical description of the vessel in 1872. Classically, RAH travels back on its parent ACA and passes above the carotid bifurcation and middle cerebral artery into the medial part of sylvian fissure before entering the anterior perforated substance. Anatomical variations are frequent.

964. "Recurrent artery of Heubner" supplies which part of internal capsule?
Journal of Neurosurgery 2000;93(6): 1084-1088, JMS 2018;1(1):5-9

A. Anterior limb
B. Genu
C. Posterior limb
D. Retrolentiform part

Lenticulostriate recurrent artery of Heubner (RAH) supplies blood to medial portion of orbitofrontal cortex, anterior portion of caudate nucleus, anterior third of putamen, external segment of globus pallidus, and anterior crus of internal capsule. RAH also supplies olfactory region, anterior hypothalamus, nucleus accumbens, parts of uncinate fasciculus, diagonal band of Broca, and the basal nucleus of Meynert.

965. "Recurrent artery of Heubner" is a branch of?
   A. Internal carotid artery
   B. Anterior cerebral artery
   C. Middle cerebral artery
   D. Posterior cerebral artery

966. Which of the following is called Heubner's disease?
   A. Carcinomatous meningitis
   B. Primary central nervous system vasculitis
   C. Syphilitic endarteritis
   D. Necrotizing arteritis

Johann Otto Leonhardt Heubner (1843-1926) described lenticulostriate recurrent artery in 1872. It can be damaged with improper clip placement during repair of aneurysms near the anterior communicating artery. He also described syphilitic endarteritis (Heubner's disease).

967. "Arteria termatica of Wilder" best relates to?
   A. Internal carotid artery
   B. Anterior cerebral artery
   C. Middle cerebral artery
   D. Posterior cerebral artery

Wilder was the first to describe fusion of both A2 segments to form a single artery & introduced the term arteria termatica of Wilder in 1885. Also known as the unpaired pericallosal stem artery, unpaired anterior cerebral artery, common anterior cerebral trunk & azygos pericallosal artery.

968. Which of the following is not supplied by the deep penetrating branches of the A1 segment of ACA?
   A. Anterior limb of internal capsule
   B. Amygdala
   C. Body of caudate nucleus
   D. Anterior hypothalamus

The A1 segment of anterior cerebral artery (ACA) gives rise to deep penetrating branches that supply the anterior limb of internal capsule, anterior perforate substance, amygdala, anterior hypothalamus, and inferior part of the head of caudate nucleus.

969. Occlusion of a single A2 segment of anterior cerebral artery (ACA) results in which of the following?
   A. Abulia
   B. Bilateral pyramidal signs with paraparesis
   C. Urinary incontinence
   D. All of the above

Occlusion of a single A2 segment of ACA results in profound abulia, bilateral pyramidal signs with paraparesis and urinary incontinence.

970. Anterior choroidal artery arises from?
   A. Internal carotid artery
   B. Middle cerebral artery
   C. Anterior cerebral artery
   D. Posterior cerebral artery

Anterior choroidal artery arises from ICA & supplies posterior limb of internal capsule & white matter posterolateral to it, through which geniculocalcarine fibers pass partly.

971. Complete syndrome of anterior choroidal artery occlusion consists of?
   A. Contralateral hemiplegia
   B. Hemianesthesia
   C. Homonymous hemianopia
   D. All of the above

The complete syndrome of anterior choroidal artery occlusion consists of contralateral hemiplegia, hemianesthesia and homonymous hemianopia.

972. Anterior choroidal strokes are usually the result of?
   A. Embolus
   B. In situ Thrombosis
   C. Vasospasm
   D. None of the above

Anterior choroidal strokes are usually the result of in situ thrombosis, and iatrogenic occlusion during surgical clipping of aneurysms of ICA.

973. "Fetal posterior cerebral artery" refers to?
   A. Single PCA
   B. Absent PCA
   C. PCA arising from internal carotid artery (ICA)
   D. PCA arising from MCA

Anatomic configuration of PCA arising from ICA is called fetal posterior cerebral artery (20%).

974. Bilateral common carotid artery occlusions at their origin may occur in?
   A. Temporal arteritis
   B. Takayasu's arteritis
   C. Kawasaki disease
   D. Polyarteritis nodosa

Bilateral common carotid artery occlusions at their origin may occur in Takayasu's arteritis.

975. The vertebral arteries join to form the basilar artery at?
   A. Foramen magnum
   B. Lower medulla oblongata
   C. Pontomedullary junction
   D. Interpeduncular fossa

Vertebral arteries join to form basilar artery at the pontomedullary junction.

976. Basilar artery divides into two posterior cerebral arteries at?
   A. Foramen magnum
   B. Lower medulla oblongata
   C. Pontomedullary junction
   D. Interpeduncular fossa

Basilar artery divides into two posterior cerebral arteries in the interpeduncular fossa.

977. Posterior circulation supplies which of the following?
   A. Hippocampus
   B. Medial temporal lobes
   C. Occipital lobes
   D. All of the above

The posterior circulation is composed of the paired vertebral arteries, the basilar artery, and the paired posterior cerebral arteries. It supplies the cerebellum, medulla, pons, midbrain, subthalamus, thalamus, hippocampus, and medial temporal and occipital lobes.

978. The artery of Percheron arises from?
Harrison's 20th Ed. Chapter 419, Page 3072

A. Anterior cerebral artery
B. Posterior cerebral artery
C. Vertebral artery
D. Basilar artery

Thalamogeniculate, Percheron and posterior choroidal arteries are the penetrating branches of the proximal P1 segment of PCA.

979. Occlusion of artery of Percheron produces?
Harrison's 20th Ed. Chapter 419, Page 3073

A. Paresis of upward gaze
B. Drowsiness
C. Abulia
D. All of the above

Occlusion of artery of Percheron produces paresis of upward gaze, drowsiness & abulia.

980. Which of the following is a penetrating artery of P1 segment of PCA?
Harrison's 20th Ed. Chapter 419, Page 3072

A. Thalamogeniculate artery
B. Percheron artery
C. Posterior choroidal artery
D. All of the above

981. P1 syndrome produces which of the following signs?
Harrison's 20th Ed. Chapter 419, Page 3072

A. Midbrain signs
B. Subthalamic signs
C. Thalamic signs
D. All of the above

P1 syndrome is due to disease of proximal P1 segment of PCA or its penetrating branches namely thalamogeniculate, Percheron, and posterior choroidal arteries. It is diagnosed by various midbrain, subthalamic, and thalamic signs.

982. Involvement of subthalamic nucleus is best related to?
Harrison's 20th Ed. Chapter 419, Page 3073

A. Upward gaze
B. Drowsiness
C. Hemiballismus
D. Abulia

If the subthalamic nucleus is involved, contralateral hemiballismus may occur.

983. Weber's syndrome results due to occlusion of?
Harrison's 20th Ed. Chapter 419, Page 3073

A. Anterior cerebral artery
B. Middle cerebral artery
C. Posterior cerebral artery
D. Basilar artery

984. Claude's syndrome results due to occlusion of?
Harrison's 20th Ed. Chapter 419, Page 3073

A. Anterior cerebral artery
B. Middle cerebral artery
C. Posterior cerebral artery
D. Basilar artery

985. In Claude's syndrome, ataxia is due to involvement of?
Harrison's 20th Ed. Chapter 419, Page 3073

A. Cerebellum
B. Superior cerebellar peduncle
C. Red nucleus
D. All of the above

III nerve palsy with contralateral ataxia is called Claude's syndrome. Ataxia is due to involvement of red nucleus or dentatorubrothalamic tract.

986. In Weber's syndrome, hemiplegia is due to involvement of?
Harrison's 20th Ed. Chapter 419, Page 3073

A. Internal capsule
B. Cerebral peduncle
C. Corpus callosum
D. Pyramidal decussation

III nerve palsy with contralateral hemiplegia is called Weber's syndrome. Hemiplegia is localized to the cerebral peduncle. Hermann Weber, German physician, 1863.

987. Complete oculomotor nerve lesion results in all except?
Harrison's 20th Ed. Chapter 419, Page 3073

A. Ipsilateral ptosis
B. Pupillary dilatation
C. Loss of pupillary & accommodation reflexes
D. Medical deviation of the eye

Complete oculomotor (III) nerve lesion results in ipsilateral ptosis, pupillary dilatation, loss of pupillary and accommodation reflexes and 'lateral' deviation of the eye. III CN supplies all extra-ocular muscles except lateral rectus and superior oblique.

988. Brown's tendon sheath syndrome simulates which of the following?
DeJong's The Neurologic Examination, 7th Ed. Page 211

A. Superior oblique palsy
B. Inferior oblique palsy
C. Superior rectus palsy
D. Inferior rectus palsy

Brown's tendon sheath syndrome, most often congenital, is limitation of free movement of superior oblique tendon through the trochlea. Restriction of movement causes an impairment of upgaze in adduction simulating inferior oblique palsy.

989. Edinger-Westphal nucleus located in?
Harrison's 20th Ed. Chapter 419, Page 3073

A. Upper mid-brain
B. Lower mid-brain
C. Pons
D. Medulla oblongata

990. Fascicles from III CN nuclei run forward & laterally through?
Harrison's 20th Ed. Chapter 419, Page 3073

A. Substantia nigra
B. Red nuclei
C. Dentate nuclei
D. Olivary nuclei

III cranial nerve nuclei are located in midbrain. They consist of Edinger-Westphal nucleus located in upper mid-brain supplying fibers to pupils and motor nucleus located in lower mid-brain supplying extra-ocular muscles, except lateral rectus and superior oblique. Fascicles from the III CN nuclei run forward & laterally through red nuclei and converge at the inter-peduncular fossa. Lesion of lower mid-brain affects extraocular muscles but spares pupils, whereas lesions involving both upper & lower parts of mid-brain are associated with pupillary dilatation.

991. Lower branch of occulomotor nerve supplies all of the following extraocular muscles except?
Harrison's 20th Ed. Chapter 419, Page 3073

A. Medial rectus
B. Levator palpebrae superioris
C. Inferior rectus
D. Inferior oblique

After emerging from mid-brain, III CN lies between posterior cerebral artery and the superior cerebellar artery. It runs forward parallel to the posterior communicating artery and enters the orbit through the superior orbital fissure, dividing into an upper and a lower branch. The upper branch supplies the levator palpebrae superioris and superior rectus muscles. The lower branch supplies three muscles: the medial rectus, the inferior rectus, and the inferior oblique muscle. The nerve to the inferior oblique muscle conveys the preganglionic parasympathetic fibers to the ciliary ganglion from which the post-ganglionic parasympathetic fibers arise to supply the ciliary muscle and the muscles of the iris (pupilloconstrictor fibers).

992. Hemiballismus is due to damage to which of the following?
Harrison's 20th Ed. Chapter 419, Page 3073

A. Substantia nigra
B. Red nucleus
C. Thalamus
D. Subthalamic nucleus

If the subthalamic nucleus is involved, contralateral hemiballismus may occur.

993. Which of the following is false about "Thalamic Dejerine-Roussy syndrome"?
Harrison's 20th Ed. Chapter 419, Page 3073

A. Contralateral hemisensory loss
B. Agonizing pain in affected area later
C. Responds poorly to analgesics
D. None of the above

Thalamic Dejerine-Roussy syndrome consists of contralateral hemisensory loss followed later by agonizing, searing or burning pain in the affected areas. Symptoms are persistent and respond poorly to analgesics. May respond to carbamazepine or gabapentin.

994. Occlusion of the posterior cerebral artery can produce which of the following?
Harrison's 20th Ed. Chapter 419, Page 3073

A. Peduncular hallucinosis
B. Contralateral homonymous hemianopia, macular sparing
C. Acute disturbance in memory
D. All of the above

All the above presentations occur due to occlusion of distal PCA causing infarction of hippocampus, medial temporal & occipital lobes. Peduncular hallucinosis means visual hallucinations of brightly colored scenes & objects. Because memory has bilateral representation, this defect clears soon.

995. Anton's syndrome results due to occlusion of?
Harrison's 20th Ed. Chapter 419, Page 3074

A. Bilateral occlusion of distal ACA
B. Bilateral occlusion of distal MCA
C. Bilateral occlusion of distal PCA
D. Bilateral occlusion of vertebral artery

Anton's syndrome is due to bilateral infarction in the distal PCAs. It produces cortical blindness with preserved pupillary light reaction.

996. In Anton's syndrome, patient is often unaware of?
Harrison's 20th Ed. Chapter 419, Page 3074

A. Smell
B. Hearing
C. Blindness
D. Colour vision

In Anton's syndrome, patient is unaware of blindness. Bilateral infarction in distal PCAs produces cortical blindness (blindness with preserved pupillary light reaction).

997. "Gun-barrel" vision is best related to?
Harrison's 20th Ed. Chapter 419, Page 3074

A. Anton's syndrome
B. Balint's syndrome
C. Claude's syndrome
D. Wallenberg's syndrome

In Anton's syndrome, rarely, only peripheral vision is lost and central vision is spared, resulting in "gun-barrel" vision.

998. Which symptom can occur in Balint's syndrome?
Harrison's 20th Ed. Chapter 419, Page 3074

A. Optic ataxia
B. Oculomotor apaxia
C. Asimultanagnosia
D. All of the above

Balint's syndrome is a disorder of the orderly visual scanning of the environment, usually resulting from infarctions secondary to low flow in "watershed" between distal PCA & MCA territories. There occurs persistence of a visual image for several minutes despite gazing at another scene (palinopsia) or an inability to synthesize whole of an image (asimultanagnosia).

999. Experiencing persistence of a visual image for several minutes despite gazing at another scene is called?
Harrison's 20th Ed. Chapter 419, Page 3074

A. Optic ataxia
B. Ocular ataxia
C. Simultagnosia
D. Palinopia

In palinopia, patients experience persistence of a visual image for several minutes despite gazing at another scene.

1000. Embolic occlusion of the top of basilar artery can produce which of the following?
Harrison's 20th Ed. Chapter 419, Page 3074

A. Ptosis
B. Pupillary asymmetry
C. Lack of reaction to light
D. All of the above

Embolic occlusion of the top of the basilar artery can produce any or all of the central or peripheral territory symptoms. The hallmark is the sudden onset of bilateral signs, ptosis, pupillary asymmetry or lack of reaction to light and somnolence.

1001. The vertebral artery enters into the transverse cervical vertebral foramen at?
Harrison's 20th Ed. Chapter 419, Page 3074

A. C7
B. C6
C. C4
D. C3

The first (V1) segment of vertebral artery extends from its origin to its entrance into the sixth or fifth transverse vertebral foramen.

1002. Branches from which segment of vertebral artery supply brainstem and cerebellum?
Harrison's 20th Ed. Chapter 419, Page 3074

A. 1
B. 2
C. 3
D. 4

Fourth (V4) segment of vertebral artery courses upward from foramen magnum to join the other vertebral artery and forms the basilar artery. Only the fourth segment gives rise to branches that supply the brainstem and cerebellum.

1003. Which segment of the vertebral artery pierce the dura at the foramen magnum?
Harrison's 20th Ed. Chapter 419, Page 3074

A. 1
B. 2
C. 3
D. 4

Third segment of vertebral artery (V3) passes through transverse foramen and circles around the arch of the atlas to pierce dura at foramen magnum.

1004. Which of the following statements about vertebral artery is false?
Harrison's 20th Ed. Chapter 419, Page 3075

A. Arises from innominate artery on right side
B. Consists of four segments
C. Atherothrombotic lesion has predilection for V3 segment
D. None of the above

Atherothrombotic lesions have a predilection for V1 & V4 segments of vertebral artery.

1005. Which of the following conditions affect the second & third segments of vertebral artery?
Harrison's 20th Ed. Chapter 419, Page 3075

A. Dissection
B. Fibromuscular dysplasia
C. Encroachment by osteophytic spurs
D. All of the above

Atheromatous disease rarely narrows second & third segments of vertebral artery, but this region is vulnerable to dissection, fibromuscular dysplasia and encroachment by osteophytic spurs within the vertebral foramina.

1006. Vertebral artery receives collateral blood supply from which of the following?
Harrison's 20th Ed. Chapter 419, Page 3075

A. Ascending cervical arteries
B. Thyrocervical arteries
C. Occipital arteries
D. All of the above

Vertebral artery receives collateral blood supply from the ascending cervical, thyrocervical or occipital arteries which is usually sufficient to prevent low-flow TIAs or stroke.

1007. "Subclavian steal" is best related to?
Harrison's 20th Ed. Chapter 419, Page 3075

A. Raynauds phenomenon
B. Posterior circulation TIA
C. Upper limb clubbing
D. All of the above

If the subclavian artery is occluded proximal to the origin of vertebral artery, there is reversal in the direction of blood flow in the ipsilateral vertebral artery. Exercise of the ipsilateral arm may increase demand on vertebral flow, producing posterior circulation TIAs, or "subclavian steal."

1008. In medial medullary syndrome, which of the following structures is involved?
Harrison's 20th Ed. Chapter 419, Page 3073 Figure 419-7

A. Ipsilateral twelfth nerve
B. Contralateral pyramidal tract
C. Contralateral medial lemniscus
D. All of the above

Medial medullary syndrome is due to occlusion of vertebral artery or branch of vertebral or lower basilar artery. Paralysis with atrophy of half tongue due to ipsilateral XII nerve occurs. On the opposite side, due to involvement of pyramidal tract & medial lemniscus, paralysis of arm & leg, impaired tactile & proprioceptive sense over half the body occur. Face is spared.

1009. Occlusion of which of the following artery is responsible for producing lateral medullary syndrome?
Harrison's 20th Ed. Chapter 419, Page 3073 Figure 419-7

A. Vertebral
B. Posterior inferior cerebellar
C. Superior lateral medullary artery
D. All of the above

Occlusion of any of the five vessels is responsible for producing lateral medullary syndrome. They are vertebral, posterior inferior cerebellar (PICA), superior, middle or inferior lateral medullary arteries.

1010. Which of the following is false for lateral medullary syndrome?
Harrison's 20th Ed. Chapter 419, Page 3073 Figure 419-7

A. Falling to side of lesion
B. Horner's syndrome
C. Impaired touch over opposite half of face
D. Loss of taste

Due to damage to descending tract and nucleus of fifth nerve, pain, numbness, impaired sensation over half the face occurs on the side of lesion.

1011. Which of the following is false for lateral medullary syndrome?
Harrison's 20th Ed. Chapter 419, Page 3073 Figure 419-7

A. Oscillopsia
B. Nystagmus
C. Strabismus
D. Dysphagia

Due to damage to vestibular nucleus, nystagmus, diplopia, oscillopsia, vertigo, nausea & vomiting occur in lateral medullary syndrome. Dysphagia, hoarseness, paralysis of palate & vocal cord, diminished gag reflex occur due to damage to issuing fibers of IX & X nerves.

1012. Loss of taste in lateral medullary syndrome is due to lesion in?
Harrison's 20th Ed. Chapter 419, Page 3073 Figure 419-7

A. Nucleus of fifth nerve
B. Vestibular nucleus
C. Nucleus and tractus solitarius
D. Cuneate and gracile nuclei

Loss of taste in lateral medullary syndrome is due to lesion in nucleus & tractus solitarius on side of lesion.

1013. Nystagmus, diplopia, oscillopsia, vertigo, nausea, vomiting in lateral medullary syndrome is due to lesion in?
Harrison's 20th Ed. Chapter 419, Page 3073 Figure 419-7

A. Descending sympathetic tract
B. Cerebellar hemisphere
C. Vestibular nucleus
D. Spinocerebellar tract

Nystagmus, diplopia, oscillopsia, vertigo, nausea, vomiting in lateral medullary syndrome is due to lesion in Vestibular nucleus.

1014. Numbness of ipsilateral arm, trunk, or leg in lateral medullary syndrome is due to lesion in?
Harrison's 20th Ed. Chapter 419, Page 3073 Figure 419-7

A. Nucleus of fifth nerve
B. Vestibular nucleus
C. Nucleus and tractus solitarius
D. Cuneate and gracile nuclei

Numbness of ipsilateral arm, trunk, or leg in lateral medullary syndrome is due to lesion in cuneate and gracile nuclei.

1015. Which of the following is not a part of lateral medullary (or Wallenberg's) syndrome?
Harrison's 20th Ed. Chapter 419, Page 3073 Figure 419-7

A. Vertigo
B. Numbness of ipsilateral face
C. Numbness of contralateral limbs
D. Contralateral Horner's syndrome

Horner's syndrome (miosis, ptosis, decreased sweating) occurs on side of lesion in lateral medullary syndrome due to damage to descending sympathetic tract.

1016. Which of the following is not a feature of vertebral artery occlusion?
Harrison's 20th Ed. Chapter 419, Page 3075

A. Vertigo
B. Diplopia
C. Quadriparesis
D. Hemiparesis

Embolic occlusion or thrombosis of a V4 segment causes ischemia of the lateral medulla. The constellation of vertigo, numbness of the ipsilateral face and contralateral limbs, diplopia, hoarseness, dysarthria, dysphagia, and ipsilateral Horner's syndrome is called the lateral medullary (or Wallenberg's) syndrome. Hemiparesis is not a feature of vertebral artery occlusion. However, quadriparesis may result from occlusion of the anterior spinal artery.

1017. Which of the following can occur in cerebellar infarction?
Harrison's 20th Ed. Chapter 419, Page 3076

A. Headache
B. Neck stiffness
C. Unilateral dysmetria
D. All of the above

Headache, neck stiffness and unilateral dysmetria favor cerebellar infarction.

1018. Which of the following are branches of the basilar artery?
Harrison's 20th Ed. Chapter 419, Page 3076

A. Paramedian
B. Short circumferential
C. Long circumferential
D. All of the above

Branches of the basilar artery supply the base of pons and superior cerebellum. The three groups are paramedian (7-10 in number supplying a wedge of pons on either side of midline), short circumferential (5-7 in number supplying lateral two-thirds of pons & middle & superior cerebellar peduncles) and bilateral long circumferential (superior cerebellar & anterior inferior cerebellar arteries coursing around pons to supply the cerebellar hemispheres).

1019. Occlusion of which of the following leads to "Top of the basilar" syndromes?
Harrison's 20th Ed. Chapter 419, Page 3076

A. Proximal basilar artery
B. Both vertebral arteries
C. Distal basilar artery
D. Any of the above

Atheromatous lesions can occur anywhere along the basilar trunk but are most frequent in the proximal basilar & distal vertebral segments. Clinical picture varies depending on the retrograde collateral flow from posterior communicating arteries. Atherothrombosis may also occlude distal portion of basilar artery (emboli from heart or proximal vertebral or basilar segments) and lead to "top of the basilar" syndromes.

1020. Which of the following can occur upon complete basilar occlusion?
Harrison's 20th Ed. Chapter 419, Page 3076

A. Bilateral long tract signs (sensory & motor)
B. Signs of cranial nerve dysfunction
C. Signs of cerebellar dysfunction
D. All of the above

1021. Corticobulbar and corticospinal tracts are damaged bilaterally due to occlusion of?
Harrison's 20th Ed. Chapter 419, Page 3076

A. Vertebral artery
B. Basilar artery
C. Anterior inferior cerebellar artery
D. Superior cerebellar artery

Basilar artery or lone vertebral artery occlusion can damage corticobulbar and corticospinal tracts bilaterally. Complete basilar occlusion leads to a constellation of bilateral long tract signs (sensory and motor) with signs of cranial nerve and cerebellar dysfunction.

1022. "Locked-in" state of preserved consciousness with quadriplegia and cranial nerve signs suggests?
Harrison's 20th Ed. Chapter 419, Page 3076

A. Complete pontine & upper midbrain infarction
B. Complete pontine & lower midbrain infarction
C. Complete pontine & medulla oblongata infarction
D. Any of the above

"Locked-in" state of preserved consciousness with quadriplegia and cranial nerve signs suggests complete pontine and lower midbrain infarction. Atherothrombotic occlusion of basilar artery with infarction causes bilateral brainstem signs, gaze paresis or internuclear ophthalmoplegia with ipsilateral hemiparesis, or unequivocal signs of bilateral pontine disease.

1023. TIAs in the proximal basilar distribution produces which of the following?
Harrison's 20th Ed. Chapter 419, Page 3077

A. Vertigo
B. Diplopia
C. Facial or circumoral numbness
D. All of the above

TIAs in the proximal basilar distribution produces vertigo, diplopia, dysarthria, facial or circumoral numbness and hemisensory symptoms.

1024. Constellation of bilateral long tract signs with signs of cranial nerve and cerebellar dysfunction is suggestive of?
Harrison's 20th Ed. Chapter 419, Page 3073 Figure 419-7

A. Complete basilar artery occlusion
B. Complete posterior cerebral artery occlusion
C. Complete middle cerebral artery occlusion
D. Complete anterior cerebral artery occlusion

Constellation of bilateral long tract signs (sensory and motor) with signs of cranial nerve and cerebellar dysfunction is suggestive of complete basilar artery occlusion.

1025. Which of the following syndromes occur due to occlusion of vertebral artery?
Harrison's 20th Ed. Chapter 419, Page 3073 Figure 419-7

A. Medial medullary syndrome
B. Lateral medullary syndrome
C. Total unilateral medullary syndrome
D. All of the above

Occlusion of vertebral artery can produce medial and lateral and total unilateral medullary syndrome. The last one being a combination of medial and lateral syndromes.

1026. Lateral pontomedullary syndrome is due to occlusion of which of the following vessel?
Harrison's 20th Ed. Chapter 419, Page 3073 Figure 419-7

A. Vertebral artery
B. Basilar artery
C. Anterior inferior cerebellar artery
D. Superior cerebellar artery

Lateral pontomedullary syndrome is due to occlusion of vertebral artery. It is a combination of lateral medullary and lateral inferior pontine syndrome.

1027. Which of the following syndromes occur due to occlusion of anterior inferior cerebellar artery?
Harrison's 20th Ed. Chapter 419, Page 3074 Figure 419-8

A. Medial medullary syndrome
B. Medial inferior pontine syndrome
C. Lateral inferior pontine syndrome
D. All of the above

Occlusion of anterior inferior cerebellar artery produces lateral inferior pontine syndrome.

1028. Which of the following syndrome occurs due to occlusion of superior cerebellar artery?
Harrison's 20th Ed. Chapter 419, Page 3076 Figure 419-10

A. Lateral midpontine syndrome
B. Medial superior pontine syndrome
C. Lateral superior pontine syndrome
D. Total unilateral medullary syndrome

Lateral superior pontine syndrome occurs due to occlusion of superior cerebellar artery - a branch of basilar artery.

1029. Horner's syndrome is produced by occlusion of which of the following arteries?
Harrison's 20th Ed. Chapter 419, Page 3077

A. Anterior inferior cerebellar artery
B. Superior cerebellar artery
C. Vertebral artery
D. All of the above

In lateral medullary syndrome due to occlusion of vertebral artery, Horner's syndrome occurs due to damage to descending sympathetic tract. Lateral inferior pontine syndrome due to occlusion of anterior inferior cerebellar artery produces Horner's syndrome. Lateral superior pontine syndrome due to occlusion of superior cerebellar artery sometimes produces Horner's syndrome.

1030. Deafness is produced by occlusion of which of the following arteries?
Harrison's 20th Ed. Chapter 419, Page 3077

A. Anterior inferior cerebellar artery
B. Upper basilar artery
C. Anterior cerebral artery
D. Any of the above

1031. Which of the following is a common presentation in both medial midbrain syndrome and lateral midbrain syndrome?
Harrison's 20th Ed. Chapter 419, Page 3077 Figure 419-11

A. Paralysis of face, arm and leg
B. Hemiataxia
C. Tremor
D. Eye "down and out" on side of lesion

1032. Which of the following is not reliably detected by CT radiographic images?
Harrison's 20th Ed. Chapter 419, Page 3078

A. Cerebral infarction for first 24 to 48 hours
B. Ischemic strokes in posterior fossa
C. Small cortical infarcts
D. All of the above

Cerebral infarction infarct may not be seen reliably for 24 to 48 hours. Also, CT may fail to show small ischemic strokes in posterior fossa and small infarcts on cortical surface.

1033. "Insular ribbon sign" is an earliest indicator of?
Harrison's 16th Ed. 2386

A. Meningitis
B. Subarachnoid hemorrhage
C. Cerebral infarction
D. All of the above

"Insular ribbon sign" is caused by edema within insular cortex and basal ganglia and is an earliest indicator of cerebral infarction in MCA territory.

1034. Which of the following is used to visualize extra- or intracranial arterial dissection?
Harrison's 20th Ed. Chapter 419, Page 3078

A. MR angiography
B. MRI with fat saturation
C. MRI with IV gadolinium contrast
D. All of the above

MRI with fat saturation is used to visualize extra- or intracranial arterial dissection as it images clotted blood within dissected vessel wall.

1035. Which of the following statements is false?
Harrison's 20th Ed. Chapter 419, Page 3079

A. Transcranial Doppler (TCD) can measure success of thrombolysis following rtPA administration
B. CT perfusion imaging increases sensitivity for detecting ischemic penumbra
C. MR perfusion studies can measure ischemic penumbra
D. None of the above

Ischemic Stroke

1036. A fall in cerebral blood flow to zero causes death of brain tissue within?
Harrison's 20th Ed. Chapter 420, Page 3079
- A. 30 seconds to 1 minute
- B. 1 to 4 minutes
- C. 4 to 10 minutes
- D. 10 to 15 minutes

A fall in cerebral blood flow to zero causes death of brain tissue within 4 to 10 minutes.

1037. When cerebral blood flow falls to <16 to 18 mL/100 gram per minute, how long would it take for brain infarction?
Harrison's 20th Ed. Chapter 420, Page 3079
- A. 1 hour
- B. 2 hours
- C. 3 hours
- D. 4 hours

When cerebral blood flow falls to <16–18 mL/100 gram/minute, brain infarction occurs in 1 hour.

1038. Decrease in cerebral blood flow to what extent causes cerebral ischemia without infarction?
Harrison's 20th Ed. Chapter 420, Page 3079
- A. < 50 mL/I00 grams tissue per minute
- B. < 40 mL/I00 grams tissue per minute
- C. < 30 mL/I00 grams tissue per minute
- D. < 20 mL/I00 grams tissue per minute

Cerebral blood flow of < 20 mL/I00 grams tissue per minute causes ischemia without infarction unless prolonged for several hours or days.

1039. Location of "Ischemic penumbra" is?
Harrison's 20th Ed. Chapter 420, Page 3079
- A. Center of the core region of infarction
- B. Within the core region of infarction
- C. Surrounding the core region of infarction
- D. Any of the above

Tissue surrounding the core region of infarction is ischemic but reversibly dysfunctional and is called as the ischemic penumbra.

1040. Which of the following is false about ischemic penumbra?
Harrison's 20th Ed. Chapter 420, Page 3079
- A. Ischemic tissue around core region of infarction
- B. Reversibly dysfunctional
- C. Imaged by perfusion-diffusion imaging with MRI or CT
- D. None of the above

In ischemic penumbra, cellular death occurs by apoptosis days to weeks later. Saving the ischemic penumbra is the goal of revascularization therapies.

1041. If no improvement in cerebral flow occurs, what will happen to ischemic penumbra?
Harrison's 20th Ed. Chapter 420, Page 3079
- A. Will improve
- B. Will infarct
- C. Will continue to remain the same
- D. Any of the above

The ischemic penumbra will eventually infarct if no change in flow occurs.

1042. In ischemic penumbra, mechanism of cell death is?
Harrison's 20th Ed. Chapter 420, Page 3079
- A. Apoptosis
- B. Necrotic
- C. Mechanical
- D. Toxicity due to free radicals

In Ischemic penumbra, apoptotic cellular death occurs days to weeks later.

1043. Cerebral ischemia produces necrosis due to?
Harrison's 20th Ed. Chapter 420, Page 3079
- A. Lack of oxygen & glucose
- B. Excess extracellular glutamate
- C. Generation of free radicals
- D. All of the above

1044. Which of the following dramatically worsens brain injury during ischemia?
Harrison's 20th Ed. Chapter 420, Page 3079
- A. Fever
- B. Headache
- C. Seizure
- D. Vomiting

1045. Which of the following worsens brain injury during ischemia?
Harrison's 20th Ed. Chapter 420, Page 3079
- A. Fever
- B. Hyperglycemia
- C. Hypovolemia
- D. All of the above

Fever dramatically worsens brain injury during ischemia as does hyperglycemia. Hypovolemia should be avoided as it contributes to hypotension and worsening infarction.

1046. Which of the following favour the diagnosis of cerebral hemorrhage rather than ischemia?
Harrison's 20th Ed. Chapter 420, Page 3080
- A. Lower initial blood pressure
- B. Higher initial blood pressure
- C. Fluctuating blood pressure
- D. Any of the above

1047. Which of the following favour the diagnosis of cerebral hemorrhage rather than ischemia?
Harrison's 20th Ed. Chapter 420, Page 3080
- A. A more depressed level of consciousness
- B. Higher initial blood pressure
- C. Worsening of symptoms after onset
- D. Any of the above

A more depressed level of consciousness, higher initial blood pressure, or worsening of symptoms after onset favor hemorrhage, and a deficit that is maximal at onset or remits suggests ischemia.

1048. BP should not be lowered acutely in acute ischemic stroke because it affects blood flow in?
Harrison's 20th Ed. Chapter 420, Page 3080

A. Cerebral arteries
B. Cerebral veins
C. Collateral channels
D. All of the above

Because collateral blood flow within the ischemic brain is blood pressure dependent, blood pressure should not be lowered acutely.

1049. In acute ischemic stroke, BP should be lowered if it is?
Harrison's 20th Ed. Chapter 420, Page 3080

A. > 140/90 mm Hg
B. > 150/100 mm Hg
C. > 165/110 mm Hg
D. > 185/110 mm Hg

1050. In acute ischemic stroke, BP should be lowered if?
Harrison's 20th Ed. Chapter 420, Page 3080

A. Malignant hypertension is present
B. Concomitant myocardial ischemia present
C. Thrombolytic therapy is planned
D. All of the above

In acute ischemic stroke, BP should be lowered if there is malignant hypertension, concomitant myocardial ischemia or if BP is >185/110 mm Hg or if thrombolytic therapy is anticipated. Routine lowering of blood pressure worsens outcome.

1051. In acute ischemic stroke, serum glucose should be kept at?
Harrison's 20th Ed. Chapter 420, Page 3080

A. < 100 mg/dL
B. < 120 mg/dL
C. < 160 mg/dL
D. < 180 mg/dL

Serum glucose should be monitored and kept at < 180 mg/dL using an insulin infusion if necessary, and above 60 mg/dL.

1052. In acute ischemic stroke, what percentage of patients develop cerebral edema to cause obtundation or brain herniation?
Harrison's 20th Ed. Chapter 420, Page 3080

A. 0.5 to 1%
B. 1 to 2%
C. 2 to 4%
D. 5 to 10%

5 to 10% of patients develop enough cerebral edema to cause obtundation or brain herniation.

1053. In acute ischemic stroke, cerebral edema peaks on?
Harrison's 20th Ed. Chapter 420, Page 3080

A. Day 1
B. Day 2–3
C. Day 4–5
D. Day 5–6

In acute ischemic stroke, cerebral edema peaks on day 2 - 3 & cause mass effect for ~10 days.

1054. Which of the following point towards the diagnosis of cerebellar infarction?
Harrison's 20th Ed. Chapter 420, Page 3080

A. Vertigo
B. Vomiting
C. Head or neck pain
D. All of the above

Cerebellar infarction due to vertebral artery dissection mimics labyrinthitis because of prominent vertigo and vomiting. Head or neck pain favour the diagnosis.

1055. The time of acute ischemic stroke onset is defined as?
Harrison's 20th Ed. Chapter 420, Page 3081

A. Time the patient's symptoms began
B. Time the patient was last seen as normal
C. Time to bed in those who awaken with stroke
D. All of the above

Time of stroke onset is defined as the time patient's symptoms began or time patient was last seen as normal. A patient who awakens with stroke has the onset defined as when they went to bed.

1056. Which of the following investigation is necessary prior to IV rtPA therapy?
Harrison's 20th Ed. Chapter 420, Page 3081

A. Brain imaging
B. Blood glucose
C. PTT/International normalized ratio (INR)
D. All of the above

Only brain imaging, blood glucose and perhaps PTT/international normalized ratio (INR) are necessary prior to IV rtPA therapy.

1057. In acute ischemic stroke, rtPA is approved in US for which of the following time window?
Harrison's 20th Ed. Chapter 420, Page 3081

A. 0 to 1 hour
B. 0 to 3 hours
C. 0 to 6 hours
D. 0 to 12 hours

In acute ischemic stroke, rtPA is approved in the 3 to 4.5 hours time window in Europe and Canada, but is still only approved for 0–3 hours in United States and Canada.

1058. Following administration of rtPA, no other antithrombotic treatment must be given for?
Harrison's 20th Ed. Chapter 420, Page 3081 Table 420-1

A. 6 hours
B. 12 hours
C. 24 hours
D. 48 hours

Following administration of rtPA, no other antithrombotic treatment must be given for 24 hours.

1059. The established dose of rtPA to be administered within 3 hours of acute ischemic stroke is?
Harrison's 20th Ed. Chapter 420, Page 3081 Table 420-1

A. 0.1 mg/kg
B. 0.3 mg/kg
C. 0.9 mg/kg
D. 1.2 mg/kg

The National Institute of Neurological Disorders and Stroke (NINDS) recombinant tPA (rtPA) Stroke Study used IV rtPA (0.9 mg/kg to a 90-mg max; 10% as a bolus, then the remainder over 60 min) in patients with ischemic stroke within 3 hours of onset.

1060. Which of the following studied the value of thrombolytics via an intraarterial route in acute ischemic stroke?
Harrison's 20th Ed. Chapter 420, Page 3081

- A. PROACT II
- B. ECASS
- C. ATLANTIS
- D. NINDS

Prolyse in Acute Cerebral Thromboembolism (PROACT) II trial found benefit for intraarterial pro-urokinase for acute middle cerebral artery (MCA) occlusions up to 6th hour following onset of stroke. Intraarterial administration of a thrombolytic agent for acute ischemic stroke (AIS) is not approved by U.S. FDA.

1061. In Chinese Acute Stroke Trial (CAST), dose of aspirin was?
Harrison's 20th Ed. Chapter 420, Page 3082

- A. 75 mg/day
- B. 160 mg/day
- C. 300 mg/day
- D. 625 mg/day

In CAST, patients with ischemic stroke received 160 mg/day of aspirin for up to 4 weeks. In International Stroke Trial (IST), dose of aspirin was 300 mg/day.

1062. Neuroprotection is the concept related to?
Harrison's 20th Ed. Chapter 420, Page 3082

- A. Preventing reinfarction
- B. Prolonging brain's tolerance to ischemia
- C. Checking the risk factors
- D. All of the above

Neuroprotection refers to providing a treatment that prolongs brain's tolerance to ischemia.

1063. What percentage of strokes remain unexplained despite extensive evaluation?
Harrison's 20th Ed. Chapter 420, Page 3082

- A. 5%
- B. 20%
- C. 30%
- D. 50%

Nearly 30% of strokes remain unexplained despite extensive evaluation.

1064. Emboli in 'Hollenhorst plaque' are composed of?
Harrison's 20th Ed. Chapter 420, Page 3082

- A. Cholesterol
- B. Calcium
- C. Platelet-fibrin debris
- D. Bacteria

American ophthalmologist Dr Robert Hollenhorst (1913-2008) who first described Hollenhorst plaque as a cholesterol embolus that originated from an atheromatous plaque in a more proximal vessel, usually internal carotid artery. It is a sign of severe atherosclerosis & is seen in a blood vessel of retina on ophthalmoscopy as a bright, glistening, refractile plaque at bifurcation of a retinal arteriole. These may break up & move, and may not be present at subsequent visits.

1065. What proportion of all ischemic strokes are due to cardioembolism?
Harrison's 20th Ed. Chapter 420, Page 3082

- A. ~ 10%
- B. ~ 20%
- C. ~ 30%
- D. ~ 40%

Cardioembolism is responsible for ~20% of all ischemic strokes.

1066. Sudden onset of neurologic dysfunction in embolic stroke is usually maximum at?
Harrison's 20th Ed. Chapter 420, Page 3082

- A. Onset
- B. At 12 hours
- C. At 24 hours
- D. At 48 hours

Embolic strokes tend to be sudden in onset, with maximum neurologic deficit at the onset.

1067. Which of the following vessels is infrequently involved in embolization from heart?
Harrison's 20th Ed. Chapter 420, Page 3082

- A. Anterior cerebral artery (ACA)
- B. Middle cerebral artery (MCA)
- C. Posterior cerebral artery (PCA)
- D. Branches of posterior cerebral artery

Emboli from heart most often lodge in MCA, the PCA, or one of their branches. Anterior cerebral artery (ACA) territory is involved infrequently.

1068. Emboli of what size are large enough to occlude stem of MCA?
Harrison's 20th Ed. Chapter 420, Page 3082

- A. 0.5–1 mm
- B. 1–2 mm
- C. 2–3 mm
- D. 3–4 mm

Emboli of the size of 3 - 4 mm are large enough to occlude stem of MCA.

1069. Which of the following is the most common cause of cerebral cardioembolism?
Harrison's 20th Ed. Chapter 420, Page 3082

- A. Rheumatic heart disease with atrial fibrillation
- B. Nonrheumatic atrial fibrillation
- C. Recent MI
- D. Mitral valve prolapse

Nonrheumatic atrial fibrillation is the most common cause of cerebral embolism. Others are mural thrombus, myocardial infarction, dilated cardiomyopathy, mitral stenosis, mechanical valve, bacterial endocarditis. Mitral valve prolapse is not a source of emboli unless prolapse is severe.

1070. Patients with atrial fibrillation have an average annual risk of stroke of?
Harrison's 20th Ed. Chapter 420, Page 3082

- A. ~ 1%
- B. ~ 5%
- C. ~ 10%
- D. ~ 15%

Patients with atrial fibrillation have an average annual risk of stroke of ~ 5%.

1071. CHA_2DS_2-VASc score is calculating risk of stroke in?
Harrison's 20th Ed. Chapter 420, Page 3085 Table 420-3

- A. Nonvalvular atrial fibrillation
- B. Mitral valve prolapse
- C. Patent foramen ovale
- D. Mechanical heart value

1072. Maximum points in CHA$_2$DS$_2$-VASc score is for?
Harrison's 20th Ed. Chapter 420, Page 3085 Table 420-3

A. Diabetes mellitus
B. Hypertension
C. Congestive heart failure
D. Stroke or TIA

CHA$_2$DS$_2$-VASc score is a calculator for anticoagulation for atrial fibrillation. It is calculated by summing of points for age >75 years (2), hypertension (1), congestive heart failure (1), diabetes (1), and stroke or TIA (2). Anticoagulation is recommended for a score of ≥2.

1073. Which of the following location of recent transmural myocardial infarction is mostly the source of cerebral emboli?
Harrison's 20th Ed. Chapter 420, Page 3083

A. Anteroapical ventricular wall
B. Inferior ventricular wall
C. Posterior ventricular wall
D. Lateral ventricular wall

Recent transmural MI involving anteroapical ventricular wall is a source of cerebral emboli.

1074. Which of the following is usually not a source of cerebral emboli?
Harrison's 20th Ed. Chapter 420, Page 3083

A. Prosthetic valves
B. Mitral valve prolapse
C. Ischemic cardiomyopathy
D. Myocardial infarction

Mitral valve prolapse is usually not a source of cerebral emboli unless the prolapse is severe.

1075. Patent foramen ovale (PFO) is present in what percentage of the general population?
Harrison's 20th Ed. Chapter 420, Page 3083

A. ~ 1%
B. ~ 5%
C. ~ 10%
D. ~ 15%

Patent foramen ovale (PFO) are present in ~15% of the general population. Besides venous clot, fat, tumor emboli, bacterial endocarditis, IV air and amniotic fluid emboli at childbirth may be responsible for paradoxical embolization. Risk is elevated in the presence of a coexisting atrial septal aneurysm. However, there is no evidence for percutaneous PFO closure for stroke prevention.

1076. Most common source of artery-to-artery embolic stroke is?
Harrison's 20th Ed. Chapter 420, Page 3083

A. Aortic arch
B. Common carotid bifurcation
C. Common carotid
D. Vertebral arteries

Common carotid bifurcation and proximal internal carotid artery atherosclerosis is the most common source of artery-to-artery embolus.

1077. What proportion of all ischemic strokes are due to carotid atherosclerosis?
Harrison's 20th Ed. Chapter 420, Page 3083

A. ~ 10%
B. ~ 20%
C. ~ 30%
D. ~ 40%

10% of ischemic stroke are due to carotid atherosclerosis.

1078. Which of the following degrees of arterial narrowing is at lower risk of stroke?
Harrison's 20th Ed. Chapter 420, Page 3083

A. 50%
B. 75%
C. 90%
D. Near occlusion

Greater degrees of arterial narrowing are generally associated with a higher risk of stroke. Those with near occlusions are at lower risk of stroke.

1079. Which of the following is associated with dissections of the internal carotid or vertebral arteries?
Harrison's 20th Ed. Chapter 420, Page 3085

A. Marfan's disease
B. Cystic medial necrosis
C. Fibromuscular dysplasia
D. All of the above

Ehlers-Danlos type IV, Marfan's disease, cystic medial necrosis, and fibromuscular dysplasia are associated with dissections of the internal carotid or vertebral arteries.

1080. What proportion of all strokes are due to small-vessel disease?
Harrison's 20th Ed. Chapter 420, Page 3085

A. ~ 10%
B. ~ 20%
C. ~ 30%
D. ~ 40%

Small-vessel strokes account for ~20% of all strokes.

1081. The underlying pathology in lacunar stroke is?
Harrison's 20th Ed. Chapter 420, Page 3085

A. Congenital anomaly
B. Embolism
C. Lipohyalinosis
D. All of the above

Lacunar infarction refers to infarction following atherothrombotic or lipohyalinotic occlusion of a small artery in the brain. Lipohyalinosis appears as an eosinophilic deposit in the connective tissue of the vessel wall.

1082. In lacunar infarction, what size of a small artery is occluded in brain?
Harrison's 20th Ed. Chapter 420, Page 3085

A. 10 to 100 μm
B. 20 to 200 μm
C. 30 to 300 μm
D. 40 to 400 μm

Lacunar infarction refers to infarction following atherothrombotic or lipohyalinotic occlusion of a small artery (30 to 300 μm) in brain. These vessels are too small to be visualized on CT angiography.

1083. "Lacune" in Latin means?
Harrison's 20th Ed. Chapter 420, Page 3085

A. Deficit
B. Lake
C. River
D. Stone

Lacunes in Latin mean "lake". Clinically, lacunae are "small, deep cerebral infarcts".

1084. Lacunar infarcts range in size from?
Harrison's 20th Ed. Chapter 420, Page 3085

A. 1 mm to 5 mm
B. 1 mm to 10 mm
C. 2 mm to 10 mm
D. 3 mm to 20 mm

Lacunar infarcts range in size from 3 mm to 20 mm.

1085. The principal risk factor for lacunar infarcts is?
Harrison's 20th Ed. Chapter 420, Page 3085

A. Hypertension
B. Diabetes mellitus
C. Cigarette smoking
D. Stress

Hypertension and age are the principal risk factors for lacunar infarcts.

1086. Which of the following is not a lacunar syndrome?
Harrison's 20th Ed. Chapter 420, Page 3085

A. Pure motor hemiparesis due to infarct in posterior limb of the internal capsule or pons
B. Pure sensory stroke due to infarct in ventral thalamus
C. Ataxic hemiparesis due to infarct in ventral pons or internal capsule
D. Dysarthria and clumsy hand due to infarction in medulla

Lacunar syndrome dysarthria and a clumsy hand or arm due to infarction in the ventral pons or in the genu of the internal capsule.

1087. Lenticulostriate arteries originate from?
Harrison's 20th Ed. Chapter 420, Page 3086 Figure 420-3

A. Anterior cerebral arteries
B. Middle cerebral arteries
C. Vertebral arteries
D. All of the above

In the anterior circulation, small penetrating arteries called "lenticulostriates" arise from the proximal portion of anterior & middle cerebral arteries to supply deep subcortical structures. In the posterior circulation, similar arteries arise directly from vertebral & basilar arteries to supply brainstem.

1088. Which of the following increases risk of venous thrombosis and arterial thrombosis?
Harrison's 20th Ed. Chapter 420, Page 3085

A. Antiphospholipid syndrome
B. Systemic malignancy
C. Homocysteinemia
D. Factor V Leiden mutation

Besides increasing risk of venous thrombosis, Protein S deficiency and homocysteinemia may cause arterial thromboses as well.

1089. Which of the following can be a cause of embolic stroke?
Harrison's 20th Ed. Chapter 420, Page 3085

A. Polycythemia vera
B. Libman-Sacks endocarditis
C. Nephrotic syndrome
D. Sickle cell anemia

Systemic lupus erythematosus with Libman-Sacks endocarditis can be a cause of embolic stroke.

1090. Cerebral veins contain how much of the total cerebral blood volume?
Semin Cerebrovasc Dis Stroke. 2004;4:2-17

A. 30%
B. 50%
C. 70%
D. 90%

Cerebral veins contain 70% of the total cerebral blood volume.

1091. Veins that connect superior sagittal sinus with the scalp veins are called?
Semin Cerebrovasc Dis Stroke. 2004;4:2-17

A. Representative veins
B. Envoy veins
C. Emissary veins
D. Messenger veins

Superior sagittal sinus (SSS) drains major part of the cortex. It also receives diploic veins, themselves connected to scalp veins by emissary veins, which explains the occurrence of SSS thrombosis after scalp infection or minor head trauma.

1092. Lateral sinuses (LS) drain blood from which of the following?
Semin Cerebrovasc Dis Stroke. 2004;4:2-17

A. Cerebellum
B. Brainstem
C. Posterior part of cerebral hemispheres
D. All of the above

The lateral sinuses (LS) drain blood from the cerebellum, brainstem, and posterior part of the cerebral hemispheres. They also receive some of the diploic veins and some small veins from the middle ear, another classic source of septic thrombosis.

1093. Which of the following is a feature of superficial cerebral veins or cortical veins?
Semin Cerebrovasc Dis Stroke. 2004;4:2-17

A. Thin walls
B. No muscle fibers
C. No valves
D. All of the above

The superficial cerebral veins or cortical veins have thin walls, no muscle fibers, and no valves, thereby permitting both dilation & reversal of the direction of blood flow when the sinus into which they drain is occluded.

1094. Which of the following drain into cavernous sinuses?
Semin Cerebrovasc Dis Stroke. 2004;4:2-17

A. Superior and inferior ophthalmic veins
B. Sphenoparietal sinus
C. Middle cerebral vein
D. All of the above

Cavernous sinuses drain the blood flow from the orbits through the superior & inferior ophthalmic veins, and from the anterior part of the base of brain by the sphenoparietal sinus and the middle cerebral vein.

1095. The cavernous sinuses empty into which of the following?
Semin Cerebrovasc Dis Stroke. 2004;4:2-17

A. Superior petrosal sinus
B. Straight sinus
C. Great vein of Galen
D. Superior sagittal sinus

The cavernous sinuses empty into both the superior and the inferior petrosal sinuses and ultimately into the internal jugular veins.

1096. Thrombosis of which of the following venous sinuses mostly manifests as cranial nerve palsies?
Semin Cerebrovasc Dis Stroke. 2004;4:2-17

A. Petrosal sinuses
B. Straight sinus
C. Superior sagittal sinus
D. Transverse sinus

Because of the close relationship of the petrosal sinuses to cranial nerves, thrombosis of petrosal sinuses (with or without thrombosis of transverse sinus) may produce cranial nerve palsies, especially cranial nerves III, V, VI, VII, and VIII. Thrombosis of the petrosal sinuses is characterized mainly by a fifth nerve palsy for the superior petrosal sinus and by a sixth nerve palsy for the inferior sinus.

1097. Which of the following statements about thrombosis of cerebral venous sinuses is false?
N Engl J Med. 2005;352:1791-8

A. In most patients, thrombosis occurs in > one sinus
B. Hypoplasia & atresia of transverse sinuses frequent
C. A prothrombotic risk factor or a direct cause is identified in ~85% of patients
D. None of the above

1098. Most common pattern of clinical presentation of CVT is?
Semin Cerebrovasc Dis Stroke. 2004;4:2-17

A. Focal deficits
B. Isolated intracranial hypertension
C. Subacute diffuse encephalopathy
D. Acute painful ophthalmoplegia

The most common pattern of clinical presentations of CVT (~75%) is characterized by the presence of focal signs such as focal deficits or partial seizures. Any neurological symptoms such as aphasia, hemiparesis, hemianopsia, and amnesia can occur with CVT. CVT can be totally asymptomatic.

1099. The most frequent but least specific symptom of sinus thrombosis is?
N Engl J Med. 2005;352:1791-8

A. Severe headache
B. Ophthalmoplegia
C. Focal deficits
D. Partial seizures

The most frequent but least specific symptom of sinus thrombosis is severe headache, which is present in >90% of adult patients.

1100. Classic picture of deep cerebral venous thrombosis is?
Semin Cerebrovasc Dis Stroke. 2004;4:2-17

A. Intracranial hypertension
B. Progressive cerebellar incoordination & cranial N. palsies
C. Acute coma, decerebration & extrapyramidal hypertonia
D. Partial seizures

Classic picture of deep cerebral venous thrombosis is that of an acute coma with decerebration and extrapyramidal hypertonia leading to death within a few days, or complicated by akinetic mutism and dementia when resolving. Thrombosis of the deep venous system, the straight sinus and its branches, causes centrally located, often bilateral thalamic lesions, with behavioral symptoms such as delirium, amnesia, and mutism, which can be the only manifestation of sinus thrombosis. Thalamic edema is the imaging hallmark.

1101. Venous sinus thrombosis pertains to which of the following?
Harrison's 20th Ed. Chapter 420, Page 3085

A. Thrombosis of lateral sinus
B. Thrombosis of sagittal sinus
C. Thrombosis of small cortical veins
D. All of the above

Thrombosis of lateral or sagittal sinus or of small cortical veins fall under the category of venous sinus thrombosis.

1102. Which of the following mutation carries a high risk of venous sinus thrombosis in women who take oral contraceptives?
Harrison's 20th Ed. Chapter 420, Page 3085

A. Thrombin G20210 mutation
B. Prothrombin G20210 mutation
C. Antiprothrombin G20210 mutation
D. Antithrombin G20210 mutation

1103. Venous sinus thrombosis as a complication of which of the following?
Harrison's 20th Ed. Chapter 420, Page 3085

A. Syphilis
B. Inflammatory bowel disease
C. Rheumatoid arthritis
D. Pancreatic carcinoma

Women who take oral contraceptives and have the prothrombin G20210 mutation are at a high risk for sinus thrombosis. Also, it occurs as a complication of pregnancy and postpartum period, inflammatory bowel disease, intracranial infections (meningitis), and dehydration. It is also seen with increased incidence in patients with laboratory-confirmed thrombophilia including polycythemia, sickle cell anemia, deficiencies of proteins C and S, factor V Leiden mutation (resistance to activated protein C), antithrombin III deficiency, and homocysteinemia. Some patients with CVT carry more than one congenital thrombophilia factors. Extensive etiologic and complete coagulation work-up should be systematically performed in patients of CVT.

1104. Which of the following investigation is normal in patients with venous sinus thrombosis?
Harrison's 20th Ed. Chapter 420, Page 3085

A. CT
B. MR-venography
C. CT-venography
D. Conventional X-ray angiography

CT imaging is normal in patients with venous sinus thrombosis unless an intracranial venous hemorrhage has occurred, but the venous sinus occlusion is readily visualized using MR- or CT-venography or conventional X-ray angiography.

1105. Which of the following is the brain CT finding in a case of superior sagittal sinus thrombosis?
Semin Cerebrovasc Dis Stroke. 2004;4:2-17

A. Dense triangle sign
B. Empty delta sign
C. Cord sign
D. All of the above

Brain CT findings in CVT include the "dense triangle sign" (occlusion of SSS by fresh clot on noncontrast CT), the "empty delta sign" (filling of collateral veins in SSS wall after contrast injection, contrasting with the nonenhancement of clot inside the thrombosed sinus), and the "cord sign" (visualization of a thrombosed cortical vein on noncontrast CT). The same radiologic signs have been described on MRI. Normal brain CT scan does not rule out CVT.

1106. Use of which of the following has no proven value in intracranial hypertension management in CVT?
Semin Cerebrovasc Dis Stroke. 2004;4:2-17

A. Acetazolamide
B. Glycerol
C. Mannitol
D. Corticosteroids

Intracranial hypertension is common in CVT and should be treated immediately. Definitive treatment is establishing reperfusion of the venous structures (Heparin, Intravenous thrombolysis, thrombectomy). Elevating head of the bed by 30° improves venous drainage. Good pain control and thermal regulation, acetazolamide, glycerol, or mannitol, surgical ventricular drainage, and surgical decompression are useful. Corticosteroids should be avoided. They increase the risk of systemic infections and are of no proven value in CVT. Moreover, there is concern about their thrombogenic risk.

1107. Recurrent sinus thrombosis within one year occurs in what percentage of patients?
N Engl J Med. 2005;352:1791-8

A. 2%
B. 4%
C. 6%
D. 8%

Recurrent sinus thrombosis occurs in 2% of patients and ~4% of patients have an extracranial thrombotic event within one year.

1108. Usually, vitamin K antagonists are given for what length of time after a first episode of sinus thrombosis?
N Engl J Med. 2005;352:1791-8

A. Six months
B. One year
C. Five years
D. Life long

Optimal duration of oral anticoagulant treatment after the acute phase is unknown. Usually, vitamin K antagonists are given for six months after a first episode of sinus thrombosis, or longer in the presence of predisposing factors, with a target INR of 2.5.

1109. Anticoagulation in patients with venous sinus thrombosis is often continued indefinitely if?
Harrison's 20th Ed. Chapter 420, Page 3085

A. Hypercoagulable state is found
B. Thrombophilia is diagnosed
C. Patient has a h/o coma
D. Patient has a h/o seizure

Intravenous heparin reduces morbidity & mortality, regardless of the presence of intracranial hemorrhage. If an underlying hypercoagulable state is not found, vitamin K antagonists (VKAs) are given for 3–6 months then switch over to aspirin. Anticoagulation is often continued indefinitely if thrombophilia is diagnosed.

1110. Mortality after treatment with anticoagulant drugs in patients of cerebral venous sinus thrombosis (CVST) is?
J Neurol Neurosurg Psychiatry 2001;70:105 - 108

A. 2% to 5%
B. 5% to 10%
C. 10% to 15%
D. 15% to 20%

Treatment with anticoagulant drugs leads to a moderate benefit for patients with CVST compared with placebo treatment, but mortality after treatment with anticoagulant drugs is still 5% to 10%.

1111. Sickle cell anemia (SS disease) is a common cause of stroke in?
Harrison's 20th Ed. Chapter 420, Page 3085

A. Infants
B. Children
C. Adults
D. Old

Sickle cell anemia (SS disease) is a common cause of stroke in children.

1112. Which of the following is a common cause of stroke in children?
Harrison's 20th Ed. Chapter 420, Page 3085

A. Temporal (giant cell) arteritis
B. Hypercoagulable disorders
C. Fibromuscular dysplasia
D. Sickle cell anemia

Sickle cell anemia (SS disease) is a common cause of stroke in children.

1113. Which of the following investigation is useful in predicting stroke in childhood in SS disease carriers?
Harrison's 20th Ed. Chapter 420, Page 3085

A. MR-venography
B. CT-venography
C. Conventional X-ray angiography
D. Transcranial Doppler ultrasonography

Documenting high-velocity blood flow within MCAs using transcranial Doppler ultrasonography can predict the chances of stroke in childhood in SS disease carriers.

1114. Which of the following diseases affects cervical arteries and occurs mainly in women?
Harrison's 20th Ed. Chapter 420, Page 3085

A. Temporal (giant cell) arteritis
B. Fibromuscular dysplasia
C. Moyamoya disease
D. Binswanger's disease

Fibromuscular dysplasia affects the cervical arteries & occurs mainly in women. Carotid or vertebral arteries show multiple rings of segmental narrowing alternating with dilatation. Involvement of the renal arteries is common and may cause hypertension.

1115. Which of the following about fibromuscular dysplasia is false?
Harrison's 20th Ed. Chapter 420, Page 3085

A. Affects carotid or vertebral arteries
B. Occurs mainly in women
C. Involvement of renal arteries is common
D. None of the above

1116. Which of the following is false about Temporal (giant cell) arteritis?
Harrison's 20th Ed. Chapter 420, Page 3086

A. Affects elderly persons
B. Affects internal & external carotid system
C. May cause blindness
D. Rarely causes stroke

Temporal (giant cell) arteritis rarely causes stroke as internal carotid artery is usually not inflamed.

1117. Which is the most common form of vasculitis that affects the carotid artery?
Harrison's 20th Ed. Chapter 420, Page 3086

A. Temporal arteritis
B. Takayasu's arteritis
C. Kawasaki disease
D. Polyarteritis nodosa

1118. Moyamoya disease results from progressive stenosis and occlusion of?
Harrison's 20th Ed. Chapter 420, Page 3086

A. Distal Basilar artery
B. Distal vertebral artery
C. Distal internal carotid artery
D. None of the above

Moyamoya disease is an occlusive disease involving large intracranial arteries, especially distal internal carotid artery and stem of middle and anterior cerebral arteries.

1119. 'Moyamoya' in Japanese language means?
Harrison's 20th Ed. Chapter 420, Page 3087

A. Cotton ball
B. Pin head
C. Puff of smoke
D. Needle

Lenticulostriate arteries (anterior circulation) develop a rich collateral circulation around the occlusive lesion, which on conventional X-ray angiography appears like a "puff of smoke" (moyamoya in Japanese).

1120. In Moyamoya disease, vascular inflammation is?
Harrison's 20th Ed. Chapter 420, Page 3087

A. Absent
B. Mild
C. Moderate
D. Severe

In Moyamoya disease, vascular inflammation is absent.

1121. Posterior reversible encephalopathy syndrome (PRES) can occur with?
Harrison's 20th Ed. Chapter 420, Page 3087

A. Head injury
B. Seizure
C. Eclampsia
D. Any of the above

Posterior reversible encephalopathy syndrome (PRES) can occur with head injury, seizure, migraine, sympathomimetic drug use, eclampsia and in the postpartum period.

1122. Reversible cerebral vasoconstriction syndrome (RCVS) closely resembles which of the following?
Harrison's 20th Ed. Chapter 420, Page 3087

A. Migraine
B. Amaurosis Fugax
C. Subarachnoid hemorrhage
D. Benign positional vertigo

Reversible cerebral vasoconstriction syndrome (RCVS) typically presents with sudden, severe headache closely mimicking SAH. Patients may experience ischemic infarction and intracerebral hemorrhage and typically have new-onset severe hypertension.

1123. CADASIL is due to mutations in which gene?
Harrison's 20th Ed. Chapter 420, Page 3087

A. Notch-1
B. Notch-2
C. Notch-3
D. Notch-4

CADASIL is caused by mutations in Notch-3 gene. Notch-3 is a member of a highly conserved gene family characterized by epidermal growth factor repeats in its extracellular domain.

1124. Which of the following is categorized under monogenic disorders as a cause of stroke?
Harrison's 20th Ed. Chapter 420, Page 3087

A. CADASIL
B. CARASIL
C. HERNS
D. All of the above

Stroke due to monogenic disorders represent <1% of all stroke patients. They are cerebral autosomal-dominant arteriopathy with subcortical infarcts and leukoencephalopathy (CADASIL), cerebral autosomal-recessive arteriosclerosis with subcortical infarcts and leukoencephalopathy (CARASIL), hereditary endotheliopathy with retinopathy, nephropathy, and stroke (HERNS), Fabry disease, pseudoxanthoma elasticum, Neurofibromatosis type 1, familial MoyaMoya disease, Ehlers-Danlos syndrome type IV, Marfan syndrome.

1125. Which of the following is false about CADASIL?
Harrison's 20th Ed. Chapter 420, Page 3087

A. Onset is in IV or V decade of life
B. Autosomal recessive condition
C. Presents as small-vessel strokes, progressive dementia
D. Extensive symmetric white matter changes in MRI

CADASIL (cerebral autosomal dominant arteriopathy with subcortical infarcts and leukoencephalopathy) is an autosomal dominant inherited disorder.

1126. Which of the following is a monogenic ischemic stroke syndrome?
Harrison's 20th Ed. Chapter 420, Page 3087

A. Moyamoya disease
B. Binswanger's disease
C. CADASIL
D. None of the above

CADASIL (cerebral autosomal dominant arteriopathy with subcortical infarcts and leukoencephalopathy) is a monogenic ischemic stroke syndrome. Genetic testing is available. Other monogenic ischemic stroke syndromes include cerebral autosomal recessive arteriopathy with subcortical infarcts and leukoencephalopathy (CARASIL) and hereditary endotheliopathy, retinopathy, nephropathy, and stroke (HERNS).

1127. In Greek, word "mitos" means?
N Engl J Med. 2013;369:2236-51

A. Lamp
B. Thread
C. Tail
D. Baloon

Word mitochondrion is derived from Greek words mitos (meaning thread) and chondrion (meaning granule).

1128. Which of the following is a mitochondrial syndrome?
N Engl J Med. 2013;369:2236-51

A. Joubert syndrome
B. Senior-Loken syndrome
C. Leigh's disease
D. Caroli's syndrome

Mitochondrial syndromes include MELAS syndrome (mitochondrial encephalomyopathy, lactic acidosis, and strokelike episodes caused by mutation of mitochondrial transfer RNAs), and Leigh's disease (caused by mutations in genes related to oxidative phosphorylation).

1129. Which of the following disorders can mimic multiple sclerosis?
Harrison's 20th Ed. Page 3194 Table 436-4

A. Acute disseminated encephalomyelitis (ADEM)
B. Mitochondrial encephalopathy with lactic acidosis and stroke (MELAS)
C. Cerebral autosomal dominant arteriopathy, subcortical infarcts, and leukoencephalopathy (CADASIL)
D. All of the above

1130. Chronic progressive subcortical arteriosclerotic leukoencephalopathy is called?
Harrison's 20th Ed. Chapter 420, Page 3087

A. Moyamoya disease
B. Binswanger's disease
C. CADASIL
D. None of the above

Binswanger's disease is also called chronic progressive subcortical encephalopathy. It is one of the most common causes of dementia. The term Binswanger's disease should be used with caution, because it does not clearly identify a single entity.

1131. Small-vessel strokes, progressive dementia, and extensive symmetric white matter changes in MRI is suggestive of which of the following?
Harrison's 20th Ed. Chapter 420, Page 3087

A. Moyamoya disease
B. Binswanger's disease
C. CADASIL
D. None of the above

CADASIL (cerebral autosomal dominant arteriopathy with subcortical infarcts and leukoencephalopathy) is an inherited disorder that presents as small-vessel strokes, progressive dementia, and extensive symmetric white matter changes visualized by MRI in the fourth or fifth decade of life. It is caused by one of several mutations in Notch-3 gene.

1132. In CADASIL, which of the following is a prominent manifestation?
Harrison's 20th Ed. Chapter 420, Page 3087

A. Transient blindness
B. Migraine with aura
C. Vertigo
D. Amnesia

In CADASIL, ~40% of patients have migraine with aura.

1133. Which of the following mutation is associated with multiple small vessel strokes with hemorrhagic transformation?
Harrison's 20th Ed. Chapter 420, Page 3087

A. COL4A1
B. COL4A2
C. COL4A3
D. COL4A4

COL4A1 mutation is associated with multiple small vessel strokes with hemorrhagic transformation.

1134. In the first 3 months after TIA, risk of stroke is?
Harrison's 20th Ed. Chapter 420, Page 3087

A. ~10–15%
B. ~20–35%
C. ~40–60%
D. ~60–85%

Risk of stroke after TIA is ~10–15% in first 3 months, with most events occurring in first 2 days.

1135. Most neurologic events occur within what duration after a TIA?
Harrison's 20th Ed. Chapter 420, Page 3087

A. First 2 days
B. First 7 days
C. First 15 days
D. First 30 days

Most neurologic events occur in first 2 days after TIA. Risk of stroke is ~10% in first 3 months.

1136. Which of the following estimates risk of stroke following TIA?
Harrison's 20th Ed. Chapter 420, Page 3087 Table 420-5

A. ABCD2 Score
B. SAPS II Score
C. IPI score
D. Modified Child-Pugh classification

APACHE (acute physiology and chronic health evaluation) system and SAPS (simplified acute physiology score) system are severity-of-illness (SOI) scoring systems. International Prognostic Index (IPI) is for NHL. Modified Child-Pugh classification is a staging system for cirrhosis.

1137. Which of the following is not a part of ABCD2 Scoring system for TIA?
Harrison's 20th Ed. Chapter 420, Page 3087 Table 420-5

A. Age
B. Sex
C. Hypertension
D. Diabetes

ABCD2 Scoring system for TIA includes age, blood pressure (SBP & DBP), clinical symptoms (unilateral weakness, speech disturbance without weakness), duration and diabetes. 2 points are for unilateral weakness and duration >60 minutes each, rest have one point.

1138. Which of the following leads to poor metabolism of clopidogrel into its active form?
Harrison's 20th Ed. Chapter 420, Page 3087

A. Decreased CYP2D6 activity
B. Decreased CYP2C19 activity
C. Decreased CYP2C9 activity
D. All of the above

Failure to respond to the combination of aspirin & clopidogrel is linked to carriage of a common CYP2C19 polymorphism (common in Asians) that leads to poor metabolism of clopidogrel into its active form (clopidogrel hypometabolism).

1139. Which of the following is the most significant of the modifiable risk factors to reduce the burden of stroke?
Harrison's 20th Ed. Chapter 420, Page 3088

A. Hypertension
B. Older age
C. Diabetes mellitus
D. Dyslipidemia

1140. The average duration of a TIA is?
Harrison's 20th Ed. Chapter 420, Page 3088

A. ~1 minute
B. ~12 minutes
C. ~35 minutes
D. ~56 minutes

The average duration of a TIA is ~12 minutes.

1141. Brain infarction occurs in what percentage of TIAs even when neurologic signs and symptoms are absent?
Harrison's 18th Ed. 3280

A. 1–5%
B. 3–20%
C. 10–20%
D. 15–50%

Even in absence of neurologic signs & symptoms, infarcts of brain occur in 15 - 50% of TIAs.

1142. Systolic Blood Pressure Intervention Trial (SPRINT), recommends that all hypertension should be treated to a target of?
Harrison's 20th Ed. Chapter 420, Page 3088

A. < 120/80 mm Hg
B. < 130/80 mm Hg
C. < 140/90 mm Hg
D. < 150/90 mm Hg

1143. SPRINT trial suggests that lowering SBP to <120 mm Hg reduces stroke & heart attack by?
Harrison's 20th Ed. Chapter 420, Page 3088

A. 13%
B. 23%
C. 33%
D. 43%

SPRINT trial suggests that lowering systolic blood pressure to <120 mm Hg reduces stroke & heart attack by 43% compared to systolic blood pressure <140 mm Hg, without an increased risk of syncope or falls.

1144. Out of the following, which drug is of least importance in reducing the risk of stroke in hypertensives with TIA?
Harrison's 20th Ed. Chapter 420, Page 3088

A. Thiazide diuretics
B. Calcium channel blockers
C. Angiotensin-converting enzyme inhibitors
D. Angiotensin receptor blockers

Lowering BP to normotensive levels reduces risk of stroke in hypertensives with TIA. Drugs of value are thiazide diuretics, ACE inhibitors & ARBs. Statins reduce it by 16–30%. In diabetics, pioglitazone is effective.

1145. Which of the following is related to the trial 'SPARCL'?
Harrison's 20th Ed. Chapter 420, Page 3088

A. Aspirin
B. Pioglitazone
C. Atorvastatin
D. Clopidogrel

1146. Which of the following is false about Stroke Prevention by Aggressive Reduction in Cholesterol Levels (SPARCL) trial?
Harrison's 20th Ed. Chapter 420, Page 3088

A. Done on patients with recent stroke or TIA
B. Secondary stroke reduction
C. Dose of atorvastatin used was 80 mg/day
D. None of the above

SPARCL (Stroke Prevention by Aggressive Reduction in Cholesterol Levels) trial showed benefit in secondary stroke reduction for patients with recent stroke or TIA who were prescribed atorvastatin, 80 mg/day.

1147. Which of the following is a primary prevention trial advocating use of statins to reduce the risk of stroke?
Harrison's 20th Ed. Chapter 420, Page 3088

A. SPARCL
B. CAPRIE
C. JUPITER
D. MATCH

Justification for the Use of Statins in Prevention: An Intervention Trial Evaluating Rosuvastatin (JUPITER) was a primary prevention trial. It found that patients with low LDL (<130 mg/dL) caused by elevated C-reactive protein benefitted by daily use of rosuvastatin. Primary stroke occurrence was reduced by 51% with no increase in rates of intracranial hemorrhage.

1148. Which of the following platelet antiaggregation agents is least preferred to prevent atherothrombotic events?
Harrison's 20th Ed. Chapter 420, Page 3088

A. Aspirin
B. Clopidogrel
C. Dipyridamole
D. Ticlopidine

Though Ticlopidine is more effective than aspirin, it has been abandoned because of its adverse effects like diarrhea, skin rash, neutropenia and thrombotic thrombocytopenic purpura (TTP).

1149. Which of the following about aspirin is false?
Harrison's 20th Ed. Chapter 420, Page 3088

A. Aspirin acetylates platelet cyclooxygenase
B. Irreversibly inhibits formation of thromboxane A2 in platelets
C. Action lasts for the usual 8 day life of platelets
D. None of the above

1150. Which of the following about aspirin is false?
Harrison's 20th Ed. Chapter 420, Page 3088

A. Inhibits formation in endothelial cells of prostacyclin
B. Inhibition of prostacyclin is transient
C. Higher doses of aspirin are not more effective than lower doses
D. None of the above

1151. Which of the following about Clopidogrel is false?
Harrison's 20th Ed. Chapter 420, Page 3088

A. Clopidogrel is a prodrug
B. Thienopyridine derivative
C. Blocks adenosine diphosphate (ADP) receptor on platelets
D. None of the above

Thienopyridine derivatives include clopidogrel & prasugrel.

1152. Which of the following is an ADP receptor?
Harrison's 20th Ed. Chapter 113, Page 840

A. P2X1
B. P2Y1
C. P2Y12
D. All of the above

ADP receptors include P2X1, P2Y1, and P2Y12.

1153. Which of the following is an inhibitor of ADP P2Y12 receptor?
Harrison's 20th Ed. Chapter 114, Page 845 Figure 114-3

A. Clopidogrel
B. Prasugrel
C. Ticagrelor
D. All of the above

Clopidogrel & prasugrel irreversibly block ADP receptor on platelet surface P2Y12., Cangrelor & ticagrelor are reversible inhibitors of P2Y12.

1154. Which of the following is responsible for bioactivation of clopidogrel?
Harrison's 20th Ed. Chapter 113, Page 841

A. CYP2C9
B. DPYD
C. CYP2D6
D. CYP2C19

CYP2C19 is responsible for bioactivation of antiplatelet drug clopidogrel. Omeprazole phenocopy this effect by inhibiting CYP2C19. Loss-of-function polymorphisms in CYP2C19 is the strongest individual variable affecting pharmacokinetics & antiplatelet response to clopidogrel.

1155. Which of the following is an antiplatelet drug?
Harrison's 20th Ed. Chapter 420, Page 844

A. Cangrelor
B. Ticagrelor
C. Vorapaxar
D. All of the above

1156. Which of the following drug was studied in the CAPRIE, MATCH and CHARISMA trials?
Harrison's 20th Ed. Chapter 420, Page 3088

- A. Ticlopidine
- B. Dipyridamole
- C. Clopidogrel & Aspirin
- D. Statins

These three trials concluded that use of clopidogrel in combination with aspirin is not recommended for stroke prevention. But, may be beneficial in acute period.

1157. Which of the following trials was done for cerebral small-vessel disease?
Harrison's 20th Ed. Chapter 420, Page 3088, N Engl J Med. 2012;367:817-25

- A. SPS3 trial
- B. CHARISMA
- C. CURRENT–OASIS 7
- D. CURE

The Secondary Prevention of Small Subcortical Strokes (SPS3) trial investigators concluded that among patients with recent lacunar strokes, addition of clopidogrel to aspirin did not significantly reduce risk of recurrent stroke & did significantly increase the risk of bleeding & death.

1158. Which of the following drug was studied in the ESPS II, ESPRIT and PRoFESS trials?
Harrison's 20th Ed. Chapter 420, Page 3088

- A. Ticlopidine & Aspirin
- B. Dipyridamole & Aspirin
- C. Clopidogrel & Aspirin
- D. Statins & Aspirin

Dipyridamole with aspirin combination drug was studied in three trials.

1159. Which of the following about Dipyridamole is false?
Harrison's 20th Ed. Chapter 420, Page 3088

- A. Inhibits uptake of adenosine by vascular endothelium
- B. Potentiates antiaggregatory effects of prostacyclin
- C. Its erratic absorption depends on stomach pH
- D. None of the above

Antiplatelet agent Dipyridamole inhibits uptake of adenosine by vascular endothelium. Consequently, accumulated adenosine acts as an inhibitor of platelet aggregation. It also potentiates the antiaggregatory effects of prostacyclin. Dipyridamole is erratically absorbed depending on stomach pH.

1160. Which of the following is the principal side effect of dipyridamole?
Harrison's 20th Ed. Chapter 420, Page 3088

- A. Diarrhea
- B. Headache
- C. Skin rash
- D. Neutropenia

The principal side effect of dipyridamole is headache.

1161. What is the overall 'relative' reduction in risk of all vascular events with antiplatelet agents?
Harrison's 20th Ed. Chapter 420, Page 3088

- A. 5%
- B. 10%
- C. 18%
- D. 25%

Antiplatelet agents produce an overall relative reduction in risk of nonfatal stroke of about 25–30% and of all vascular events of about 25%.

1162. Individuals with a 10–15% risk of vascular events per year have a reduction to how much with use of antiplatelet agents?
Harrison's 20th Ed. Chapter 420, Page 3088

- A. ~ 1.5–5%
- B. ~ 7.5–11%
- C. ~ 14.5–21%
- D. ~ 27.5–41%

Individuals with a 10–15% risk of vascular events per year experience a reduction in stroke to ~ 7.5–11% with use of antiplatelet agents.

1163. How much is the average annual risk of another stroke in a patient who has experienced atherothrombotic stroke or TIA?
Harrison's 20th Ed. Chapter 420, Page 3089

- A. 3–6%
- B. 8–10%
- C. 12–20%
- D. 28–40%

Every patient who has experienced atherothrombotic stroke or TIA should take antiplatelet agent regularly, because average annual risk of another stroke is 8–10%.

1164. In chronic nonvalvular, nonrheumatic AF (NVAF), anticoagulation with warfarin reduces risk of cerebral embolism by?
Harrison's 20th Ed. Chapter 420, Page 3089

- A. ~ 17%
- B. ~ 27%
- C. ~ 47%
- D. ~ 67%

In chronic nonvalvular, nonrheumatic atrial fibrillation (NVAF), warfarin (a vitamin K antagonist - VKA) reduces the risk of cerebral embolism by ~67% both for primary & secondary prevention of stroke or TIA. The risk of a major bleeding complication is 1–3% per year.

1165. Which of the following agents was used in ARISTOTLE trial?
Harrison's 20th Ed. Chapter 420, Page 3089

- A. Apixaban
- B. Aspirin
- C. Atorvastatin
- D. Abciximab

In Apixaban for Reduction in Stroke and Other Thromboembolic Events in Atrial Fibrillation (ARISTOTLE) trial, patients were randomized between apixaban, 5 mg twice daily, and dose-adjusted warfarin (INR 2-3).

1166. Which of the following agents was used in ROCKET-AF trial?
Harrison's 20th Ed. Chapter 420, Page 3089

- A. Rivaroxaban
- B. Ramipril
- C. Rosuvastatin
- D. Recombinant tPA

Rivaroxaban Once Daily Oral Direct Factor Xa Inhibition Compared with Vitamin K Antagonism for Prevention of Stroke and Embolism Trial in Atrial Fibrillation (ROCKET-AF).

1167. Which of the following statements is false?
Harrison's 20th Ed. Chapter 420, Page 3089

- A. Intermittent AF carries the same risk of stroke as chronic AF
- B. Dabigatran requires no blood monitoring to titrate its dose
- C. Dabigatran is less effective than warfarin in patients with prosthetic heart valve implantation
- D. None of the above

1168. In ACTIVE-A trial, which of the following drugs was not used?
Harrison's 20th Ed. Chapter 420, Page 3089

A. Clopidogrel
B. Aspirin
C. Ticlopidine
D. Irbesartan

In Atrial Fibrillation Clopidogrel Trial with Irbesartan for Prevention of Vascular Events (ACTIVE-A) trial, patients who cannot take anticoagulants, clopidogrel plus aspirin was compared to aspirin alone.

1169. NASCET and ECST trials advocate carotid endarterectomy when carotid artery stenosis is more than?
Harrison's 20th Ed. Chapter 420, Page 3090

A. 30%
B. 50%
C. 70%
D. 90%

North American Symptomatic Carotid Endarterectomy Trial (NASCET) & European Carotid Surgery Trial (ECST) showed benefit for carotid endarterectomy when stenosis of ≥70%.

1170. Carotid endarterectomy is most beneficial within how many weeks of symptom onset?
Harrison's 20th Ed. Chapter 420, Page 3090

A. 2 weeks
B. 4 weeks
C. 6 weeks
D. 8 weeks

1171. Carotid endarterectomy is most beneficial in?
Harrison's 20th Ed. Chapter 420, Page 3090

A. Men
B. Those >75 years
C. When performed within 2 weeks of symptom onset
D. All of the above

Carotid endarterectomy is most beneficial when performed within 2 weeks of symptom onset. Benefits more men than women and those >75 years.

1172. Which of the following trails does not address carotid endarterectomy?
Harrison's 20th Ed. Chapter 420, Page 3090

A. ACAS
B. ECST
C. WARSS
D. NASCET

Warfarin-Aspirin Reinfarction Stroke Study (WARSS) study found no benefit of warfarin sodium over aspirin for secondary prevention of stroke. Similarly, Warfarin-Aspirin Symptomatic Intracranial Disease (WASID) study demonstrated no benefit of warfarin over aspirin in patients with symptomatic intracranial atherosclerosis. North American Symptomatic Carotid Endarterectomy Trial (NASCET) and the European Carotid Surgery Trial (ECST) showed a substantial benefit for surgery in patients with a symptomatic carotid stenosis of ≥70%. ECST found harm for patients with stenosis <30% treated surgically. Meta-analysis of NASCET and ECST trials showed that endarterectomy is most beneficial when performed within 2 weeks of symptom onset, in patients >75 years, and men appear to benefit more than women.

1173. What is the annual stroke rate in the natural history of asymptomatic carotid stenosis?
Harrison's 20th Ed. Chapter 420, Page 3090

A. ~1%
B. ~2%
C. ~3%
D. ~4%

1174. What is the annual stroke rate in the natural history of symptomatic carotid stenosis?
Harrison's 20th Ed. Chapter 420, Page 3090

A. ~10%
B. ~11%
C. ~12%
D. ~13%

The natural history of asymptomatic carotid stenosis is ~2% per year stroke rate, while symptomatic patients experience a 13% per year risk of stroke.

1175. SAPPHIRE, CREST, and ICSS pertain to which of the following?
Harrison's 20th Ed. Chapter 420, Page 3090

A. Anticoagulation in stroke
B. Use of atherothrombotics in TIA/stroke
C. Carotid artery stenting and angioplasty
D. Extracranial-to-intracranial (EC-IC) bypass surgery

Stenting and Angioplasty with Protection in Patients at High Risk for Endarterectomy (SAPPHIRE) trial was done in high risk patients with symptomatic carotid stenosis >50% or asymptomatic stenosis >80% by either stenting combined with a distal emboli-protection device or endarterectomy. Carotid Revascularization Endarterectomy versus Stenting Trial (CREST) and International Carotid Stenting (ICSS) trial also studied symptomatic patients treated with stents or endarterectomy.

1176. Which of the following has been found to be dramatically harmful in stroke treatment?
Harrison's 20th Ed. Chapter 420, Page 3091

A. Extracranial-to-intracranial (EC-IC) bypass surgery
B. Intracranial stenting of intracranial atherosclerosis
C. Balloon angioplasty coupled with stenting
D. Carotid endarterectomy

Intracranial stenting of intracranial atherosclerosis was found to be dramatically harmful as compared to aspirin in Stenting and Aggressive Medical Management for Preventing Recurrent Stroke in Intracranial Stenosis (SAMMPRIS) trial.

Intracranial Hemorrhage

1177. Bleeding into subdural and epidural spaces is principally produced by?
Harrison's 20th Ed. Chapter 421, Page 3091

- A. Trauma
- B. Coagulation disorders
- C. Hypertension
- D. Cocaine use

Bleeding into subdural and epidural spaces is principally produced by trauma.

1178. Subarachnoid hemorrhage results from?
Harrison's 20th Ed. Chapter 421, Page 3091

- A. Trauma
- B. Rupture of intracranial aneurysm
- C. Arteriovenous malformation (AVM)
- D. Any of the above

SAH results from trauma or the rupture of an intracranial aneurysm or arteriovenous malformation (AVM).

1179. Which of the following clinical trial addresses effect of acute blood pressure lowering on ICH functional outcome?
Harrison's 20th Ed. Chapter 421, Page 3091

- A. INTERACT2
- B. STICH
- C. ARUBA
- D. WASID

INTERACT2 trial is a large phase 3 clinical trial to address the effect of acute blood pressure lowering on ICH functional outcome.

1180. Which of the following is a clinical trial designed similarly to INTERACT2?
Harrison's 20th Ed. Chapter 421, Page 3091

- A. ATACH2
- B. STAR-D
- C. TACT
- D. HYVET

1181. In intraparenchymal hemorrhage, mean arterial blood pressure should be?
Harrison's 20th Ed. Chapter 421, Page 3091

- A. < 160 mm Hg
- B. < 150 mm Hg
- C. < 140 mm Hg
- D. < 130 mm Hg

1182. In patients with spontaneous ICH whose initial SBP was 150 – 220 mm Hg, systolic blood pressure can be safely lowered acutely and rapidly to?
Harrison's 20th Ed. Chapter 421, Page 3091

- A. < 110 mm Hg
- B. < 120 mm Hg
- C. < 130 mm Hg
- D. < 140 mm Hg

Systolic blood pressure (SBP) can be safely lowered acutely and rapidly to < 140 mm Hg in patients with spontaneous ICH whose initial SBP was 150 - 220 mm Hg (INTERACT2).

1183. In intraparenchymal hemorrhage, cerebral perfusion pressure should be maintained above?
Harrison's 20th Ed. Chapter 421, Page 3091

- A. 20–40 mm Hg
- B. 40–50 mm Hg
- C. 50–70 mm Hg
- D. 70–80 mm Hg

Current recommendation in hypertensive patients of intraparenchymal hemorrhage is to maintain the cerebral perfusion pressure (mean arterial pressure [MAP] minus ICP) at 50–70 mm Hg.

1184. Which of the following drugs is useful in lowering blood pressure in intraparenchymal hemorrhage?
Harrison's 20th Ed. Chapter 421, Page 3092

- A. Nicardipine
- B. Labetalol
- C. Esmolol
- D. All of the above

Intraparenchymal hemorrhage is exacerbated by acutely elevated BP & should be lowered to a mean arterial BP of <130 mm Hg by nonvasodilating IV drugs like nicardipine, labetalol or esmolol.

1185. Intraparenchymal hemorrhage accounts for what proportion of all strokes?
Harrison's 20th Ed. Chapter 421, Page 3092

- A. ~ 1%
- B. ~ 5%
- C. ~ 10%
- D. ~ 15%

1186. Out of the following hemorrhagic stroke subtypes, which has the maximum frequency of occurrence?
Harrison's 20th Ed. Chapter 421, Page 3092

- A. Intraparenchymal
- B. Subdural
- C. Epidural
- D. Subarachnoid

Intraparenchymal hemorrhage is the most common type of intracranial hemorrhage. It accounts for ~10% of all strokes and is associated with a 35–45% case fatality rate within the first month. Hypertension, coagulopathy, sympathomimetic drugs (cocaine, methamphetamine), and cerebral amyloid angiopathy (CAA) cause most of intraparenchymal hemorrhages.

1187. Which of the following is the most important cause of intraparenchymal hemorrhage in the young?
Harrison's 20th Ed. Chapter 421, Page 3092

- A. Hypertension
- B. Cerebral amyloid angiopathy
- C. Cocaine use
- D. Heavy alcohol consumption

Advanced age & heavy alcohol consumption increase risk of intraparenchymal hemorrhage. Cocaine & methamphetamine use is one of the most important cause in young (<45 years).

1188. Which of the following is associated with cocaine use?
Harrison's 20th Ed. Chapter 421, Page 3092

A. Intracerebral hemorrhage (ICH)
B. Ischemic stroke (IS)
C. Subarachnoid hemorrhage (SAH)
D. All of the above

Intracerebral hemorrhage, ischemic stroke, and SAH are all associated with cocaine use.

1189. Hypertensive intraparenchymal hemorrhage is due to spontaneous rupture of?
Harrison's 20th Ed. Chapter 421, Page 3092

A. Penetrating artery
B. Bifurcation of artery
C. Aneurysm of artery
D. Any of the above

Hypertensive intraparenchymal hemorrhage usually results from spontaneous rupture of a small penetrating artery deep in the brain.

1190. Which of the following is not a common site for hypertensive intraparenchymal hemorrhage?
Harrison's 20th Ed. Chapter 421, Page 3092

A. Basal ganglia
B. Cerebellum
C. Pons
D. Medulla oblongata

The most common sites of hypertensive intraparenchymal hemorrhage are basal ganglia (esp. putamen), thalamus, cerebellum and pons.

1191. Out of the following, which is the most common site for hypertensive intraparenchymal hemorrhage?
Harrison's 20th Ed. Chapter 421, Page 3092

A. Thalamus
B. Putamen
C. Caudate nucleus
D. Globus pallidus

Putamen is the most common site for hypertensive intraparenchymal hemorrhage.

1192. In hypertensive intraparenchymal hemorrhage, if blood dissects into the ventricular space, the morbidity?
Harrison's 20th Ed. Chapter 421, Page 3092

A. Remains the same
B. Increases
C. Decreases
D. Any of the above

In hypertensive intraparenchymal hemorrhage, blood may dissect into the ventricular space which substantially 'increases' morbidity and may cause hydrocephalus.

1193. Most hypertensive intraparenchymal hemorrhages develop over what period of time?
Harrison's 20th Ed. Chapter 421, Page 3092

A. 1 to 10 minutes
B. 10 to 30 minutes
C. 30 to 90 minutes
D. 90 to 180 minutes

Most hypertensive intraparenchymal hemorrhages develop over 30 to 90 minutes.

1194. Which of the following statements about intracerebral hemorrhages is false?
Harrison's 20th Ed. Chapter 421, Page 3092

A. Almost always occur in awake state
B. Abrupt onset of focal neurologic deficit
C. Seizures are common
D. Focal deficit worsens steadily over 30 to 90 minutes

Intracerebral hemorrhages almost always occur in awake state. Hemorrhage presents as abrupt onset of focal neurologic deficit. Seizures are uncommon. Focal deficit worsens steadily over 30–90 minutes with a diminishing level of consciousness & signs of raised ICP (headache/vomiting).

1195. In hypertensive putaminal hemorrhage, the eyes deviate towards which side?
Harrison's 20th Ed. Chapter 421, Page 3092

A. Away from the side of hemiparesis
B. Towards the side of hemiparesis
C. Remain in the center
D. Rotate upwards

In putaminal hypertensive hemorrhage, contralateral hemiparesis is the sentinel sign. Eyes deviate away from the side of hemiparesis.

1196. In hypertensive intraparenchymal hemorrhage, if there is a downward & inward deviation of eyes, the location of hemorrhage is in?
Harrison's 20th Ed. Chapter 421, Page 3092

A. Putamen
B. Thalamus
C. Pons
D. Cerebellum

Thalamic hemorrhages may extend inferiorly into upper midbrain and cause deviation of eyes downward and inward.

1197. In thalamic hemorrhage, which of the following sensory modality is affected?
Harrison's 20th Ed. Chapter 421, Page 3092

A. Exteroceptive
B. Proprioceptive
C. Cortical
D. All of the above

Thalamic hemorrhages also produce contralateral hemiplegia due to involvement of adjacent internal capsule. Prominent sensory deficit involving all modalities is usually present.

1198. Which of the following is true in thalamic hemorrhage?
Harrison's 20th Ed. Chapter 421, Page 3092

A. Unequal pupils with absence of light reaction
B. Absence of convergence
C. Ipsilateral Horner's syndrome
D. All of the above

Thalamic hemorrhages by extension inferiorly into upper midbrain may lead to homonymous visual field defect, unequal pupils with absence of light reaction, skew deviation with eye opposite hemorrhage displaced downward & medially, ipsilateral Horner's syndrome, absence of convergence, paralysis of vertical gaze, and retraction nystagmus.

1199. Contralateral pain3 syndrome is also called?
Harrison's 20th Ed. Chapter 421, Page 3092

A. Cogan's syndrome
B. Brugada syndrome
C. Wallenberg's syndrome
D. Déjérine-Roussy syndrome

Thalamic Déjérine-Roussy syndrome consists of contralateral hemisensory loss followed later by persistent agonizing, searing, or burning pain in the affected areas. It is responds poorly to analgesics. Carbamazepine, gabapentin or tricyclic antidepressants may be beneficial.

1200. In hypertensive intraparenchymal hemorrhage, if there is impairment of doll's head or oculocephalic maneuver, the location of hemorrhage is in?
Harrison's 20th Ed. Chapter 421, Page 3092

A. Putamen
B. Thalamus
C. Pons
D. Cerebellum

In pontine hemorrhages, there is impairment of reflex horizontal eye movements evoked by head turning (doll's head or oculocephalic maneuver).

1201. Which of the following is a feature of pontine hemorrhages?
Harrison's 20th Ed. Chapter 421, Page 3092

A. Hyperpnea
B. Severe hypertension
C. Hyperhidrosis
D. All of the above

1202. Excessive sweating (hyperhidrosis) is a feature of which of the following CVAs?
Harrison's 20th Ed. Chapter 421, Page 3092

A. Basal ganglia hemorrhage
B. Thalamic hemorrhage
C. Pontine hemorrhage
D. Cerebellar hemorrhage

Presentation of pontine hemorrhage include sudden onset, pinpoint pupils (1 mm) reactive to light, loss of reflex eye movements and corneal responses, ocular bobbing, posturing, hyperventilation, severe hypertension and excessive sweating.

1203. Decerebrate rigidity is most frequent which of the following hypertensive intraparenchymal hemorrhage?
Harrison's 20th Ed. Chapter 421, Page 3092

A. Basal ganglia hemorrhage
B. Thalamic hemorrhage
C. Pontine hemorrhage
D. Cerebellar hemorrhage

In pontine hemorrhages, deep coma with quadriplegia usually occurs over a few minutes with prominent decerebrate rigidity.

1204. Cerebellar hemorrhages are characterized by?
Harrison's 20th Ed. Chapter 421, Page 3092

A. Occipital headache
B. Repeated vomiting
C. Ataxia of gait
D. All of the above

Cerebellar hemorrhages develop over several hours & are characterized by occipital headache, repeated vomiting, and ataxia of gait.

1205. In mild cases of cerebellar hemorrhage, there may be no other neurologic sign other than?
Harrison's 20th Ed. Chapter 421, Page 3092

A. Gait ataxia
B. Occipital headache
C. Repeated vomiting
D. Seizure

In mild cases of cerebellar hemorrhage, there may be no other neurologic signs other than gait ataxia.

1206. Which of the following about cerebellar hemorrhage is false?
Harrison's 20th Ed. Chapter 421, Page 3092

A. Forced deviation of eyes to opposite side
B. Paresis of conjugate lateral gaze toward side of hemorrhage
C. Usually develop over several hours
D. None of the above

In cerebellar hemorrhage, dizziness or vertigo may be prominent. There is paresis of conjugate lateral gaze toward the side of hemorrhage, forced deviation of eyes to opposite side, or an ipsilateral sixth nerve palsy.

1207. Which of the following lobar hemorrhage causes arm weakness?
Harrison's 20th Ed. Chapter 421, Page 3093

A. Occipital hemorrhage
B. Left temporal hemorrhage
C. Parietal hemorrhage
D. Frontal hemorrhage

Major neurologic deficit with occipital hemorrhage is hemianopia, with left temporal hemorrhage, it is aphasia and delirium, with parietal hemorrhage, it is a hemisensory loss and with frontal hemorrhage, it is arm weakness.

1208. Which of the following is uncommon in lobar hemorrhages?
Harrison's 20th Ed. Chapter 421, Page 3093

A. Focal headaches
B. Vomiting
C. Drowsiness
D. Stiff neck

Most patients with lobar hemorrhages have focal headaches and more than half vomit or are drowsy. Stiff neck and seizures are uncommon.

1209. Which of the following is mainly affected in cerebral amyloid angiopathy?
Harrison's 20th Ed. Chapter 421, Page 3093

A. Arterioles
B. Venules
C. Capillaries
D. All of the above

1210. Cerebral amyloid angiopathy affects mainly?
Harrison's 20th Ed. Chapter 421, Page 3093

A. Children
B. Adults
C. Elderly
D. All of the above

Cerebral amyloid angiopathy is a disease of the elderly in which arteriolar degeneration occurs and amyloid is deposited in the walls of the cerebral arteries.

1211. Cerebral amyloid angiopathy cause which of the following?
Harrison's 20th Ed. Chapter 421, Page 3093

A. Intraparenchymal hemorrhage
B. Lobar hemorrhage
C. Cerebellar hemorrhage
D. Subarachnoid hemorrhage

Cerebral amyloid angiopathy causes both single and recurrent lobar hemorrhages and is the most common cause of lobar hemorrhage in elderly.

1212. Intracranial hemorrhages associated with anticoagulant therapy occur in?
Harrison's 20th Ed. Chapter 421, Page 3093

A. Lobar hemorrhage
B. Thalamic hemorrhage
C. Pontine hemorrhage
D. Any location

Intracranial hemorrhages associated with anticoagulant therapy & hematologic disorders can occur at any location (lobar or subdural) and may present as multiple intracerebral hemorrhages. Skin and mucous membrane bleeding is usually evident and offers a diagnostic clue.

1213. Which of the following hematologic disorders can cause ICH?
Harrison's 20th Ed. Chapter 421, Page 3093

A. Leukemia
B. Aplastic anemia
C. Thrombocytopenic purpura
D. All of the above

ICH associated with hematologic disorders like leukemia, aplastic anemia and thrombocytopenic purpura. Any site is possible and may present as multiple ICHs.

1214. Which of the following is a cause of stroke in young?
Harrison's 20th Ed. Chapter 421, Page 3093

A. Cocaine use
B. Moyamoya disease
C. Dissection of the internal carotid or vertebral arteries
D. All of the above

1215. Which of the following is associated with stimulant use?
Harrison's 20th Ed. Chapter 421, Page 3093

A. ICH
B. Ischemic stroke
C. Subarachnoid hemorrhage (SAH)
D. All of the above

Cocaine enhances sympathetic activity causing acute, sometimes severe, hypertension, and this may lead to hemorrhage. Over 50% of stimulant-related intracranial hemorrhages are intracerebral & rest are subarachnoid when a saccular aneurysm is usually identified. Acute hypertension causes aneurysmal rupture.

1216. Which of the following worsens the prognosis in intracerebral hemorrhage?
Harrison's 20th Ed. Chapter 421, Page 3093

A. Extension into the ventricular system
B. Advanced age
C. Location within the posterior fossa
D. All of the above

Extension into ventricular system, advanced age, location within posterior fossa & depressed level of consciousness at initial presentation worsens prognosis in intracerebral hemorrhage.

1217. Which of the following metastatic tumors is associated with ICH?
Harrison's 20th Ed. Chapter 421, Page 3093

A. Choriocarcinoma
B. Renal cell carcinoma
C. Bronchogenic carcinoma
D. All of the above

Choriocarcinoma, malignant melanoma, renal cell carcinoma and bronchogenic carcinoma are among the most common metastatic tumors associated with ICH.

1218. What volume of supratentorial hematomas due to hypertensive intracerebral hemorrhage have a good prognosis?
Harrison's 20th Ed. Chapter 421, Page 3094

A. < 30 mL
B. < 60 mL
C. < 90 mL
D. < 120 mL

1219. What volume of supratentorial hematomas due to hypertensive intracerebral hemorrhage have a poor prognosis?
Harrison's 20th Ed. Chapter 421, Page 3094

A. > 10 mL
B. > 25 mL
C. > 40 mL
D. > 60 mL

Volume and location of hematoma determine prognosis. Supratentorial hematomas due to hypertensive intracerebral hemorrhage with volumes <30 mL have a good prognosis 30 to 60 mL, an intermediate prognosis and >60 mL, a poor prognosis during initial hospitalization.

1220. What diameter of cerebellar hematoma will require surgical evacuation?
Harrison's 20th Ed. Chapter 421, Page 3094

A. > 0.5 cm
B. > 1.5 cm
C. > 2 cm
D. > 3 cm

Most cerebellar hematomas >3 cm in diameter require surgical evacuation.

1221. Reversible posterior leukoencephalopathy best relates to which of the following?
Harrison's 20th Ed. Chapter 421, Page 3093

A. Hypertensive encephalopathy
B. Intracranial hemorrhages due to anticoagulant therapy
C. Head injury
D. Primary intraventricular hemorrhage

MRI brain imaging shows a pattern of typically posterior (occipital > frontal) brain edema that is reversible and termed reversible posterior leukoencephalopathy.

1222. Hemorrhages into the spinal cord are usually the result of?
Harrison's 20th Ed. Chapter 421, Page 3093

A. AVM
B. Cavernous malformation
C. Metastatic tumor
D. All of the above

Hemorrhages into spinal cord are the result of an AVM, cavernous malformation or metastatic tumor.

1223. Spot sign best relates to?
Harrison's 20th Ed. Chapter 421, Page 3094

A. Subdural hematoma
B. Intraventricular leak
C. Ongoing bleeding within a hematoma
D. Hemangioma

CT angiography (CTA) or postcontrast CT imaging may reveal one or more small areas of enhancement within a hematoma. This "spot sign" represents ongoing bleeding. Presence of a spot sign is associated with an increased risk of hematoma expansion, increased mortality and lower likelihood of favorable functional outcome.

1224. Which is the agent of first choice in reversing warfarin induced coagulopathy in intracerebral hemorrhage?
Harrison's 20th Ed. Chapter 421, Page 3094

A. Prothrombin complex concentrate infusion
B. Fresh-frozen plasma
C. Vitamin K
D. Any of the above

Agent of first choice in reversing warfarin induced coagulopathy in intracerebral hemorrhage is prothrombin complex concentrate (PCCs). Fresh frozen plasma (FFP) is an alternative.

1225. Which of the following is an effective antidote to oral thrombin inhibitor dabigatran?
Harrison's 20th Ed. Chapter 421, Page 3094

A. Vitamin K
B. Prothrombin complex concentrates (PCC)
C. Fresh frozen plasma
D. None of the above

There is no effective antidote to ICH associated with oral thrombin inhibitor dabigatran. PCC may partially reverse the effects of oral factor Xa inhibitors and are reasonable to administer if available.

1226. Which of the following is a monoclonal antibody to dabigatran?
Harrison's 20th Ed. Chapter 421, Page 3094

A. Andexanet alfa
B. Idarucizumab
C. Ciraparantag
D. All of the above

Idarucizumab is a monoclonal antibody to dabigatran and is a specific reversal agent for dabigatran. It binds dabigatran with high affinity to form a 1:1 complex that is then cleared by kidneys. Idarucizumab is given as an intravenous bolus of 5 gram.

1227. Which of the following is a universal anti-Xa antidote?
Harrison's 20th Ed. Chapter 273, Page 1915

A. Eptinezumab
B. Fremanezumab
C. Andexanet
D. Galcanezumab

Andexanet is a universal anti-Xa antidote for betrixaban, rivaroxaban, apixaban, and edoxaban.

1228. Which of the following is not helpful for the edema from intracerebral hematoma?
Harrison's 20th Ed. Chapter 421, Page 3094

A. Glucocorticoids
B. Osmotic agents
C. Induced hyperventilation
D. Ventriculostomy

Glucocorticoids are not helpful for the edema from intracerebral hematoma.

1229. Largest AVMs are most frequently found in?
Harrison's 20th Ed. Chapter 421, Page 3095

A. Anterior half of hemispheres
B. Posterior half of hemispheres
C. Brainstem
D. Spinal cord

AVMs occur in all parts of cerebral hemispheres, brainstem & spinal cord. The largest ones are mostly located in posterior half of the hemispheres, commonly forming a wedge-shaped lesion extending from cortex to the ventricle.

1230. Bleeding, headache and seizures due to AVMs are most common between the ages of?
Harrison's 20th Ed. Chapter 421, Page 3095

A. 1 and 10 years
B. 10 and 30 years
C. 30 and 50 years
D. 50 and 75 years

Bleeding, headache and seizures due to AVMs are most common between the ages of 10 & 30 years.

1231. Which of the following is a familial AVM?
Harrison's 20th Ed. Chapter 421, Page 3095

A. Sagging brain syndrome
B. Osler-Rendu-Weber syndrome
C. Posterior cortical atrophy syndrome
D. Capgras' syndrome

Familial AVM may be a part of the autosomal dominant syndrome of hereditary hemorrhagic telangiectasia called Osler-Rendu-Weber syndrome. It is due to mutations in either endoglin or activin receptor-like kinase 1, both involved in transforming growth factor (TGF) signaling & angiogenesis.

1232. Which of the following statements about AVM bleed is false?
Harrison's 20th Ed. Chapter 421, Page 3095

A. Hemorrhage is mainly intraparenchymal
B. Symptomatic cerebral vasospasm is rare
C. Smaller lesions have a higher hemorrhage rate
D. MRI is gold standard for evaluating anatomy of AVM

Hemorrhage is mainly intraparenchymal. Symptomatic cerebral vasospasm is rare. Smaller lesions have a higher hemorrhage rate. Conventional X-ray angiography is the gold standard for evaluating precise anatomy of AVM.

1233. Which of the following increases risk of AVM rupture?
Harrison's 20th Ed. Chapter 421, Page 3095

A. Presence of deep venous drainage
B. Presence of venous outflow stenosis
C. Presence of intranidal aneurysms
D. All of the above

Paradoxically, smaller AVM lesions have a higher hemorrhage rate.

1234. Which of the following is a common location of capillary telangiectasias in brain?
Harrison's 20th Ed. Chapter 421, Page 3095

A. Pons
B. Mid brain
C. Medulla oblongata
D. Cerebellum

Capillary telangiectasias are true capillary malformations located typically in pons and deep cerebral white matter as in hereditary hemorrhagic telangiectasia (Osler-Rendu-Weber) syndrome. Bleeding rarely produces mass effect or significant symptoms.

1235. Intracranial hemorrhage located usually in brainstem is due to which of the following?
Harrison's 20th Ed. Chapter 421, Page 3092 Table 421-1

A. Hypertensive hemorrhage
B. Cocaine abuse
C. Capillary telangiectasias
D. Arteriovenous malformation

Capillary telangiectasias are true capillary malformations in normal brain structure. Pons & deep cerebral white matter are typical locations. Hereditary hemorrhagic telangiectasia (Osler-Rendu-Weber) syndrome is an example.

1236. Lobar intracranial Hemorrhage is due to?
Harrison's 20th Ed. Chapter 421, Page 3092 Table 421-1

A. Metastatic brain tumor
B. Amyloid angiopathy
C. Arteriovenous malformation
D. All of the above

1237. Which of the following is not an acquired vascular lesions?
Harrison's 20th Ed. Chapter 421, Page 3095

A. Dural arteriovenous fistulas
B. Cavernous angiomas
C. Capillary telangiectasias
D. None of the above

Capillary telangiectasias are true capillary malformations. Dural AV fistulas are acquired connections from a dural artery to dural sinus. Cavernous angiomas are tufts of capillary sinusoids in deep hemispheric white matter & brainstem with no normal intervening neural structures.

1238. Which of the following gene is responsible in causing cavernous angiomas?
Harrison's 20th Ed. Chapter 421, Page 3095, N Engl J Med. 2002;347:1711

A. NOTCH3
B. APP
C. BRI
D. KRIT1

KRIT1, CCM2 and PDCD10 have been identified as genes causing cavernous angiomas. KRIT1 and CCM2 have a role in blood vessel formation. PDCD10 is an apoptotic gene.

1239. Pulse-synchronous cephalic bruit ("pulsatile tinnitus") is a feature of?
Harrison's 20th Ed. Chapter 421, Page 3095

A. Dural arteriovenous fistulas
B. Cavernous angiomas
C. Capillary telangiectasias
D. All of the above

1240. Which of the following genes can cause autosomal dominant amyloid angiopathies?
N Engl J Med. 2002;347:1711

A. APP
B. CST3
C. BRI
D. All of the above

APP, CST3, BRI genes cause autosomal dominant amyloid angiopathies.

1241. Primary class of antibody that is associated with antiphospholipid antibody syndrome is?
Harrison's 20th Ed. Chapter 350, Page 2526

A. Anticardiolipin antibodies (aCL)
B. Lupus anticoagulant (LA)
C. Antibodies against β2GP1 (anti-β2GPI)
D. All of the above

1242. Thrombotic events associated with antiphospholipid antibodies include?
Harrison's 20th Ed. Chapter 350, Page 2526

A. Deep vein thrombosis (DVT)
B. Pulmonary embolus
C. Placental vascular thrombosis
D. All of the above

1243. The lupus anticoagulants prolong which of the following coagulation test results?
Disease-a-Month. 2003;49:696-741

A. Activated partial thromboplastin time (aPTT)
B. Prothrombin time
C. Dilute Russell viper venom time (dRVVT)
D. All of the above

1244. Which of these is a natural anticoagulant?
Disease-a-Month. 2003;49:696-741

A. Beta2-Gp1
B. Activated protein C
C. Annexin V
D. All of the above

1245. Sneddon syndrome consists of?
Disease-a-Month. 2003;49:696-741

A. Stroke
B. Livido reticularis
C. Hypertension
D. All of the above

1246. Obstetric complications in antiphospholipid syndrome are usually seen at?
Disease-a-Month. 2003;49:696-741

A. 10 or more weeks of gestation
B. 8 or more weeks of gestation
C. 6 or more weeks of gestation
D. 4 or more weeks of gestation

1247. Which of the following is the preferred test for diagnosis of antiphospholipid antibody?
Disease-a-Month. 2003;49:696-741

A. aPTT
B. KCT
C. dRVVT
D. Bleeding time

1248. Antiphospholipid syndrome is a disorder characterized by?
Disease-a-Month. 2003;49:696-741

A. Recurrent arterial thrombosis
B. Spontaneous abortions
C. Thrombocytopenia
D. All of the above

Subarachnoid Hemorrhage

1249. Which of the following is false about idiopathic SAHs localized to perimesencephalic cisterns?
Harrison's 20th Ed. Chapter 302, Page 2084

A. Benign
B. Venous or capillary source
C. Angiography is unrevealing
D. None of the above

Some idiopathic SAHs are localized to perimesencephalic cisterns and are benign with a venous or capillary source. Angiography is unrevealing.

1250. Which of the following is the most common cause of SAH?
Harrison's 20th Ed. Chapter 302, Page 2084

A. Rupture of a saccular aneurysm
B. Bleeding from a vascular anomaly
C. Extension into subarachnoid space from a primary intracerebral hemorrhage
D. Idiopathic

After head trauma, the most common cause of SAH is rupture of a saccular aneurysm.

1251. What percentage of adults harbor intracranial aneurysms?
Harrison's 20th Ed. Chapter 302, Page 2084

A. 1%
B. 2%
C. 3%
D. 4%

Autopsy & angiography studies show that ~2% of adults harbor intracranial aneurysms.

1252. In SAH, the mortality rate over the first month is?
Harrison's 20th Ed. Chapter 302, Page 2084

A. ~15%
B. ~25%
C. ~35%
D. ~45%

SAH patients who arrive alive at hospital, the mortality rate over the next month is ~45%.

1253. In SAH, the rate of rebleeding in the first month is about?
Harrison's 20th Ed. Chapter 302, Page 2084

A. 20%
B. 30%
C. 40%
D. 50%

In SAH, if the patient survives but aneurysm is not obliterated, the rate of rebleeding is about 20% in first 2 weeks, 30% in first month.

1254. Annual risk of rupture for aneurysms ≥10 mm in size is?
Harrison's 20th Ed. Chapter 302, Page 2084

A. ~0.1–0.5%
B. ~0.5–1%
C. ~1.0–1.5%
D. ~1.5–2%

Annual risk of rupture for aneurysms <10 mm size is ~0.1%, for aneurysms ≥10 mm in size it is ~0.5–1%.

1255. An aneurysm is termed 'Giant' when its diameter is?
Harrison's 20th Ed. Chapter 302, Page 2084

A. >0.5 cm
B. >1.0 cm
C. >1.5 cm
D. >2.5 cm

Berry aneurysms >2.5 cm in diameter are called giant aneurysms, and account for 5% of cases.

1256. Most common location of an intracranial aneurysm is?
Harrison's 20th Ed. Chapter 302, Page 2084

A. Anterior communicating artery
B. Posterior communicating artery
C. Terminal internal carotid artery
D. Vertebral artery

1257. Most common location of an intracranial aneurysm is?
Harrison's 20th Ed. Chapter 302, Page 2084

A. Anterior communicating artery
B. MCA bifurcation
C. Posterior communicating artery
D. Middle of basilar artery

1258. Most common location of an intracranial aneurysm is?
Harrison's 20th Ed. Chapter 302, Page 2084

A. Anterior communicating artery
B. Posterior communicating artery
C. Top of basilar artery
D. Middle of basilar artery

The three most common locations of berry aneurysms are the terminal internal carotid artery, MCA bifurcation, and top of basilar artery. Their risk of rupture is ~6% in the first year.

1259. Mycotic aneurysms are best related to?
Harrison's 20th Ed. Chapter 302, Page 2084

A. Hypertension
B. Diabetes mellitus
C. Bacterial endocarditis
D. Trauma

Mycotic aneurysms are usually located distal to the first bifurcation of major arteries of the circle of Willis. Most result from infected emboli due to bacterial endocarditis.

1260. Mycotic aneurysms are usually located distal to which bifurcation of major arteries of circle of Willis?
Harrison's 20th Ed. Chapter 302, Page 2084

A. 1st
B. 2nd
C. 3rd
D. 4th

Mycotic aneurysms due to infected emboli are usually located distal to the first bifurcation of major arteries of the circle of Willis.

1261. Anterior circulation accounts for what percentage of all intracranial aneurysms?
Harrison's 20th Ed. Chapter 302, Page 2084

A. 25%
B. 45%
C. 65%
D. 85%

~85% of aneurysms occur in the anterior circulation, mostly on the circle of Willis.

1262. What percentage of all intracranial aneurysms are multiple?
Harrison's 20th Ed. Chapter 302, Page 2084

A. 5%
B. 10%
C. 20%
D. 40%

~20% of patients have multiple aneurysms, many at mirror sites bilaterally.

1263. Which of the following characteristics of a berry aneurysm make it at greater risk of rupture?
Harrison's 20th Ed. Chapter 302, Page 2084

A. >7 mm in diameter
B. At the top of basilar artery
C. At the origin of posterior communicating artery
D. Any of the above

Those >7 mm in diameter and those at the top of the basilar artery and at the origin of the posterior communicating artery are at greater risk of rupture.

1264. The site of rupture of a berry aneurysm is?
Harrison's 20th Ed. Chapter 302, Page 2084

A. Base of the neck
B. Top of the neck
C. Dome
D. Any of the above

The site of rupture of a berry aneurysm most often is the dome. As an aneurysm develops, it typically forms a neck with a dome. Arterial internal elastic lamina disappears at the base of neck. Media thins & connective tissue replaces smooth-muscle cells. Most often, the dome is the site of rupture.

1265. Patients first complaint upon regaining consciousness in SAH is?
Harrison's 20th Ed. Chapter 302, Page 2084

A. Blurred vision
B. Headache
C. Thirst
D. Nausea

Most patients first complain of headache upon regaining consciousness.

1266. The location of headache in SAH is?
Harrison's 20th Ed. Chapter 302, Page 2084

A. Frontal
B. Occipital
C. Temporal
D. Generalized

In SAH, headache is sudden, usually generalized, often with neck stiffness and vomiting.

1267. Which of the following is a feature of headache in SAH?
Harrison's 20th Ed. Chapter 302, Page 2084

A. Sudden onset
B. Severe headache associated with exertion
C. A change in the patient's usual headache pattern
D. All of the above

1268. Which of the following is a feature of aneurysmal rupture SAH?
Harrison's 20th Ed. Chapter 302, Page 2084

A. Sudden headache
B. Absence of focal neurologic symptoms
C. Generalized headache with neck stiffness and vomiting
D. All of the above

1269. Common deficits that result due to middle cerebral bifurcation aneurysmal rupture include all except?
Harrison's 20th Ed. Chapter 302, Page 2084

A. Hemiparesis
B. Aphasia
C. Abulia
D. Acalculia

ACA or MCA bifurcation aneurysms may rupture into adjacent brain or subdural space and form a hematoma large enough to produce mass effect resulting in hemiparesis, aphasia and abulia.

1270. III cranial nerve palsy, with pupillary dilatation, loss of ipsilateral light reflex and focal pain above or behind the eye suggests what location of an aneurysm?
Harrison's 20th Ed. Chapter 302, Page 2084

A. Posterior communicating artery aneurysm
B. Aneurysm in the cavernous sinus
C. Anterior cerebral artery aneurysm
D. Anterior inferior cerebellar artery aneurysm

1271. VI cranial nerve palsy suggests what location of an aneurysm?
Harrison's 20th Ed. Chapter 302, Page 2084

A. Posterior communicating artery aneurysm
B. Aneurysm in the cavernous sinus
C. Anterior cerebral artery aneurysm
D. Anterior inferior cerebellar artery aneurysm

1272. Occipital and posterior cervical pain suggests what location of an aneurysm?
Harrison's 20th Ed. Chapter 302, Page 2084

A. Posterior communicating artery aneurysm
B. Aneurysm in the cavernous sinus
C. Anterior cerebral artery aneurysm
D. Anterior inferior cerebellar artery aneurysm

1273. Visual field defects suggests what location of an aneurysm?
Harrison's 20th Ed. Chapter 302, Page 2084

A. Posterior communicating artery aneurysm
B. Aneurysm in the cavernous sinus
C. Anterior cerebral artery aneurysm
D. Anterior inferior cerebellar artery aneurysm

1274. Occipital and posterior cervical pain suggests what location of an aneurysm?
Harrison's 20th Ed. Chapter 302, Page 2084

A. Posterior communicating artery aneurysm
B. Aneurysm in the cavernous sinus
C. Anterior cerebral artery aneurysm
D. Posterior inferior cerebellar artery aneurysm

1275. Pain in or behind the eye and in the low temple suggests what location of an aneurysm?
Harrison's 20th Ed. Chapter 302, Page 2084

A. Posterior communicating artery aneurysm
B. Aneurysm in the cavernous sinus
C. Anterior cerebral artery aneurysm
D. MCA aneurysm

III cranial nerve palsy associated with pupillary dilatation, loss of ipsilateral light reflex and focal pain above or behind the eye, may occur with an expanding aneurysm at the junction of posterior communicating artery and internal carotid artery. VI cranial nerve palsy may indicate an aneurysm in cavernous sinus, and visual field defects can occur with an anterior cerebral artery aneurysm. Occipital and posterior cervical pain may signal a posterior inferior cerebellar artery or anterior inferior cerebellar artery aneurysm. Pain in or behind the eye and in the low temple can occur with an expanding MCA aneurysm.

1276. 'Sentinel bleed' is the term used for small aneurysmal rupture into?
Harrison's 20th Ed. Chapter 302, Page 2085

A. Subarachnoid space
B. White matter
C. Gray matter
D. Thalamus

Aneurysms with small ruptures & leaks of blood into subarachnoid space are sentinel bleeds. "Sentinel" or "warning" headache is a sudden, severe headache that resolves & that is retrospectively identified to have occurred days to weeks before the SAH.

1277. 'Wide-neck aneurysms' are those in which the ratio of neck diameter to that of the largest dome is?
N Engl J Med. 2006;354:387-96

A. > 0.2
B. > 0.3
C. > 0.4
D. > 0.5

1278. In a case of SAH who also has third-nerve palsy, which artery is possibly involved?
N Engl J Med. 2006;354:387-96

A. Anterior communicating artery
B. Posterior communicating artery
C. Anterior cerebral artery
D. Middle cerebral artery

1279. In a case of SAH who also has bilateral weakness in legs or abulia, which artery is possibly involved?
N Engl J Med. 2006;354:387-96

A. Anterior communicating artery
B. Posterior communicating artery
C. Anterior cerebral artery
D. Middle cerebral artery

1280. In a case of SAH who also has aphasia, hemiparesis, or visuospatial neglect, which artery is possibly involved?
N Engl J Med. 2006;354:387-96

A. Anterior communicating artery
B. Posterior communicating artery
C. Anterior cerebral artery
D. Middle cerebral artery

1281. In a case of SAH who also has retinal and subhyaloid hemorrhage, which artery is possibly involved?
N Engl J Med. 2006;354:387-96

A. Anterior communicating artery
B. Posterior communicating artery
C. Anterior cerebral artery
D. Any of the above

1282. Clinical scale of Hunt and Hess is used in?
Harrison's 20th Ed. Chapter 302, Page 2085, N Engl J Med. 2006;354:387-96

A. Bacterial meningitis
B. HIV dementia
C. Subarachnoid hemorrhage
D. Multiple sclerosis

Initial clinical manifestations of SAH can be graded by Hunt-Hess or World Federation of Neurosurgical Societies (WFNS) classification.

1283. Which of the following grading systems is related to SAH?
CCJM 2015;82(3):177-192

A. Hunt and Hess
B. World Federation of Neurological Surgeons (WFNS)
C. Fisher or its modified version
D. All of the above

Different grading systems used for SAH are based on the findings on initial neurologic examination and on initial noncontrast CT (thickness of blood and intraventricular hemorrhage) are those developed by Hunt and Hess and by the World Federation of Neurosurgical Surgeons (WFNS), and the CT grading scales (Fisher or its modified version).

1284. Which of the following is not a cause of delayed neurologic deficit in SAH?
Harrison's 20th Ed. Chapter 302, Page 2085

A. Infection
B. Hydrocephalus
C. Vasospasm
D. Hyponatremia

There are four major causes of delayed neurologic deficits in SAH. They are rerupture, hydrocephalus, vasospasm, and hyponatremia.

1285. Peak incidence of rerupture of an untreated aneurysm following SAH is within?
Harrison's 20th Ed. Chapter 302, Page 2085

A. 1 day
B. 3 days
C. 7 days
D. 14 days

Incidence of rerupture of an untreated aneurysm in the first month following SAH is ~30% with the peak in the first 7 days. Rerupture is associated with a 50% mortality rate and poor outcome.

1286. Chronic hydrocephalus after SAH manifests as?
Harrison's 20th Ed. Chapter 302, Page 2085

A. Gait difficulty
B. Incontinence
C. Impaired mentation
D. All of the above

Hydrocephalus is the most common early neurologic complication after aneurysmal subarachnoid hemorrhage, with an overall incidence of 50%. Chronic hydrocephalus may develop weeks to months after SAH and manifest as gait difficulty, incontinence, or impaired mentation.

1287. Delayed vasospasm in SAH is due to?
Harrison's 20th Ed. Chapter 302, Page 2085

A. Hypertension
B. Hyperviscosity
C. Clotted blood & its breakdown products on artery
D. All of the above

Delayed vasospasm is due to direct effects of clotted blood & its breakdown products on arteries within subarachnoid space.

1288. Signs of cerebral ischemia due to vasospasm following SAH is most often on which day?
Harrison's 20th Ed. Chapter 302, Page 2085

A. Day 1
B. Day 3
C. Day 7
D. Day 14

Signs of cerebral ischemia appear 4 to 14 days after SAH, most often at 7 days.

1289. In most cases of SAH, focal vasospasm is preceded by?
Harrison's 20th Ed. Chapter 302, Page 2085

A. Headache
B. Seizure
C. Decline in mental status
D. Vomiting

In most SAH cases, focal vasospasm is preceded by decline in mental status.

1290. Hyponatremia following SAH is due to?
Harrison's 20th Ed. Chapter 302, Page 2085

A. Inappropriate secretion of vasopressin
B. Secretion of atrial natriuretic factors
C. Secretion of brain natriuretic factors
D. All of the above

Hyponatremia following SAH or "cerebral salt-wasting syndrome" develop in first 2 weeks due to inappropriate secretion of vasopressin & secretion of atrial and brain natriuretic peptides. It should not be treated with free-water restriction as this may increase risk of stroke. It clears over 1 to 2 weeks.

1291. Xanthochromic CSF in SAH usually lasts for?
Harrison's 20th Ed. Chapter 302, Page 2085

A. 1 to 4 days
B. 1 to 2 weeks
C. 1 to 3 weeks
D. 1 to 4 weeks

Xanthochromic CSF in SAH is due to lysis of RBCs & subsequent conversion of hemoglobin to bilirubin which stains spinal fluid yellow within 6 to 12 hours. It peaks in intensity at 48 hours and lasts for 1 to 4 weeks.

1292. Incidence of symptomatic vasospasm in MCA & ACA is high when early CT scans show subarachnoid clots of what size in basal cisterns?
Harrison's 20th Ed. Chapter 302, Page 2086

A. > 2 x 3 mm
B. > 3 x 3 mm
C. > 4 x 3 mm
D. > 5 x 3 mm

1293. Incidence of symptomatic vasospasm in MCA & ACA is high when early CT scans show blood layer of what thickness in the cerebral fissures?
Harrison's 20th Ed. Chapter 302, Page 2086

A. > 0.1 mm
B. > 0.25 mm
C. > 0.6 mm
D. > 1 mm

High incidence of symptomatic vasospasm in MCA & ACA is observed when early CT scans show subarachnoid clots >5 x 3 mm in basal cisterns or layers of blood >1 mm thick in cerebral fissures. CT scans less reliably predict vasospasm in vertebral, basilar or posterior cerebral arteries.

1294. Secondary to intracranial hemorrhage, which of the following ECG finding is unusual?
Harrison's 20th Ed. Chapter 302, Page 2086

A. Prolonged QRS complex
B. Increased QT interval
C. "Peaked" or deeply inverted symmetric T waves
D. Serious ventricular dysrhythmias

Prolonged QRS, increased QT interval & prominent "peaked" or deeply inverted symmetric T waves occur secondary to intracranial hemorrhage. Serious ventricular dysrhythmias are unusual.

1295. Echocardiography in a case of SAH reveals relative sparing of?
Harrison's 20th Ed. Chapter 302, Page 2086

A. Apex
B. Inferior wall
C. Anterior wall
D. Posterior wall

In SAH, echocardiography shows regional wall motion abnormalities (RWMA) that follow distribution of sympathetic nerves rather than major coronary arteries, with relative sparing of ventricular wall apex.

1296. In endovascular treatment of aneurysms, coils are made of?
Harrison's 20th Ed. Chapter 302, Page 2086, N Engl J Med. 2006;354:387-96

A. Platinum
B. Silver
C. Gold
D. Steel

Newer endovascular technique involves placing platinum coils within aneurysm via a femoral artery catheter to enhance thrombosis & over time is walled-off from circulation.

1297. Intracranial hypertension following aneurysmal rupture occurs secondary to all except?
Harrison's 20th Ed. Chapter 302, Page 2086

A. Subarachnoid blood
B. Parenchymal hematoma
C. Systemic hypertension
D. Loss of vascular autoregulation

Intracranial hypertension following aneurysmal rupture occurs secondary to subarachnoid blood, parenchymal hematoma, acute hydrocephalus, or loss of vascular autoregulation.

1298. Which of the following are poor prognostic signs in SAH?
Harrison's 20th Ed. Chapter 302, Page 2086

A. High ICP refractory to treatment
B. Rerupture of untreated aneurysm in 1st month of SAH
C. Vasospasm causing symptomatic ischemia & infarction
D. All of the above

High ICP refractory to treatment is a poor prognostic sign. Rerupture is associated with a 60% mortality and poor outcome. Vasospasm following SAH causes symptomatic ischemia and infarction and is a major cause of delayed morbidity and death.

1299. In treatment of SAH, intracranial pressure should be maintained at?
Harrison's 20th Ed. Chapter 302, Page 2077

A. < 5 mm Hg
B. < 10 mm Hg
C. < 15 mm Hg
D. < 20 mm Hg

In general, ICP should be maintained at <20 mm Hg.

1300. In treatment of SAH, cerebral perfusion pressure (CPP) should be maintained at?
Harrison's 20th Ed. Chapter 302, Page 2086

A. 30–40 mm Hg
B. 40–50 mm Hg
C. 50–60 mm Hg
D. 60–70 mm Hg

In treatment of SAH, cerebral perfusion pressure should be maintained at 60–70 mm Hg.

1301. Which of the following drugs is most suited to lower raised blood pressure in patients with acute SAH?
Harrison's 20th Ed. Chapter 302, Page 2086

A. Nifedipine
B. Amlodipine
C. Nicardipine
D. Any of the above

1302. Which of the following drugs is most suited to lower raised blood pressure in patients with acute SAH?
Harrison's 20th Ed. Chapter 302, Page 2086

A. Labetalol
B. Esmolol
C. Nicardipine
D. Any of the above

Patients with acute SAH should have blood pressure lowered to a normal range with nonvasodilating agents such as nicardipine, labetalol, or esmolol.

1303. "Triple-H" therapy in SAH refers to all except?
Cleveland Clinic Journal of Medicine. 2015;82(3):177-192

A. Hypertension
B. Hemodilution
C. Hypervolemia
D. Hyperventilation

"Triple-H" therapy in SAH includes hypertension, hemodilution and hypervolemia and is achieved by volume expansion. However, clinical data supporting this intervention, to prevent delayed cerebral ischemia due to vasospasm, have been called into question.

1304. In SAH, if symptomatic vasospasm persists despite optimal medical therapy, which drug is then used?
Harrison's 20th Ed. Chapter 302, Page 2086

A. Intravenous nitroglycerine
B. Intra-arterial papaverine
C. EACA
D. Intravenous phenylephrine

If symptomatic vasospasm persists despite optimal medical therapy, intra-arterial vasodilators & percutaneous transluminal angioplasty are considered. Vasodilators like verapamil & nicardipine do not last > 8-24 hours. Intra-arterial papaverine is an effective vasodilator, but neurotoxic.

1305. Which of the following drugs is preferred for reducing vasospasm in SAH?
Harrison's 20th Ed. Chapter 302, Page 2086

A. Nifedipine
B. Amlodipine
C. Nicardipine
D. Nimodipine

1306. Which of the following is a complication of correction of marked hyponatremia of several days' duration?
Harrison's 20th Ed. Chapter 302, Page 2086

A. Cortical venous thrombosis
B. Hydrocephalus
C. Osmotic demyelination syndrome
D. All of the above

Care must be taken not to correct serum sodium too quickly in patients with marked hyponatremia of several days' duration as osmotic demyelination syndrome may occur.

1307. "Pentobarb coma" refers to?
Harrison's 20th Ed. Chapter 302, Page 2077

A. Coma due to accidental ingestion of barbiturates
B. Coma due to barbiturates given for induction of anesthesia
C. High-dose barbiturates for refractory elevated ICP
D. Any of the above

High-dose barbiturate therapy for refractory elevated ICP is termed "pentobarb coma".

1308. Emergent treatment of elevated ICP is most quickly achieved by which of the following?
Harrison's 20th Ed. Chapter 302, Page 2077

A. Ventriculostomy
B. Hyperventilation
C. High-dose barbiturates
D. Hypothermia

Emergent treatment of elevated ICP is most quickly achieved by intubation and hyperventilation to bring $PaCO_2$ level to 30–35 mm Hg.

1309. Heritable connective-tissue disorders associated with presence of intracranial aneurysm & subarachnoid hemorrhage include?
N Engl J Med. 2006;354:387-96

A. Polycystic kidney disease
B. Ehlers–Danlos syndrome (type IV)
C. Pseudoxanthoma elasticum
D. All of the above

Alzheimer's Disease

1310. Alois Alzheimer belonged to which nation?
JAMA. 1969;208(6):1017-1018
A. Spain
B. Germany
C. Poland
D. Sweden

Alzheimer's disease (AD) was first described by German psychiatrist Alois Alzheimer (14 June 1864 - 19 December 1915) in a patient at Frankfurt asylum named Mrs. Auguste Deter.

1311. Which of the following President of United States of America suffered from Alzheimer's disease?
A. Richard Nixon
B. Lyndon B Johnson
C. Gerald Ford
D. Ronald Reagan

1312. Cognitive changes of AD characteristically begin with?
Harrison's 20th Ed. Chapter 423, Page 3108
A. Memory impairment
B. Language deficit
C. Visuospatial deficit
D. Any of the above

Cognitive changes of AD follow a characteristic pattern, beginning with memory impairment and going on to language and visuospatial deficits, followed by executive dysfunction.

1313. The nonmemory complaints in a patient of AD include?
Harrison's 20th Ed. Chapter 423, Page 3108
A. Word-finding difficulty
B. Organizational difficulty
C. Navigational difficulty
D. All of the above

~ 20% of patients with AD patients present with non-memory complaints like word finding, organizational or navigational difficulty.

1314. Which of the following can be a primary manifestations of AD?
Harrison's 20th Ed. Chapter 423, Page 3108
A. Posterior cortical atrophy syndrome
B. Progressive "logopenic" aphasia
C. Asymmetric akinetic rigid-dystonic syndrome
D. All of the above

Upstream visual processing dysfunction (referred to as posterior cortical atrophy syndrome), a progressive "logopenic" aphasia, an asymmetric akinetic rigid-dystonic ("corticobasal") syndrome or a dysexecutive "frontal variant" of AD are the primary manifestations of AD for years before progressing to involve memory and other cognitive domains.

1315. Term mild cognitive impairment (MCI) is applied when memory loss falls how many standard deviations below normal on standardized memory tests?
Harrison's 20th Ed. Chapter 423, Page 3108
A. 0.5
B. 1.0
C. 1.5
D. 2.0

Term mild cognitive impairment (MCI) is applied when memory loss falls 1.5 standard deviations below normal on standardized memory tests.

1316. What percentage of mild cognitive impairment individuals will progress to Alzheimer's disease (AD) in 4 years?
Harrison's 20th Ed. Chapter 423, Page 3108
A. ~ 20%
B. ~ 30%
C. ~ 40%
D. ~ 50%

Approximately 50% of patients with mild cognitive impairment (MCI) will progress to AD over 4 years (roughly 12% per year).

1317. "Prodromal AD" refers to a person with?
Harrison's 20th Ed. Chapter 423, Page 3108
A. Amyloid imaging positive with PET
B. Low cerebrospinal Ab42
C. Mildly elevated cerebrospinal tau
D. All of the above

"Prodromal AD" refers to a person with biomarker evidence of AD (amyloid imaging positive with positron emission tomography or low cerebrospinal Ab42 and mildly elevated tau) in the absence of symptoms.

1318. In the middle and later stages of AD, which of the following remains intact?
Harrison's 20th Ed. Chapter 423, Page 3108
A. Social graces
B. Routine behavior
C. Superficial conversation
D. All of the above

In middle stages of AD, social graces, routine behavior & superficial conversation remain surprisingly intact, even in the later stages of AD illness.

1319. In AD, which of the following in language becomes impaired first?
Harrison's 20th Ed. Chapter 423, Page 3108
A. Naming
B. Comprehension
C. Fluency
D. Any of the above

In AD, language becomes impaired. It affects naming first, then comprehension, and finally fluency.

1320. In AD, which of the following is the first to become impaired?
Harrison's 20th Ed. Chapter 423, Page 3108
A. Word-finding difficulties
B. Naming
C. Loss of judgment and reasoning
D. Fluency

Word-finding difficulties & circumlocution is evident in early stages, even when naming & fluency are intact. Apraxia emerges, and patients have trouble performing learned sequential motor tasks. Visuospatial deficits interfere with dressing, eating or even walking and patients fail to solve simple puzzles or copy geometric figures. Simple calculations and clock reading become difficult in parallel.

1321. Which of the following develop in the late stages of AD?
Harrison's 20th Ed. Chapter 423, Page 3108
A. Loss of judgment and reasoning
B. Shuffling gait with generalized muscle rigidity
C. Capgras' syndrome
D. All of the above

1322. Which of the following is rare in AD?
Harrison's 20th Ed. Chapter 423, Page 3108

- A. Hyperactive tendon reflexes
- B. Myoclonic jerks
- C. Resting tremor
- D. Delusion

Patients of AD often look parkinsonian but rarely have a high-amplitude, low-frequency rhythmic, resting tremor. Hyperactive tendon reflexes and myoclonic jerks develop in the end stages of AD.

1323. Of the following, which is the most common cause of death in AD?
Harrison's 20th Ed. Chapter 423, Page 3108

- A. Secondary infections
- B. Pulmonary emboli
- C. Heart disease
- D. Aspiration

Aspiration is the most common cause of death in AD. Others include malnutrition, secondary infections, pulmonary emboli, and heart disease.

1324. The typical duration of Alzheimer's disease is?
Harrison's 20th Ed. Chapter 423, Page 3108

- A. 2–3 years
- B. 4–6 years
- C. 6–8 years
- D. 8–10 years

The typical duration of AD is 8 to 10 years, but the course can range from 1 to 25 years.

1325. Neuroimaging studies in AD may show atrophy in?
Harrison's 20th Ed. Chapter 423, Page 3108

- A. Medial temporal lobes
- B. Lateral and medial parietal lobes
- C. Lateral frontal cortex
- D. All of the above

As AD progresses, posterior predominant cortical atrophy becomes apparent, along with atrophy of medial temporal memory structures. In typical amnestic AD, neuroimaging studies (CT & MRI) show atrophy that begins in medial temporal lobes before spreading to lateral and medial parietal lobes and lateral frontal cortex.

1326. On neuroimaging studies (CT and MRI), which of the following is a single specific finding for the diagnosis of AD?
Harrison's 20th Ed. Chapter 423, Page 3108

- A. Posterior-predominant cortical atrophy
- B. Atrophy of medial temporal memory structures
- C. Hydrocephalus
- D. None of the above

Neuroimaging studies (CT & MRI) do not show a single specific pattern with AD and may be normal early in the disease.

1327. Which of the following PET finding is required for entry into treatment trials for AD?
Harrison's 20th Ed. Chapter 423, Page 3109

- A. Amyloid positivity
- B. Temporal-parietal hypometabolism
- C. Temporal-parietal hypoperfusion
- D. Lower activity of FDG in the parietal lobes

Amyloid binding with PET is typical for AD and amyloid PET positivity is becoming required for entry into treatment trials for AD.

1328. At autopsy, AD is misdiagnosed with?
Harrison's 20th Ed. Chapter 423, Page 3109

- A. Frontotemporal lobar degeneration (FTLD)
- B. DLB
- C. Hippocampal sclerosis of elderly
- D. All of the above

1329. Early prominent gait disturbance with only mild memory loss suggests?
Harrison's 20th Ed. Chapter 423, Page 3109

- A. Vascular dementia
- B. Parkinson's disease (PD)
- C. Dementia with Lewy bodies (DLB)
- D. Creutzfeldt-Jacob disease (CJD)

Early prominent gait disturbance with only mild memory loss suggests vascular dementia or, rarely, NPH.

1330. Resting tremor with stooped posture, bradykinesia and masked facies suggests?
Harrison's 20th Ed. Chapter 423, Page 3109

- A. Vascular dementia
- B. Parkinson's disease (PD)
- C. Alzheimer's disease (AD)
- D. Creutzfeldt-Jacob disease (CJD)

Resting tremor with stooped posture, bradykinesia and masked facies suggest PD or DLB.

1331. Which of the following features suggests Dementia with Lewy bodies?
Harrison's 20th Ed. Chapter 423, Page 3109

- A. Early appearance of parkinsonian features
- B. Visual hallucinations
- C. Delusional misidentification
- D. All of the above

Early appearance of parkinsonian features in association with fluctuating alertness, visual hallucinations or delusional misidentification suggests DLB.

1332. Which of the following features suggests CJD?
Harrison's 20th Ed. Chapter 423, Page 3109

- A. Rapid progression over a few weeks or months
- B. Rigidity
- C. Myoclonus
- D. All of the above

Rapid progression over a few weeks or months associated with rigidity and myoclonus suggests CJD.

1333. Which of the following features suggests frontotemporal dementia (FTD)?
Harrison's 20th Ed. Chapter 423, Page 3109

- A. Prominent behavioral changes
- B. Intact navigation
- C. Focal anterior-predominant atrophy
- D. All of the above

Prominent behavioral changes with intact navigation and focal anterior-predominant atrophy on brain imaging are typical of FTD.

1334. Which of the following clinical features of Alzheimer's disease occurs in the later phases of the disease?
N Engl J Med. 2004;351:56-67

A. Amnesic type of memory impairment
B. Deterioration of language
C. Visuospatial deficits
D. Gait disturbances

1335. Which of the following is a genetic disorder associated with dementia?
Harrison's 20th Ed. Chapter 423, Page 3109

A. Frontotemporal dementia (FTD)
B. Huntington's disease (HD)
C. Prion disease
D. All of the above

A positive family history of dementia suggests either one of the familial forms of AD or one of the other genetic disorders associated with dementia, such as FTD, HD, prion disease or rare hereditary ataxias.

1336. Risk factors for AD are?
Harrison's 20th Ed. Chapter 423, Page 3109

A. Old age
B. Positive family history
C. Female gender
D. All of the above

Risk factors for AD are old age, positive family history, female gender, past history of head trauma with concussion, very low educational attainment, exposure to aluminum, mercury & viruses, elevated homocysteine & cholesterol levels, hypertension, diminished serum folic acid, low levels of exercise, low dietary intake of fruits, vegetables, red wine & diabetes. Use of NSAID's & capacity to express complex written language in early adulthood reduces risk of AD.

1337. Most severe pathology in Alzheimer's disease is found in?
Harrison's 20th Ed. Chapter 423, Page 3109

A. Hippocampus
B. Lateral temporal cortex
C. Nucleus basalis of Meynert
D. All of the above

Most severe pathology is found in medial temporal lobe (entorhinal/perirhinal cortex and hippocampus), lateral temporal cortex and nucleus basalis of Meynert (lateral septum), the last being a major source of cholinergic input to cerebral cortex.

1338. Which of the following statements is true about microscopic findings in Alzheimer's disease?
Harrison's 20th Ed. Chapter 423, Page 3109

A. Neuritic plaques contain Ab amyloid
B. Silver staining neurofibrillary tangles in cytoplasm
C. Aβ amyloid in arterial walls of cerebral blood vessels
D. All of the above

In AD, microscopic examination of brain shows neuritic plaques containing Aβ amyloid, silver-staining neurofibrillary tangles (NFTs) in neuronal cytoplasm, and accumulation of Aβ amyloid in arterial walls of cerebral arterioles (amyloid angiopathy).

1339. In Alzheimer's disease, the neuritic plaque contains?
Harrison's 20th Ed. Chapter 423, Page 3109

A. Aβ amyloid
B. Apo ε4
C. α antichymotrypsin
D. All of the above

Neuritic plaques contain a central core that includes Aβ amyloid, proteoglycans, Apo ε4 and α-antichymotrypsin.

1340. Which of the following statements is true about Aβ amyloid in Alzheimer's disease?
Harrison's 20th Ed. Chapter 423, Page 3109

A. Neuritic plaques contains Aβ amyloid
B. It is a protein of 39–42 amino acids
C. Derived proteolytically from amyloid precursor protein
D. All of the above

Aβ amyloid is a protein of 39-42 amino acids that is derived proteolytically from a larger transmembrane protein, amyloid precursor protein (APP).

1341. Amyloid precursor protein (APP) is catabolized by?
Harrison's 20th Ed. Chapter 423, Page 3110 Figure 423-2

A. α secretase
B. β secretase
C. γ secretase
D. All of the above

Amyloid precursor protein (APP) is catabolized by α, β and γ secretases.

1342. Ab peptide results from cleavage of amyloid precursor protein (APP) by?
Harrison's 20th Ed. Chapter 423, Page 3110 Figure 423-2

A. β secretase
B. δ secretase
C. ε secretase
D. All of the above

Aβ peptide results from cleavage of APP by β-and γ-secretases.

1343. Which of the following products of Amyloid precursor protein (APP) is neurotoxic?
Harrison's 20th Ed. Chapter 423, Page 3110 Figure 423-2

A. Aβ42
B. Aβ40
C. P3
D. All of the above

A key initial step is the digestion of APP by either β secretase (BASE) or α secretase (ADAM10 or ADAM17 [TACE]), producing smaller nontoxic products. Cleavage of APP by α and β secretases results in two products i.e. α secretase product and β secretase product. γ secretase acts on α secretase product to produce nontoxic P3 peptide. Similarly, γ secretase acts on β secretase product to produce nontoxic Aβ40 and toxic Aβ42 peptide. Excess production of Aβ42 is a key initiator of cellular damage in Alzheimer's disease. Therapeutics for AD have focussed on attempts to reduce accumulation of Aβ42 by antagonizing β or γ secretases, promoting α secretase, or clearing Aβ42 that has already formed by use of specific antibodies.

1344. In familial early-onset Alzheimer's disease, increased production of which peptide is most neurotoxic?
Harrison's 20th Ed. Chapter 423, Page 3109, N Engl J Med. 2003;349:1056-63

A. Aβ36
B. Aβ38
C. Aβ40
D. Aβ42

Soluble amyloid fibrils (oligomers) lead to dysfunction of neural cells in AD. Misfolded Aβ42 molecules may be the most toxic form of this protein. Accumulation of oligomers eventually leads to formation of neuritic plaques.

1345. In Alzheimer's disease, neuritic plaque is surrounded by?
Harrison's 20th Ed. Chapter 423, Page 3109

A. Dystrophic, tau-immunoreactive neurites
B. Activated microglia
C. Macrophages
D. All of the above

In AD, neuritic plaque core is surrounded by debris of degenerating neurons, microglia & macrophages.

1346. In Alzheimer's disease, amyloid angiopathy may lead to?
Harrison's 20th Ed. Chapter 423, Page 3109

A. Microhemorrhages
B. Large lobar hemorrhages
C. Ischemic infarctions
D. All of the above

Accumulation of Aβ amyloid in cerebral arterioles, termed amyloid angiopathy, can lead to microhemorrhages, large lobar hemorrhages, or ischemic infarctions.

1347. Neurofibrillary tangles (NFTs) in Alzheimer's disease is characterized by all except?
Harrison's 20th Ed. Chapter 423, Page 3109

A. Found in neuronal cytoplasm
B. Paired helical & twisted neurofilaments
C. Represent abnormally phosphorylated tau protein
D. Gold staining

NFTs are silver-staining, twisted neurofilaments in neuronal cytoplasm that represent abnormally phosphorylated tau protein and appear as paired helical filaments by electron microscopy.

1348. Tau protein is characterized by all except?
Harrison's 20th Ed. Chapter 423, Page 3109

A. It is a microtubule associated protein
B. Functions to assemble and stabilize microtubules
C. In Alzheimer's disease, it is hypophosphorylated
D. Progressive supranuclear palsy may represent a tau pathologic process

Tau (t) is a microtubule-associated protein that assembles & stabilizes microtubules that convey cell organelles, glycoproteins through neuron. A 'hyperphosphorylated' state of tau impairs its capacity to bind to microtubules.

1349. Tau protein has pathological significance in which of the following disorders?
Harrison's 20th Ed. Chapter 423, Page 3111

A. Alzheimer's disease
B. Frontotemporal dementia
C. Progressive supranuclear palsy
D. All of the above

Tau plays a major role in the pathogenesis of FTD, PSP and Cortical Basal Degeneration (CBD).

1350. In Alzheimer's disease, which of the following neurotransmitters in cerebral cortex is decreased?
Harrison's 20th Ed. Chapter 423, Page 3109

A. Acetylcholine
B. Norepinephrine
C. Serotonin
D. All of the above

AD is associated with decreased levels of acetylcholine, its synthetic enzyme choline acetyltransferase and nicotinic cholinergic receptors in cerebral cortex due to degeneration of cholinergic neurons in nucleus basalis of Meynert. There is also reduction in norepinephrine levels in brainstem nuclei like locus coeruleus.

1351. APP gene implicated in the pathogenesis of Alzheimer's disease is present on which chromosome?
Harrison's 20th Ed. Chapter 423, Page 3109

A. Chromosome 9
B. Chromosome 11
C. Chromosome 18
D. Chromosome 21

APP gene implicated in the pathogenesis of Alzheimer's disease is present on chromosome 21.

1352. Adults with which of the following consistently develop typical neuropathologic hallmarks of AD?
Harrison's 20th Ed. Chapter 423, Page 3109

A. Klienfelter syndrome
B. Turner syndrome
C. Down's syndrome (trisomy 21)
D. All of the above

Adults with trisomy 21 (Down's syndrome) consistently develop the typical neuropathologic hallmarks of AD if they survive beyond age 40.

1353. Presenilin-1 (PSEN-1) gene implicated in the pathogenesis of Alzheimer's disease is present on which chromosome?
Harrison's 20th Ed. Chapter 423, Page 3110

A. Chromosome 9
B. Chromosome 11
C. Chromosome 14
D. Chromosome 21

Presenilin-1 (PSEN-1) gene implicated in the pathogenesis of Alzheimer's disease is present on chromosome 14 and encodes a presenilin-1 protein called S182.

1354. Presenilin-2 (PSEN-2) gene implicated in the pathogenesis of Alzheimer's disease is present on which chromosome?
Harrison's 20th Ed. Chapter 423, Page 3110

A. Chromosome 1
B. Chromosome 11
C. Chromosome 14
D. Chromosome 21

Presenilin-2 (PSEN-2) gene implicated in the pathogenesis of Alzheimer's disease is present on chromosome 1 and encodes presenilin-2 protein called STM2 (seven transmembrane domains).

1355. Which of the following about S182 & STM2 is false?
Harrison's 20th Ed. Chapter 423, Page 3110

A. Cytoplasmic neuronal proteins
B. Widely expressed throughout nervous system
C. Homologous to cell-trafficking protein - sel 12
D. None of the above

S182 and STM2 are cytoplasmic neuronal proteins, widely expressed in the nervous system and are homologous to a cell-trafficking protein - sel 12 found in the nematode Caenorhabditis elegans.

1356. Mutations in which of the following gene causes early age-of-onset Familial Alzheimer's disease (FAD)?
Harrison's 20th Ed. Chapter 423, Page 3110

A. APP
B. Presenilin-1 (PS-1)
C. Presenilin-2 (PS-2)
D. Apo e gene

Mutations in Presenilin-1 (PS-1) gene cause an early-onset AD (onset before age 60) transmitted in an autosomal dominant, highly penetrant fashion.

1357. Apo ε gene implicated in the pathogenesis of Alzheimer's disease is present on which chromosome?
Harrison's 20th Ed. Chapter 423, Page 3110

A. Chromosome 1
B. Chromosome 11
C. Chromosome 19
D. Chromosome 21

Apo ε gene implicated in the pathogenesis of Alzheimer's disease is present on chromosome 19.

1358. Gene implicated in pathogenesis of Alzheimer's disease is?
Harrison's 20th Ed. Chapter 423, Page 3110

A. APP
B. Presenilin-1 (PSEN-1) & Presenilin-2 (PSEN-2)
C. Apo ε gene
D. All of the above

AD genes include APP, Presenilin-1 (PSEN-1), Presenilin-2 (PSEN-2) and Apo ε gene.

1359. Mutations in which gene is the most common cause of late-onset familial & sporadic forms of Alzheimer's disease?
Harrison's 20th Ed. Chapter 423, Page 3110

A. APP
B. Presenilin-1 (PS-1)
C. Presenilin-2 (PS-2)
D. Apo ε gene

Apo ε gene on chromosome 19 leads to late onset familial and sporadic forms of AD.

1360. Age of onset of sporadic & familial forms of AD is modulated by which allelic variants of apolipoprotein e?
Harrison's 20th Ed. Chapter 423, Page 3110, N Engl J Med. 2001;344:1516

A. ε 2
B. ε 3
C. ε 4
D. All of the above

Apo e4 allele has a strong association with sporadic and late-onset familial cases of AD. Apo ε4 remains the single most important biologic marker associated with risk for AD.

1361. For Alzheimer's disease, which allelic variant of apolipoprotein ε is protective?
Harrison's 20th Ed. Chapter 423, Page 3111

A. ε 2
B. ε 3
C. ε 4
D. All of the above

There is evidence that the Apo ε2 allele may be "protective" against Alzheimer's disease.

1362. Carrying of which APO ε allele nearly doubles the lifetime risk of Alzheimer's disease?
N Engl J Med. 2003;349:1056-63

A. APO ε2
B. APO ε3
C. APO ε4
D. None of the above

Apo ε4 allele is an important risk factor for AD.

1363. Apo ε4 allele associated with which of the following diseases?
Harrison's 20th Ed. Chapter 423, Page 3111

A. AD
B. FTD
C. DLB
D. CJD

Apo ε4 allele is not associated with FTD, DLB, or CJD.

1364. Which of the following gene is implicated in AD pathogenesis?
Harrison's 20th Ed. Chapter 423, Page 3111

A. Clusterin (CLU)
B. Phosphatidylinositol-binding clathrin assembly protein (PICALM)
C. Complement component (3b/4b) receptor 1 (CR1)
D. All of the above

Recent genome-wide association studies have implicated the clusterin (CLU), phosphatidylinositol-binding clathrin assembly protein (PICALM), and complement component (3b/4b) receptor 1 (CR1) genes in AD pathogenesis. CLU may play a role in synapse turnover, PICALM participates in clathrin-mediated endocytosis & CR1 may be involved in amyloid clearance through complement pathway.

1365. Polycystic lipomembranous osteodysplasia with sclerosing leukoencephalopathy (PLOSL) is also called?
Neurol India. 2018;66:538-41

A. Nasu–Hakola disease
B. Motohashi-Shinohara disease
C. Akai-Tateishi disease
D. Nakamagoe-Shioya disease

PLOSL or Nasu–Hakola disease is an autosomal recessive disease due to mutations in TYROBP and TREM2 that are expressed in microglia & osteoclasts (both derived from monocyte–macrophage lineage). There occurs delayed differentiation of osteoclasts & microgliosis, resulting in an imbalance of bone-remodeling capability leading to bony cysts formation. Inflammatory & immunological imbalance in brain result in brain atrophy and dementia.

1366. TREM stands for?
N Engl J Med. 2013;368:182

A. Triggering receptor expressed on myeloma cells
B. Triggering receptor expressed on macrophage cells
C. Triggering receptor expressed on myeloid cells
D. Triggering receptor expressed on monocyte cells

1367. Which of the following about TREM2 is false?
N Engl J Med. 2013;368:182

A. TREM2 is a member of immunoglobulin family
B. TREM2 is an innate immune receptor
C. TREM2 signals through TYROBP
D. None of the above

TREM2 is an innate immune receptor expressed on cell membrane of a subset of myeloid cells like immature dendritic cells, osteoclasts, tissue macrophages & microglia. TREM2 is a member of immunoglobulin family and acts as a phagocytic receptor of bacteria. It recognizes anionic lipopolysaccharides in cell wall of bacteria and signals through a transmembrane adapter protein called TYROBP (also called DAP12). When a bacterium binds to TREM2 on macrophages, activation of the signaling pathway triggers the phagocytic uptake of bacteria and the release of reactive oxygen species (ROS). Heterozygous rare variants in TREM2 are associated with a significant increase in the risk of Alzheimer's disease.

1368. Which of the under mentioned drug for Alzheimer's disease is a cholinesterase inhibitor?
Harrison's 20th Ed. Chapter 423, Page 3111

A. Galantamine
B. Donepezil
C. Rivastigmine
D. All of the above

Pharmacologic action of donepezil, rivastigmine, and galantamine is inhibition of cholinesterase primarily acetylcholinesterase, with a resulting increase in cerebral acetylcholine levels.

1369. Which of the following drug has been discarded due to hepatotoxicity?
Harrison's 20th Ed. Chapter 423, Page 3111

A. Donepezil
B. Rivastigmine
C. Tacrine
D. Galantamine

1370. **Which of the following acts on N-methyl-D-aspartate (NMDA) channels?**

Harrison's 20th Ed. Chapter 423, Page 3111

A. Donepezil
B. Rivastigmine
C. Memantine
D. Galantamine

Memantine acts by blocking overexcited N-methyl-D-aspartate (NMDA) channels. It is used along with cholinesterase inhibitors and is not approved for mild AD.

1371. **Which of the following drugs is contraindicated in patients with Parkinson's disease?**

N Engl J Med. 2003;349:1056-63

A. Galantamine
B. Donepezil
C. Rivastigmine
D. Haloperidol

1372. **Which of the following drugs is associated with an increased risk of stroke?**

N Engl J Med. 2003;349:1056-63

A. Galantamine
B. Donepezil
C. Rivastigmine
D. Risperidone

1373. **Tarenflurbil and Semagacestat are?**

Harrison's 20th Ed. Chapter 423, Page 3111

A. Estrogen analogues
B. Vaccines
C. Gamma secretase inhibitors
D. HMG-CoA reductase inhibitors

Tarenflurbil and Semagacestat are gamma secretase inhibitors. Their use is being explored in AD treatment with a hypothesis that they would diminish the production of Aβ42.

1374. **EEG studies are most useful for the diagnosis of?**

N Engl J Med. 2001;344:1516, Harrison's 17th Ed. 2542

A. Alzheimer's disease
B. Frontotemporal dementia
C. Parkinson's disease
D. Creutzfeldt - Jakob disease

Abnormal periodic EEG discharges & cortical/basal ganglia abnormalities on diffusion-weighted MRI are unique diagnostic features of CJD.

1375. **"Leukoaraiosis" refers to?**

Harrison's 20th Ed. Chapter 423, Page 3087

A. White skin tags
B. White lines around umbilicus
C. Diffuse white matter disease
D. White nails

Leukoaraiosis or subcortical arteriosclerotic leukoencephalopathy or Binswanger's disease is a diffuse white matter disease which presents with dementia with lacunar infarctions found on MRI. Term Binswanger's disease should be used with caution, because it does not clearly identify a single entity.

Frontotemporal Dementia

1376. Which of the following statements about frontotemporal dementia (FTD) is false?
Harrison's 20th Ed. Chapter 424, Page 3115

A. Begins in fifth to seventh decade
B. Family history of dementia is common
C. Behavioral symptoms predominate in early stages
D. None of the above

FTD begins in V to VII decades. Unlike AD, behavioral symptoms predominate in early stages of FTD.

1377. Primary progressive aphasia is related to?
Harrison's 20th Ed. Chapter 424, Page 3115

A. FTD
B. PSP
C. CBD
D. Motor neuron disease

The left-hemisphere presentation of FTD is called primary progressive aphasia with nonfluent and semantic variants.

1378. Which of the following clinical variant is seen in familial and sporadic FTD?
Harrison's 20th Ed. Chapter 424, Page 3115

A. Behavioral variant
B. Semantic variant
C. Nonfluent/agrammatic variant
D. All of the above

Three core clinical syndromes seen in familial and sporadic FTD are behavioral variant (bvFTD), semantic variant and nonfluent/agrammatic variant. The last two are forms of primary progressive aphasia (PPA).

1379. Which of the following FTD variant may be most often accompanied by motor neuron disease (MND)?
Harrison's 20th Ed. Chapter 424, Page 3115

A. Behavioral variant (bvFTD)
B. Semantic variant (svPPA)
C. Nonfluent/agrammatic variant (nfvPPA)
D. All of the above

Most often bvFTD, but other two can be accompanied by motor neuron disease (MND), and is called FTD-MND.

1380. Which of the following is considered part of the FTLD clinical spectrum?
Harrison's 20th Ed. Chapter 424, Page 3115

A. Corticobasal syndrome (CBS)
B. Progressive supranuclear palsy syndrome (PSP-S)
C. Primary progressive aphasia (PPA)
D. All of the above

1381. Degeneration in which of the following areas of brain predicts bvFTD?
Harrison's 20th Ed. Chapter 424, Page 3115 Figure 424-1

A. Anterior cingulate atrophy
B. Frontoinsular atrophy
C. Orbital & dorsolateral prefrontal cortex atrophy
D. All of the above

Right hemisphere-predominant or symmetric anterior cingulate/medial prefrontal, orbital and anterior insular degeneration predicts bvFTD. Patients with nonfluent/agrammatic PPA show left (dominant) frontal opercular, dorsalinsula and precentral gyrus degeneration, whereas left anterior temporal (temporopolar) atrophy presents with semantic variant PPA.

1382. Which of the following statements about frontotemporal dementia is false?
Harrison's 20th Ed. Chapter 424, Page 3115 Figure 424-1

A. Memory and visuospatial skills relatively spared
B. Cholinergic system is relatively spared
C. Marked atrophy of temporal and/or frontal lobes
D. None of the above

Visuoconstructive ability, arithmetic calculations and navigation may remain normal late in any FTD syndrome. Distinguishing anatomic hallmark of FTD is a focal atrophy of frontal, insular, and/or temporal cortex. Cholinergic system is spared in FTD.

1383. In FTD, mutations occur in which of the following genes?
Harrison's 20th Ed. Chapter 424, Page 3115

A. C9ORF72
B. MAPT
C. GRN
D. All of the above

The most common autosomal dominantly inherited mutations causing FTD involve the C9ORF72 on chromosome 9, GRN on chromosome 17, altering progranulin protein gene and MAPT onchromosome 17, causing loss of function in tau molecule genes. Both MAPT & GRN mutations are associated with parkinsonian features. Mutations in valosin-containing protein (VCP, chromosome 9), TANK binding kinase 1 (TBK-1), T cell-restricted intracellular antigen-1 (TIA1), and charged multivesicular body protein 2b (CHMP2b, chromosome 3) genes also lead to autosomal dominant familial FTD.

1384. In ALS, mutations occur in which of the following genes?
Harrison's 20th Ed. Chapter 424, Page 3115

A. C9ORF72
B. TARDBP
C. MAPT
D. GRN

Mutations in the TARDBP (encoding TDP-43) and FUS (encoding fused in sarcoma [FUS]) genes cause familial ALS, sometimes in association with an FTD syndrome.

1385. TDP-43 stands for?
Harrison's 20th Ed. Chapter 424, Page 3043

A. TAR DNA binding protein 43
B. TAR depleted protein 43
C. TAR dense protein 43
D. TAR divided protein 43

TDP-43 stands for TAR DNA binding protein 413.

1386. Most common genetic cause of familial or sporadic FTD is?
Harrison's 20th Ed. Chapter 424, Page 3115

A. Trinucleotide expansions
B. Pentanucleotide expansions
C. Hexanucleotide expansions
D. Heptanucleotide expansions

Hexanucleotide (GGGGCC) expansions in the noncoding portion of C9ORF72 represent the most common genetic cause of familial or sporadic FTD (usually presenting as bvFTD with or without MND) and amyotrophic lateral sclerosis (ALS) leading to reduced C9ORF72 mRNA expression, nuclear mRNA foci containing transcribed portions of the expansion and other mRNAs, neuronal cytoplasmic inclusions containing dipeptide repeat proteins translated from the repeat mRNA and transactive response DNA-binding protein of 43 kDa (TDP-43) neuronal cytoplasmic and glial inclusions.

1387. Progranulin binds to which of the following?
Harrison's 20th Ed. Chapter 424, Page 3115

A. NMDA receptor
B. Tumor necrosis factor (TNF) receptors
C. Interleukin (IL) 7 receptor (CD 127)
D. ACh receptor

Progranulin is a growth factor that binds to tumor necrosis factor (TNF) receptors and participates in tissue repair and tumor growth.

1388. The gross pathologic hallmark of FTLD is a focal atrophy of?
Harrison's 20th Ed. Chapter 424, Page 3115

A. Frontal cortex
B. Insular cortex
C. Temporal cortex
D. Any of the above

Gross pathologic hallmark of FTLD is a focal atrophy of frontal, insular and/or temporal cortex. Atrophy often begins focally in one hemisphere before spreading to anatomically interconnected regions, including basal ganglia.

1389. Microscopic findings seen across all patients with FTLD include which of the following?
Harrison's 20th Ed. Chapter 424, Page 3115

A. Gliosis
B. Microvacuolation
C. Neuronal loss
D. All of the above

Microscopic findings seen across all patients with FTLD include gliosis, microvacuolation and neuronal loss. Protein composition of neuronal & glial inclusions contain either tau or TDP-43 in ~90% of patients (FTLD-TDP), remaining ~10% showing inclusions containing FUS (FTLD-FUS).

1390. Frontotemporal lobar degeneration pathology is divided according to presence of which inclusions in neurons & glia?
Harrison's 20th Ed. Chapter 424, Page 3116 Figure 424-2

A. Tau
B. TDP-43
C. FUS
D. All of the above

Frontotemporal dementia syndromes have in common the underlying frontotemporal lobar degeneration pathology. It can be divided according to the presence of tau, TDP-43, or FUS-containing inclusions in neurons and glia.

1391. Which of the following is not a member of FTLD-tau category?
Harrison's 20th Ed. Chapter 424, Page 3116 Figure 424-2

A. Pick's disease
B. Corticobasal degeneration (CBD)
C. Neuronal intermediate filament inclusion disease (NIFID)
D. Progressive supranuclear palsy (PSP)

1392. Which of the following is not a member of FTLD-FUS category?
Harrison's 20th Ed. Chapter 424, Page 3116 Figure 424-2

A. Neuronal intermediate filament inclusion disease (NIFID)
B. Basophilic inclusion body disease (BIBD)
C. Atypical frontotemporal lobar degeneration with ubiquitin-positive inclusions (aFTLD-U)
D. Frontotemporal dementia with parkinsonism linked to chromosome 17 (FTDP-17)

1393. Which of the following best relates to Pick bodies?
Harrison's 20th Ed. Chapter 424, Page 3116

A. Astrocytic plaque
B. Intraneuronal cytoplasmic inclusions
C. Ballooned neurons
D. All of the above

Pick's disease is characterized by selective involvement of anterior frontal & temporal neocortex and pathologically by intraneuronal cytoplasmic inclusions (Pick bodies) which are argyrophilic, staining positively with the Bielschowsky silver method (but not with the Gallyas method) and also with immunostaining for hyperphosphorylated tau.

1394. According to immunohistochemistry, tufted astrocyte is characteristic of?
Harrison's 20th Ed. Chapter 424, Page 3117 Figure 424-3

A. Pick's disease
B. Progressive supranuclear palsy
C. Corticobasal degeneration
D. FTLD-TDP, type A

1395. According to immunohistochemistry, astrocytic plaque is characteristic of?
Harrison's 20th Ed. Chapter 424, Page 3117 Figure 424-3

A. Pick's disease
B. Progressive supranuclear palsy
C. Corticobasal degeneration
D. FTLD-TDP, type A

1396. Which of the following drugs is effective in FTD?
Harrison's 20th Ed. Chapter 424, Page 3116

A. L-dopa
B. Selegiline
C. Pramipexole
D. None of the above

Treatment is symptomatic and there are currently no therapies known to slow progression or improve symptoms.

1397. Which of the following is also called Richardson syndrome?
Harrison's 20th Ed. Chapter 424, Page 3116

A. Corticobasal syndrome (CBS)
B. Frontotemporal dementia syndrome
C. Progressive supranuclear palsy syndrome (PSP-S)
D. Frontotemporal dementia with motor neuron disease

Progressive supranuclear palsy syndrome (PSP-S) is also known as Steele-Richardson-Olszewski syndrome or Richardson syndrome.

1398. Which of the following structures of brain is involved in PSP-S?
Harrison's 20th Ed. Chapter 424, Page 3116

A. Brainstem
B. Basal ganglia
C. Diencephalon
D. All of the above

PSP-S is a degenerative disorder that involves the brainstem, basal ganglia, diencephalon and selected areas of cortex.

1399. PSP begins with which of the following?
Harrison's 20th Ed. Chapter 424, Page 3116

A. Frequent falls
B. Symmetrical axial rigidity
C. Dementia
D. Seizure

Clinically, PSP-S begins with unexplained falls (frequently backwards) and executive or subtle personality changes (mental rigidity, impulsivity or apathy). Frequent unexplained falls are common secondary to a combination of axial rigidity, inability to look down, and bad judgment.

1400. Which of the following diseases cause ophthalmoparesis?
Harrison's 20th Ed. Chapter 424, Page 3116, 3156, 3279, 1055

A. Myotonic dystrophy
B. Metronidazole therapy
C. Machado-Joseph disease
D. All of the above

Besides PSP, Wernicke's syndrome, Myotonic dystrophy, Machado-Joseph disease, SCA7 and prolonged Metronidazole therapy can cause ophthalmoparesis.

1401. Which of the following diseases can cause supranuclear ophthalmoplegia?
Harrison's 20th Ed. Chapter 424, Page 1225

A. Whipple's disease
B. Multiple sclerosis
C. Wernicke's encephalopathy
D. All of the above

1402. Which of the following controls vertical gaze?
Harrison's 20th Ed. Chapter 424, Page 192

A. Nucleus basalis of Meynert
B. Nucleus locus coeruleus
C. Nucleus of Cajal
D. Nucleus of the solitary tract (NTS)

Vertical gaze is controlled at the level of midbrain. Lesions of rostral interstitial nucleus of medial longitudinal fasciculus and interstitial nucleus of Cajal cause supranuclear paresis of upgaze, downgaze or all vertical eye movements.

1403. Which of the following is an ocular finding in PSP?
Harrison's 20th Ed. Chapter 424, Page 3116

A. Slow ocular saccades
B. Eyelid apraxia
C. Impairment of downward gaze
D. All of the above

Progressive oculomotor syndrome in PSP begins with square wave jerks, followed by slowed saccades (vertical worse than horizontal) before resulting in progressive supranuclear ophthalmoparesis. In PSP, oculomotor disorder is supranuclear because oculocephalic reflexes (vertical doll's head maneuver) are preserved.

1404. "Hummingbird sign" on MRI is typical of which of the following?
Harrison's 20th Ed. Chapter 427, Page 3122

A. Corticobasal syndrome (CBS)
B. Frontotemporal dementia syndrome
C. Progressive supranuclear palsy syndrome (PSP-S)
D. Frontotemporal dementia with motor neuron disease

MRI may reveal a characteristic atrophy of the midbrain with relative preservation of the pons, the "hummingbird sign" on midsagittal images.

1405. Globose tangles best relate to?
Harrison's 20th Ed. Chapter 424, Page 3116

A. HD
B. PSP
C. CBD
D. AD

In PSP, accumulation of hyperphosphorylated 4-repeat tau is seen within neurons and glia. Neuronal inclusions often take the form of NFTs, which may be large, spherical ("globose") and coarse in brainstem, cerebellar dentate and diencephalic neurons.

1406. PSP is characterized by degeneration of which of the following?
Harrison's 20th Ed. Chapter 424, Page 3116

A. Substantia nigra
B. Globus pallidus
C. Subthalamic nucleus
D. All of the above

In PSP, the most prominent involvement (degeneration) is in subthalamic nucleus, globus pallidus, substantia nigra, locus coeruleus, periaqueductal gray, tectum, oculomotor nuclei and dentate nucleus of cerebellum.

1407. Which of the following is a neuropathological feature in PSP?
Harrison's 20th Ed. Chapter 424, Page 3117

A. Tufted astrocytes
B. Thorny astrocytes
C. Coiled oligodendroglial inclusions ("coiled bodies")
D. All of the above

PSP is associated with prominent tau-positive glial pathologies, such as tufted astrocytes, thorny astrocytes and coiled oligodendroglial inclusions ("coiled bodies").

1408. In PSP, neurofibrillary tangles are histochemically positive for which of the following?
Harrison's 20th Ed. Chapter 424, Page 3117

A. Tau
B. Amyloid
C. α-synuclein
D. All of the above

Pathologically, PSP is characterized by deposition of neurofibrillary tangles histochemically positive for tau and negative for amyloid or α-synuclein.

1409. "Alien hand" phenomenon is a feature of?
Harrison's 20th Ed. Chapter 424, Page 3117

A. PSP
B. DLB
C. CBS
D. AD

In corticobasal syndrome (CBS), apraxia of one arm and hand is called the alien hand. The limb exhibits unintended motor actions like grasping, groping, drifting or undoing.

1410. Corticobasal syndrome (CBS) can be due to?
Harrison's 20th Ed. Chapter 424, Page 3117

A. CBD
B. PSP
C. FTLD-TDP
D. All of the above

CBS refers to the clinical syndrome while CBD refers to a specific histopathologic FTLD-tau entity. CBS can be due to CBD, PSP, FTLD-TDP or even AD.

1411. Severe tauopathy burden in subcortical white matter is pathognomonic of?
Harrison's 20th Ed. Chapter 424, Page 3117

A. PSP
B. DLB
C. CBD
D. AD

In CBD, microscopic features include ballooned & achromatic tau-positive neurons, astrocytic plaques and dystrophic glial tau pathomorphologies that overlap with those seen in PSP. Most specifically, CBD features a severe tauopathy burden in the subcortical white matter, consisting of threads and oligodendroglial coiled bodies.

1412. Which of the following is a characteristic feature of dementia with Lewy Bodies (DLB)?
Harrison's 20th Ed. Chapter 424, Page 3117

A. Seizure
B. Symmetrical axial rigidity
C. Visual hallucinations
D. Auditory hallucinations

DLB is characterized by visual hallucinations, parkinsonism, fluctuating alertness, falls and REM sleep behavior disorder (RBD).

1413. Often, the first manifestation of illness in PDD and DLB is?
Harrison's 20th Ed. Chapter 424, Page 3117

A. Blindness
B. Seizure
C. Loss of memory
D. Delirium

PDD and DLB are highly sensitive to metabolic perturbations, and in some patients, the first manifestation of illness is a delirium, often precipitated by an infection, new medicine or other systemic disturbance. In DLB, there is relative preservation of memory.

1414. In DLB, Lewy bodies are found in?
Harrison's 20th Ed. Chapter 424, Page 3117

A. Cingulate gyrus
B. Amygdala
C. Substantia nigra
D. All of the above

Key neuropathologic feature of DLB is the presence of Lewy bodies in specific brainstem nuclei, substantia nigra, amygdala, cingulate gyrus and ultimately neocortex.

1415. Which of the following about Lewy bodies is false?
Harrison's 20th Ed. Chapter 424, Page 3117

A. Intraneuronal cytoplasmic inclusions
B. Stain with periodic acid–Schiff (PAS) & ubiquitin
C. Composed of straight neurofilaments 7 to 20 nm long
D. None of the above

Lewy bodies are intraneuronal cytoplasmic inclusions that stain with periodic acid-Schiff (PAS) & ubiquitin. They are composed of straight neurofilaments 7–20 nm long with surrounding amorphous material.

1416. In idiopathic PD, Lewy bodies are typically found in?
Harrison's 20th Ed. Chapter 424, Page 3117

A. Substantia nigra
B. Amygdala
C. Cingulate gyrus
D. All of the above

Lewy bodies are typically found in the substantia nigra of patients with idiopathic PD, where they can be readily seen with hematoxylin-and-eosin staining.

1417. Which of the following is a rapidly progressive dementing condition?
Harrison's 20th Ed. Chapter 423, Page 3112

A. Hashimoto's encephalopathy
B. Viral or bacterial encephalitides
C. Creutzfeldt-Jakob disease
D. All of the above

Besides Creutzfeldt-Jakob disease (CJD), viral or bacterial encephalitides, Hashimoto's encephalopathy, central nervous system (CNS) vasculitis, lymphoma, or paraneoplastic/autoimmune syndromes are other rapidly progressive dementing conditions.

1418. George Huntington belonged to which country?

A. Great Britain
B. America
C. Australia
D. Canada

Huntington's disease (HD) was described by George Huntington, an American physician in 1872. Huntington's gene is single, causal gene and an accurate genetic test for HD is available.

1419. Huntington's disease (HD) is caused by mutations in the Huntington's gene on the?
Harrison's 20th Ed. Chapter 428, Page 3137

A. Short arm of chromosome 4
B. Long arm of chromosome 4
C. Short arm of chromosome 5
D. Long arm of chromosome 5

HD is caused by mutations in the Huntington's gene on the short arm of chromosome 4.

1420. "Huntingtin" is a?
Harrison's 20th Ed. Chapter 428, Page 3137

A. Cell membrane protein
B. Cytoplasmic protein
C. Nuclear protein
D. Nuclear membrane protein

Huntingtin gene (HTT) encodes the highly conserved cytoplasmic protein huntingtin which is present in all neurons.

1421. Chorea is a characteristic feature of which of the following?
Harrison's 20th Ed. Chapter 423, Page 3112

A. Dementia with Lewy Bodies (DLB)
B. Huntington's disease (HD)
C. Cortical basal degeneration (CBD)
D. Creutzfeldt-Jakob disease (CJD)

HD is an autosomal dominant, degenerative brain disorder characterized by chorea, behavioral disturbance & frontal executive disorder in IV or V decade. Memory is frequently not impaired.

1422. In Huntington's disease (HD), which of the following is predominantly atrophied?
Harrison's 20th Ed. Chapter 423, Page 3112

A. Striatum
B. Cerebellum
C. Hippocampus
D. Mamillary bodies

Neuropathology of HD consists of widespread cerebral atrophy with prominent involvement of striatum and cerebral cortex.

1423. Which of the following is not a feature of normal-pressure hydrocephalus (NPH)?
Harrison's 20th Ed. Chapter 423, Page 3112

A. Abnormal gait
B. Dementia
C. Chorea
D. Urinary incontinence

Clinical triad of normal-pressure hydrocephalus (NPH) includes abnormal gait (ataxic or apractic), mild to moderate dementia and urinary incontinence.

1424. Cortical atrophy is not a feature of?
Harrison's 20th Ed. Chapter 423, Page 3112

- A. AD
- B. FTD
- C. NPH
- D. CJD

In NPH, neuroimaging shows enlarged lateral ventricles (hydrocephalus) with little or no cortical atrophy with a patent aqueduct of Sylvius suggesting communicating hydrocephalus.

1425. Which of the following is not a MRI feature of normal-pressure hydrocephalus?
Harrison's 20th Ed. Chapter 423, Page 3112

- A. Stretching of corpus callosum
- B. Elevation of the floor of third ventricle
- C. Enlargement of the aqueduct
- D. Dilation of the lateral ventricle

MRI feature of normal-pressure hydrocephalus (NPH) include dilation of lateral ventricle, stretching of corpus callosum, depression of the floor of third ventricle, enlargement of the patent aqueduct (communicating hydrocephalus).

1426. Which of the following is a feature of gait abnormality in NPH?
Harrison's 20th Ed. Chapter 423, Page 3112

- A. External hip rotation
- B. Low foot clearance
- C. Short strides
- D. All of the above

Characteristic "magnetic" gait with external hip rotation, low foot clearance and short strides, along with prominent truncal sway or instability, favors NPH.

1427. Dementia & seizures in Marchiafava-Bignami disease is related to?
Harrison's 20th Ed. Chapter 423, Page 3112

- A. Male
- B. Italian
- C. Drinkers of red wine
- D. All of the above

1428. Which of the following degenerates in Marchiafava-Bignami disease?
Harrison's 20th Ed. Chapter 423, Page 3112

- A. Caudate nucleus
- B. Thalamus
- C. Corpus callosum
- D. Substantia nigra

Marchiafava-Bignami disease consists of dementia and seizures with degeneration of corpus callosum in male Italian drinkers of red wine.

1429. Which of the following is not related to Wernicke's encephalopathy?
Harrison's 20th Ed. Chapter 423, Page 3113

- A. Confusion
- B. Seizure
- C. Ataxia
- D. Diplopia

Clinical presentation of Wernicke's encephalopathy include confusion, ataxia, & diplopia due to ophthalmoplegia.

1430. Thiamine deficiency damages which of the following?
Harrison's 20th Ed. Chapter 423, Page 3113

- A. Thalamus
- B. Mammillary bodies
- C. Midline cerebellum
- D. All of the above

Thiamine (vitamin B1) deficiency damages thalamus, mammillary bodies, midline cerebellum, periaqueductal grey matter of midbrain, peripheral nerves and trochlear & abducens nuclei.

1431. In Thiamine deficiency, damage to which of the following correlates most closely with memory loss?
Harrison's 20th Ed. Chapter 423, Page 3113

- A. Dorsomedial thalamus
- B. Mammillary bodies
- C. Midline cerebellum
- D. Periaqueductal grey matter of midbrain

In thiamine deficiency, damage to dorsomedial thalamus correlates most closely with memory loss.

1432. Which of the following is related to Korsakoff's psychosis?
Harrison's 20th Ed. Chapter 423, Page 3113

- A. Prolonged untreated thiamine deficiency
- B. Irreversible dementia
- C. Amnestic syndrome
- D. All of the above

Prolonged untreated thiamine deficiency results in irreversible dementia/amnestic syndrome (Korsakoff's psychosis) or even death.

1433. In Vitamin B_{12} deficiency, damage occurs to?
Harrison's 20th Ed. Chapter 423, Page 3113

- A. Posterior columns
- B. Corticospinal tracts
- C. Peripheral nerves
- D. All of the above

In Vitamin B_{12} deficiency, damage occur to posterior columns, corticospinal tracts, peripheral nerves and cerebral myelinated fibers (dementia).

1434. In Vitamin B_{12} deficiency, neurologic damage is related to?
Harrison's 20th Ed. Chapter 423, Page 3113

- A. Inhibition of δ-aminolevulinic acid dehydrase
- B. Deficiency of S-adenosyl methionine
- C. Elevated plasma levels of Aβ amyloid
- D. All of the above

Mechanism of neurologic damage in Vitamin B_{12} deficiency is related to deficiency of S-adenosyl methionine which is required for methylation of myelin phospholipids.

1435. Limbic encephalitis best relates to?
Harrison's 20th Ed. Chapter 423, Page 3113

- A. Primary neoplasms of CNS
- B. Metastatic neoplasms of CNS
- C. Paraneoplastic syndrome
- D. Isolated vasculitis of CNS

A paraneoplastic syndrome of dementia associated with occult carcinoma (small cell lung cancer) is termed limbic encephalitis in which confusion, agitation, seizures, poor memory, emotional changes, and frank dementia may occur.

1436. Which of the following chronic metal exposure can lead to choreoathetosis?
Harrison's 20th Ed. Chapter 423, Page 3113

A. Chronic mercury poisoning
B. Aluminum poisoning
C. Chronic arsenic intoxication
D. Chronic lead poisoning

Chronic mercury poisoning produces dementia, peripheral neuropathy, ataxia, and tremulousness that may progress to choreoathetosis.

1437. Mees' lines are best related to?
Harrison's 20th Ed. Chapter 423, Page 3113

A. Chronic mercury poisoning
B. Aluminum poisoning
C. Chronic arsenic intoxication
D. Chronic lead poisoning

Mees' lines are transverse white lines of the fingernails seen in chronic arsenic intoxication.

1438. Which of the following chronic metal exposure can lead to myoclonic jerks?
Harrison's 20th Ed. Chapter 423, Page 3113

A. Chronic mercury poisoning
B. Aluminum poisoning
C. Chronic arsenic intoxication
D. Chronic lead poisoning

Dialysis dementia syndrome due to aluminum overexposure is associated with confusion, aphasia, memory loss, agitation, and, later, lethargy and stupor. Speech arrest and myoclonic jerks are common and associated with severe and generalized EEG changes.

1439. "Dementia pugilistica" is related to which of the following?
Harrison's 20th Ed. Chapter 423, Page 3113

A. Nonconvulsive seizure disorder
B. Transient global amnesia (TGA)
C. Chronic metal exposure
D. Recurrent head trauma in professional boxers

Recurrent head trauma in professional boxers may lead to dementia, called the "punch drunk" syndrome or dementia pugilistica.

1440. In Transient global amnesia (TGA), which of the following memory types is lost?
Harrison's 20th Ed. Chapter 423, Page 3113

A. Working
B. Episodic
C. Remote
D. All of the above

Transient global amnesia is characterized by sudden onset of a severe episodic memory deficit in the setting of an emotional stimulus or physical exertion, in persons over age 50 years.

1441. Along with dementia, myoclonus is a feature of which of the following disease?
Harrison's 20th Ed. Chapter 423, Page 3113

A. Neuronal cerebrolipofuscinoses
B. Creutzfeldt - Jakob disease
C. Corticobasal degeneration (CBD)
D. All of the above

Vascular Dementia

1442. Which of the following can disrupt structural cognitive networks in Vascular cognitive impairment and vascular dementia (VCI-VaD)?
Harrison's 20th Ed. Chapter 425, Page 3118

- A. Chronic progressive white matter degeneration
- B. Disrupted cerebrovascular autoregulation
- C. Blood brain barrier dysfunction
- D. All of the above

Microinfarcts, microbleeds, macroinfarcts, large hemorrhages, chronic progressive white matter degeneration, altered cerebral hemodynamics, disrupted cerebrovascular autoregulation, neurovascular decoupling (loss of normal hemodynamic responses to neural activity), and blood brain barrier dysfunction can disrupt structural cognitive networks in Vascular cognitive impairment and vascular dementia (VCI-VaD).

1443. On neuroimaging, by the age of 70 years, what proportion of population has white matter disease & lesions?
Harrison's 20th Ed. Chapter 425, Page 3118

- A. 30%
- B. 50%
- C. 70%
- D. 90%

By the age of 70 years, 70% of the population has white matter disease & lesions on neuroimaging, with small infarcts (lacunar infarcts) found in 11–24% of the population.

1444. Which of the following statements is false?
Harrison's 20th Ed. Chapter 425, Page 3118

- A. Hemorrhages account for ~20% of all strokes
- B. Ischemic strokes compose 80% of all strokes
- C. Chronic cerebral small vessel disease (SVD) has the strongest association with cognitive impairment
- D. None of the above

SVD typically causes occlusion of deep-penetrating arterioles and disease of draining venules, causing damage to subcortical structures such as the basal ganglia, thalami, and white matter tracts.

1445. Average volume of lacunes is?
Harrison's 20th Ed. Chapter 425, Page 3118

- A. 2 mm
- B. 4 mm
- C. 6 mm
- D. 8 mm

Lacunes average 2 mm in volume, but can range from 0.2 to 15 mm.

1446. Which of the following about small vessel disease (SVD) is false?
Harrison's 20th Ed. Chapter 425, Page 3118

- A. Sporadic
- B. CADASIL is a genetic SVD-related VaD syndrome
- C. SVD accounts for 36–67% of all VaDs
- D. None of the above

1447. Which of the following abnormality is associated with SVD?
Harrison's 20th Ed. Chapter 425, Page 3118

- A. Blood-brain-barrier compromise
- B. Chronic cerebral hypoperfusion
- C. Hippocampal atrophy & sclerosis
- D. All of the above

SVD is associated with blood-brain-barrier (BBB) compromise, accumulating white matter disease, and a state of chronic cerebral hypoperfusion, hippocampal atrophy & sclerosis.

1448. Which of the following increase the risk of dementia?
Harrison's 20th Ed. Chapter 425, Page 3118

- A. White matter hyperintensities (WMH)
- B. Cortical microinfarcts
- C. Enlarged Virchow-Robin spaces (eVRS)
- D. All of the above

Neuroimaging markers of SVD include white matter hyperintensities (WMH) of presumed vascular origin, microbleeds, cortical microinfarcts and enlarged Virchow-Robin spaces (eVRS). They increase the risk of dementia.

1449. Subcortical arteriosclerotic encephalopathy is also called?
Harrison's 20th Ed. Chapter 425, Page 3118

- A. Lewy body disease
- B. Binswanger's disease
- C. Huntington's disease
- D. Prion disease

Binswanger's disease is also called subcortical arteriosclerotic encephalopathy. It is considered a prototypical clinical syndrome of vascular cognitive impairment (VCI) and a pathologically homogenous subgroup.

1450. Which of the following neuroimaging technique is used for assessment of blood brain barrier integrity?
Harrison's 20th Ed. Chapter 425, Page 3118

- A. Functional MRI (fMRI)
- B. Magnetic resonance angiography (MRA)
- C. Magnetic resonance venography (MRV)
- D. Dynamic contrast-enhanced MRI (DCE-MRI)

Novel neuroimaging technique for assessment of blood brain barrier integrity is dynamic contrast-enhanced MRI (DCE-MRI).

1451. Which of the following about Binswanger's disease is false?
Harrison's 20th Ed. Chapter 425, Page 3118

- A. Progressive confluent subcortical & periventricular white matter disease
- B. Extensive demyelination & destruction of white matter with relative sparing of subcortical U fibers
- C. Gradual accumulation of focal neurological deficits
- D. None of the above

Subcortical U-fibers have a relatively slower rate of myelin turnover and are spared in Binswanger's disease & Neuromyelitis Optica (NMO). Multiple sclerosis (MS) & progressive multifocal leukoencephalopathy (PML) typically demonstrate early U-fiber involvement.

1452. **Subcortical U fibers are involved in which of the following?**
Harrison's 20th Ed. Chapter 425, Page 3118

   A. CADASIL
   B. Multiple sclerosis (MS)
   C. Acute Disseminated Encephalomyelitis (ADEM)
   D. All of the above

1453. **Infarct in which of the following locations results in marked cognitive dysfunction & dementia?**
Harrison's 20th Ed. Chapter 425, Page 3118

   A. Thalamus
   B. Basal ganglia
   C. Angular gyrus
   D. All of the above

A strategically placed infarct, usually in the thalamus, basal ganglia or angular gyrus can also result in marked cognitive dysfunction & dementia.

1454. **Occlusion of which of the following artery can lead to bilateral infarction of dorsomedial nucleus & mammillothalamic tracts?**
Harrison's 20th Ed. Chapter 425, Page 3118

   A. Recurrent artery of Heubner
   B. Artery of Percheron (AOP)
   C. Artery of Adamkiewicz
   D. Marginal artery of Drummond

Single paramedian artery (artery of Percheron) supplies both anteromedial thalamic regions, and its occlusion results in altered mental status, vertical gaze palsy, and memory impairment.

Dementia with Lewy Bodies

1455. Lewy body and Lewy neurite pathology most often begins in?
Harrison's 20th Ed. Chapter 426, Page 3119

A. Enteric and autonomic nervous systems
B. Optic nerve
C. Somatic nerves
D. All of the above

Lewy body & Lewy neurite pathology begins in the enteric & autonomic nervous systems before ascending through the brainstem to substantia nigra, limbic system, and ultimately cerebral cortex. Disease may also begin in the olfactory bulb & spread inward through olfactory system connections.

1456. "Neurons release the same neurotransmitters at all of their synapses" is called?
Proc. R. Soc. Med.28. ; 1935: 319-332

A. Bloch's law
B. Bell - Magendie law
C. Bunsen - Roscoe law
D. Dale's principle

Formulated by Henry Dale (1875 - 1968), British neurophysiologist in the 1940's, the original hypothesis was that each neuron releases only one type of neurotransmitter.

1457. DLB is a progressive dementia syndrome characterised by?
Harrison's 20th Ed. Chapter 426, Page 3119

A. Spontaneous parkinsonism
B. Visual hallucinations
C. Fluctuating cognition
D. All of the above

1458. DLB syndrome is characterized by?
Harrison's 20th Ed. Chapter 426, Page 3119

A. Neuroleptic sensitivity
B. Hyposmia
C. Rapid eye movement (REM) sleep behavior disorder (RBD)
D. All of the above

DLB syndrome is characterized by visual hallucinations, parkinsonism, fluctuating alertness, neuroleptic sensitivity, rapid eye movement (REM) sleep behavior disorder (RBD), and often hyposmia and excessive daytime sleepiness. The side-effects of neuroleptics (drowsiness, parkinsonism, and falls) are more prominent in dementia with Lewy bodies (DLB).

1459. Which of the following best relates to DLB syndrome?
Harrison's 20th Ed. Chapter 426, Page 3119

A. Déjà entendu
B. Jamais vu
C. Reduplicative paramnesia
D. Cryptomnesia

Reduplicative paramnesia (RP) is a subset of delusional misidentification syndromes. It is marked by a delusional belief that a place or location has been duplicated, existing in two or more places simultaneously, or that it has been 'relocated' to another site.

1460. Which of the following symptoms referable to brainstem pathology may accompany or precede DLB?
Harrison's 20th Ed. Chapter 426, Page 3119

A. Constipation
B. Orthostatic lightheadedness
C. Depression/anxiety
D. All of the above

Both PDD & DLB may be accompanied or preceded by symptoms referable to brainstem pathology below substantia nigra including constipation, orthostatic lightheadedness, depression/anxiety and RBD.

1461. Which of the following is false about DLB and PDD?
Harrison's 20th Ed. Chapter 426, Page 3119

A. Highly sensitive to metabolic disturbances
B. Marked day-to-day variation in cognitive functioning
C. Relative preservation of episodic memory
D. None of the above

1462. In Lewy body disease (LBD), Lewy bodies and Lewy neurites are found in?
Harrison's 20th Ed. Chapter 426, Page 3119

A. Substantia nigra
B. Amygdala
C. Cingulate gyrus
D. All of the above

Presence of Lewy bodies & Lewy neurites is the key neuropathological feature in Lewy body disease (LBD). They are present throughout specific brainstem nuclei, substantia nigra, amygdala, cingulate gyrus and ultimately, the neocortex causing profound cholinergic deficit.

1463. Patients with DLB are extremely sensitive to which of the following medications?
Harrison's 20th Ed. Chapter 426, Page 3119

A. Oral anticoagulant medication
B. Antiplatelet medication
C. Dopaminergic medication
D. All of the above

Patients with DLB are extremely sensitive to dopaminergic medications and atypical antipsychotics.

Parkinson's Disease

1464. Paralysis agitans was described in Ayurveda (Charaka Samhita) centuries ago by the name of?
N Engl J Med. 1998;339:1049

A. Adhyashana
B. Kampavata
C. Jatharagni
D. Shalmali

Paralysis agitans described by James Parkinson is an independent description of Kampavata (Kampa:tremor, Vata:metabolic derangement predisposing to neurologic and mental diseases) described in Ayurveda (Charaka Samhita) centuries ago. Several preparations containing Mucuna pruriens (Kapikachu) were described for treatment of patients with Kampavata. The major active compound present in Mucuna pruriens is levodopa.

1465. The first name of Parkinson was?
Harrison's 20th Ed. Chapter 427, Page 3120

A. John
B. James
C. Jack
D. George

Parkinson disease was first described by English physician James Parkinson in 1817.

1466. Corpus Luysii is the name given to?
Principles of Neurology, Adams RD, 5th Ed. 57

A. Claustrum
B. Subthalamic nucleus
C. Globus pallidus
D. Substantia nigra

Corpus Luysii is the name given to subthalamic nucleus (STN) which is the only glutamatergic nucleus in the "basal ganglia".

1467. Which of the following is commonest neurodegenerative disease?
Harrison's 20th Ed. Chapter 427, Page 3120

A. Alzheimer's disease (AD)
B. Parkinson's disease (PD)
C. Wilson's disease (WD)
D. SCA 3 (spinocerebellar ataxia)

Parkinson's disease (PD) is the second commonest neurodegenerative disease, exceeded only by Alzheimer's disease (AD).

1468. In patients under the age of 65 years, which of the following is the most common cause of dementia?
Harrison's 20th Ed. Chapter 427, Page 153

A. Frontotemporal lobar degeneration
B. Multisystem atrophy
C. Parkinson's disease
D. Huntington's disease

In patients under the age of 65 years, FTD rivals AD as the most common cause of dementia.

1469. Which of the following is not included in the cardinal features of PD?
Harrison's 20th Ed. Chapter 427, Page 3120

A. Rest tremor
B. Masked facies (hypomimia)
C. Bradykinesia
D. Gait dysfunction with postural instability

Cardinal features of PD include rest tremor, rigidity, bradykinesia and gait impairment with postural instability. Nondopaminergic features (as they do not fully respond to dopaminergic therapy) include freezing of gait, speech difficulty, autonomic disturbances, sensory alterations, mood disorders, sleep dysfunction, cognitive impairment, and dementia.

1470. The whistle-smile sign is also called?
DeJong's The Neurologic Examination, 7th Ed. Page 253

A. Levine's sign
B. Comet sign
C. Hanes sign
D. Gower sign

Because of their paucity of facial expression, patients with Parkinson's disease may fail to smile after being asked to whistle—the whistle-smile (Hanes) sign.

1471. Non-motor features of PD include all except?
Harrison's 20th Ed. Chapter 427, Page 3120 Table 427-1

A. Sleep disturbances
B. Cognitive impairment
C. Loss of taste
D. Loss of smell

Non-motor aspects of PD include depression and anxiety, cognitive impairment, sleep disturbances, sensory abnormalities and pain, loss of smell (anosmia) and disturbances of autonomic function.

1472. Clinicopathologic correlation is better if which of the following is included to define Parkinson's Disease?
Harrison's 20th Ed. Chapter 427, Page 3120

A. Rest tremor
B. Asymmetry of motor impairment
C. Good response to levodopa
D. All of the above

Clinicopathologic correlation studies have determined that parkinsonism associated with rest tremor, asymmetry of motor impairment, and a good response to levodopa is more likely to predict the correct pathologic diagnosis of PD (International Parkinson's Disease and Movement Disorder Society (MDS)).

1473. Decreased smell function is among the first signs of which of the following diseases?
Harrison's 20th Ed. Chapter 25, Page 153

A. Wilson's disease
B. Parkinson's disease
C. Progressive supranuclear palsy
D. All of the above

1474. Decreased smell function is found in which of the following diseases?
Harrison's 20th Ed. Chapter 29, Page 194, 197

A. iRBD
B. Parkinson's disease
C. Alzheimer's disease
D. All of the above

Decreased smell function is among the first signs, if not the first sign, of such neurodegenerative diseases as Parkinson's disease (PD) and Alzheimer's disease (AD), signifying their "presymptomatic" phase. Olfactory impairment in PD often predates the clinical diagnosis by at least 4 years. Others include Huntington's disease, Down's syndrome, parkinsonism-dementia complex of Guam, dementia with Lewy bodies (DLB), multiple system atrophy, corticobasal degeneration, frontotemporal dementia, multiple sclerosis (MS) and idiopathic rapid eye movement (REM) behavioral sleep disorder (iRBD). Smell loss is minimal or nonexistent in progressive supranuclear palsy and MPTP-induced parkinsonism.

1475. Pathological hallmark feature of PD is?
Harrison's 20th Ed. Chapter 427, Page 3120

A. Degeneration of dopaminergic neurons in SNc
B. Reduced striatal dopamine
C. Intracytoplasmic proteinaceous inclusions (Lewy bodies)
D. All of the above

Pathologically, the hallmark features of PD are degeneration of dopaminergic neurons in the substantia nigra pars compacta (SNc), reduced striatal dopamine, and intracytoplasmic proteinaceous inclusions known as Lewy bodies. There is relative sparing of caudate nucleus.

1476. Cholinergic neurons are present in?
Harrison's 20th Ed. Chapter 427, Page 3120

A. Locus coeruleus (LC)
B. Nucleus basalis of Meynert (NBM)
C. Raphe nuclei of the brainstem
D. All of the above

1477. Norepinephrine neurons are present in?
Harrison's 20th Ed. Chapter 427, Page 3120

A. Locus coeruleus (LC)
B. Nucleus basalis of Meynert (NBM)
C. Raphe nuclei of the brainstem
D. All of the above

Cholinergic neurons are present in nucleus basalis of Meynert (NBM). Norepinephrine neurons are present in locus coeruleus (LC) and serotonin neurons in raphe nuclei of the brainstem, and neurons of the olfactory system, cerebral hemispheres, spinal cord, and peripheral autonomic nervous system.

1478. Pathological changes in PD (Lewy body pathology) begin in?
Harrison's 20th Ed. Chapter 427, Page 3120

A. Peripheral autonomic nervous system
B. Olfactory system
C. Dorsal motor nucleus of vagus nerve in lower brainstem
D. All of the above

In PD, pathology begins in peripheral autonomic nervous system, olfactory system & dorsomotor nucleus of vagus nerve in lower brainstem, and then spreads in a sequential manner to affect the upper brainstem and cerebral hemispheres. Thus, dopamine neurons are affected in midstage disease (Braak staging).

1479. Which of the following is mostly responsible for signs of parkinsonism?
Harrison's 20th Ed. Chapter 427, Page 3120

A. Decreased traffic in indirect striato-pallidal pathway
B. Increased traffic in direct striato-nigral pathway
C. Decreased ability of thalamus to activate frontal cortex
D. All of the above

Striatal dopamine denervation results in increased traffic in indirect striato-pallidal pathway and decreased traffic in direct pathway. Downstream consequence of this is increased activity in striatal outflow stemming from the increased activity of STN and ultimately GPi/SNr neurons. Because striatal outflow is inhibitory to the thalamus (GABA), there is a decrease in the ability of thalamus to activate frontal cortex leading to signs of parkinsonism.

1480. Which of the following is not a component of basal ganglia?
Harrison's 20th Ed. Chapter 427, Page 3120

A. Striatum (putamen & caudate nucleus)
B. Subthalamic nucleus (STN)
C. Globus pallidus pars externa (GPe)
D. Claustrum

Basal ganglia are subcortical nuclei that include striatum (putamen & caudate nucleus), subthalamic nucleus (STN), globus pallidus pars externa (GPe), globus pallidus pars interna (GPi) & SNc. Symptom complex of Parkinsonism reflect damage to different components of basal ganglia.

1481. Which of the following is the revised criteria for the clinical diagnosis of PD?
Harrison's 20th Ed. Chapter 427, Page 3120

A. UK brain bank criteria
B. UK brain store criteria
C. UK brain support criteria
D. UK brain diagnosis criteria

UK brain bank criteria is the revised criteria for the clinical diagnosis of PD.

1482. In PD, metabolic imaging (PET/SPECT) shows which of the following?
Harrison's 20th Ed. Chapter 427, Page 3121

A. Reduced uptake in posterior putamen
B. Increased activity in GPi
C. Decreased activity in thalamus
D. All of the above

Imaging of brain dopamine system in PD with positron emission tomography (PET) or single-photon emission computed tomography (SPECT) shows reduced uptake of striatal dopaminergic markers, particularly in posterior putamen, increased activity in the GPi with decreased activity in thalamus.

1483. Commonest cause of familial PD is due to mutations of?
Harrison's 20th Ed. Chapter 427, Page 3121

A. LRRK1 gene
B. LRRK2 gene
C. LRRK3 gene
D. LRRK4 gene

Mutations of LRRK2 (leucine rich repeat kinase 2) gene are the commonest cause of familial PD and are responsible for ~1% of typical sporadic cases of the disease.

1484. Familial Parkinson's disease is associated with mutations in which of the following genes?
Harrison's 20th Ed. Chapter 427, Page 3043

A. PINK1
B. DJ-1
C. Parkin
D. All of the above

Familial Parkinson's disease is associated with mutations in leucine rich repeat kinase 2 (LRRK2, α-synuclein, parkin, PINK1 and DJ-1. PINK1 is a mitochondrial kinase and DJ-1 is a protein involved in protection from oxidative stress. Parkin, which causes autosomal recessive early-onset Parkinson's disease, is a ubiquitin ligase.

1485. Atypical parkinsonism group of neurodegenerative conditions include?
Harrison's 20th Ed. Chapter 427, Page 3122

A. Multiple System Atrophy (MSA)
B. Progressive Supranuclear Palsy (PSP)
C. Corticobasal syndrome (CBS)
D. All of the above

1486. Diagnosis of atypical Parkinsonism is favoured by all except?
Harrison's 20th Ed. Chapter 427, Page 3122

A. Early speech impairment
B. Early gait impairment
C. Absence of rest tremor
D. Asymmetry

Atypical Parkinsonism is characterized by early speech and gait impairment, absence of rest tremor, no asymmetry, poor or no response to levodopa, and an aggressive clinical course. Pathologically, neurodegeneration occurs without Lewy bodies. Metabolic imaging of basal ganglia/thalamus network shows decreased activity in GPi with increased activity in thalamus, reverse of what is seen in PD.

1487. Manifestations of multiple-system atrophy (MSA) include all except?
Harrison's 20th Ed. Chapter 427, Page 3122

A. Parkinsonian features
B. Cerebellar features
C. Sensory features
D. Autonomic features

Multiple-system atrophy (MSA) manifests as a combination of parkinsonian, cerebellar, and autonomic features. When parkinsonian features are predominant, term MSA-p is used and when cerebellar features are predominant, term MSA-c is used.

1488. Degeneration of which of the following is found in MSA?
Harrison's 20th Ed. Chapter 427, Page 3122

A. SNc
B. Striatum
C. Inferior olivary nuclei
D. All of the above

1489. Glial cytoplasmic inclusions (GCIs) characteristic of MSA stain positive for?
Harrison's 20th Ed. Chapter 427, Page 3122

A. Tau
B. α-synuclein
C. UCHL-1
D. Parkin

Pathologically, MSA is characterized by degeneration of SNc, striatum, cerebellum & inferior olivary nuclei coupled with characteristic glial cytoplasmic inclusions (GCIs) that stain for α-synuclein.

1490. "Hot cross buns" sign relates to which of the following?
Harrison's 20th Ed. Chapter 427, Page 3122

A. MSA
B. PSP
C. Corticobasal ganglionic degeneration
D. All of the above

The pontine "hot cross buns" sign is a MRI feature of MSA-c.

1491. PSP is characterized by?
Harrison's 20th Ed. Chapter 427, Page 3122

A. Slow ocular saccades
B. Eyelid apraxia
C. Restricted vertical eye movements
D. All of the above

1492. Which of the following eye movements is impaired in PSP?
Harrison's 20th Ed. Chapter 427, Page 3122

A. Upward gaze
B. Downward gaze
C. Lateral gaze
D. Medial gaze

PSP is a form of atypical parkinsonism, characterized by slow ocular saccades, eyelid apraxia & restricted vertical eye movements particularly impairment of downward gaze.

1493. Which of the following is associated with PSP?
Harrison's 20th Ed. Chapter 427, Page 3122

A. Hyperextension of neck with early gait disturbance & falls
B. Swallowing difficulty & cognitive impairment
C. Little or no response to levodopa therapy
D. All of the above

In PSP (Richardson), hyperextension of neck with early gait disturbance & falls occurs. Speech & swallowing difficulty and cognitive impairment become obvious in later stages. There is usually little or no response to levodopa. In the "Parkinson" form of PSP, resemblance to PD is observed in early stages including a positive response to levodopa. The gait of PSP is typically more erect compared with stooped posture of typical Parkinson's disease, and toppling falls within the first year also suggest the possibility of PSP.

1494. "Hummingbird sign" on mid sagittal MRI images relates to which of the following?
Harrison's 20th Ed. Chapter 427, Page 3122

A. MSA
B. PSP
C. Corticobasal ganglionic degeneration
D. All of the above

The "hummingbird sign" on mid sagittal MRI images is a feature of progressive supranuclear palsy (PSP) and is due to atrophy of midbrain with relative preservation of pons.

1495. Pathologically, PSP is characterized by?
Harrison's 20th Ed. Chapter 427, Page 3122

A. Degeneration of SNc, striatum, STN, midline thalamic nuclei & pallidum
B. Neurofibrillary tangles
C. Inclusions positive for tau protein
D. All of the above

Pathologically, PSP is characterized by degeneration of SNc, striatum, STN, midline thalamic nuclei & pallidum, along with neurofibrillary tangles & inclusions that stain positive for tau protein.

1496. Corticobasal syndrome (CBS) presents with?
Harrison's 20th Ed. Chapter 427, Page 3123

A. Asymmetric dystonic contractions
B. Clumsiness of one hand
C. Apraxia, agnosia, focal limb myoclonus, or alien limb phenomenon
D. All of the above

CBS, least common of the three atypical parkinsonisms, presents with both cortical & basal ganglia features. These include asymmetric dystonic contractions & clumsiness of one hand along with cortical sensory disturbances like apraxia, agnosia, focal limb myoclonus, or alien limb phenomenon (where the limb assumes a position in space without patient being aware of the position or recognizing that limb belongs to him/her). Dementia may occur at any stage of the disease.

1497. Carbon monoxide or manganese damage which of the following?
Harrison's 20th Ed. Chapter 427, Page 3123

A. Substantia nigra
B. Subthalamic nucleus (STN)
C. Globus pallidus
D. All of the above

Carbon monoxide or manganese damage globus pallidus & presentation resembles atypical parkinsonism.

1498. Most common cause of secondary parkinsonism is?
Harrison's 20th Ed. Chapter 427, Page 3123

A. Calcium channel blockers (flunarizine, cinnarizine)
B. Amiodarone
C. Lithium
D. Dopamine-blocking agents like neuroleptics

Dopamine-blocking agents like neuroleptics are the most common cause of secondary parkinsonism. Metoclopramide is neuroleptic agent also.

1499. Which of the following is false about Dopa-Responsive Dystonia?
Harrison's 20th Ed. Chapter 427, Page 3123

A. Due to impaired production of dopa & dopamine in brain
B. No abnormalities on FD-PET, no neurodegeneration
C. Responds to levodopa
D. None of the above

Dopa-Responsive Dystonia should be considered in dystonia individuals aged <20 years who present with a clinical picture resembling PD. It is due to a mutation in GTP-Cyclohydrolase 1 gene leading to impaired production of dopa & dopamine. It responds to levodopa and is not associated with abnormalities on fluoro-dopa positron emission tomography (FD-PET). There is no evidence of neurodegeneration.

1500. Parkinsonism can be seen as a feature of?
Harrison's 20th Ed. Chapter 427, Page 3123

A. Wilson's disease
B. Huntington's disease
C. Hallervorden-Spatz disease
D. All of the above

Parkinsonism is a feature of Wilson's disease, Huntington's disease (Westphal variant), dopa-responsive dystonia and pantothenate kinase (PANK)–associated neurodegeneration (formerly called Hallervorden Spatz disease).

1501. Which of the following is the cause of PD in majority?
Harrison's 20th Ed. Chapter 427, Page 3123

A. Sporadic
B. Genetic
C. Cerebrovascular disease
D. Drugs

Most PD cases occur sporadically (85–90%) and are of unknown cause. Gene mutations are the only known causes of PD in younger-onset patients.

1502. Which of the following is a primary autonomic degenerative disorder?
Harrison's 20th Ed. Chapter 18, Page 126

A. Multiple system atrophy (Shy-Drager syndrome)
B. Dementia with Lewy bodies
C. Pure autonomic failure
D. All of the above

1503. α-synuclein, aggregates predominantly in the cytoplasm of neurons in all of the following except?
Harrison's 20th Ed. Chapter 18, Page 126

A. Parkinson's disease
B. Dementia with Lewy bodies
C. Pure autonomic failure
D. Multiple system atrophy

1504. Which of the following is a Lewy body disorder?
Harrison's 20th Ed. Chapter 18, Page 126

A. Parkinson's disease
B. Dementia with Lewy bodies
C. Pure autonomic failure
D. All of the above

Primary autonomic degenerative disorders are multiple system atrophy (Shy-Drager syndrome), Parkinson's disease, dementia with Lewy bodies, and pure autonomic failure. These are also called "synucleinopathies" due to the presence of α-synuclein that aggregates predominantly in cytoplasm of neurons in Lewy body disorders (Parkinson's disease, dementia with Lewy bodies & pure autonomic failure) and in the glia in multiple system atrophy (MSA).

1505. Peak age of onset of Sporodic Parkinson's disease (PD) is in which decade of life?
Harrison's 20th Ed. Chapter 427, Page 3123

A. 50s
B. 60s
C. 70s
D. 80s

Most cases of PD begin after the age of 60 years and the incidence increases up to the age of ~80 years (range is 35 to 85 years) and the course of the illness ranges between 10 and 25 years.

1506. Factors linked to a reduced incidence of PD include all except?
Harrison's 20th Ed. Chapter 427, Page 3123

A. Coffee drinking
B. Smoking
C. Use of NSAIDs
D. Alcohol use

Factors linked to a reduced incidence of PD include coffee drinking, smoking, use of nonsteroidal anti-inflammatory drugs, and estrogen replacement in postmenopausal women.

1507. Environmental risk factors for PD include all except?
Harrison's 20th Ed. Chapter 427, Page 3123

A. Exposure to pesticides
B. Consumption of well water
C. Rural living
D. Urban living

Risk factors include a positive family history, male gender, head injury, exposure to pesticides, consumption of well water, and rural living.

1508. Which of the following neurotoxin produces parkinsonism?
Harrison's 20th Ed. Chapter 427, Page 3123

A. Apamin
B. Botulinum
C. MPTP
D. Tetanospasmin

MPTP (1-methyl-4-phenyl-1,2,5,6-tetrahydropyridine) is a byproduct of the illicit manufacture of a heroin-like drug, causes a PD-like syndrome in addicts. MPTP is transported to CNS, where it is metabolized to form MPP$^+$, a mitochondrial toxin that is selectively taken up by, and damages, dopamine neurons. MPTP toxicity can be prevented by coadministration of a MAO-B inhibitor that blocks its conversion to the toxic pyridinium ion MPP$^+$.

1509. Toxins that can produce secondary Parkinsonism include all except?
Harrison's 20th Ed. Chapter 427, Page 3121 Table 427-2

A. 1-Methyl-1,2,4,6 tetrahydropyridine (MPTP)
B. Manganese
C. Cyanide
D. Carbon dioxide

1510. Toxins that can produce secondary PD include all except?
Harrison's 20th Ed. Chapter 427, Page 3121 Table 427-2

A. Methanol
B. Ethanol
C. Carbon monoxide
D. Carbon disulfide

1-Methyl-1,2,4,6 tetrahydropyridine (MPTP), Manganese, Cyanide, Methanol, Carbon monoxide, Carbon disulfide, Hexane produce parkinsonism.

1511. Drug that can cause secondary parkinsonism is?
Harrison's 20th Ed. Chapter 427, Page 3123

A. Amiodarone
B. Lithium
C. Cinnarizine
D. All of the above

Drugs that can cause secondary parkinsonism include metoclopramide, flunarizine, cinnarizine, tetrabenazine, amiodarone, and lithium.

1512. Drugs that can produce secondary PD include all except?
Harrison's 20th Ed. Chapter 427, Page 3123

A. Metoclopramide
B. Reserpine
C. Methyldopa
D. Clonidine

1513. Drugs that can produce secondary PD include all except?
Harrison's 20th Ed. Chapter 427, Page 3123

A. Lithium carbonate
B. Valproic acid
C. Phenytoin
D. Fluoxetine

Drugs that can produce secondary PD include neuroleptics (typical antipsychotics), some atypical antipsychotics, antiemetics (compazine, metoclopramide), dopamine-depleting agents (reserpine, tetrabenazine), alpha methyldopa, lithium carbonate, valproic acid, fluoxetine.

1514. Mutations in which of the following gene numerically represent the most important risk factor for the development of PD?
Harrison's 20th Ed. Chapter 427, Page 3125

A. Glucocerebrosidase
B. α-glucosidase
C. α-galactosidase A
D. Hexosaminidase A

Mutations in the glucocerebrosidase (GBA) gene associated with Gaucher's disease numerically represent the most important risk factor for the development of PD. There is a reciprocal interaction between glucocerebrosidase and α-synuclein. In sporadic PD, glucocerebrosidase concentrations & enzymatic activity are reduced in substantia nigra. α-synuclein is degraded by chaperone-mediated & macro autophagy. α-synuclein inhibits activity of glucocerebrosidase, therefore there is bidirectional feedback between α-synuclein & glucocerebrosidase.

1515. Autophagy is impaired in which of the following diseases?
Harrison's 20th Ed. Chapter 417, Page 3044

A. Alzheimer's disease
B. Parkinson's disease
C. Huntington's disease
D. All of the above

Autophagy is the degradation of cystolic components in lysosomes. Autophagy plays an important role in degradation of protein aggregates in neurodegenerative diseases and it is impaired in AD, Parkinson's disease and Huntington's disease.

1516. Which of the following drug induces autophagy?
Harrison's 20th Ed. Chapter 417, Page 3044

A. Resveratrol
B. Spermidine
C. Rapamycin
D. Metformin

Rapamycin induces autophagy.

1517. As a cause of PD, which LRRK2 mutation is the commonest?
Harrison's 20th Ed. Chapter 427, Page 3125

A. p.G2017S
B. p.G2018S
C. p.G2019S
D. p.G2020S

Seven different LRRK2 mutations have been linked to PD, with p.G2019S being the commonest.

1518. The protein LRRK2 is also called?
Brain.2005;128(12):2786-96

A. Kardarin
B. Mardarin
C. Dardarin
D. Pardarin

The protein LRRK2 is also called "dardarin" from the Basque term "dardara" which means "to tremble."

1519. Confirmed genes responsible for the autosomal dominant form of PD are?
Harrison's 20th Ed. Chapter 427, Page 3124 Table 427-4

A. SNCA (PARK1)
B. LRRK2 (PARK8)
C. VPS35 (PARK17)
D. All of the above

1520. Phenotype of LRRK2 p.G2019S mutations is distinguished from that of sporadic PD by?
Harrison's 20th Ed. Chapter 427, Page 3125

A. Mask like face
B. Leg tremor
C. Frequent falls
D. Dementia

Phenotype of LRRK2 p.G2019S mutations is indistinguishable from that of sporadic PD, although tremor appears to be more common, and leg tremor may be a useful diagnostic clue. In G2019S mutation, glycine to serine substitution (G2019S) occurs within the protein kinase domain encoded by exon 41.

1521. Which of the following gene leads to an autosomal dominant form of PD?
Harrison's 20th Ed. Chapter 427, Page 3124 Table 427-4

A. SNCA (PARK1)
B. LRRK2 (PARK8)
C. VPS35 (PARK17)
D. All of the above

1522. Which of the following gene leads to an autosomal recessive form of PD?
Harrison's 20th Ed. Chapter 427, Page 3124 Table 427-4

A. PARK-Parkin (PARK2)
B. PARK-PINK1 (PARK6)
C. PARK-DJ1 (PARK7)
D. All of the above

1523. Which of the following about Kufor-Rakeb syndrome (KRS) is false?
Harrison's 20th Ed. Chapter 427, Page 3124 Table 427-4

A. Autosomal-recessive form of juvenile-onset PD
B. Caused by ATP13A2 gene mutations
C. Supranuclear upgaze paresis, facial-faucial-finger minimyoclonus
D. None of the above

Kufor-Rakeb syndrome (KRS; PARK 9) is a rare autosomal-recessive form of nigro-striatal-pallidal-pyramidal neurodegeneration caused by ATP13A2 gene mutations presenting as juvenile-onset Parkinson's disease (PD). Rapidly progressive symptoms of parkinsonism, spasticity, supranuclear upgaze paresis, facial-faucial-finger minimyoclonus, visual hallucinations, oculogyric dystonic spasms, and dementia, usually noted between 12 & 16 years, leads to severe motor handicap.

1524. Which of the following genes is mutated in PARK7 Parkinson's disease?
Harrison's 20th Ed. Chapter 427, Page 3124 Table 427-4

A. PINK1
B. DJ-1
C. Parkin
D. UCHL-1

1525. Which of the following about PD due to mutations in Parkin & PINK1 is false?
Harrison's 20th Ed. Chapter 427, Page 3125

A. Autosomal recessive and early-onset PD
B. Commonly complicated by dystonia
C. Lewy bodies are typically absent
D. None of the above

1526. Which of the following is false for familial Parkinson's disease?
Harrison's 20th Ed. Chapter 427, Page 3125

A. Mutations in a-synuclein and ubiquitin carboxy-terminal hydroxylase L1 (UCH-L1)
B. Characteristic histopathologic feature is Lewy body
C. Lewy body is eosinophilic cytoplasmic inclusion that contains neurofilaments and α-synuclein
D. None of the above

1527. Which of the following about basal ganglia is false?
Harrison's 20th Ed. Chapter 427, Page 3125

A. Striatum is the major input region of basal ganglia and receives its major input from cortex
B. GPi & SNr are the major output regions
C. Output of basal ganglia provides inhibitory (GABAergic) tone to thalamic & brainstem neurons
D. None of the above

1528. Glutamate is the neurotransmitter for which of the following pathways?
Harrison's 20th Ed. Chapter 427, Page 3126 Figure 427-5

A. Globus pallidus externa—subthalamic nucleus
B. Substantia nigra compacta—striatum
C. Subthalamic nucleus—Substantia nigra reticulata
D. Globus pallidus interna—thalamus

1529. Gamma aminobutyric acid (GABA) is the neurotransmitter for which of the following pathways?
Harrison's 20th Ed. Chapter 427, Page 3126 Figure 427-5

A. Globus pallidus externa—subthalamic nucleus
B. Striatum—Globus pallidus interna
C. Globus pallidus interna—thalamus
D. All of the above

1530. Which of the following pathways is excitatory?
Harrison's 20th Ed. Chapter 427, Page 3126 Figure 427-5

A. Globus pallidus externa—subthalamic nucleus
B. Striatum—Globus pallidus externa
C. Globus pallidus interna—thalamus
D. Subthalamic nucleus—Globus pallidus interna

1531. Which of the following pathways is inhibitory?
Harrison's 20th Ed. Chapter 427, Page 3126 Figure 427-5

A. Globus pallidus externa—subthalamic nucleus
B. Striatum—Globus pallidus externa
C. Globus pallidus interna—thalamus
D. All of the above

1532. Which of the following is false in PD?
Harrison's 20th Ed. Chapter 427, Page 3125

A. Increased firing of neurons in STN
B. Increased firing of neurons in GPi
C. Excessive inhibition of thalamus
D. None of the above

In PD, dopamine denervation causes increased firing of neurons in STN & GPi, resulting in excessive inhibition of thalamus with consequent reduced activation of cortical motor systems & development of parkinsonian features.

1533. Which of the following is most frequently present in patients with true PD?
Harrison's 20th Ed. Chapter 427, Page 3125

A. Rest tremor
B. Rigidity
C. Bradykinesia
D. Masked facies

Three cardinal signs of PD are rest tremor, rigidity & bradykinesia. Tremor is present in 85% of patients with true PD and diagnosis of PD is difficult if tremor is absent.

1534. Most disabling motor feature of PD is?
Harrison's 20th Ed. Chapter 427, Page 3125

A. Rest tremor
B. Rigidity
C. Bradykinesia
D. Stooped posture

The most disabling motor feature of PD is bradykinesia.

1535. Which of the following is false about 'rest tremor' in PD?
Harrison's 20th Ed. Chapter 427, Page 3125

A. Frequency of 4 to 6 Hz
B. Appear bilaterally, first distally
C. May appear in lips, tongue and jaw
D. Spares head and neck

Rest tremor, at a frequency of 4 to 6 Hz, typically appears unilaterally, first distally, involving the digits and wrist with a "pill-rolling" character. Tremor usually spreads proximally, ipsilaterally, and occasionally to the leg before crossing to the other side. It may appear later in lips, tongue and jaw but spares the head and neck.

1536. Testing for postural instability in PD is done by?
Harrison's 20th Ed. Chapter 427, Page 147

A. Swing test
B. Push test
C. Pull test
D. Lift test

In advanced PD, postural instability is one of the most disabling feature. It can be tested in office with the "pull test". A Tai Chi exercise program has been demonstrated to reduce the risk of falls and injury in patients with Parkinson's disease.

1537. Term used to describe gait in PD is?
Harrison's 20th Ed. Chapter 427, Page 146

A. Pigeon gait
B. Antalgic gait
C. Scissor gait
D. Festinating gait

Festinating gait is a classic sign of parkinsonism due to a combination of flexed posture and loss of postural reflexes. The patient accelerates to "catch up" with body's center of gravity. In Parkinson's disease, the fall due to freezing of gait. Feet stick to floor & center of mass keeps moving, resulting in a disequilibrium & a forward fall. Gait freezing can also occur as the patient attempts to turn & change direction.

1538. In Latin "festino" means?

A. "to fall"
B. "to freeze"
C. "to hurry"
D. "to swing"

In Latin "festino" means "to hurry".

1539. Manifestation that may be present long before the onset of motor signs in PD include?
Harrison's 20th Ed. Chapter 427, Page 3120, 3131

A. Anosmia
B. Depression
C. Sleep disorders
D. All of the above

1540. Which of the following symptom precedes onset of PD?
Harrison's 20th Ed. Chapter 427, Page 154, 3131

A. Rapid eye movement - behavioral disorder (RBD)
B. Micrographia
C. Hypophonia
D. All of the above

Epidemiologic studies suggest that clinical symptoms reflecting this nondopaminergic degeneration, such as constipation, anosmia, rapid eye movement (REM) behavior sleep disorder, restless legs and rapid eye movement–behavioral disorder (RBD) and cardiac denervation can precede the onset of the classic motor features of PD.

1541. Cardiac postganglionic adrenergic innervation is markedly impaired in?
Harrison's 20th Ed. Chapter 427, Page 3163

A. Multiple system atrophy (MSA)
B. Parkinson's disease (PD)
C. Guillain Barre syndrome
D. Diabetes Mellitus

Cardiac postganglionic adrenergic innervation, measured by uptake of fluorodopamine on positron emission tomography, is markedly impaired in the dysautonomia of Parkinson's disease (PD) but is usually normal in MSA.

1542. Neurogenic dysphagia results from?
Harrison's 20th Ed. Chapter 427, Page 251

A. Cerebrovascular accidents
B. Parkinson's disease
C. Amyotrophic lateral sclerosis
D. All of the above

1543. Constipation is common in?
Harrison's 20th Ed. Chapter 427, Page 269, 3131

A. Parkinson's disease
B. Multiple sclerosis
C. Diabetic neuropathy
D. All of the above

1544. 'Early appearance of hallucinations' favours which of the following diagnosis?
DeJong's The Neurologic Examination, 7th Ed. Page 488

A. Parkinson's disease
B. Wilson's disease
C. Cortical dementia with Lewy bodies (DLB)
D. Alzheimer's disease

In DLB, parkinsonian features are compounded by early appearance of hallucinations or drug-induced hallucinations and disturbances in arousal and behavior.

1545. 'Early imbalance & falls' favours the diagnosis of?
DeJong's The Neurologic Examination, 7th Ed. Page 488

A. Parkinson's disease
B. Progressive supranuclear palsy (PSP)
C. Cortical dementia with Lewy bodies (DLB)
D. Multiple system atrophy (MSA)

The development of early imbalance and falls suggests progressive supranuclear palsy (PSP).

1546. 'Early urinary incontinence, orthostatic hypotension, and dysarthria' favours which of the following diagnosis?
DeJong's The Neurologic Examination, 7th Ed. Page 488

A. Parkinson's disease
B. Progressive supranuclear palsy (PSP)
C. Cortical dementia with Lewy bodies (DLB)
D. Multiple system atrophy (MSA)

The development of early urinary incontinence, orthostatic hypotension and dysarthria suggest multiple system atrophy (MSA).

1547. Parkinsonian symptoms develop when striatal dopamine depletion reaches how much of normal?
Harrison's 20th Ed. Chapter 427, Page 3122

A. 10 to 30%
B. 30 to 50%
C. 50 to 70%
D. 70 to 90%

Symptoms develop when striatal dopamine depletion reaches 50 to 70% of normal.

1548. Which of the following symptoms respond poorly to therapy in PD?
Harrison's 20th Ed. Chapter 427, Page 3129

A. Bradykinesia
B. Abnormal posture
C. Balance difficulties
D. Rigidity

1549. Which of the following symptoms respond poorly to therapy in PD?
Harrison's 20th Ed. Chapter 427, Page 3129

A. Cognitive symptoms
B. Abnormal posture
C. Tremor
D. Rigidity

Cognitive symptoms, hypophonia, autonomic dysfunction & balance difficulties respond poorly to symptomatic therapy. While, bradykinesia, tremor, rigidity & abnormal posture respond well.

1550. Dopamine agonists act directly on which of the following postsynaptic dopamine receptor?

Harrison's 17th Ed. 2554

A. D1 type
B. D2 type
C. D3 type
D. D4 type

Dopamine agonists readily cross the blood-brain barrier and act directly on postsynaptic dopamine receptors - primarily D2 type.

1551. Which of the following statements is false?

Harrison's 20th Ed. Chapter 427, Page 3126

A. Levodopa is a dopamine precursor
B. Dopamine does not cross blood-brain barrier (BBB)
C. Domperidone is a peripheral dopamine-blocking agent
D. None of the above

1552. Which of the following area of the brain is not protected by the blood-brain barrier (BBB)?

Harrison's 20th Ed. Chapter 427, Page 3126, J Neuroinflammation 2010;7:70

A. Posterior pituitary gland
B. Pineal gland
C. Area postrema
D. All of the above

Four areas of brain are not protected by the blood-brain barrier. These areas include posterior pituitary gland, pineal gland, median eminence of hypothalamus and area postrema. Area postrema (a paired circumventricular organ & vomiting center in medulla) is not covered by BBB because it senses toxins in blood that other parts of brain are protected from. Area postrema triggers nausea & vomiting to prevent further ingestion of toxins.

1553. "No on" effect refers to?

Harrison's 20th Ed. Chapter 427, Page 3126

A. Loss of benefit following an individual dose
B. Delay in turning on the response
C. No response at all to a given dose
D. None of the above

With continued levodopa therapy, duration of benefit following an individual dose becomes progressively shorter. This loss of benefit is known as "wearing off effect". Patients may experience a delay in turning on (delayed-on) or no response at all to a given dose (no-on).

1554. Which of the following is false for Dyskinesias in PD?

Harrison's 20th Ed. Chapter 427, Page 3126

A. Choreiform and dystonic movements
B. Occur as a peak dose effect
C. Occur at the beginning or end of the dose
D. None of the above

Dyskinesias refer to choreiform and dystonic movements that can occur as a peak dose effect or at the beginning or end of the dose (diphasic dyskinesias).

1555. Nature of dyskinesia due to levodopa therapy is?

Harrison's 20th Ed. Chapter 427, Page 3126

A. Choreiform
B. Dystonia
C. Myoclonus
D. Any of the above

Nature of dyskinesia due to levodopa therapy can be choreiform in nature but can manifest as dystonic movements, myoclonus or other movement disorders predominantly involving the lower extremities, relieved by increasing the dose of levodopa. Dyskinesias tend to occur at the time of levodopa peak plasma concentration and maximal clinical benefit (peak-dose dyskinesia). "Diphasic dyskinesias" occur as the levodopa dose begins to take effect and again as it wears off.

1556. Which of the following is false about levodopa-induced motor complications?

Harrison's 20th Ed. Chapter 427, Page 3127

A. More likely to occur in females
B. More likely to occur in younger individuals with more severe disease
C. More likely to occur with higher doses of levodopa
D. None of the above

Levodopa-induced motor complications are more likely to occur in female, younger individuals with more severe disease and with the use of higher doses (mg/kg) of levodopa.

1557. Punding refers to?

Harrison's 20th Ed. Chapter 427, Page 3127

A. Hypersexuality
B. Meaningless assembly & disassembly of objects
C. Phobic cry
D. Craving for levodopa

PD patients taking high doses of levodopa can develop purposeless, stereotyped behaviors such as the meaningless assembly and disassembly or collection and sorting of objects. This is known as punding. This term is taken from Swedish description of meaningless behaviors seen in chronic amphetamine users.

1558. Dopamine dysregulation syndrome refers to?

Harrison's 20th Ed. Chapter 427, Page 3127

A. Hypersexuality
B. Meaningless assembly & disassembly of objects
C. Phobic cry
D. Craving for levodopa

In dopamine dysregulation syndrome, patients have a craving for levodopa and take frequent and unnecessary doses of the drug in an addictive manner.

1559. Levodopa can be combined with?

Harrison's 20th Ed. Chapter 427, Page 3127

A. Carbidopa
B. Benserazide
C. Entacapone
D. All of the above

To prevent peripheral metabolism of levodopa to dopamine & development of nausea & vomiting due to activation of dopamine receptors in area postrema, levodopa is used in combination with peripheral decarboxylase inhibitor (carbidopa or benserazide) or COMT inhibitor (tolcapone or entacapone).

1560. Which of the following statements about Levodopa is false?

Harrison's 20th Ed. Chapter 427, Page 3127

A. Is a precursor of dopamine
B. It is not metabolized centrally by dopa-decarboxylase
C. It is metabolized peripherally by dopa-decarboxylase
D. It is metabolized by COMT & MAO

Levodopa is a precursor of dopamine and is metabolized centrally & peripherally by dopa-decarboxylase, catechol-O-methyltransferase (COMT) and monoamine oxidase. Inhibitors of monoamine oxidase type B (MAO-B) block central dopamine metabolism & increase synaptic concentrations of the neurotransmitter.

1561. Which of the following is not a 'Dopamine agonist'?
Harrison's 20th Ed. Chapter 427, Page 3127

A. Levodopa
B. Pergolide
C. Bromocriptine
D. Pramipexole

Levodopa is a precursor of dopamine.

1562. Which of the following dopamine agonist is an ergot derivative?
Harrison's 20th Ed. Chapter 427, Page 3127

A. Bromocriptine
B. Pergolide
C. Cabergoline
D. All of the above

1563. Which of the following dopamine agonist is a nonergot derivative?
Harrison's 20th Ed. Chapter 427, Page 3127

A. Pramipexole
B. Ropinirole
C. Rotigotine
D. All of the above

Dopamine agonists include ergot alkaloids like bromocriptine, cabergoline, lisuride and pergolide and second generation non-ergot alkaloids like pramipexole, ropinirole and rotigotine.

1564. Which of the following antiparkinsonian drug is associated with valvular disease?
Harrison's 20th Ed. Chapter 427, Page 3127

A. Levodopa
B. Pergolide
C. Pramipexole
D. Rotigotine

Pergolide is associated with asymptomatic valvular disease on chronic administration.

1565. Which of the following is administered as a transdermal patch?
Harrison's 20th Ed. Chapter 427, Page 3127

A. Pramipexole
B. Ropinirole
C. Rotigotine
D. Levodopa

Rotigotine is administered as a once-daily transdermal patch.

1566. Which of the following is used as a rescue agent for treatment of severe "off" episodes?
Harrison's 20th Ed. Chapter 427, Page 3127

A. Apomorphine
B. Ropinirole
C. Pramipexole
D. Levodopa

Apomorphine is a dopamine agonist but must be administered parenterally (SC/continuous infusion) and is used as a rescue agent for the treatment of severe "off" episodes.

1567. Which of the following is an impulse-control disorder?
Harrison's 20th Ed. Chapter 427, Page 3127

A. Pathologic gambling
B. Hypersexuality
C. Compulsive eating
D. All of the above

1568. What amount of carbidopa is necessary to block peripheral levodopa decarboxylation into dopamine?
Harrison's 17th Ed. 2556

A. 10 mg/day
B. 25 mg/day
C. 50 mg/day
D. 75 mg/day

Mostly, 75 mg/day of carbidopa is necessary to block peripheral levodopa decarboxylation into dopamine.

1569. MAO is responsible for the deactivation of?
Cleveland Clinic Journal of Medicine 2010:77;860

A. Norepinephrine
B. 5-hydroxytryptamine
C. Dopamine
D. All of the above

Intramitochondrial enzyme MAO is responsible for the deactivation of norepinephrine, 5-hydroxytryptamine, and dopamine.

1570. With MAO inhibitors, tyramine-induced hypertensive crisis is named as?
Harrison's 20th Ed. Chapter 427, Page 3128

A. Alcohol effect
B. Diet effect
C. Cheese effect
D. Wine effect

Inhibition of MAO-A prevents metabolism of tyramine in gut, leading to a potentially fatal hypertensive reaction known as a "cheese effect" as it can be precipitated by foods rich in tyramine (some cheeses, aged meats & red wine).

1571. Which of the following is a monoamine oxidase (MAO) B inhibitor?
Harrison's 20th Ed. Chapter 427, Page 3128

A. Pramipexole
B. Pergolide
C. Selegiline
D. Entacapone

Selegiline & rasagiline are selective & irreversible monoamine oxidase (MAO) B inhibitor that block central dopamine metabolism & increase its synaptic concentration. They do not functionally inhibit MAO-A.

1572. Which of the following is a monoamine oxidase (MAO) inhibitor?
Harrison's 20th Ed. Chapter 427, Page 1563

A. Furazolidone
B. Cycloserine
C. Clarithromycin
D. Amikacin

Furazolidone inhibits monoamine oxidase (MAO) gradually over several days.

1573. Which of the following is a monoamine oxidase (MAO) inhibitor?
Harrison's 20th Ed. Chapter 427, Page 1055

A. Linezolid
B. Rifapentine
C. Clarithromycin
D. Capreomycin

Linezolid is a weak MAO inhibitor and can be associated with the serotonin syndrome when given concomitantly with serotonergic drugs (SSRI). Iproniazid was the first antidepressant introduced and is a MAOI anti-tuberculous drug.

1574. Which of the following is a reversible MAO-B inhibitor?
Harrison's 20th Ed. Chapter 427, Page 3128

A. Glycinamide
B. Safinamide
C. N-acetylprocainamide (NAPA)
D. Dichlorphenamide

1575. Which of the following is not a MAO inhibitor?
Harrison's 20th Ed. Chapter 427, Page 3308 Table 450-4

A. Isocarboxazid
B. Phenelzine
C. Tetrabenazine
D. Tranylcypromine

MAO inhibitors include selegiline, isocarboxazid, phenelzine and tranylcypromine. The last three are irreversible enzyme inhibitors that binds to MAO covalently, destroying its function forever.

1576. MAO catabolizes which of the following?
Cleveland Clinic Journal of Medicine 2010;77;860

A. Norepinephrine
B. Serotonin
C. Dopamine
D. All of the above

MAO is a flavin-containing enzyme critical for regulating neurotransmitter levels by catabolizing endogenous monoamines (NE, serotonin & dopamine) & exogenous amines (dietary tyramine). MAO exists in two subtypes, A & B. MAO-A preferentially metabolizes serotonin (5-HT) & NE. MAO-B preferentially metabolizes trace amines, including phenethylamine. MAO-A & MAO-B metabolize DA & tyramine.

1577. Which of the following have only MAO-B?
Cleveland Clinic Journal of Medicine 2010;77;860

A. Intestine
B. Brain
C. Platelets
D. Liver

MAO-A is the major enzyme outside of brain, with the exception of platelets and lymphocytes, which have only MAO-B. Ratio of MAO-A to MAO-B in human brain is 25%:75%, whereas in liver, ratio is 50%:50%, in intestine, ratio is 80%:20% & in peripheral adrenergic neurons, ratio is 90%:10%.

1578. Which of the following is a selective MAO-A inhibitor?
Cleveland Clinic Journal of Medicine 2010;77;860

A. Phenelzine
B. Isocarboxazid
C. Clorgyline
D. Moclobemide

Nonselective MAO inhibitors are phenelzine, isocarboxazid & tranylcypromine. Selegiline is selective for MAO-B. Clorgyline is selective for MAO-A. Moclobemide is a reversible MAO inhibitor.

1579. Which of the following is a Catechol O-methyltransferase (COMT) inhibitor?
Harrison's 20th Ed. Chapter 427, Page 3128

A. Selegiline
B. Entacapone
C. Bromocriptine
D. Pergolide

Entacapone and tolcapone are catechol-O-methyl transferase (COMT) inhibitors. They augment the effects of levodopa by blocking peripheral enzymatic degradation of levodopa and dopamine.

1580. Which of the following is a long-acting, once daily COMT inhibitor?
Harrison's 20th Ed. Chapter 427, Page 3128

A. Tolcapone
B. Entacapone
C. Opicapone
D. All of the above

1581. Discoloration of urine can be due to which of the following drugs?
Harrison's 20th Ed. Chapter 427, Page 3128

A. Selegiline
B. Entacapone
C. Bromocriptine
D. Pergolide

Though not of clinical concern, discoloration of urine can be seen with both COMT inhibitors (tolcapone and entacapone) due to accumulation of a metabolite.

1582. Which of the following is a side effect of tolcapone?
Harrison's 20th Ed. Chapter 427, Page 3128

A. Severe diarrhea
B. Hepatic toxicity
C. Discoloration of urine
D. All of the above

1583. Which of the following clinical studies relate to treatment of PD?
Harrison's 20th Ed. Chapter 427, Page 3128

A. DATATOP study
B. ADAGIO study
C. STRIDE-PD study
D. All of the above

1584. The only oral agent that reduces dyskinesia while improving parkinsonian features is?
Harrison's 20th Ed. Chapter 427, Page 3128

A. Selegiline
B. Amantadine
C. Bromocriptine
D. Pergolide

Amantadine, an antiviral agent, is the only oral agent that reduces dyskinesia while improving parkinsonian features.

1585. Livedo reticularis is the side effect of?
Harrison's 20th Ed. Chapter 427, Page 3128

A. Selegiline
B. Amantadine
C. Bromocriptine
D. Pergolide

Amantadine is a weak NMDA-receptor antagonist. Its side effects are livido reticularis, weight gain, and impaired cognitive function.

1586. Which of the following about Amantadine is false?
Harrison's 20th Ed. Chapter 427, Page 3128

A. Withdrawal-like symptoms on discontinuation
B. Antiviral agent

C. Potent anti-dyskinesia agent
D. None of the above

1587. Which of the following anticonvulsant has antiparkinsonian effects?
Harrison's 20th Ed. Chapter 427, Page 3128

A. Oxcarbazepine
B. Tiagabine
C. Felbamate
D. Zonisamide

1588. Which of the following is a A_{2A} antagonist?
Harrison's 20th Ed. Chapter 427, Page 3129

A. Rolofylline
B. Istradefylline
C. Pentifylline
D. Pentoxifylline

The A_{2A} antagonist Istradefylline is approved in Japan.

1589. Which of the following drugs has neuroprotective function in PD?
Harrison's 20th Ed. Chapter 427, Page 3129

A. Levodopa
B. Bromocryptine
C. Selegiline
D. Amantadine

Selegiline in addition to a mild symptomatic effect has a neuroprotective function. High doses of coenzyme Q_{10}, intrastriatal infusion of neurotrophic factors and exercise may be beneficial.

1590. Which of the following drugs have the potential of a neuroprotective therapy in PD?
Harrison's 20th Ed. Chapter 427, Page 3129

A. Rasagiline
B. Pramipexole
C. Ropinirole
D. All of the above

Rasagiline, selegiline, pramipexole, ropinirole & coenzyme Q_{10} are promising neuroprotection or disease modification agents in PD.

1591. Deep brain stimulation (DBS) for PD primarily targets which of the following?
Harrison's 20th Ed. Chapter 427, Page 3129

A. Ventrolateral thalamus
B. Subthalamic nucleus (STN)
C. Substantia nigra, pars compacta
D. Motor cortex

DBS for PD primarily targets subthalamic nucleus (STN) or internal segment of globus pallidus (GPi). GPi stimulation may be associated with a reduced frequency of depression.

1592. Trophic factors with beneficial effects on dopamine neurons include?
Harrison's 20th Ed. Chapter 427, Page 3130

A. Ciliary neurotrophic factor (CNTF)
B. Brain-derived neurotrophic factor (BDNF)
C. Neurturin
D. All of the above

Trophic factors that have beneficial effects on dopamine neurons in laboratory studies include Glial-derived neurotrophic factor (GDNF) and neurturin.

1593. In gene therapy for PD, which of the following is used as viral vector?
Harrison's 20th Ed. Chapter 427, Page 3130

A. AAV1
B. AAV2
C. AAV3
D. AAV4

Gene therapy involves viral vector delivery of DNA of a therapeutic protein to specific target regions. The AAV2 virus is used as viral vector as it does not cause inflammatory response, is not incorporated into host genome, and is associated with long-lasting transgene expression.

1594. Which of the following may be helpful for both depression & PD motor features?
Harrison's 20th Ed. Chapter 427, Page 3130

A. Selegiline
B. Rasagiline
C. Pramipexole
D. Ropinirole

1595. In patients of PD with psychotic symptoms, which of the following drug is preferred?
Harrison's 20th Ed. Chapter 427, Page 3130

A. Quetiapine
B. Clozapine
C. Risperidone
D. Olanzapine

Quetiapine is recommended because it lacks the risk of agranulocytosis associated with clozapine. Risperidone, olanzapine and aripiprazole are not well tolerated by most patients with PD due to a higher incidence of drug-induced parkinsonism (DIP) and akathisia.

1596. Which of the following in PD patients is a harbinger of a developing dementia?
Harrison's 20th Ed. Chapter 427, Page 3130

A. Panic attacks
B. Sweating
C. Constipation
D. Hallucinations

Hallucinations in PD patients are often a harbinger of a developing dementia. In contrast to AD, hallucinations are typically visual, formed and nonthreatening.

1597. Which atypical neuroleptic is also an inverse agonist of serotonin 5-HT2A receptor?
Harrison's 20th Ed. Chapter 427, Page 3130

A. Pimavanserin
B. Quetiapine
C. Clozapine
D. All of the above

Atypical neuroleptic Pimavanserin is also an inverse agonist of the serotonin 5-HT2A receptor.

1598. Cause of neuropsychiatric symptoms in PD can be?
Harrison's 20th Ed. Chapter 427, Page 3130

A. Accompanying Alzheimer's disease (AD)
B. Accompanying cortical dementia with Lewy bodies (DLB)
C. Side effect of pharmacotherapy
D. All of the above

Neuropsychiatric symptoms of later stages of PD may be direct result of PD or accompanying Alzheimer's disease, cortical dementia with Lewy bodies or as a side effect of its drugs.

1599. In dementia in PD (PDD), which of the following is relatively spared?

Harrison's 20th Ed. Chapter 427, Page 3130

- A. Language
- B. Memory
- C. Calculation
- D. All of the above

In contrast to AD, PDD primarily affects executive functions & attention, with relative sparing of language, memory, and calculation domains.

1600. To preserve or regain cognitive functions in PD, which of the following drug is withdrawn first?

Harrison's 20th Ed. Chapter 427, Page 3130

- A. Anticholinergics
- B. Dopamine agonists
- C. COMT inhibitors
- D. MAO-B inhibitors

To preserve or regain cognitive functions in PD, drugs are discontinued in the following sequence: anticholinergics, amantadine, dopamine agonists, COMT inhibitors, and MAO-B inhibitors. Patients are managed with lowest dose of standard levodopa.

1601. Which of the following drugs reduce the rate of deterioration of cognitive function in PD?

Harrison's 20th Ed. Chapter 427, Page 3130

- A. Memantine
- B. Rivastigmine
- C. Donepezil
- D. All of the above

Anticholinesterase agents (memantine, rivastigmine & donepezil) reduce the rate of deterioration of cognitive function and can improve attention in PD.

1602. Which of the following is typical of REM behavior disorder (RBD)?

Harrison's 20th Ed. Chapter 427, Page 3131

- A. Violent movements & vocalizations during REM sleep
- B. Orthostatic hypotension & fainting on awakening
- C. Visual hallucinations
- D. All of the above

REM behavior disorder (RBD) is a syndrome comprised of violent movements and vocalizations during REM sleep possibly representing acting out of dreams due to a failure of normal inhibition of motor movements that typically accompanies REM sleep.

Tremor, Chorea, and Other Movement Disorders

1603. Which of the following best relate to hyperkinetic movement disorders?
Harrison's 20th Ed. Chapter 428, Page 3132

A. Voluntary
B. Involuntary
C. Seizure
D. Passive

Hyperkinetic movement disorders are characterized by involuntary movements occurring in isolation or in combination, unaccompanied by weakness.

1604. Which of the following is not a kind of tremor?
Harrison's 20th Ed. Chapter 428, Page 3132

A. Rest tremor
B. Kinetic tremor
C. Akinetic tremor
D. Postural tremor

Tremor consists of alternating contractions of agonist & antagonist muscles in an oscillating, rhythmic manner. It can be most prominent at rest (rest tremor), on assuming a posture (postural tremor), on actively reaching for a target (kinetic tremor) or on carrying out a movement (action tremor).

1605. PD is characterized by which of the following tremor?
Harrison's 20th Ed. Chapter 428, Page 3132

A. Rest tremor
B. Kinetic tremor
C. Postural tremor
D. All of the above

1606. Essential tremor (ET) is characterized by which of the following tremor?
Harrison's 20th Ed. Chapter 428, Page 3132

A. Rest tremor
B. Kinetic tremor
C. Postural tremor
D. All of the above

1607. Cerebellar disease is characterized by which of the following tremor?
Harrison's 20th Ed. Chapter 428, Page 3132

A. Rest tremor
B. Kinetic tremor
C. Postural tremor
D. All of the above

PD is characterized by a resting tremor, essential tremor (ET) by a postural tremor, and cerebellar disease by an intention or kinetic tremor associated with hypotonia & past pointing.

1608. Which of the following about physiologic tremor is false?
Harrison's 20th Ed. Chapter 428, Page 3133

A. High-frequency (10 - 12 Hz)
B. Postural or action tremor
C. Affecting the upper extremities
D. None of the above

1609. Enhanced physiologic tremor (EPT) can be seen with the use of?
Harrison's 20th Ed. Chapter 428, Page 3133

A. Valproate
B. Lithium
C. Alcohol
D. All of the above

Enhanced physiologic tremors (EPT) are mild, high-frequency, postural or action tremors usually of no clinical consequence seen in anxiety, fatigue, hyperthyroidism, electrolyte abnormalities, valproate, lithium, smoking, caffeine or alcohol.

1610. Which of the following is the most common movement disorder?
Harrison's 20th Ed. Chapter 428, Page 3133

A. Myoclonus
B. Tic
C. Essential tremor (ET)
D. Dystonia

ET is the most common movement disorder, affecting ~5% of the population.

1611. Which of the following is not a feature of essential tremor?
Harrison's 20th Ed. Chapter 428, Page 3133

A. Bilaterality
B. Frequency of 6 to 10 Hz
C. Postural dependency
D. Aggravation with alcohol

Essential tremor (ET) presentation includes bilaterality, higher frequency (6 to 10 Hz), and postural dependency and significant relief with alcohol.

1612. Which part of body is affected most in essential tremor (ET)?
Harrison's 20th Ed. Chapter 428, Page 3133

A. Arms
B. Head
C. Legs
D. Tongue

Essential tremor (ET) is the most common movement disorder characterized by 6- to 10-Hz postural & kinetic tremor affecting the upper extremities mostly. Tremor involves head in ~30%, voice in ~20%, tongue in ~20%, face/jaw in ~10%, and lower limbs in ~10% of cases. Multiple body parts are involved in ~50% of cases.

1613. Which of the following about ET is false?
Harrison's 20th Ed. Chapter 428, Page 3133

A. Bilateral & symmetric
B. Improved by alcohol & worsened by stress
C. Patients have relatively large handwriting
D. None of the above

1614. All of the following can aggravate essential tremors except?
Harrison's 20th Ed. Chapter 428, Page 3133

A. Valproic acid
B. Tricyclic antidepressants
C. Alcohol
D. Serotonin reuptake blockers

Alcohol consumption reduces ET. Stress and drugs that can aggravate any tremor include valproic acid, lithium, beta-adrenergic agonists, methylxanthines, thyroxin, glucocorticoids, tricyclic antidepressants, and serotonin reuptake blockers.

1615. Drugs that have usefulness in treatment of essential tremors include all except?

Harrison's 20th Ed. Chapter 428, Page 3133

- A. Primidone
- B. Propranolol
- C. Valproic acid
- D. Gabapentin

Primidone and propranolol are the first-line treatments for ET. Additional useful medications, with or without the primary agents, include benzodiazepines, gabapentin, topiramate, and botulinum toxin injections to affected muscle groups. Surgical therapies targeting the VIM nucleus of the thalamus can be very effective for severe and drug-resistant cases.

1616. Criteria for Essential Tremor of the International Parkinson and Movement Disorder Society (2017) includes all except?

N Engl J Med. 2018;378:1802-10

- A. Bilateral upper-limb action tremor
- B. Duration of at least 5 years
- C. With or without tremor in head, voice, or lower limbs
- D. Absence of other neurologic signs

According to International Parkinson and Movement Disorder Society (2017), criteria for isolated tremor syndrome include bilateral upper-limb action tremor, duration of at least 3 years, with or without tremor in other locations (head, voice, or lower limbs) and absence of other neurologic signs, such as dystonia, ataxia, or parkinsonism.

1617. Criteria for Essential Tremor plus of the International Parkinson and Movement Disorder Society (2017) includes characteristics of essential tremor with?

N Engl J Med. 2018;378:1802-10

- A. Impaired tandem gait
- B. Questionable dystonic posturing
- C. Memory impairment
- D. Any of the above

According to International Parkinson and Movement Disorder Society (2017), besides characteristics of essential tremor, criteria for essential tremor plus includes additional neurologic signs of uncertain clinical significance such as impaired tandem gait, questionable dystonic posturing, memory impairment, or other mild neurologic signs that do not suffice to make an additional syndrome classification or diagnosis. Essential tremor with additional tremor at rest should be classified as essential tremor plus.

1618. Association with which of the following gene is found in patients with young-onset ET?

N Engl J Med. 2018;378:1802-10

- A. PLOD1 gene
- B. LINGO1 gene
- C. COL1A1 gene
- D. TNXB gene

Association with LINGO1 gene is found in patients with young-onset ET.

1619. Which of the following about LINGO1 protein is false?

N Engl J Med. 2018;378:1802-10

- A. Inhibits cell differentiation during development
- B. Inhibits axonal regeneration
- C. Inhibits synaptic plasticity
- D. None of the above

1620. Which of the following is noted in the cerebellum of persons with essential tremor?

N Engl J Med. 2018;378:1802-10

- A. Decreased levels of N-acetylaspartate on Magnetic resonance spectroscopy
- B. Increased LINGO1 levels
- C. γ-aminobutyric acid (GABA) dysfunction
- D. All of the above

In ET, cerebellar metabolism is high at rest, increases with arm extension & decreases with administration of ethanol. Cellular bursts in cerebellar receiving zone of thalamus (ventral intermediate nucleus, VIM) correlate strongly with tremor itself.

1621. Which of the following is included in "Essential tremor plus"?

N Engl J Med. 2018;378:1802-10

- A. Impaired tandem gait
- B. Questionable dystonic posturing
- C. Impaired memory
- D. Any of the above

In "Essential tremor plus" additional "soft" or mild neurologic signs of uncertain clinical significance like impaired tandem gait, questionable dystonic posturing, or impaired memory are included.

1622. Which of the following is best related to essential tremor?

N Engl J Med. 2018;378:1802-10

- A. Killian's triangle
- B. Triangle of Koch
- C. Guillain–Mollaret triangle
- D. Calot triangle

The Guillain–Mollaret triangle comprises of the ipsilateral red nucleus in midbrain, inferior olive in medulla and contralateral dentate nucleus in cerebellum. Together, these form the dentato-rubro-olivary pathway. Pathology in this triangle disinhibits (and so activates) inferior olivary nucleus.

1623. Which of the following about essential tremor is false?

N Engl J Med. 2018;378:1802-10

- A. Often familial, with autosomal dominant pattern
- B. Related to gene that encodes LINGO1
- C. Rhythmic activity in cortico–ponto–cerebello–thalamo–cortical loop
- D. None of the above

Pathophysiology of essential tremor almost certainly involves rhythmic activity in the cortico-ponto-cerebello-thalamo-cortical loop.

1624. Swollen axons of Purkinje's cells are called?

N Engl J Med. 2018;378:1802-10

- A. Missiles
- B. Torpedoes
- C. Gun barrels
- D. Cannons

Swollen axons of Purkinje's cells seen in pathological studies are called Torpedoes.

1625. Potential tremor-inducing drugs include all except?

N Engl J Med. 2018;378:1802-10

- A. Valproate
- B. Sympatholytic agents
- C. Selective serotonin-reuptake inhibitors
- D. Lithium and toxins like mercury, lead, or manganese.

Potential tremor-inducing drugs include valproate, selective serotonin-reuptake inhibitors, sympathomimetic agents, or lithium and toxins like mercury, lead, or manganese.

1626. Differential diagnoses of isolated tremor syndromes without other neurologic signs include?
N Engl J Med. 2018;378:1802-10

A. Enhanced physiologic tremor
B. Isolated focal tremors
C. Orthostatic tremors
D. All of the above

Differential diagnoses of isolated tremor syndromes without other neurologic signs include enhanced physiologic tremor, isolated focal tremors (isolated tremors of head, voice, or palate), and orthostatic tremors.

1627. Tremor syndromes with prominent additional neurologic signs include?
N Engl J Med. 2018;378:1802-10

A. Dystonic tremors
B. Holmes tremor
C. Myorhythmia
D. All of the above

Tremor syndromes with prominent additional neurologic signs include dystonic tremors, tremors combined with parkinsonism, intention tremor syndromes, Holmes tremor (combined low-frequency rest, posture, and intention tremor due to lesions in the cerebellar outflow tract), & myorhythmia.

1628. Which of the following about Holmes tremor is false?
N Engl J Med. 2018;378:1802-10

A. Resting, postural & intention tremor
B. Caused by lesions in brainstem, thalamus and cerebellum
C. Stereotactic thalamotomy & DBS in VIM effective
D. None of the above

1629. Primidone is metabolized to phenobarbital and?
N Engl J Med. 2018;378:1802-10

A. Phenylpropanolamine
B. Phenylhydrazine
C. L-dihydroxyphenylserine
D. Phenylethylmalonamide

Primidone is metabolized to phenylethylmalonamide (PEMA) and phenobarbital.

1630. Rating scale assessment of essential tremor is?
N Engl J Med. 2018;378:1802-10

A. WHIGET scale
B. TETRAS
C. Fahn-Tolosa-Marin scale
D. All of the above

The Essential Tremor Rating Assessment Scale (TETRAS) was developed by the Tremor Research Group to quantify essential tremor severity & its impact on activities of daily living.

1631. Which of the following statements is false about dystonia?
Harrison's 20th Ed. Chapter 428, Page 3133

A. Co-contraction of agonist and antagonist muscles
B. Appear during attempted voluntary movement
C. Exacerbated by stress and fatigue
D. None of the above

Co-contraction of agonist and antagonist muscles is a fundamental feature of dystonia and characteristically present during attempted voluntary movement. Dystonia is exacerbated by stress and fatigue and attenuated by sensory inputs [touching affected body part or sensory trick (geste antagoniste)]. The geste antagoniste sign is a legacy of Paris Neurological School. The term was introduced by Meige & Feindel in their 1902 book on tics while mentioning Brissaud, who first described this sign in 1893.

1632. Most of the genetic forms of dystonia belong to which phenotypic group?
Harrison's 20th Ed. Chapter 428, Page 3133

A. Isolated dystonia
B. Combined dystonia
C. Complex dystonia
D. Any of the above

When dystonia is the only disease manifestation with the exception of tremor, its grouped in "isolated dystonia". When dystonia co-occurs with another movement disorder like parkinsonism or myoclonus, its grouped in "combined dystonia" and when dystonia is only one of several clinical manifestations and may be a less prominent or even inconsistent feature, it is in the "complex dystonia" phenotypic group.

1633. Which of the following is a clinical phenotype of focal dystonia?
Harrison's 20th Ed. Chapter 428, Page 3134

A. Spasmodic dysphonia
B. Blepharospasm
C. Oromandibular dystonia (OMD)
D. All of the above

Focal dystonia can be focal, multifocal or segmental. The major clinical phenotypes of focal dystonia are cervical dystonia, blepharospasm, oromandibular dystonia (OMD), spasmodic dysphonia and limb dystonia.

1634. Which of the following is a combination of oromandibular dystonia (OMD) and blepharospasm?
Harrison's 20th Ed. Chapter 428, Page 3134

A. Dopa responsive dystonia (DRD)
B. Idiopathic torsion dystonia (ITD)
C. Meige's syndrome
D. Lubag form of dystonia-parkinsonism

1635. Which of the following best relates to Meige's syndrome?
Harrison's 20th Ed. Chapter 428, Page 3134

A. Cervical dystonia
B. Limb dystonia
C. Oromandibular dystonia (OMD)
D. Spasmodic dysphonia

Meige's syndrome is a combination of OMD and blepharospasm that predominantly affects women aged >60 years.

1636. Which of the following is a focal dystonia?
Harrison's 20th Ed. Chapter 428, Page 3134

A. Blepharospasm
B. Torticollis
C. Laterocollis
D. All of the above

Most common forms of dystonia are in adults - blepharospasm, cervical dystonias (torticollis, laterocollis, anterocollis, retrocollis), oromandibular dystonia, spasmodic dysphonia.

1637. Which of the following is the least common dystonia?
Harrison's 20th Ed. Chapter 428, Page 3134

A. Cervical dystonia
B. Oromandibular dystonia (OMD)
C. Blepharospasm
D. Spasmodic dysphonia

Frequency of focal dystonias is cervical dystonia (~50%), blepharospasm (~20%), Focal hand or leg dystonia (~5%), spasmodic dysphonia (~2%), musician's dystonia (~3%), or OMD (~1%).

1638. Which of the following is a gene for isolated dystonia?
Harrison's 20th Ed. Chapter 428, Page 3134

A. TOR1A
B. THAP1
C. ANO3
D. All of the above

Well established genes for isolated dystonia are TOR1A, THAP1, ANO3, GNAL and KMT2B.

1639. Which of the following is called Dopa-responsive dystonia (DRD)?
Harrison's 20th Ed. Chapter 428, Page 3134

A. Boerhaave syndrome
B. Segawa syndrome
C. Reye's syndrome
D. Sweet syndrome

Dopa-responsive dystonia (DRD is also called Segawa syndrome).

1640. Segawa syndrome is caused by mutations in which of the following gene?
Harrison's 20th Ed. Chapter 428, Page 3134

A. TAF1 gene
B. ATP1A3 gene
C. SGCE gene
D. GCH1 gene

Segawa syndrome is caused by mutations in GCH1 gene (GTP cyclohydrolase-1) that encodes for the rate-limiting enzyme in biosynthesis of dopamine via the biopterin pathway without nigral cell loss.

1641. Any patient suspected of having a childhood-onset dystonia should receive a trial of?
Harrison's 20th Ed. Chapter 428, Page 3134

A. Valproate
B. Lithium
C. Levodopa
D. Serotonin reuptake blockers

Any patient suspected of having a childhood-onset dystonia should receive a trial of levodopa to exclude Dopa responsive dystonia (DRD) or the Segawa variant (DYT5).

1642. Dystonia frequently accompanied by psychiatric disturbances goes in favour of?
Harrison's 20th Ed. Chapter 428, Page 3134

A. Idiopathic torsion dystonia (ITD)
B. Myoclonic dystonia
C. X-linked dystonia-parkinsonism (Lubag)
D. Dopa responsive dystonia (DRD)

Myoclonic dystonia results from mutations in SGCE gene (sarcoglycan epsilon) which codes for the ε member of sarcoglycan family. It typically manifests as a combination of dystonia and action-induced, alcohol-responsive myoclonic jerks predominantly involving the upper body half, frequently accompanied by psychiatric disturbances such as depression, anxiety-related disorders, and alcohol dependence.

1643. Which of the following is an X-linked recessive dystonia parkinsonism?
Harrison's 20th Ed. Chapter 428, Page 3134

A. Huntington's disease
B. X-linked dystonia-parkinsonism (Lubag)
C. Leigh's disease
D. All of the above

X-linked dystonia-parkinsonism (Lubag) affects Filipino men originating principally from the Panay Island. Retrotransposon insertion in TAF1 (TATA-Box Binding Protein Associated Factor 1) gene is the most likely cause of disease.

1644. Which of the following is a complex dystonia?
Harrison's 20th Ed. Chapter 428, Page 3134

A. Wilson's disease (WD)
B. Huntington's disease (HD)
C. Lesh Nyhan syndrome
D. All of the above

In complex dystonias, dystonia is one part (usually non-dominant neurologic feature) of a syndrome with multiple different manifestations. Wilson's disease (WD), Huntington's disease (HD) & Lesh Nyhan syndrome belong to complex dystonias.

1645. Most effective treatment for generalized primary dystonia is?
Harrison's 20th Ed. Chapter 428, Page 3135

A. Primidone
B. Propranolol
C. Valproic acid
D. Anticholinergic drugs

Anticholinergic drugs are the most effective forms of treatment for generalized primary dystonia.

1646. Dystonic storm can occur in response to?
Harrison's 20th Ed. Chapter 428, Page 3136

A. Anticholinergic drug overdose
B. Inadequate anticholinergic drug dose
C. Stress situation
D. All of the above

1647. George Huntington belonged to which country?
Harrison's 20th Ed. Chapter 428, Page 3136

A. Great Britain
B. America
C. Australia
D. Canada

Huntington's disease (HD) was described by George Huntington, an American physician in 1872. Huntington's gene is single, causal gene and an accurate genetic test for HD is available.

1648. Which of the following is most characteristic feature of HD?
Harrison's 20th Ed. Chapter 428, Page 3136

A. Gait disturbance
B. Chorea
C. Oculomotor abnormalities
D. Myoclonus

HD is characterized by rapid, nonpatterned, semi-purposeful, involuntary choreiform movements. Dysarthria, gait disturbance, and oculomotor abnormalities are common features. As disease progresses, chorea is reduced & dystonia, rigidity, bradykinesia, myoclonus, and spasticity emerge.

1649. Westphal variant of Huntington's disease (HD) relates to which of the following?
Harrison's 20th Ed. Chapter 428, Page 3136

A. Alzheimer's disease
B. Parkinsonian syndrome
C. Orthostatic hypotension
D. Dementia

HD can present as an akinetic-rigid or parkinsonian syndrome (Westphal variant).

1650. Which of the following is a typical MRI finding in Huntington's Disease (HD)?
Harrison's 20th Ed. Chapter 428, Page 3136

- A. Atrophy of the thalamus
- B. Progressive atrophy of head of the caudate nucleus
- C. Iron accumulation in striatum
- D. Atrophy of the midbrain

HD predominantly strikes striatum. Progressive atrophy of head of the caudate nucleus and consequent enlargement of lateral ventricles is seen in MRI. Putamen can be equally or even more severely affected.

1651. Huntington's disease (HD) is caused by mutations in the Huntington's gene on the?
Harrison's 20th Ed. Chapter 428, Page 3137

- A. Short arm of chromosome 4
- B. Long arm of chromosome 4
- C. Short arm of chromosome 5
- D. Long arm of chromosome 5

HD is caused by mutations in the Huntington's gene on the short arm of chromosome 4. Alleles from normal individuals have between 12 and 37 CAG repeats. HD is caused by an increase in the number of polyglutamine (CAG) repeats (>40) in the coding sequence of the huntingtin gene. The larger the number of repeats, the earlier the disease is manifest.

1652. Phenomenon referred to as 'anticipation' is relevant to which of the following?
Harrison's 20th Ed. Chapter 428, Page 3137

- A. Huntington's disease (HD)
- B. Wilson's disease
- C. Tourette's syndrome (TS)
- D. Restless legs syndrome

In Huntington's disease, acceleration of disease process occur, particularly in males, with subsequent generations having larger numbers of repeats & earlier age of disease onset, a phenomenon referred to as anticipation.

1653. Which of the following about huntingtin is false?
Harrison's 20th Ed. Chapter 428, Page 3137

- A. Cytoplasmic protein
- B. Widely distributed in neurons
- C. Function is not known
- D. None of the above

1654. Which of the following drug is useful in the treatment of Huntington's disease?
Harrison's 20th Ed. Chapter 428, Page 3137

- A. Levodopa
- B. Trihexyphenidyl
- C. Tetrabenazine
- D. All of the above

Tetrabenazine is a presynaptic dopamine depleting agent & is approved for the treatment of chorea.

1655. Which of the following HD-like (HDL) disorders is an autosomal dominant condition?
Harrison's 20th Ed. Chapter 428, Page 3137

- A. HDL-1
- B. HDL-2
- C. HDL-4
- D. All of the above

HD-like (HDL) disorders 1, 2 and 4 are inherited autosomal dominant conditions that typically present in adulthood and closely mimic HD.

1656. Which of the following is a prion disease?
Harrison's 20th Ed. Chapter 428, Page 3137

- A. HD-like (HDL) disorders 1
- B. α-Synuclein Parkinson's disease (PD)
- C. Creutzfeldt-Jakob disease (CJD)
- D. All of the above

1657. Which of the following HD-like (HDL) disorders 1 is related to PRNP gene?
Harrison's 20th Ed. Chapter 428, Page 3137

- A. HDL-1
- B. HDL-2
- C. HDL-4
- D. All of the above

HDL-1, a prion disease, is due to expansion of an octapeptide repeat in PRNP, the gene encoding the prion protein. Patients exhibit personality change in third or fourth decade, followed by chorea, rigidity, myoclonus, ataxia & epilepsy.

1658. Which of the following HD-like (HDL) disorders 1 is related to acanthocytosis?
Harrison's 20th Ed. Chapter 428, Page 3137

- A. HDL-1
- B. HDL-2
- C. HDL-4
- D. All of the above

HDL-2 manifests in the third or fourth decade with chorea, dystonia or parkinsonism and dementia and acanthocytosis.

1659. Which of the following HD-like (HDL) disorders 1 is related to junctophilin-3 (JPH3) gene?
Harrison's 20th Ed. Chapter 428, Page 3137

- A. HDL-1
- B. HDL-2
- C. HDL-4
- D. All of the above

HDL-2 is caused by an abnormally expanded CTG/CAG trinucleotide repeat expansion in the junctophilin-3 (JPH3) gene.

1660. Which of the following HD-like (HDL) disorders is related to TBP gene?
Harrison's 20th Ed. Chapter 428, Page 3137

- A. HDL-1
- B. HDL-2
- C. HDL-4
- D. All of the above

HDL-4, the most common HDL, is caused by expansion of trinucleotide repeats in TBP, the gene that encodes the TATA box binding protein involved in regulating transcription.

1661. Which of the following HD-like (HDL) disorders 1 is identical to spinocerebellar ataxia (SCA) 17?
Harrison's 20th Ed. Chapter 428, Page 3137

- A. HDL-1
- B. HDL-2
- C. HDL-4
- D. All of the above

HDL-4 is identical to spinocerebellar ataxia (SCA) 17 and most patients present primarily with ataxia rather than chorea.

1662. Mutations in which of the following gene causes Chorea-acanthocytosis (neuroacanthocytosis)?
Harrison's 20th Ed. Chapter 428, Page 3137

- A. TCF7L2
- B. PRC1
- C. VPS13C
- D. VPS13A

Chorea-acanthocytosis (neuroacanthocytosis) is a progressive and fatal autosomal recessive disorder characterized by chorea with red cell abnormalities on peripheral blood smear (acanthocytes). Chorea can be severe with self mutilating behavior, dystonia, tics, seizures and polyneuropathy. Mutations in VPS13A gene encoding chorein is documented.

1663. Sydenham's choreas responds to which of the following?
Harrison's 20th Ed. Chapter 428, Page 3137

- A. Dopamine-blocking agents
- B. Valproic acid
- C. Carbamazepine
- D. All of the above

Sydenham's chorea (St. Vitus' dance) is of acute onset and responds to dopamine-blocking agents, valproic acid, and carbamazepine. Chorea may recur in later life, particularly in association with pregnancy (chorea gravidarum) or treatment with sex hormones.

1664. Chorea may be associated with which of the following?
Harrison's 20th Ed. Chapter 428, Page 3137

- A. Cryptococcal encephalitis
- B. Progressive rubella panencephalitis
- C. Herpes simplex virus encephalitis
- D. Limbic encephalitis

Chorea may be associated with NMDA receptor antibody-positive encephalitis following herpes simplex virus encephalitis.

1665. Most common systemic disorder that causes chorea is?
Harrison's 20th Ed. Chapter 428, Page 3137

- A. Hyperthyroidism
- B. HIV disease
- C. Systemic lupus erythematosus (SLE)
- D. Polycythemia rubra vera

Systemic lupus erythematosus is the most common systemic disorder that causes chorea. Choreas can also be seen with hyperthyroidism, Sjögren's syndrome, HIV disease, metabolic alterations, polycythemia rubra vera, with many medications (anticonvulsants, cocaine, CNS stimulants, estrogens, lithium) and paraneoplastic syndromes associated with anti-CRMP-5 or anti-Hu antibodies.

1666. Which of the following is X-linked disorder?
Harrison's 20th Ed. Chapter 456, Page 3361

- A. Rett's syndrome
- B. Danon's disease
- C. Hunter disease (MPS II)
- D. All of the above

1667. Which of the following is X-linked disorder?
Harrison's 20th Ed. Chapter 456, Page 3361

- A. Fabry disease
- B. Alport's syndrome
- C. Ehlers-Danlos syndrome Type V
- D. All of the above

1668. Which of the following is X-linked disorder?
Harrison's 20th Ed. Chapter 456, Page 3361

- A. Dent's disease
- B. IPEX syndrome
- C. Wiskott-Aldrich syndrome (WAS)
- D. All of the above

1669. Which of the following is X-linked disorder?
Harrison's 20th Ed. Chapter 428, Page 3361

- A. Adrenomyeloneuropathy
- B. Kennedy's syndrome
- C. McLeod syndrome
- D. All of the above

1670. Disorder having excess brain iron accumulation on MRI is?
Harrison's 20th Ed. Chapter 428, Page 3141

- A. Autosomal dominant neuroferritinopathy
- B. Hallervorden-Spatz disease
- C. Neuroacanthocytosis
- D. Aceruloplasminemia

Neurodegenerative diseases with brain iron accumulation (NBIA) manifesting with chorea include autosomal dominant neuroferritinopathy, autosomal recessive pantothenate-kinase-associated neurodegeneration (PKAN; Hallervorden-Spatz disease), and aceruloplasminemia. Iron accumulation in globus pallidus provides on MRI the characteristic "eye of the tiger" appearance.

1671. Which of the following best relates to hemiballismus?
Harrison's 20th Ed. Chapter 428, Page 3138

- A. Chorea
- B. Athetosis
- C. Choreoathetosis
- D. Any of the above

Hemiballismus is a violent form of chorea composed of wild, flinging, large-amplitude movements of proximal limb muscles on one side of the body.

1672. Which of the following is a violent form of chorea?
Harrison's 20th Ed. Chapter 428, Page 3138

- A. Hemiballismus
- B. Monoballism
- C. Paraballism
- D. All of the above

In hemiballismus proximal limb muscles are predominantly affected. These movements may affect just one limb (monoballism) or, more exceptionally, both upper or lower limbs (paraballism).

1673. In hemiballismus, most often the lesion is in?
Harrison's 20th Ed. Chapter 428, Page 3138

- A. Globus pallidus
- B. Cerebellum
- C. Subthalamic nucleus
- D. Pedunculopontine nucleus

Most common cause of hemiballismus is a lesion (infarct or hemorrhage) of subthalamic nucleus (STN), but cases can also be seen with lesions in the putamen, thalamus and parietal cortex.

1674. Phonic (or vocal) tic with expression of obscene words is called?
Harrison's 20th Ed. Chapter 428, Page 3138

- A. Grunting
- B. Echolalia
- C. Palilalia
- D. Coprolalia

1675. Which of the following is a kind of vocal tic?
Harrison's 20th Ed. Chapter 428, Page 3138

A. Echolalia
B. Palilalia
C. Coprolalia
D. All of the above

Vocal tics include grunting, echolalia (repeating other people's words), palilalia (repeating one's own words), and coprolalia (expression of obscene words).

1676. Tics may present in adulthood with?
Harrison's 20th Ed. Chapter 428, Page 3138

A. PD
B. HD
C. Levodopa therapy
D. All of the above

Tics may present in adulthood and can also be seen with PD, HD, trauma, dystonia, drugs (levodopa, neuroleptics) and toxins.

1677. Which of the following is a neurobehavioral disorder?
Harrison's 20th Ed. Chapter 428, Page 3138

A. Essential tremor (ET)
B. Wilson's disease
C. Huntington's disease (HD)
D. Tourette's syndrome (TS)

Tourette's syndrome (TS) is a neurobehavioral disorder named after French neurologist Georges Gilles de la Tourette.

1678. Associated behavioral disturbance with Tourette's syndrome (TS) include?
Harrison's 20th Ed. Chapter 428, Page 3138

A. Anxiety, depression
B. Attention deficit hyperactivity disorder
C. Obsessive-compulsive disorder
D. All of the above

Associated behavioral disturbances with Tourette's syndrome (TS) include anxiety, depression, attention deficit hyperactivity disorder, and obsessive-compulsive disorder.

1679. Which of the following gene is implicated in Tourette's syndrome?
Harrison's 20th Ed. Chapter 428, Page 3138

A. VPS13A
B. BHC2
C. C9Orf
D. None of the above

TS is considered as a genetic disorder, but no specific gene mutation has been identified. The risk of a family with one affected child having a second is about 25%.

1680. PANDAS is best related to?
Harrison's 20th Ed. Chapter 428, Page 3138

A. Trauma
B. β-hemolytic streptococcal infection
C. Obsessive-compulsive disorder
D. Levodopa

PANDAS refers to pediatric autoimmune neuropsychiatric disorder associated with streptococcal infection.

1681. Effective medication in treatment of Tourette's syndrome is?
Harrison's 20th Ed. Chapter 428, Page 3138

A. Clonidine
B. Guanfacine
C. Olanzapine
D. All of the above

Clonidine, Guanfacine, Atypical neuroleptics (risperidone, olanzapine, ziprasidone) and classical neuroleptics (haloperidol, fluphenazine, or pimozide) are useful in treatment of TS.

1682. Which of the following about myoclonus is false?
Harrison's 20th Ed. Chapter 428, Page 3138

A. Rapid, jerky movement of <100 msec duration
B. Asterixis is a negative myoclonus
C. Interferes with normal movement
D. Suppressible

Myoclonus is a rapid, jerky movement of <100 msec. duration due to single or repetitive muscle discharges. It occur spontaneously, in association with voluntary movement (action myoclonus) or in response to an external stimulus (reflex or startle myoclonus).

1683. Myoclonic jerks can be?
Harrison's 20th Ed. Chapter 428, Page 3138

A. Focal
B. Multifocal
C. Generalized
D. Any of the above

Myoclonic jerks can be focal, multifocal, segmental or generalized and can occur spontaneously, in association with voluntary movement (action myoclonus) or in response to an external stimulus (reflex or startle myoclonus).

1684. Which of the following is an example of negative myoclonus?
Harrison's 20th Ed. Chapter 428, Page 3138

A. Tic
B. Dystonia
C. Asterixis
D. Hypnagogic jerks

Negative myoclonus consists of a brief loss of muscle activity (asterixis in hepatic failure). Myoclonic jerks differ from tics in that they interfere with normal movement and are not suppressible.

1685. Myoclonus can be seen in association with pathology in?
Harrison's 20th Ed. Chapter 428, Page 3138

A. Cortical region
B. Subcortical region
C. Spinal cord region
D. All of the above

Myoclonus can be seen in association with pathology in cortical, subcortical, brainstem or spinal cord regions and associated with hypoxemic damage, encephalopathy, and neurodegeneration.

1686. Reversible myoclonus can be seen with which of the following?
Harrison's 20th Ed. Chapter 428, Page 3138

A. Renal failure
B. Electrolyte imbalance
C. Hypocalcemia
D. All of the above

Reversible myoclonus can be seen with metabolic disturbances (renal failure, electrolyte imbalance, hypocalcemia), toxins and many medications.

1687. Which of the following is false about essential myoclonus?
Harrison's 20th Ed. Chapter 428, Page 3138

A. Focal
B. Very brief lightning-like movements
C. Alcohol sensitive
D. Benign familial condition

Essential myoclonus is a relatively benign familial condition characterized by multifocal, very brief, lightning-like movements that are frequently alcohol sensitive.

1688. Which of the following is useful in the treatment of myoclonus?
Harrison's 20th Ed. Chapter 428, Page 3139

A. Valproic acid
B. Piracetam
C. Levetiracetam
D. All of the above

Treatment primarily consists of treating the underlying condition or removing offending agent. Valproic acid, piracetam, clonazepam, primidone and levetiracetam may be effective.

1689. Which of the following is an example of Dystonia?
Harrison's 20th Ed. Chapter 428, Page 3139

A. Blepharospasm
B. Torticollis
C. Oromandibular dystonia
D. All of the above

Dystonia is the most common acute hyperkinetic drug reaction. It is typically generalized in children and focal in adults like blepharospasm, torticollis, or oromandibular dystonia.

1690. Which of the following about tardive dyskinesia (TD) is false?
Harrison's 20th Ed. Chapter 428, Page 3139

A. Choreiform movements
B. Mouth, lips, and tongue mostly involved
C. Valbenazine helpful in refractory cases
D. None of the above

Valbenazine is an ester of tetrabenazine useful in the treatment of tardive dyskinesia. It acts as a vesicular monoamine transporter type 2 (VMAT-2) inhibitor & blocks storage of dopamine.

1691. Use of metoclopramide for more than how many weeks increases the risk of tardive dyskinesia (TD)?
Harrison's 20th Ed. Chapter 428, Page 3139

A. 2 weeks
B. 4 weeks
C. 6 weeks
D. 12 weeks

FDA has warned that use of metoclopramide for more than 12 weeks increases the risk of TD.

1692. Which of the following may occur after chronic neuroleptic exposure?
Harrison's 20th Ed. Chapter 428, Page 3139

A. Tardive akathisia
B. Tardive TS
C. Tardive tremor syndrome
D. All of the above

1693. Levels of which of the following is markedly elevated in neuroleptic malignant syndrome (NMS)?
Harrison's 20th Ed. Chapter 428, Page 3139

A. Creatine kinase
B. Lactic dehydrogenase
C. Lactic acid
D. All of the above

Neuroleptic malignant syndrome (NMS) is characterized by muscle rigidity, elevated temperature, altered mental status, hyperthermia, tachycardia, labile blood pressure, renal failure, and markedly elevated creatine kinase levels. Myoclonus is not a feature of NMS but of serotonin syndrome.

1694. Myoclonus can result with the use of which of the following drugs?
Harrison's 20th Ed. Chapter 428, Page 3139

A. Phenytoin
B. Fluoxetine
C. Buspirone
D. All of the above

Drugs can be associated with parkinsonism & hyperkinetic movement disorders like phenytoin (chorea, dystonia, tremor, myoclonus), carbamazepine (tics and dystonia), tricyclic antidepressants (dyskinesias, tremor, myoclonus), fluoxetine (myoclonus, chorea, dystonia), oral contraceptives (dyskinesia), adrenergics (tremor), buspirone (akathisia, dyskinesias, myoclonus), and digoxin, cimetidine, diazoxide, lithium, methadone, and fentanyl (dyskinesias).

1695. Which of the following is a paroxysmal dyskinesia?
Harrison's 20th Ed. Chapter 428, Page 3140

A. Paroxysmal kinesigenic dyskinesia (PKD)
B. Paroxysmal nonkinesigenic dyskinesias (PNKD)
C. Paroxysmal exertion-induced dyskinesia (PED)
D. All of the above

1696. Which of the following gene is associated with paroxysmal PED?
Harrison's 20th Ed. Chapter 428, Page 3140

A. SLC2A1
B. SLC2A2
C. SLC2A3
D. SLC2A4

1697. Restless Legs Syndrome was first described by?
Harrison's 20th Ed. Chapter 428, Page 3140

A. Christopher Ross
B. Micheal Emre
C. Thomas Willis
D. James Hardy

Restless legs syndrome (RLS) is a neurologic disorder and was first described in seventeenth century by English physician Thomas Willis.

1698. The restless legs syndrome (RLS) is also known as?
N Engl J Med. 2003;348:2103-9

A. Earley's syndrome
B. Hening's syndrome
C. Wetter's syndrome
D. Ekbom's syndrome

The restless legs syndrome (RLS) is also known as Ekbom's syndrome (Ekbom KA. Restless legs syndrome. Acta Med. Scand 1945;158(suppl):1–123).

1699. Which of the following is not a core symptom required for diagnosis of RLS?
Harrison's 20th Ed. Chapter 428, Page 3140

A. Urge to move the legs
B. Symptoms begin or worsen with rest
C. Partial or complete relief by movement
D. Worsening during daytime

According to International RLS Study Group (1995), the four core symptoms required for diagnosis of RLS are an urge to move the legs, symptoms begin or worsen with rest, partial or complete relief by movement and worsening during the evening or night. Paresthesias secondary to peripheral neuropathy persist with activity.

1700. Which of the following is false about periodic leg movements (PLMs) associated with RLS?
Harrison's 20th Ed. Chapter 428, Page 3140, N Engl J Med. 2003;348:2103-9

A. Occur during sleep
B. Brief involuntary movements
C. Recur every 5–90 seconds
D. None of the above

RLS is usually associated with semirhythmic leg movements during sleep that are referred to as periodic limb movements of sleep.

1701. Periodic leg movements can be observed in which of the following conditions?
N Engl J Med. 2003;348:2103-9

A. Sleep apnea
B. Spinal cord lesions
C. Stroke
D. All of the above

Periodic leg movements that are apparent on polysomnography. Apart from RLS, they are observed in sleep apnea, neurodegenerative diseases, spinal cord lesions, stroke, narcolepsy, and with treatment with antidepressant or neuroleptic agents.

1702. Which of the following description best relate to RLS?
BMJ 2012;344:e3056

A. Tearing of the skin
B. Legs immersed in ice cold water
C. Insects crawling under the skin
D. Tight rope around the legs

Urge to move legs is typical of RLS accompanied by abnormal sensations described as burning, tingling, aching, or "insects crawling under the skin".

1703. Which of the following description best relate to RLS?
N Engl J Med. 2003;348:2103-9

A. "Creepy-crawly" sensation
B. "Like ants marching in my legs"
C. "Like soda water in the veins"
D. All of the above

The sensation in RLS may be described as a muscle ache or tension. Other patients describe a "creepy-crawly" sensation or a feeling "like ants marching in my legs" or "like soda water in the veins."

1704. Which of the following about primary restless legs syndrome is false?
Harrison's 20th Ed. Chapter 428, Page 3140

A. Genetic with autosomal dominant pattern of inheritance
B. Mean age of onset is 27 years
C. Neurologic examination is normal
D. None of the above

1705. Which of the following about restless legs syndrome is false?
BMJ 2012;344:e3056

A. More prevalent in women than in men
B. Prevalence increases with age
C. Most common movement disorder in pregnancy
D. None of the above

1706. Secondary RLS may be associated with?
Harrison's 20th Ed. Chapter 428, Page 3140

A. Pregnancy
B. Peripheral neuropathy
C. Renal failure
D. All of the above

Secondary RLS may be associated with pregnancy, anemia, ferritin deficiency, renal failure, and peripheral neuropathy.

1707. Factor that may exacerbate RLS symptoms is?
Cleveland Clinic Journal of Medicine. 2005;72 (9):773

A. Cold & heat
B. Fatigue
C. Stress
D. All of the above

Factors other than immobility that may exacerbate RLS include cold, heat, fatigue & stress.

1708. Secondary RLS may be associated with?
Harrison's 20th Ed. Chapter 428, Page 3140, BMJ 2012;344:e3056

A. Ferritin deficiency
B. Renal failure
C. Peripheral neuropathy
D. All of the above

Secondary RLS may be associated with pregnancy, anemia, ferritin deficiency, renal failure, and peripheral neuropathy. Restless legs syndrome may also be associated with cardiovascular disease, obesity, diabetes, rheumatological disorders, radiculopathy, Parkinson's disease, multiple sclerosis, Charcot-Marie-Tooth disease, and spinal cord lesions.

1709. RLS has been reported to occur with which of the following?
N Engl J Med. 2003;348:2103-9

A. During pregnancy
B. In patients undergoing dialysis
C. Iron deficiency
D. All of the above

1710. Restless legs syndrome (RLS) is related to which of the following?
Harrison's 20th Ed. Chapter 428, Page 3140

A. Iron metabolism
B. Copper metabolism
C. Zinc metabolism
D. Magnesium metabolism

Pathogenesis of RLS probably involves disordered dopamine function (peripheral or central), in association with an abnormality of iron metabolism. Low serum ferritin (<50 μg/L) favours its diagnosis. Serum ferritin correlates inversely with symptom severity. Iron is an essential cofactor for tyrosine hydroxylase and seems to have a crucial role in dopamine metabolism.

1711. Severity of RLS can be exacerbated by?
BMJ 2012;344:e3056

A. Dopamine agonists
B. Serotonergic antidepressants
C. Anticonvulsants
D. Opiates

RLS is characterised by upregulation of dopaminergic transmission, with postsynaptic desensitisation. Dopamine agonists (pramipexole, ropinirole & rotigotine), Levodopa, anticonvulsants, analgesics, gabapentin and opiates can be effective in RLS. Symptoms can be exacerbated by sleep deprivation, caffeine, alcohol, serotonergic antidepressants (selective serotonin reuptake inhibitors and serotonin noradrenaline reuptake inhibitors), and pregnancy.

1712. Treatment of choice for RLS is with?
Harrison's 20th Ed. Chapter 428, Page 3140

A. Opioids
B. Benzodiazepines
C. Pramipexole
D. Gabapentin

Symptoms of RLS are exquisitely sensitive to dopaminergic drugs (pramipexole or ropinirole), which are the treatments of choice. Opioids, benzodiazepines, and gabapentin may also be of therapeutic value.

1713. Vesper's curse best relates to?
Cleveland Clinic Journal of Medicine. 2005;72 (9):773

A. Congestive heart failure + Lumbar spinal stenosis
B. Congestive heart failure + OSA
C. Congestive heart failure + Parkinsonism
D. Congestive heart failure + Blindness

Vesper's curse refers to lumbosacral and associated leg pain and paresthesias arousing patients from a sound sleep occurring in patients with congestive heart failure in association with lumbar spinal stenosis. An increase in right atrial filling pressure reflected in elevated paraspinal venous volumes within the reduced confines of a stenotic lumbar spine is believed to be the precipitating cause of this syndrome.

1714. Polymorphism in which of the following genes has been linked to RLS?
Harrison's 20th Ed. Chapter 428, Page 174

A. BTBD9
B. MEIS1
C. PTPRD
D. All of the above

Polymorphisms in BTBD9, MEIS1, MAP2K5/LBXCOR and PTPRD genes have been linked to RLS.

1715. Which of the following conditions may have a common pathophysiology as of RLS?
Harrison's 20th Ed. Chapter 428, Page 174

A. Somnambulism
B. Sleep enuresis
C. Periodic limb movement disorder (PLMD)
D. REM sleep behavior disorder (RBD)

Most patients with restless legs also experience PLMD, although the reverse is not the case.

1716. Wilson's disease is caused by mutations in?
Harrison's 20th Ed. Chapter 428, Page 3140

A. ATP5B gene
B. ATP6B gene
C. ATP7B gene
D. ATP8B gene

Wilson's disease is caused by mutations in the ATP7B gene encoding a P-type ATPase.

1717. What was the first name of Wilson who described Wilson's disease?
Harrison's 20th Ed. Chapter 428, Page 3140

A. Camelo
B. Hebert
C. Charles
D. Kinnier

Wilson's disease was first described by English neurologist Kinnier Wilson at the beginning of twentieth century. At around the same time, German physicians Kayser & Fleischer separately noted the characteristic association of corneal pigmentation with hepatic and neurologic features.

1718. Which of the following in Wilson's disease can manifest alone?
Harrison's 20th Ed. Chapter 428, Page 3140

A. Neurologic disorders
B. Psychiatric disorders
C. Liver disorders
D. Any of the above

Wilson's disease (WD) is an autosomal recessive inherited disorder of copper metabolism that may manifest with neurologic, psychiatric, and liver disorders, alone or in combination. About half of WD patients (esp. younger patients) manifest with liver abnormalities.

1719. Which of the following marks the onset of neurologic manifestations in WD?
Harrison's 20th Ed. Chapter 428, Page 3140

A. Bradykinesia
B. Tremor
C. Dystonia
D. Dysarthria

Neurologic onset usually manifests in the second decade with tremor and rigidity. Tremor is usually in upper limbs, bilateral, and asymmetric.

1720. Kayser-Fleischer (KF) rings are seen in nearly what proportion of WD patients with hepatic presentations?
Harrison's 20th Ed. Chapter 428, Page 3140

A. 20%
B. 40%
C. 80%
D. 100%

Kayser-Fleischer (KF) rings are seen in 80% of WD patients with hepatic presentations.

1721. Kayser-Fleischer (KF) rings are seen in nearly what proportion of WD patients with neurologic features?
Harrison's 20th Ed. Chapter 428, Page 3140

A. 20%
B. 40%
C. 80%
D. 100%

Kayser-Fleischer (KF) rings are seen in nearly all WD patients with neurologic features. It is very rare for WD patients with neurologic features not to have KF rings.

1722. Which of the following statements about Kayser-Fleischer (KF) rings is false?
Harrison's 20th Ed. Chapter 428, Page 3140

A. Represent deposition of copper in Descemet's membrane
B. Grayish discoloration of the peripheral cornea
C. Best detected by slit-lamp examination
D. None of the above

Kayser-Fleischer rings (KF rings) represent the deposition of copper in Descemet's membrane producing grayish discoloration of peripheral cornea. They are best detected by slit-lamp examination.

1723. The neuropathologic lesion in WD is in?
Harrison's 20th Ed. Chapter 428, Page 3140

A. Substantia nigra
B. Striatum
C. Globus pallidus
D. Thalamus

Neuropathologic examination is characterized by neurodegeneration and astrogliosis in the basal ganglia, particularly in the striatum.

1724. In WD, which of the following is false?
Harrison's 20th Ed. Chapter 428, Page 3141

A. Low levels of blood copper
B. Low levels of blood ceruloplasmin
C. High levels of urinary copper
D. None of the above

In WD, low levels of blood copper and ceruloplasmin and high levels of urinary copper are found but normal levels do not exclude the diagnosis.

1725. In WD, MRI shows symmetric hyperintensity on T2-weighted images in?
Harrison's 20th Ed. Chapter 428, Page 3141

A. Putamen
B. Caudate
C. Globus pallidus
D. All of the above

In WD, MRI shows symmetric hyperintensity on T2-weighted images in putamen, caudate & pallidum.

1726. Which of the following is the gold standard for the diagnosis of WD?
Harrison's 20th Ed. Chapter 428, Page 3141

A. Kayser-Fleischer (KF) rings
B. Generalized atrophy on CT brain scan
C. Hyperintensity of putamen on T2-weighted MRI images
D. High copper levels in liver biopsy

Liver biopsy with demonstration of high copper levels is the gold standard for diagnosis of WD.

1727. Which of the following blocks the absorption of copper?
Harrison's 20th Ed. Chapter 428, Page 3141

A. Penicillamine
B. Tetrathiomolybdate
C. Trientine
D. Zinc

Tetrathiomolybdate blocks absorption of copper. Penicillamine increases copper excretion. Trientine & zinc are useful drugs for maintenance therapy.

1728. Which of the following statements about Penicillamine is false?
Harrison's 20th Ed. Chapter 428, Page 3141

A. Worsens symptoms in initial stages of therapy
B. Increases copper excretion
C. Should be coadministered with pyridoxine
D. None of the above

1729. What time after therapy, KF rings may disappear?
Harrison's 20th Ed. Chapter 428, Page 3141

A. 6 months
B. 1 year
C. 2 years
D. Never disappear

KF rings tend to decrease after 3–6 months of therapy and disappear by 2 years.

1730. In neurodegeneration with brain iron accumulation (NBIA), the iron accumulates in?
Harrison's 20th Ed. Chapter 428, Page 3141

A. Pineal gland
B. Basal ganglia
C. Corpus callosum
D. Cerebral cortex

Neurodegeneration with brain iron accumulation (NBIA) represents a group of inherited disorders characterized by iron accumulation in the basal ganglia.

1731. NBIA can manifest as which of the following?
Harrison's 20th Ed. Chapter 428, Page 3141

A. Parkinsonism
B. Neuropsychiatric abnormalities
C. Retinal degeneration
D. Any of the above

NBIA can manifest as a progressive neurologic disorder that may manifest as parkinsonism, dystonia, neuropsychiatric abnormalities, retinal degeneration, cognitive disorders and cerebellar dysfunction.

1732. Most common form of NBIA is?
Harrison's 20th Ed. Chapter 428, Page 3141

A. Restless legs syndrome
B. Wilson's disease
C. Pantothenate kinase-associated neurodegeneration
D. Machado-Joseph disease

1733. "Eye of the tiger" sign in MRI best relates with?
Harrison's 20th Ed. Chapter 428, Page 3141

A. Restless legs syndrome
B. Wilson's disease
C. Hallervorden-Spatz disease
D. Machado-Joseph disease

Pantothenate kinase-associated neurodegeneration (PKAN) known earlier as Hallervorden-Spatz disease (HSD) is the most common form of NBIA. It is caused by a mutation in PANK2 gene. Onset is in early childhood & manifests as a combination of dystonia, parkinsonism & spasticity. MRI shows a characteristic low signal abnormality in center of globus pallidus on T2-weighted scans known as the "eye of the tiger" sign caused by iron accumulation. Systemic & CSF iron levels, as well as plasma ferritin, transferrin, and ceruloplasmin, all are normal.

1734. The most common psychogenic movement disorder is?
Harrison's 20th Ed. Chapter 428, Page 3141

A. Tremor affecting the upper limbs
B. Tremor affecting the lower limbs
C. Tremor affecting the lips & tongue
D. Tremor affecting the body

Tremor affecting the upper limbs is the most common psychogenic movement disorder.

1735. Astasia-abasia is best related to?
Harrison's 20th Ed. Chapter 428, Page 3141

A. Parkinsonism
B. Cerebellar degeneration
C. Psychogenic movement disorder
D. Nystagmus

Astasia-abasia refers to odd gyrations of posture with wastage of muscular energy, extreme slow motion, and dramatic fluctuations over time observed in patients with somatoform disorders and conversion reaction with no underlying pathology.

Amyotrophic Lateral Sclerosis and Other Motor Neuron Diseases

1736. Lou Gehrig's disease is the other name of?
N Engl J Med. 2001;344:1688

- A. Amyotrophic lateral sclerosis
- B. Myasthenia gravis
- C. Multiple sclerosis
- D. Subacute combined degeneration of cord

ALS is often called Lou Gehrig's disease after Lou Gehrig (1903-1941), a hall-of-fame baseball player for New York Yankees who suffered with ALS. People in England and Australia call ALS as Motor Neurone Disease (MND). The French refer to it as Maladie de Charcot, after the French doctor Jean-Martin Charcot, who first wrote about ALS in 1869.

1737. Which of the following is the most common form of progressive motor neuron disease?
Harrison's 20th Ed. Chapter 429, Page 3141

- A. Amyotrophic lateral sclerosis
- B. Primary lateral sclerosis
- C. Progressive muscular atrophy
- D. Familial spastic paraplegia

Amyotrophic lateral sclerosis (ALS) is the most common form of progressive motor neuron disease.

1738. Which of the following is the most devastating of the neurodegenerative disorders?
Harrison's 20th Ed. Chapter 429, Page 3141

- A. Amyotrophic lateral sclerosis
- B. Primary lateral sclerosis
- C. Progressive muscular atrophy
- D. Familial spastic paraplegia

Amyotrophic lateral sclerosis is a neurodegenerative disease & is the most devastating of the neurodegenerative disorders.

1739. Which of the following is involved in motor neuron degenerative disorders?
Harrison's 20th Ed. Chapter 429, Page 3142

- A. Anterior horn cells in spinal cord
- B. Brainstem nuclei innervating bulbar muscles
- C. Corticospinal motor neurons
- D. All of the above

Pathologic hallmark of motor neuron degenerative disorders is death of lower motor neurons. These include anterior horn cells in spinal cord, brainstem nuclei innervating bulbar muscles, upper or corticospinal motor neurons originating in layer five of motor cortex and descending via the pyramidal tract to synapse with lower motor neurons, either directly or indirectly via interneurons. Characteristically, in ALS, upper or lower motor neurons both will eventually be involved.

1740. Acute sporadic motor neuron diseases include?
Harrison's 20th Ed. Chapter 429, Page 3143 Table 429-2

- A. Poliomyelitis
- B. Herpes zoster
- C. Coxsackie virus
- D. All of the above

Acute sporadic motor neuron diseases include Poliomyelitis, Herpes zoster, West Nile virus and Coxsackie virus.

1741. Chronic sporadic motor neuron disease with predominant involvement of upper motor neurons is?
Harrison's 20th Ed. Chapter 429, Page 3143 Table 429-2

- A. Amyotrophic lateral sclerosis
- B. Multifocal motor neuropathy with conduction block
- C. Motor neuropathy with paraproteinemia
- D. Primary lateral sclerosis

Chronic sporadic MND with predominant involvement of UMN is primary lateral sclerosis. Upper and lower motor neuron are involved in Amyotrophic lateral sclerosis (ALS).

1742. Chronic sporadic motor neuron disease with predominant involvement of lower motor neurons are?
Harrison's 20th Ed. Chapter 429, Page 3143 Table 429-2

- A. Multifocal motor neuropathy with conduction block
- B. Motor neuropathy with paraproteinemia or cancer
- C. Motor-predominant peripheral neuropathies
- D. All of the above

In Amyotrophic lateral sclerosis, both upper & lower motor neurons are involved. In Primary lateral sclerosis, predominantly upper motor neurons are involved. In Multifocal motor neuropathy with conduction block, Motor neuropathy with paraproteinemia or cancer and Motor-predominant peripheral neuropathies, predominantly lower motor neurons are affected.

1743. Disease that affect lower motor neurons of spinal cord is?
Harrison's 20th Ed. Chapter 429, Page 3142

- A. Pseudobulbar palsy
- B. Primary lateral sclerosis (PLS)
- C. Familial spastic paraplegia (FSP)
- D. Progressive muscular atrophy

In spinal muscular atrophy (SMA), also called progressive muscular atrophy, the lower motor neurons of spinal cord are most severely involved.

1744. Diseases that affect only upper motor neurons innervating the brainstem and spinal cord are?
Harrison's 20th Ed. Chapter 429, Page 3142

- A. Pseudobulbar palsy
- B. Primary lateral sclerosis (PLS)
- C. Familial spastic paraplegia (FSP)
- D. All of the above

Pseudobulbar palsy, primary lateral sclerosis (PLS), and familial spastic paraplegia (FSP) affect only upper motor neurons innervating the brainstem and spinal cord.

1745. Lipofuscin accumulation in motor neurons is seen in which of the following diseases?
Harrison's 20th Ed. Chapter 429, Page 3142

- A. Amyotrophic lateral sclerosis
- B. Spinal muscular atrophy (SMA)
- C. Primary lateral sclerosis (PLS)
- D. All of the above

Lipofuscin, the age pigment, gets accumulated in motor neurons in ALS, pseudobulbar palsy, primary lateral sclerosis (PLS), familial spastic paraplegia (FSP), bulbar palsy and spinal muscular atrophy (SMA).

1746. Which of the following is a marker for degeneration?
Harrison's 20th Ed. Chapter 429, Page 3142

A. Phosphorylated tau
B. β-amyloid
C. Ubiquitin
D. α-synuclein

Ubiquitin is a marker for degeneration.

1747. In sporadic and familial amyotrophic lateral sclerosis, the affected neurons ultrastructurally demonstrate which of the following?
Harrison's 20th Ed. Chapter 429, Page 3142

A. Ubiquitin (+)ve aggregates associated with protein TDP41
B. Ubiquitin (+)ve aggregates associated with protein TDP42
C. Ubiquitin (+)ve aggregates associated with protein TDP43
D. Ubiquitin (+)ve aggregates associated with protein TDP44

In sporadic & familial ALS, affected neurons demonstrate ubiquitin-positive aggregates, typically associated with protein TDP43 along with proliferation of astroglia and microglia that are inevitable accompaniment of all degenerative processes in the central nervous system (CNS).

1748. In amyotrophic lateral sclerosis, the structures that are left intact include?
Harrison's 20th Ed. Chapter 429, Page 3142

A. Sensory apparatus
B. Centers for control & coordination of movement
C. Centers for cognitive processes
D. All of the above

A remarkable feature of ALS is the selectivity of neuronal cell death. Entire sensory apparatus, regulatory mechanisms for the control and coordination of movement and the components of brain that are needed for cognitive processes remain intact.

1749. Until late in the disease, ALS spares neurons that innervate?
N Engl J Med. 2017;377:162-72

A. Diaphragm muscles
B. Sphincter muscles
C. Tongue muscles
D. Neck muscles

ALS typically begins in limbs. ~ One third of cases are bulbar causing difficulty chewing, speaking, or swallowing. Until late in the disease, ALS spares neurons that innervate eye & sphincter muscles (bladder).

1750. In amyotrophic lateral sclerosis, the structures that are left intact include?
Harrison's 20th Ed. Chapter 429, Page 3142

A. Motor neurons for ocular motility
B. Parasympathetic neurons in sacral spinal cord
C. Sensory apparatus
D. All of the above

In ALS, within motor system, there is selectivity of involvement. Motor neurons required for ocular motility remain unaffected, as do the parasympathetic neurons in the sacral spinal cord (the nucleus of Onufrowicz, or Onuf) that innervate the sphincters of the bowel and bladder.

1751. Which of the following is affected in the very late stages of the ALS?
Harrison's 20th Ed. Chapter 429, Page 3142

A. Sensory functions
B. Ocular motility
C. Cognitive functions
D. Bowel and bladder functions

Even in the late stages of the illness, sensory, bowel and bladder, and cognitive functions are preserved. Even when there is severe brainstem disease, ocular motility is spared until the very late stages of the illness.

1752. In ALS, the cause leading to death is?
Harrison's 20th Ed. Chapter 429, Page 3143

A. Infections
B. Depression and suicide
C. Respiratory paralysis
D. Cardiovascular event

In ALS, the cause leading to death is respiratory paralysis.

1753. In ALS, the median survival is from?
Harrison's 20th Ed. Chapter 429, Page 3143

A. 3 months to 12 months
B. 1 to 3 years
C. 3 to 5 years
D. 6 to 8 years

In ALS, the median survival is from 3 to 5 years.

1754. Which of the following is a risk factor for ALS?
Harrison's 20th Ed. Chapter 429, Page 3143

A. Exposure to pesticides & insecticides
B. Smoking
C. Service in the military
D. All of the above

The strongest risk factor for ALS is military service.

1755. Familial ALS (FALS) is due to mutations in which of the following genes?
Harrison's 20th Ed. Chapter 429, Page 3143

A. Gene encoding protein C90rf72
B. Gene encoding cytosolic enzyme SOD1
C. Gene encoding RNA binding proteins TDP43
D. Any of the above

Familial ALS (FALS) is inherited as autosomal dominant trait. It is due to mutations in multiple genes, including those encoding the protein C90rf72 (open reading frame 72 on chromosome 9), cytosolic enzyme SOD1 (superoxide dismutase), the RNA binding proteins TDP43 (encoded by the TAR DNA binding protein gene) and FUS/TLS (fused in sarcoma/translocated in liposarcoma).

1756. Familial ALS (FALS) is most commonly due to mutations in which of the following genes?
Harrison's 20th Ed. Chapter 429, Page 3143

A. Gene encoding protein C90rf72
B. Gene encoding cytosolic enzyme SOD1
C. Gene encoding RNA binding proteins TDP43
D. Gene encoding proteins optineuron, TBK1 & profilin-1

Most common cause of FALS is mutation in C90rf72 (~45–50%). Mutations in SOD1 account for 20% of cases of FALS, whereas TDP43 and FUS/TLS each represent about 5% of familial cases. Minority of cases (~1–2%) are caused by mutations in genes encoding proteins optineuron, TBK1 and profilin-1.

1757. Which of the following gene is implicated in childhood onset motor neuron disease?

Harrison's 20th Ed. Chapter 429, Page 3143

A. Alsin
B. Senataxin
C. Dynactin
D. All of the above

Predominantly lower motor neuron disease with early hoarseness due to laryngeal dysfunction is due to mutations in the gene encoding cellular accessory motor protein dynactin. Mutations in senataxin, a helicase, cause an early adult-onset, slowly evolving ALS variant. Slowly disabling degenerative, predominantly upper motor neuron disease that starts in first decade is caused by mutations in a gene that expresses a novel signaling molecule with properties of a guanine exchange factor, termed alsin.

1758. Which of the following is not a feature of ALS?

Harrison's 20th Ed. Chapter 429, Page 3143

A. Absence of pain or of sensory changes
B. Normal bowel and bladder function
C. Normal roentgenographic studies of spine
D. Raised proteins in cerebrospinal fluid (CSF)

Absence of pain or of sensory changes, normal bowel & bladder function, normal roentgenographic studies of the spine, and normal cerebrospinal fluid (CSF), all favor ALS.

1759. Involuntary excess in weeping or laughing (pseudobulbar affect) is a feature of?

Harrison's 20th Ed. Chapter 429, Page 3143

A. Multifocal motor neuropathy with conduction block
B. Amyotrophic lateral sclerosis
C. Kennedy's disease
D. Adult Tay-Sachs disease

In ALS, degeneration of corticobulbar projections innervating brainstem results in dysarthria and exaggeration of motor expressions of emotion which leads to involuntary excess in weeping or laughing (pseudobulbar affect).

1760. Which of the following antibiotics has neuroprotective properties?

N Engl J Med. 2003;348:1365-75

A. Azithromycin
B. Minocycline
C. Spiramycin
D. Vancomycin

Minocycline is a second-generation tetracycline with neuroprotective properties. Minocycline inhibits ischemia-induced up-regulation of nitric oxide synthase, caspase 1, and reactive microgliosis. Neuroprotection by minocycline has been observed in Huntington's disease, ALS, brain injury, Parkinson's disease, and multiple sclerosis.

1761. Differential diagnosis of amyotrophic lateral sclerosis is?

Harrison's 20th Ed. Chapter 429, Page 3146

A. Compression of cervical spinal cord
B. Thyrotoxicosis
C. Chronic lead poisoning
D. All of the above

D/D of ALS includes cervical spinal cord compression, cervicomedullary junction tumors, cervical or foramen magnum tumors, cervical spondylosis, chronic lead poisoning, thyrotoxicosis, hexosaminidase A, or alpha-glucosidase deficiency, multifocal motor neuropathy with conduction block (MMCB), Lyme disease.

1762. Fasciculations may be taken as benign, if?

Harrison's 20th Ed. Chapter 429, Page 3146

A. There is absence of weakness
B. There is absence of atrophy
C. There is no denervation phenomena electrophysiologically.
D. All of the above

1763. Amyotrophic lateral sclerosis may develop concurrently with which of the following?

Harrison's 20th Ed. Chapter 429, Page 3146

A. Parkinsonism
B. Frontotemporal dementia
C. Chronic traumatic encephalopathy
D. All of the above

1764. The most commonly mutated gene in ALS is?

N Engl J Med. 2017;377:162-72

A. NOD2
B. NLRP3
C. C9ORF72
D. CERCR1

1765. Which of the following genes are involved in RNA processing, transport and metabolism?

Harrison's 20th Ed. Chapter 429, Page 3146

A. C9orf73
B. TDP43
C. FUS
D. All of the above

Genes involved in RNA processing, transport and metabolism are C9Orf73, TDP43 and FUS.

1766. Which of the following is an intronic repeat disorder?

Harrison's 20th Ed. Chapter 429, Page 3146

A. Amyotrophic lateral sclerosis
B. Myotonic dystrophy
C. Spinocerebellar atrophy type 8
D. All of the above

1767. Mutations in gene encoding which of the following protein cause an aggressive, infantile motor neuron disease?

Harrison's 20th Ed. Chapter 429, Page 3146

A. Tyrosine phosphatase non-receptor 22
B. GLE1
C. Lymphoid tyrosine phosphatase
D. Cryopyrin

1768. Riluzole - a glutamate antagonist is useful in treatment of?

Harrison's 20th Ed. Chapter 429, Page 3146

A. Amyotrophic lateral sclerosis
B. Multiple sclerosis
C. Subacute combined degeneration of cord
D. Myasthenia gravis

Riluzole is approved for ALS. Riluzole reduces excitotoxicity by diminishing glutamate release.

1769. Which of the following drug is useful in the treatment of amyotrophic lateral sclerosis?
Harrison's 20th Ed. Chapter 429, Page 3146

A. Nusinersen
B. Edaravone
C. IV immunoglobulin
D. All of the above

1770. Disease in which peripheral motor neurons are affected without involvement of corticospinal motor system is?
Harrison's 20th Ed. Chapter 429, Page 3146

A. X-Linked spinobulbar muscular atrophy (Kennedy's disease)
B. Adult Tay-Sachs disease
C. Spinal muscular atrophy
D. All of the above

Diseases in which peripheral motor neurons are affected without involvement of corticospinal motor system include X-Linked spinobulbar muscular atrophy (Kennedy's disease), adult tay-sachs disease, spinal muscular atrophy, Multifocal Motor Neuropathy with Conduction Block, Fazio-Londe syndrome, Machado-Joseph disease and olivopontocerebellar degenerations.

1771. Which of the following is false for Kennedy's Disease?
Harrison's 20th Ed. Chapter 429, Page 3147

A. X-linked spinobulbar muscular atrophy
B. Lower motor neuron disorder
C. Gynecomastia and reduced fertility
D. None of the above

Azoospermia & male-factor infertility occurs in association with mild loss of function mutations in androgen receptor. Trinucleotide (CAG) repeat expansion, from a mean of 22 repeats to greater than 40 repeats, within a highly polymorphic region of androgen receptor is associated with spinal & bulbar muscular atrophy (Kennedy disease). These patients may show evidence of partial androgen insensitivity in adolescence or adulthood (gynecomastia).

1772. Which of the following diseases is caused by deficiency of enzyme β-hexosaminidase (hex A)?
Harrison's 20th Ed. Chapter 429, Page 3147

A. Familial spastic paraplegia
B. Werdnig-Hoffmann disease
C. Adult Tay-Sachs disease
D. Kugelberg-Welander disease

1773. Which of the following is false about Adult Tay-Sachs Disease?
Harrison's 20th Ed. Chapter 429, Page 3147

A. Very slowly progressive
B. Dysarthria
C. Cerebellar atrophy
D. None of the above

1774. Intraneuronal inclusions "Bunina bodies" are a pathognomonic feature of?
N Engl J Med. 2001;344:1688

A. Motor neuron disease
B. Multiple sclerosis
C. Subacute combined degeneration of cord
D. Myasthenia gravis

1775. Which of the following is false about spinal muscular atrophy?
Harrison's 20th Ed. Chapter 429, Page 3147

A. Genetic lower motor neuron disease
B. Early onset
C. Locus on chromosome 5
D. None of the above

Spinal muscular atrophy (SMA) maps to a locus on chromosome 5 encoding a putative motor neuron survival protein (SMN, for survival motor neuron) that is important in the formation & trafficking of RNA complexes across nuclear membrane.

1776. Which of the following is false about spinal muscular atrophy?
Harrison's 20th Ed. Chapter 429, Page 3147

A. Extensive loss of large motor neurons
B. Evidence of denervation atrophy on muscle biopsy
C. Electrophysiologic evidence of denervation
D. None of the above

1777. Werdnig-Hoffmann Disease is the name given to?
Harrison's 20th Ed. Chapter 429, Page 3147

A. SMA I
B. SMA II
C. SMA III
D. None of the above

1778. Kugelberg-Welander disease is the name given to?
Harrison's 20th Ed. Chapter 429, Page 3147

A. SMA I
B. SMA II
C. SMA III
D. None of the above

1779. Which out of the following carries the worst prognosis?
Harrison's 20th Ed. Chapter 429, Page 3147

A. SMA I
B. SMA II
C. SMA III
D. None of the above

Infantile SMA or SMA I is known as Werdnig-Hoffmann disease with earliest onset & most rapidly fatal course. Chronic childhood SMA (SMA II) begins later in childhood & evolves with slowly progressive course. Juvenile SMA (SMA III or Kugelberg-Welander disease) manifests in late childhood & has a slow course. EP studies distinguish SMA III from myopathic syndromes.

1780. Which of the following drug is useful in the treatment of spinal muscular atrophy?
Harrison's 20th Ed. Chapter 429, Page 3146

A. Nusinersen
B. Edaravone
C. IV immunoglobulin
D. All of the above

1781. Which of the following is false about 'Multifocal Motor Neuropathy with Conduction Block' (MMCB)?
Harrison's 20th Ed. Chapter 429, Page 3147

A. Elevated serum titers of mono- & polyclonal antibodies to ganglioside GM1
B. No corticospinal tract signs
C. Respond to intravenous immunoglobulin therapy
D. None of the above

1782. Multifocal motor neuropathy with conduction block (MMCB) evolves in association with which of the following?

Harrison's 20th Ed. Chapter 429, Page 3146

A. Tuberculosis
B. Lymphoma
C. Syphilis
D. All of the above

MMCB is a diffuse, lower motor axonal neuropathy mimicking ALS which sometimes evolves in association with lymphoma or multiple myeloma.

1783. Which of the following is true for Fazio-Londe syndrome?

Harrison's 20th Ed. Chapter 429, Page 3147

A. ALS variant
B. Juvenile onset
C. Involves musculature innervated by brainstem mainly
D. All of the above

Fazio-Londe syndrome is an ALS variant of juvenile onset that involves mainly the musculature innervated by the brainstem.

1784. Which of the following about primary lateral sclerosis is false?

Harrison's 20th Ed. Chapter 429, Page 3147

A. Affects adults in mid to late life
B. Combined involvement of corticospinal & corticobulbar tracts
C. Progressive spastic weakness of limbs, dysarthria & dysphagia
D. None of the above

1785. Which of the following is absent in primary lateral sclerosis?

Harrison's 20th Ed. Chapter 429, Page 3147

A. Fasciculations
B. Amyotrophy
C. Sensory changes
D. All of the above

In primary lateral sclerosis, fasciculations, amyotrophy, and sensory changes are absent. Neither electromyography nor muscle biopsy shows denervation. There occurs a selective loss of large pyramidal cells in precentral gyrus & degeneration of corticospinal & corticobulbar projections. Peripheral motor neurons & other neuronal systems are spared.

1786. Which of the following is false for Hereditary Spastic Paraplegia (HSP) in adults?

Harrison's 20th Ed. Chapter 429, Page 3147

A. X-linked transmission
B. Presents in third or fourth decade
C. Progressive spastic weakness in lower extremities
D. Long survival

In its pure form, most adult-onset HSP are transmitted as an autosomal dominant trait. HSP has long survival because respiratory function is spared.

1787. Which of the following is false for Hereditary Spastic Paraplegia (HSP)?

Harrison's 20th Ed. Chapter 429, Page 3147

A. Sexual function preserved
B. Spastin and atlastin gene mutations common
C. Degeneration of corticospinal tracts
D. None of the above

In HSP, sexual function tends to be preserved. Gene implicated is spastin & atlastin in dominantly inherited and childhood-onset dominant HSP respectively. Degeneration of corticospinal tracts (dying-back or distal axonopathy) occurs in HSP, most severe at more caudal levels in spinal cord. Posterior column (vibration & position) abnormalities and disturbance of bowel & bladder function happen.

1788. Which of the following is a disorder of CNS myelin?

Harrison's 20th Ed. Chapter 429, Page 3147

A. Fragile X syndrome
B. Pelizaeus-Merzbacher syndrome
C. Prader-Willi syndrome
D. Rett syndrome

Pelizaeus-Merzbacher disease is a widespread dysmyelinating disorder of CNS myelin caused by mutations in the gene for proteolipid protein (PLP) that normally promotes extracellular compaction between adjacent myelin lamellae.

Prion Diseases

1789. Scrapie agent is synonym of?
Harrison's 20th Ed. Chapter 430, Page 3148

A. Amyloid
B. Prion
C. Myelin
D. None of the above

Prions cause scrapie in sheep & goats & Creutzfeldt-Jakob disease in humans. Prions are abnormal proteins that propagate & cause disease by altering the structure of a normal cell protein.

1790. Prions play a key role in which of the following illnesses?
Harrison's 20th Ed. Chapter 430, Page 3148

A. Creutzfeldt-Jakob disease (CJD)
B. Alzheimer's disease (AD)
C. Parkinson's disease (PD)
D. All of the above

Prions play a key role in Alzheimer's disease (AD) and Parkinson's disease (PD).

1791. Which of the following about prions is false?
Harrison's 20th Ed. Chapter 430, Page 3148

A. Infectious proteins
B. Self-propagating
C. Lacks nucleic acid
D. None of the above

Prions are the only known 'transmissible pathogens' that are devoid of nucleic acid (RNA or DNA).

1792. Which of the following is a prion protein?
Harrison's 20th Ed. Chapter 430, Page 3148

A. PrP^{Sc}
B. α-synuclein
C. Aβ
D. All of the above

Creutzfeldt-Jakob disease (CJD) is caused by accumulation of PrP^{Sc} prions. α-synuclein prions cause multiple system atrophy (MSA), Aβ prions contribute to AD, α-synuclein prions to PD & tau prions to some types of frontotemporal dementia (FTD).

1793. Most CJD patients are between the age of?
Harrison's 20th Ed. Chapter 430, Page 3148

A. 20 & 35 years
B. 35 & 45 years
C. 50 & 75 years
D. 75 & 90 years

Most CJD patients are between 50 & 75 years of age. CJD is relentlessly progressive & generally causes death within 9 months of onset.

1794. The fundamental event underlying prion diseases is?
Harrison's 20th Ed. Chapter 430, Page 3148

A. α-to-β structural transition in PrP
B. α-to-β structural transition in PrP^{SC}
C. α-to-γ structural transition in PrP
D. α-to-γ structural transition in PrP^{SC}

α-to-β structural transition in prion protein (PrP^{C}) is the fundamental event underlying prion diseases

1795. Prion diseases may manifest as?
Harrison's 20th Ed. Chapter 430, Page 3148

A. Infectious disorders
B. Genetic disorders
C. Sporadic disorders
D. All of the above

Prion diseases manifest as infectious, genetic & sporadic disorders. No other single etiology illness present with such wide spectrum clinical manifestations.

1796. Disease causing isoform of prion is?
Harrison's 20th Ed. Chapter 430, Page 3149 Table 430-1

A. PrP^{C}
B. PrP^{D}
C. PrP^{Sc}
D. PrP^{Sd}

Prions reproduce by binding to normal, cellular isoform of prion protein (PrP^{C}) & stimulating conversion of PrP^{C} into disease-causing isoform (PrP^{Sc}).

1797. Which of the following statements about prions is false?
Harrison's 20th Ed. Chapter 430, Page 3148

A. Devoid of nucleic acid
B. Prion diseases result from accumulation of PrP^{Sc}
C. Pathologic hallmarks of CJD are spongiform degeneration and astrocytic gliosis
D. CSF is always abnormal in CJD

In CJD, CSF is nearly always normal but may show protein elevation & rarely mild pleocytosis.

1798. Which of the following is the precursor of PrP^{Sc}?
Harrison's 20th Ed. Chapter 430, Page 3149 Table 430-1

A. PrP 27-30
B. PrP^{C}
C. PrP^{D}
D. PRNP

PrP^{C} is the precursor of PrP^{Sc}

1799. Which of the following retains prion infectivity and polymerizes into amyloid?
Harrison's 20th Ed. Chapter 430, Page 3149 Table 430-1

A. PrP 27-30
B. PrP^{C}
C. PrP^{D}
D. PRNP

PrP 27-30 retains prion infectivity and polymerizes into amyloid.

1800. In humans, PrP gene (PRNP) is located on?
Harrison's 20th Ed. Chapter 430, Page 3149 Table 430-1

A. Short arm of chromosome 12
B. Short arm of chromosome 14
C. Short arm of chromosome 16
D. Short arm of chromosome 20

In humans, PrP gene is designated PRNP and is located on the short arm of chromosome 20.

1801. Which of the following about prions is false?
Harrison's 20th Ed. Chapter 430, Page 3148

- A. Prions reproduce by binding to PrP^C
- B. PrP^C is rich in α helix & has little β structure
- C. PrP^Sc has less α helix & high amount of β structure
- D. PrP 27-30 is a fragment of PrP^C

PrP 27-30 is a fragment of PrP^Sc, generated by truncation of the NH2-terminus by limited digestion with proteinase K.

1802. Which is the most common prion disorder in humans?
Harrison's 20th Ed. Chapter 430, Page 3148

- A. Sporadic CJD (sCJD)
- B. Familial CJD (fCJD)
- C. Gerstmann-Straussler-Scheinker disease (GSS)
- D. Fatal familial insomnia (FFI)

Sporadic CJD is the most common prion disorder in humans (~85%).

1803. Inherited prion disease caused by mutations in PrP gene is?
Harrison's 20th Ed. Chapter 430, Page 3148

- A. Familial CJD (fCJD)
- B. Gerstmann-Straussler-Scheinker disease (GSS)
- C. Fatal familial insomnia (FFI)
- D. All of the above

fCJD, GSS disease & FFI are dominantly inherited prion diseases caused by mutations in PrP gene.

1804. Iatrogenic CJD can be caused by?
Harrison's 20th Ed. Chapter 430, Page 3151

- A. Corneal transplantation
- B. Contaminated EEG electrode implantation
- C. Implantation of duramater grafts
- D. All of the above

Accidental transmission of CJD to humans can occur with corneal transplantation, contaminated EEG electrode implantation, duramater/pericardium graft Transmission of CJD prions from contaminated human growth hormone (hGH) preparations derived from human pituitaries has been responsible for fatal cerebellar disorders with dementia.

1805. Which of the following is a prion disease endemic in deer & elk in regions of North America?
Harrison's 20th Ed. Chapter 430, Page 3149

- A. Mink encephalopathy
- B. Bovine spongiform encephalopathy (BSE)
- C. Chronic wasting disease (CWD)
- D. Kuru

Chronic wasting disease (CWD) is a prion disease endemic in deer and elk in regions of North America. In contrast to other prion diseases, CWD is highly communicable. Feces from asymptomatic, infected cervids contain prions that are responsible for the spread of CWD.

1806. Which of the following about PrP prion diseases is false?
Harrison's 20th Ed. Chapter 430, Page 3149

- A. Aberrant metabolism of PrP
- B. PrP isoforms are encoded by a chromosomal gene
- C. Epigenetically heritable
- D. None of the above

1807. Pathologic hallmarks of Creutzfeldt-Jakob disease (CJD) is?
Harrison's 20th Ed. Chapter 430, Page 3151

- A. Spongiform degeneration
- B. Astrocytic gliosis
- C. Lack of inflammatory response
- D. All of the above

Pathologic hallmarks of CJD are spongiform degeneration, astrocytic gliosis & lack of inflammatory response.

1808. "Florid plaques" is characteristic feature of?
Harrison's 20th Ed. Chapter 430, Page 3152

- A. sCJD (Creutzfeldt-Jakob disease)
- B. fCJD
- C. vCJD
- D. iCJD

Presence of "florid plaques" is a characteristic feature of vCJD. These are composed of a central core of PrP amyloid, surrounded by vacuoles in a pattern suggesting petals on a flower.

1809. Most patients with CJD present with?
Harrison's 20th Ed. Chapter 430, Page 3152

- A. Deficits in higher cortical function
- B. Cerebellar gait & coordination deficits
- C. Extrapyramidal dysfunction
- D. Visual impairment

Most patients with CJD present with deficits in higher cortical function.

1810. Dementia with myoclonus is seen in?
Harrison's 20th Ed. Chapter 430, Page 3152

- A. Alzheimer's disease (AD)
- B. Unverricht-Lundborg disease
- C. Creutzfeldt-Jakob disease (CJD)
- D. All of the above

Dementia with myoclonus can be due to Alzheimer's disease (AD), dementia with Lewy bodies, corticobasal degeneration, cryptococcal encephalitis, or myoclonic epilepsy disorder—Unverricht-Lundborg disease.

1811. Which of the following about myoclonus in CJD is false?
Harrison's 20th Ed. Chapter 430, Page 3152

- A. Persists during sleep
- B. Elicited by loud sounds & bright lights
- C. Occur later in the course of CJD
- D. None of the above

In CJD, myoclonus is neither specific nor confined to CJD and tends to occur later in the course. Myoclonus persists during sleep, is elicited by loud sounds or bright lights.

1812. Most patients with CJD survive for what length of time after onset of clinical signs & symptoms?
Harrison's 20th Ed. Chapter 430, Page 3152

- A. 6–12 months
- B. 12–24 months
- C. 24–48 months
- D. 48–60 months

Most patients with CJD survive for 6–12 months after the onset of clinical signs and symptoms. Some live for up to 5 years.

1813. Clinical abnormalities in CJD involve?
Harrison's 20th Ed. Chapter 430, Page 3152

- A. CNS
- B. PNS
- C. ANS
- D. All of the above

Clinical abnormalities in CJD are confined to the CNS.

1814. Which of the following is a finding in CJD?
Harrison's 20th Ed. Chapter 430, Page 3152

A. Fever
B. Leukocytosis
C. Pleocytosis in CSF
D. None of the above

Fever, elevated ESR, leukocytosis, or pleocytosis in CSF point towards another etiology to explain patient's CNS dysfunction.

1815. Which of the following is the typical MRI finding in Creutzfeldt-Jakob disease?
Harrison's 20th Ed. Chapter 430, Page 3152

A. Insular ribon
B. Basal ganglia hypointensity
C. Cortical ribboning
D. All of the above

On FLAIR sequences and diffusion-weighted imaging, ~90% of CJD patients show increased intensity in basal ganglia and cortical ribboning. This pattern is not seen with other neurodegenerative disorders but is seen infrequently with viral encephalitis, paraneoplastic syndromes or seizures.

1816. Ataxia is a prominent & presenting feature in?
Harrison's 20th Ed. Chapter 430, Page 3152

A. Familial CJD (fCJD)
B. Gerstmann-Straussler-Scheinker disease (GSS)
C. Fatal familial insomnia (FFI)
D. Sporadic Creutzfeldt-Jakob disease (sCJD)

Ataxia is a prominent & presenting feature in GSS disease, with dementia occurring late in the disease course. Early ataxia & visual hallucinations with a prominent psychiatric prodrome point towards vCJD.

1817. Insomnia & dysautonomia are a feature of?
Harrison's 20th Ed. Chapter 430, Page 3152

A. Familial CJD (fCJD)
B. Gerstmann-Straussler-Scheinker disease (GSS)
C. Fatal familial insomnia (FFI)
D. vCJD

FFI is characterized by insomnia & dysautonomia. Dementia occurs in terminal phase of illness.

1818. Prominent psychiatric prodrome is a feature of?
Harrison's 20th Ed. Chapter 430, Page 3152

A. Familial CJD (fCJD)
B. Gerstmann-Straussler-Scheinker disease (GSS)
C. Fatal familial insomnia (FFI)
D. Variant CJD (vCJD)

1819. Most common disorder to be mistaken for CJD is?
Harrison's 20th Ed. Chapter 430, Page 3152

A. AD
B. FTD
C. Progressive supranuclear palsy
D. Dementia with Lewy bodies

Dementia with Lewy bodies is the most common disorder mistaken for CJD. Absence of abnormalities on diffusion-weighted & fluid-attenuated inversion recovery (FLAIR) magnetic resonance imaging (MRI) almost always distinguishes other dementing conditions from CJD.

1820. Which of the following is false for Hashimoto's encephalopathy?
Harrison's 20th Ed. Chapter 430, Page 3152

A. Subacute progressive encephalopathy
B. Tonic-clonic seizures
C. Periodic triphasic complexes on EEG
D. Fluctuations in severity

Myoclonus & periodic triphasic complexes on EEG, high titers of antithyroglobulin or antithyroid peroxidase (antimicrosomal) antibodies and improvement with glucocorticoid therapy point towards Hashimoto's encephalopathy.

1821. On FLAIR sequences & diffusion-weighted imaging MRI, which of the following suggests sCJD?
Harrison's 20th Ed. Chapter 430, Page 3152

A. Entorhinal cortex & hippocampal atrophy
B. Frontal, insular, and/or temporal atrophy
C. Cortical ribboning
D. Posterior parietal atrophy

In diffusion/ fluid-attenuate inversion recovery MRI, cortical ribboning & increased intensity in the basal ganglia distinguishing sCJD from most other conditions. Markedly abnormal periodic complexes on EEG (repetitive, high-voltage, triphasic & polyphasic sharp discharges) provide further aid. Entorhinal cortex & hippocampal atrophy suggests AD, frontal, insular, and/or temporal atrophy suggests FTD, posterior parietal atrophy suggests DLB.

1822. In CJD, levels of which of the following is elevated in CSF?
Harrison's 20th Ed. Chapter 430, Page 3153

A. Neuron-specific enolase
B. Tau
C. Stress protein 14-3-3
D. All of the above

1823. Stress protein 14-3-3 is elevated in the CSF of?
Harrison's 20th Ed. Chapter 430, Page 3152

A. Herpes simplex virus encephalitis
B. Multi-infarct dementia
C. Stroke
D. All of the above

1824. Stress protein 14-3-3 is elevated in the CSF of all except?
Harrison's 20th Ed. Chapter 430, Page 3152

A. Herpes simplex virus encephalitis
B. Multi-infarct dementia
C. AD
D. CJD

1825. Which of the following about CJD is true?
Harrison's 20th Ed. Chapter 430, Page 3153

A. Contagious
B. Communicable
C. Transmissible
D. Vulnerable to common inactivation procedures

CJD is not contagious or communicable but it is transmissible.

1826. Sterilization for Creutzfeldt-Jakob disease (CJD) contaminated materials is done by?

Harrison's 20th Ed. Chapter 430, Page 3153

A. Hcl
B. NaOH
C. NaHCO$_3$
D. HNO$_3$

Prions are extremely resistant to common inactivation procedures. Autoclaving at 134°C for 5 hours or treatment with 2 N NaOH for several hours is recommended for sterilization of prions.

1827. Besides PrP, which of the following proteins can become prions?

Harrison's 20th Ed. Chapter 430, Page 3153

A. Amyloid beta (Aβ)
B. Huntingtin
C. α-synuclein
D. All of the above

Besides PrP, proteins like amyloid beta (Aβ), tau, α-synuclein & huntingtin can all become prions.

Ataxic Disorders

1828. Symptoms and signs of ataxia consist of?
Harrison's 20th Ed. Chapter 431, Page 3154

A. Gait impairment
B. Visual blurring due to nystagmus
C. Tremor with movement
D. All of the above

Symptoms & signs of ataxia consist of gait impairment, unclear or scanning speech, visual blurring due to nystagmus, hand incoordination & tremor with movement.

1829. Ataxia is due to involvement of?
Harrison's 20th Ed. Chapter 431, Page 3154

A. Cerebellum
B. Spinocerebellar pathway
C. Fronto-ponto-cerebellar pathway
D. All of the above

Ataxia is due to involvement of cerebellum & its afferent and efferent pathways, including spinocerebellar pathways, and frontopontocerebellar pathway originating in the rostral frontal lobe.

1830. Which of the following about true cerebellar ataxia is false?
Harrison's 20th Ed. Chapter 431, Page 3154

A. It is devoid of vertiginous complaints
B. It is an unsteady gait due to imbalance
C. Not associated with vestibular nerve or labyrinthine disease
D. None of the above

True cerebellar ataxia is clearly an unsteady gait due to imbalance and is different from ataxia associated with vestibular nerve or labyrinthine disease. Ataxia associated with vestibular nerve or labyrinthine disease results in a gait disorder associated with significant degrees of dizziness, light-headedness or perception of movement which are absent in true cerebellar ataxia.

1831. Sensory information for postural control is primarily generated by?
Harrison's 20th Ed. Chapter 431, Page 3154

A. Visual system
B. Vestibular system
C. Proprioceptive receptors in muscle spindles & joints
D. All of the above

Sensory information for postural control is primarily generated by visual system, vestibular system and by proprioceptive receptors in the muscle spindles and joints. Loss of two of the three pathways is compromises standing balance. Clinically, gait disorder must be viewed as the product of a neurologic deficit and a functional adaptation.

1832. Bilateral ataxia with symmetric involvement suggests which of the following?
Harrison's 20th Ed. Chapter 431, Page 3154

A. Genetic etiology
B. Metabolic etiology
C. Toxic etiology
D. Any of the above

A gradual & progressive increase in ataxic symptoms with bilateral & symmetric involvement suggests a genetic, metabolic, immune or toxic etiology.

1833. Acute & reversible ataxias are caused by?
Harrison's 20th Ed. Chapter 431, Page 3154

A. Intoxication with alcohol
B. Phenytoin
C. Lithium
D. All of the above

Acute & reversible ataxias are caused by intoxication with alcohol, phenytoin, lithium, barbiturates. Other agents include toluene exposure, gasoline sniffing, glue sniffing, spray painting, or exposure to methyl mercury or bismuth, treatment with cytotoxic chemotherapeutic drugs like fluorouracil & paclitaxel.

1834. "As if walking on a slippery surface" best relates to?
Harrison's 20th Ed. Chapter 23, Page 144

A. Cautious gait
B. Stiff-legged gait
C. Freezing gait
D. Frontal dait disorder

Cautious gait refers to describe a patient who walks with an abbreviated stride & lowered center of mass, as if walking on a slippery surface. This disorder is both common and nonspecific.

1835. Which of the following is the commonest etiology of gait disorders?
Harrison's 20th Ed. Chapter 431, Page 23 Table 23-1

A. Sensory deficits
B. Parkinsonism
C. Cerebellar degeneration
D. Psychogenic

1836. Stiff-legged gait category includes which of the following?
Harrison's 20th Ed. Chapter 23, Page 144

A. Spastic gait
B. Dystonia
C. Stiff-Person syndrome
D. All of the above

1837. Causes of freezing gait include?
Harrison's 20th Ed. Chapter 23, Page 144

A. Parkinson's disease
B. Progressive supranuclear palsy
C. Corticobasal degeneration
D. All of the above

Difficulty with gait initiation leads to a freezing gait seen in PD, progressive supranuclear palsy, multiple system atrophy, corticobasal degeneration & primary pallidal degeneration.

1838. Pill-rolling tremor is specific for?
Harrison's 20th Ed. Chapter 23, Page 144

A. Parkinson's disease
B. Progressive supranuclear palsy
C. Corticobasal degeneration
D. All of the above

Patients of PSP, MSA and CBD frequently present with axial stiffness, postural instability, and a shuffling gait but lack the characteristic pill-rolling tremor of Parkinson's disease.

1839. "Gait apraxia" is characteristic of?
Harrison's 20th Ed. Chapter 23, Page 144

A. Sensory ataxia
B. Cerebellar gait ataxia
C. Frontal gait disorder
D. Psychogenic gait disorder

Frontal gait disorder or "gait apraxia" features wide base of support, short stride, shuffling along floor and difficulty with starts & turns.

1840. Which of the following relate to frontal gait disorders?
Harrison's 20th Ed. Chapter 23, Page 144

A. Gait apraxia
B. "Slipping clutch" syndrome
C. Lower body parkinsonism
D. All of the above

Difficulty with gait initiation is referred to as "slipping clutch" syndrome & lower body parkinsonism.

1841. Cerebellar gait ataxia is characterized by all except?
Harrison's 20th Ed. Chapter 23, Page 144

A. Unable to walk tandem heel to toe
B. Difficulty in maintaining balance when turning
C. Narrow base of support
D. Falls is a late event

Cerebellar gait ataxia is characterized by a wide base of support, erratic foot placement, difficulty in maintaining balance on turning (an early feature) and tandem gait. Falls in daily life is a late event.

1842. Sensory ataxia is characterized by?
Harrison's 20th Ed. Chapter 23, Page 144

A. Stance destabilized by eye closure
B. Look down at their feet when walking
C. Joint position & vibration sense diminished in lower limbs
D. All of the above

In sensory ataxia, stance is destabilized by eye closure. Patient looks down at their feet when walking and do poorly in dark. Joint position & vibration sense is diminished in lower limbs.

1843. Which of the following is a feature of vestibular disorder?
Harrison's 20th Ed. Chapter 23, Page 144

A. Vertigo
B. Nystagmus
C. Poor balance
D. All of the above

Feature of vestibular disorders are vertigo (subjective appreciation or illusion of movement), nystagmus (vestibulo-oculomotor sign) & poor balance (impairment of vestibulo-spinal function).

1844. Symptoms & signs of true cerebellar ataxia consist of all except?
Harrison's 20th Ed. Chapter 23, Page 144

A. Gait impairment
B. Hand incoordination
C. Romberg sign
D. Tremor with movement

Ataxia due to vestibular nerve or labyrinthine disease results in gait disorder associated with dizziness, light-headedness or perception of movement. Cerebellar ataxia presents as gait impairment, scanning speech, visual blurring due to nystagmus, hand incoordination and tremor with movement. True cerebellar ataxia is devoid of vertiginous complaints. In sensory ataxia, imbalance worsens when visual input is removed (Romberg sign).

1845. Symptoms & signs of true cerebellar ataxia consist of all except?
Harrison's 20th Ed. Chapter 23, Page 144

A. Nystagmus
B. Scanning speech
C. Dizziness
D. Tremor with movement

Patients with hereditary ataxia or alcoholic cerebellar degeneration do not complain of dizziness.

1846. True cerebellar ataxia result from the involvement of?
Harrison's 20th Ed. Chapter 23, Page 144

A. Cerebellum
B. Spinocerebellar pathway
C. Frontopontocerebellar pathway
D. All of the above

True cerebellar ataxia result from involvement of cerebellum, spinocerebellar pathways and frontopontocerebellar pathway from rostral frontal lobe. True cerebellar ataxia is devoid of vertiginous complaints (dizziness, light-headedness or the perception of movement) and is clearly an unsteady gait due to imbalance.

1847. Which of the following may lead to development of ataxia of gait?
Harrison's 20th Ed. Chapter 431, Page 3154

A. B1 deficiency
B. B12 deficiency
C. Hyponatremia
D. All of the above

Subacute development of ataxia of gait may be due to vitamin B1 and B12 deficiency and hyponatremia.

1848. Anti-Tr autoantibody is related to which of the following?
Harrison's 20th Ed. Chapter 431, Page 3154

A. Breast cancer
B. Ovarian cancer
C. Small-cell lung cancer
D. Hodgkin's disease

Paraneoplastic cerebellar ataxia may present with various tumor states. Autoantibodies related to breast and ovarian cancers is anti-Yo, with small-cell lung cancer is anti-PQ type voltage-gated calcium channel, and with Hodgkin's disease is anti-Tr.

1849. Paraneoplastic Opsoclonus-Myoclonus Syndrome is related to which of the following?
Harrison's 20th Ed. Chapter 90, Page 672

A. Breast cancer
B. Lung cancer
C. Neuroblastoma
D. All of the above

Opsoclonus is a disorder of eye movement characterized by involuntary, chaotic saccades that occur in all directions of gaze frequently associated with myoclonus & ataxia. When the cause of opsoclonus-myoclonus is paraneoplastic, tumors involved are usually cancer of lung and breast in adults, neuroblastoma in children and ovarian teratoma in adolescents and young women.

1850. Patients with which of the following disorder fall over backwards?
Harrison's 20th Ed. Chapter 23, Page 144

A. Progressive supranuclear palsy
B. Cerebellar pathology
C. Lesions of the vestibular system
D. Patients with somatosensory deficits

Patients with cerebellar pathology may lean & topple toward side of lesion. Patients with lesions of vestibular system have lateral pulsion & toppling falls. Patients with progressive supranuclear palsy fall over backwards. Gait freezing in Parkinson's disease results in a forward fall.

1851. Which of the following is not a cause of symmetric ataxia?
Harrison's 20th Ed. Chapter 431, Page 3154 Table 431-1

A. Inherited ataxia
B. Hypothyroidism
C. Multiple sclerosis
D. Meningovascular syphilis

Demyelinating disease multiple sclerosis presents with focal and ipsilateral cerebellar signs of subacute duration (days to weeks).

1852. Paraneoplastic cerebellar ataxia is associated with?
Harrison's 20th Ed. Chapter 431, Page 3154

A. Breast cancer
B. Small-cell lung cancer
C. Hodgkin's disease
D. All of the above

Paraneoplastic cerebellar ataxia is associated with breast and ovarian cancers (anti-Yo), small-cell lung cancer (anti-PQ type voltage-gated calcium channel), and Hodgkin's disease (anti-Tr).

1853. Which of the following is best related to congenital cyst of the posterior fossa?
Harrison's 20th Ed. Chapter 431, Page 3155

A. Haw River syndrome
B. Bassen-Kornzweig syndrome
C. Chiari malformation
D. Dandy-Walker syndrome

1854. Which of the findings dominate presentation of inherited ataxias?
Harrison's 20th Ed. Chapter 431, Page 3155

A. Optic nerves & retina
B. Peripheral nerves
C. Cerebellar
D. Spinal cord

Findings of cerebellar disease dominate the clinical picture of inherited ataxias. There may also be characteristic changes in the basal ganglia, brainstem, spinal cord, optic nerves, retina and peripheral nerves.

1855. Which of the following is caused by an untranslated pentanucleotide repeat?
Harrison's 20th Ed. Chapter 431, Page 3155

A. SCA6
B. SCA7
C. SCA10
D. SCA17

Autosomal spinocerebellar ataxias (SCAs) include SCA types 1 through SCA28, dentatorubropallidoluysian atrophy (DRPLA) & episodic ataxia (EA) types 1 and 2. SCA1, SCA2, SCA3 [Machado-Joseph disease (MJD)], SCA6, SCA7, and SCA17 are caused by CAG triplet repeat expansions in different genes. SCA8 is due to an untranslated CTG repeat expansion, SCA12 is linked to an untranslated CAG repeat, and SCA10 is caused by an untranslated pentanucleotide repeat.

1856. Ataxins are?
Harrison's 20th Ed. Chapter 431, Page 3155

A. Expanded polyserine proteins
B. Expanded polyglutamine proteins
C. Expanded polyarginine proteins
D. Expanded polyleucine proteins

CAG encodes glutamine & expanded CAG triplet repeat expansions in SCA's result in expanded polyglutamine proteins, termed ataxins, that produce a toxic gain of function with autosomal dominant inheritance.

1857. About what number of glutamines due to expanded polyglutamine ataxins are potentially toxic to neurons?
Harrison's 20th Ed. Chapter 431, Page 3155

A. 10
B. 20
C. 30
D. 40

Expanded polyglutamine ataxins with more than ~40 glutamines are potentially toxic to neurons. They impair neuronal functions, alter efficiency of ubiquitin-proteosome system of protein turnover and induce neuronal apoptosis.

1858. Which of the following is a CAG repeat disease?
Harrison's 20th Ed. Chapter 431, Page 3155

A. Machado-Joseph disease (MJD)
B. Huntington's disease
C. Dentatorubral-pallidoluysian atrophy (DRPLA)
D. All of the above

Besides Machado-Joseph Disease (MJD), other CAG repeat diseases include Huntington's disease, dentatorubral-pallidoluysian atrophy (DRPLA) and X-chromosomal Spinobulbar Muscular Atrophy (SBMA or Kennedy's Disease). Other triplet repeat expansions diseases include Fragile X-syndrome (FRAXA) - CGG repeat, Fragile X-syndrome (FRAXE)–GCC repeat, Dystrophia myotonica (DM)–CTG repeat and Friedreich ataxia (FRDA1)–GAA repeat.

1859. Which of the following about increase in number of "nucleotide repeats" is false?
Harrison's 20th Ed. Chapter 431, Page 3155

A. Length correlates with severity of disease
B. Repeat length increases from one generation to next
C. Leads to anticipation
D. None of the above

Nucleotide repeat expansion disorders are associated with an increase in number of nucleotide repeats above a threshold. Repeats alter gene regulatory sequences and tends to further expand during cell division. Length of nucleotide repeat correlates with severity of disease. Repeat length increases from one generation to the next, and disease manifests severely and at an earlier age - phenomenon called anticipation.

1860. Dynamic mutation refers to?
Harrison's 20th Ed. Chapter 456, Page 3356

A. Decreasingly severe phenotype in next generation
B. Increasingly severe phenotype in next generation
C. Decreasingly severe genotype in next generation
D. Increasingly severe genotype in next generation

In subsequent generations, expanded repeat may increase further in length & result in an increasingly severe phenotype - dynamic mutation.

1861. Which of the following Trinucleotide Repeat Disorders has autosomal recessive inheritance?
Harrison's 20th Ed. Chapter 456, Page 3363 Table 456-5

A. Spinocerebellar ataxia type 1 (SCA1)
B. Machado Joseph disease (MJD)
C. Dentorubral pallidoluysiane atrophy (DRPLA)
D. Friedreich ataxia (FRDA1)

Friedreich ataxia (FRDA1) is GAA repeat autosomal recessive congenital ataxia.

1862. Which of the following was also called olivopontocerebellar atrophy?
Harrison's 20th Ed. Chapter 431, Page 3155
- A. Spinocerebellar ataxia 1
- B. Spinocerebellar ataxia 2
- C. Spinocerebellar ataxia 3
- D. Spinocerebellar ataxia 6

SCA1 was previously referred to as olivopontocerebellar atrophy.

1863. Which clinical phenotype of spinocerebellar ataxia has been described in patients from India?
Harrison's 20th Ed. Chapter 431, Page 3156
- A. Spinocerebellar ataxia 1
- B. Spinocerebellar ataxia 2
- C. Spinocerebellar ataxia 6
- D. Spinocerebellar ataxia 7

Clinical phenotype of spinocerebellar ataxia (SCA2) has been described in patients from Cuba and India.

1864. Which out of the following is the most common inherited autosomal dominant ataxia?
Harrison's 20th Ed. Chapter 431, Page 3156
- A. Spinocerebellar ataxia 1
- B. Spinocerebellar ataxia 2
- C. Spinocerebellar ataxia 3
- D. Spinocerebellar ataxia 6

In most populations, Machado-Joseph Disease (MJD) or spinocerebellar ataxias 3 is the most common autosomal dominant ataxia.

1865. Amyotrophic lateral sclerosis - parkinsonism - dystonia type presentation is in which clinical type of MJD?
Harrison's 20th Ed. Chapter 431, Page 3156
- A. Type I MJD
- B. Type II MJD
- C. Type III MJD
- D. None of the above

1866. Ataxic type presentation is seen in which type of MJD?
Harrison's 20th Ed. Chapter 431, Page 3156
- A. Type I MJD
- B. Type II MJD
- C. Type III MJD
- D. None of the above

1867. Ataxic-amyotrophic type presentation is seen in which clinical type of MJD?
Harrison's 20th Ed. Chapter 431, Page 3156
- A. Type I MJD
- B. Type II MJD
- C. Type III MJD
- D. None of the above

1868. Which is the most common clinical type of MJD?
Harrison's 20th Ed. Chapter 431, Page 3156
- A. Type I MJD
- B. Type II MJD
- C. Type III MJD
- D. All of the above

MJD is of three clinical types. Type I MJD - amyotrophic lateral sclerosis–parkinsonism–dystonia type), type II MJD - ataxic type, Type III MJD - ataxic-amyotrophic type. Type II is the most common form of MJD.

1869. The mean age of onset of symptoms in MJD is?
Harrison's 20th Ed. Chapter 431, Page 3156
- A. 5 years
- B. 10 years
- C. 15 years
- D. 25 years

The mean age of onset of symptoms in MJD is 25 years.

1870. Patients retain full intellectual function in which clinical type of MJD?
Harrison's 20th Ed. Chapter 431, Page 3156
- A. Type I MJD
- B. Type II MJD
- C. Type III MJD
- D. All of the above

Usually, MJD patients retain full intellectual function.

1871. Which of the following is spared in Machado-Joseph Disease (MJD)?
Harrison's 20th Ed. Chapter 431, Page 3156
- A. Inferior olives
- B. Corpus striatum
- C. Pars compacta of substantia nigra
- D. Dentate nucleus of cerebellum

Sparing of the inferior olives distinguishes MJD from other dominantly inherited ataxias.

1872. Which of the following spinocerebellar ataxias (SCAs) has pure cerebellar presentation?
Harrison's 20th Ed. Chapter 431, Page 3156
- A. SCA1
- B. SCA2
- C. SCA3
- D. SCA5

SCA5 (autosomal dominant type 5) maps to chromosome 11 & presentation includes ataxia & dysarthria.

1873. 'Retinal pigmentary degeneration' occurs in which of the following spinocerebellar ataxias (SCAs)?
Harrison's 20th Ed. Chapter 431, Page 3156
- A. SCA1
- B. SCA2
- C. Machado-Joseph disease
- D. SCA7

SCA7 is distinguished from all other SCAs by the presence of retinal pigmentary degeneration.

1874. The color blindness in SCA7 is for which colour?
Harrison's 20th Ed. Chapter 431, Page 3156
- A. Red-yellow
- B. Green-yellow
- C. Blue-yellow
- D. Any of the above

In SCA7, visual abnormalities first appear as blue-yellow color blindness and proceed to frank visual loss with macular degeneration.

1875. Haw River syndrome relates to which of the following?
Harrison's 20th Ed. Chapter 431, Page 3156

A. Machado-Joseph disease
B. Dentatorubropallidoluysian atrophy (DRPLA)
C. Friedreich's ataxia
D. Episodic ataxia

Haw River Syndrome (HRS) is an autosomal dominant neurodegenerative disease that has affected five generations of an African-American family in rural North Carolina. It represents a unique spectrum of multiple system degenerations resembling Huntington's disease, spinocerebellar atrophy and dentatorubropallidoluysian atrophy (DRPLA), a neurodegenerative disease that is primarily reported in Japan. Cardinal features in adults are ataxia, choreoathetosis & dementia. Cardinal features in children are mental retardation, behavioral changes, myoclonus, and epilepsy. ATN1 (DRPLA) is the only gene associated with DRPLA.

1876. Gene related to dentatorubropallidoluysian atrophy is?
Harrison's 20th Ed. Chapter 431, Page 3156

A. Dentatin
B. Quadrupin
C. Simplin
D. Atrophin

DRPLA is due to unstable CAG triplet repeats in the open reading frame of a gene "atrophin" located on chromosome 12p12-ter.

1877. Which of the following spinocerebellar ataxias (SCAs) has presentation similar to Huntington disease (HD)?
Harrison's 20th Ed. Chapter 431, Page 3156

A. SCA1
B. SCA2
C. SCA3
D. SCA17

SCAs & HD show broad phenotypic overlap including ataxia, spasticity, Parkinsonian features, dystonia, chorea, dementia & mood disorders. Later three symptoms in a hereditary context should favor a genetic test for HD. Similar phenotypes have been observed in SCA17.

1878. Episodic ataxia episodes are precipitated by?
Harrison's 20th Ed. Chapter 431, Page 3156

A. Hunger
B. Exercise
C. Sleep
D. Meals

Episodes of ataxia in EA 1 & 2, with gait imbalance & slurring of speech, occur spontaneously or are precipitated by sudden movement, excitement, stress, exercise, or excessive fatigue.

1879. Myokymia best relates to which of the following?
Harrison's 20th Ed. Chapter 431, Page 3156

A. Impaired muscle relaxation
B. Groups of fasciculations
C. Prolonged muscle contraction
D. Localized muscle pain

Myokymia refers to groups of fasciculations associated with continuous undulations of muscle.

1880. In episodic ataxia, symptoms and episodic attacks of ataxia responsive to?
Harrison's 20th Ed. Chapter 431, Page 3156

A. Lithium
B. Atypical antipsychotic drugs
C. Acetazolamide
D. Electroconvulsive therapy (ECT)

Symptoms & episodic attacks of episodic ataxia type 1 & 2 are responsive to acetazolamide (AZM) or anticonvulsants.

1881. Which of the following is not a potassium ion channelopathy?
J Neurol Neurosurg Psychiatry 2015;0:1–12

A. Episodic ataxia-1
B. Episodic ataxia-2
C. Benign neonatal familial convulsions
D. Jervell & Lange-Nielsen syndrome

Episodic ataxia-2 is a calcium ion channelopathy.

1882. Which of the following is not a sodium ion channelo-pathy?
J Neurol Neurosurg Psychiatry 2015;0:1–12

A. Paramyotonia congenita
B. Hyperkalemic periodic paralysis
C. Hypokalemic periodic paralysis
D. Generalized epilepsy with febrile convulsions plus

1883. Which of the following is not a calcium ion channelopathy?
J Neurol Neurosurg Psychiatry 2015;0:1–12

A. Episodic ataxia-2
B. Spinocerebellar ataxia-6
C. Familial hemiplegic migraine
D. Autosomal dominant progressive deafness

1884. Neurologic genetic disorders inherited in Mendelian autosomal dominant mutations include all except?
http://omim.org/

A. Huntington's disease (HD)
B. Familial Alzheimer's disease
C. Amyotrophic lateral sclerosis (ALS)
D. Friedreich's ataxia (FA)

1885. Neurologic genetic disorders inherited in Mendelian autosomal dominant mutations include all except?
http://omim.org/

A. Dystrophia myotonica (DM)
B. Ataxia telangiectasia
C. Charcot-Marie-Tooth disease 1A (CMT 1A)
D. Familial hyperkalemic periodic paralysis (HYPP)

1886. Neurologic genetic disorders inherited in Mendelian autosomal dominant mutations include all except?
http://omim.org/

A. Spinocerebellar ataxia (SCA)
B. Tuberous sclerosis
C. Wilson's disease
D. Charcot-Marie-Tooth disease 1A (CMT 1A)

1887. Neurologic genetic disorders inherited as Mendelian autosomal recessive include all except?
http://omim.org/

A. Friedreich's ataxia (FA)
B. Wilson's disease
C. Tuberous sclerosis
D. Ataxia telangiectasia

1888. Neurologic genetic disorders inherited as X-linked recessive traits include all except?

http://omim.org/

A. Duchenne muscular dystrophy (DMD)
B. Spinobulbar muscular atrophy (SBMA)
C. Fragile X syndrome
D. Friedreich's ataxia (FA)

1889. What was the nationality of Nicholaus Friedreich, after whom Friedreich's ataxia has been named?

A. British
B. French
C. German
D. Spanish

Friedreich's ataxia is named after the German physician Nicholaus Friedreich, who first described the condition in 1860s.

1890. Most common form of inherited ataxia is?

Harrison's 20th Ed. Chapter 431, Page 3157

A. Machado-Joseph Disease (MJD)
B. Friedreich's ataxia
C. Dentatorubropallidoluysian atrophy (DRPLA)
D. Episodic ataxia

Friedreich's Ataxia is the most common form of inherited ataxia, comprising half of all hereditary ataxias.

1891. Primary site of pathology in Friedreich's ataxia is?

Harrison's 20th Ed. Chapter 431, Page 3157

A. Spinal cord
B. Dorsal root ganglion cells
C. Peripheral nerves
D. All of the above

Primary pathology in Friedreich's ataxia is in spinal cord (sclerosis and degeneration in spinocerebellar tracts, lateral corticospinal tracts and posterior columns), dorsal root ganglion cells and peripheral nerves (loss of large myelinated fibers).

1892. Which of the following about Friedreich's ataxia is false?

Harrison's 20th Ed. Chapter 431, Page 3157

A. Presents before 25 years of age
B. Lower extremities more severely involved than upper
C. Flexor plantar responses
D. Absence of deep tendon reflexes

Friedreich's ataxia presents before 25 years of age. Lower extremities are more severely involved than upper. Extensor plantar responses (with normal tone in trunk & extremities), absence of deep tendon reflexes are found. Loss of vibratory & proprioceptive sensation occurs.

1893. Which of the following about Friedreich's ataxia is false?

Harrison's 20th Ed. Chapter 431, Page 3157

A. Cardiac involvement occurs in 90% of patients
B. High incidence of diabetes mellitus
C. Severe mental retardation
D. Musculoskeletal deformities are common

1894. Musculoskeletal deformities in Friedreich's ataxia are?

Harrison's 20th Ed. Chapter 431, Page 3157

A. Pes cavus
B. Pes equinovarus
C. Scoliosis
D. All of the above

Cardiomegaly, symmetric hypertrophy, murmurs & conduction defects reported in ~90% of patients. Diabetes mellitus is found in 20%. Pes cavus, pes equinovarus and progressive scoliosis common. Mental retardation is uncommon.

1895. Which of the following is a presentation of Friedreich's ataxia?

Harrison's 20th Ed. Chapter 431, Page 3157

A. Progressive staggering gait
B. Frequent falling
C. Titubation
D. All of the above

Friedreich's ataxia presents with progressive staggering gait, frequent falling and titubation. Dysarthria may be the presenting symptom. Progressive scoliosis, foot deformity, nystagmus or cardiopathy is the initial sign at times.

1896. Which of the following is a finding in Friedreich's ataxia?

Harrison's 20th Ed. Chapter 431, Page 3157

A. Nystagmus & loss of fast saccadic eye movements
B. Truncal titubation
C. Dysmetria and ataxia of trunk & limb movements
D. All of the above

Neurologic examination in Friedreich's ataxia may show nystagmus, loss of fast saccadic eye movements, truncal titubation, dysarthria, dysmetria, and ataxia of trunk & limb movements.

1897. The median age of death in Friedreich's ataxia is?

Harrison's 20th Ed. Chapter 431, Page 3157

A. 25 years
B. 35 years
C. 45 years
D. 55 years

The median age of death in Friedreich's ataxia is 35 years.

1898. In Friedreich's ataxia, sclerosis & degeneration occur in?

Harrison's 20th Ed. Chapter 431, Page 3157

A. Spinocerebellar tracts
B. Lateral corticospinal tracts
C. Posterior columns
D. All of the above

1899. In Friedreich's ataxia, which of the following is most extensively involved?

Harrison's 20th Ed. Chapter 431, Page 3157

A. Cerebral cortex
B. Peripheral nerves
C. Dorsal root ganglion cells
D. Cerebellum

The peripheral nerves are extensively involved in Friedreich's ataxia, with loss of large myelinated fibers.

1900. Which of the following is a large-fiber sensory neuropathy?

Harrison's 20th Ed. Chapter 431, Page 3157

A. Friedreich's ataxia
B. Lepromatous leprosy
C. Diabetes mellitus
D. Antiretroviral therapy neuropathy

1901. Which of the following diseases is due to genetic abnormalities of DNA mismatch/repair?
Harrison's 20th Ed. Chapter 431, Page 3350

A. Bloom's syndrome
B. Ataxia telangiectasia
C. Hereditary nonpolyposis colon cancer (HNPCC)
D. All of the above

Genetic abnormalities of DNA mismatch/repair include xeroderma pigmentosum, Bloom's syndrome, ataxia telangiectasia, and hereditary nonpolyposis colon cancer (HNPCC). They strongly predispose to neoplasia because of the rapid acquisition of additional mutations.

1902. Classic form of Friedreich's ataxia is mapped to chromosome?
Harrison's 20th Ed. Chapter 431, Page 3157

A. 4
B. 5
C. 6
D. 9

Friedreich's ataxia is an autosomal recessive congenital ataxia and is caused by a mutation in gene FXN (formerly known as X25) that codes for frataxin, located on chromosome 9q13-q21.1.

1903. Genes for which of the following are on chromosome 9?
Harrison's 20th Ed. Chapter 431, Page 3157

A. ABL oncogene
B. JAK2 gene
C. C9ORF72
D. All of the above

1904. Mutant gene in classic form of Friedreich's ataxia is?
Harrison's 20th Ed. Chapter 431, Page 3157

A. Frataxin
B. Ataxin 1
C. Ataxin 2
D. All of the above

The classic form of Friedreich's ataxia is mapped to 9q13-q21.1. Mutant gene frataxin contains expanded GAA triplet repeats in the first intron. Because the defect is located on an intron (which is removed from the mRNA transcript between transcription and translation), this mutation does not result in the production of abnormal frataxin proteins. Instead, the mutation causes gene silencing (i.e., the mutation decreases the transcription of the gene) through induction of a heterochromatin structure. In Friedreich's ataxia, patients have 200 - 900 GAA repeats (normal 7–22). Altered protein is called frataxin.

1905. Which of the following about Friedreich's ataxia is false?
Harrison's 20th Ed. Chapter 431, Page 3157

A. Frataxin is a mitochondrial protein for iron homeostasis
B. Excess oxidized intramitochondrial iron
C. Iron chelators and antioxidants are potentially harmful
D. None of the above

Frataxin mRNA and frataxin protein are low in Friedreich's ataxia. Frataxin is a mitochondrial protein involved in iron homeostasis. Mitochondrial iron accumulation due to loss of the iron transporter coded by the mutant frataxin gene results in oxidized intramitochondrial iron resulting in oxidation of cellular components & irreversible cell injury. Iron chelators and antioxidants are potentially harmful.

1906. Which of the following MRI finding is typical of Friedreich's ataxia?
Harrison's 20th Ed. Chapter 431, Page 3157

A. Brainstem atrophy
B. Cerebellar artophy
C. Spinal cord atrophy
D. Obstructive hydrocephalus

Neuroimaging reveals thinning of the cervical spinal cord.

1907. Which of the following drugs is of use in Friedreich's ataxia?
Harrison's 20th Ed. Chapter 431, Page 3158

A. Desferrioxamine
B. Idebenone
C. Ascorbic acid
D. All of the above

Idebenone, a short-chain analogue of coenzyme Q10 and a free-radical scavenger, can improve myocardial hypertrophy when used at an early stage reduces progression of cerebellar manifestation.

1908. Which of the following is a feature of Bassen-Kornzweig syndrome?
Harrison's 20th Ed. Chapter 431, Page 3157

A. Diabetes mellitus
B. Cardiomyopathy
C. Abetalipoproteinemia
D. Hypothyroidism

Bassen-Kornzweig syndrome is an autosomal recessive disorder in which a person is unable to fully absorb dietary fats through intestines. It is caused by a defect in microsomal triglyceride transfer protein (MTP) gene. Defects in MTP result in impairment of formation and secretion of VLDL in liver (abetalipoproteinemia). This defect results in a deficiency of delivery of vitamin E to tissues, including the central & peripheral nervous system, as VLDL is the transport molecule for vitamin E.

1909. Which of the following is false regarding ataxia with vitamin E deficiency (AVED)?
Harrison's 20th Ed. Chapter 431, Page 3157

A. Due to mutations in gene for a tocopherol transfer protein
B. Autosomal recessive
C. Chromosomal localization is on 8q13
D. None of the above

AVED is due to mutations in the gene for alpha-tocopherol transfer protein (a TTP). These patients have an impaired ability to bind vitamin E into the VLDL produced and secreted by the liver, resulting in a deficiency of vitamin E in peripheral tissues.

1910. Ataxia Telangiectasia is also known as?
Neurology. 2018;91(4):175-179

A. Louis-Bar syndrome
B. Nijmegen breakage syndrome (NBS1)
C. Lou Gehrig's disease
D. Pott's disease

Other names for ataxia-telangiectasia are A-T, Ataxia Telangiectasia Syndrome, ATM, Louis-Bar syndrome, Telangiectasia, cerebello-oculocutaneous.

1911. Gene responsible for Ataxia Telangiectasia is found on which chromosome?
Harrison's 20th Ed. Chapter 431, Page 3157

A. Chromosome 11
B. Chromosome 12
C. Chromosome 13
D. Chromosome 14

Ataxia Telangiectasia is inherited as an autosomal recessive disorder and offending gene is found on the long arm of chromosome 11 at 11q22-23. It controls the production of a phosphatidylinositol-3-kinase-like enzyme involved in cellular responses to stress, DNA damage and cell cycle control.

1912. Full name of ATM - the gene for Ataxia Telangiectasia is?
Harrison's 20th Ed. Chapter 68, Page 462

A. Ataxia-telangiectasia mutated kinase
B. Ataxia-telangiectasia manifested kinase
C. Ataxia-telangiectasia morphed kinase
D. Ataxia-telangiectasia magnified kinase

Ataxia-telangiectasia gene - ATM is on chromosome 11 and ATM stands for ataxia-telangiectasia mutated kinase. ATM encodes a protein that is predominantly confined to nucleus of cells and that remains constant throughout all stages of the cell cycle and participate in cell's responses to genomic damage. ATM gene is homologous to genes involved in DNA repair & control of cell cycle checkpoints. Mutations in the ATM gene give rise to defects in meiosis as well as increasing susceptibility to damage from ionizing radiation.

1913. ATM (ataxia-telangiectasia) carries an increased risk of?
Harrison's 20th Ed. Chapter 431, Page 3157

A. Breast cancer
B. Lymphoma
C. Acute T cell leukemias
D. All of the above

ATM (ataxia-telangiectasia) gene carries an increased risk of breast cancer, lymphoma and pancreatic cancer and there is an increased incidence of lymphomas, Hodgkin's disease, acute T cell leukemias, and breast cancer.

1914. A variant of AT - AT-like disease is caused by mutation in?
Harrison's 20th Ed. Chapter 344, Page 2494

A. IKBKAP gene
B. MRE11 gene
C. TRK-fused gene (TFG)
D. Serine palmitoyltransferase long-chain base 1 (SPTLC1) gene

1915. Inherited disease with defective DNA repair is?
Harrison's 20th Ed. Chapter 100, Page 740

A. Fanconi anemia
B. Bloom syndrome
C. Ataxia telangiectasia
D. All of the above

Inherited diseases with defective DNA repair are Fanconi anemia, Bloom syndrome and ataxia telangiectasia. They are also associated with AML.

1916. Mutation of which of the following gene causes a variant of AT (AT-like disease)?
Harrison's 20th Ed. Chapter 344, Page 2494

A. SBDS
B. MRE11
C. CHD7
D. STAT5b

A variant of AT (AT-like disease) is caused by mutation of the MRE11 gene.

1917. AT causes which of the following?
Harrison's 20th Ed. Chapter 344, Page 2494

A. Low IgA
B. IgG2 deficiency
C. Low antibody production
D. All of the above

AT causes a B cell immunodeficiency (low IgA, IgG2 deficiency, and low antibody production) that often requires immunoglobulin replacement therapy. Also, AT is associated with a progressive T cell immunodeficiency.

1918. Which of the following is false about Ataxia Telangiectasia?
Harrison's 20th Ed. Chapter 431, Page 3157

A. Present in first decade of life
B. Progressive telangiectatic lesions with deficits in cerebellar function & nystagmus
C. High incidence of recurrent pulmonary infections and neoplasms of lymphatic and reticuloendothelial system
D. None of the above

1919. In Ataxia Telangiectasia (AT), the most consistent defect of the lymphoid system is?
Harrison's 20th Ed. Chapter 431, Page 3157

A. Poorly developed or absent thymus gland
B. Generalised lymphadenopathy
C. Splenomegaly
D. Lymphedema

Poorly developed or absent thymus gland is the most consistent defect of the lymphoid system.

1920. Telangiectasia in Ataxia telangiectasia usually occur on?
Harrison's 20th Ed. Chapter 431, Page 3157

A. Bulbar conjunctiva
B. Nail bed
C. Intracranial
D. All of the above

Telangiectasia in AT usually occur on the white portion of eye (bulbar conjunctiva) but may also be found on the ears, neck and extremities.

1921. Neurologic manifestation in AT is?
Harrison's 20th Ed. Chapter 431, Page 3157

A. Truncal and limb ataxia
B. Extensor plantar responses & areflexia
C. Myoclonic jerks
D. All of the above

1922. Neuropathologic change seen in ataxia telangiectasia is?
Harrison's 20th Ed. Chapter 431, Page 3157

A. Loss of Purkinje, granule & basket cells in cerebellar cortex and loss of neurons in the deep cerebellar nuclei
B. Loss of anterior horn neurons in spinal cord
C. Loss of dorsal root ganglion cells
D. All of the above

The most striking neuropathologic change in AT is loss of Purkinje, granule, and basket cells in cerebellar cortex as well as of neurons in the deep cerebellar nuclei.

1923. Which of the following laboratory tests is useful in the diagnosis of Ataxia Telangiectasia?
Harrison's 20th Ed. Chapter 431, Page 3157

A. Cryofibrinogen
B. Ceruloplasmin level in blood
C. Alpha-fetoprotein level in blood
D. Apolipoprotein A-1

Alpha-fetoprotein levels in the blood are elevated (> 10 ng/ml) in >95% of patients of AT. AFP is produced only during fetal development. Immunoglobulin deficiency is noted.

1924. Which of the following statements about Ataxia-telangiectasia is false?

Harrison's 20th Ed. Chapter 431, Page 3157

A. Affected child has normal intelligence
B. Hypersensitivity to ionizing radiation
C. Predisposition to malignancy
D. None of the above

AT causes large telangiectatic lesions of face, cerebellar ataxia, immunologic defects & hypersensitivity to ionizing radiation. Affected child has normal or above normal intelligence. Insulin-resistant diabetes mellitus associated with anti-insulin antibodies occurs in patients with ataxia-telangiectasia.

1925. Hereditary forms of mitochondrial cytopathies include?

Harrison's 20th Ed. Chapter 431, Page 3251

A. Kearns-Sayre syndrome
B. Myoclonus epilepsy with ragged red fibers (MERRF)
C. Mitochondrial encephalopathy with lactic acidosis and stroke-like episodes (MELAS)
D. All of the above

Since mtDNA is transmitted exclusively by the mother, mitochondrial cytopathies show maternal inheritance and can be excluded when paternal transmission of the disease occurs in the family.

Disorders of the Autonomic Nervous System

1926. Autonomic nervous system (ANS) regulates which of the following?
Harrison's 20th Ed. Chapter 432, Page 3158
- A. Sleep function
- B. Glandular function
- C. Pupillary function
- D. All of the above

Autonomic nervous system (ANS) innervates the entire neuraxis & influences all organ systems. It regulates blood pressure, heart rate, sleep, glandular, pupillary, bladder & bowel function.

1927. Connections between cerebral cortex and autonomic centers occurs in?
Harrison's 20th Ed. Chapter 432, Page 3158
- A. Cerebral cortex
- B. Brainstem
- C. Spinal cord
- D. All of the above

Connections between cerebral cortex & autonomic centers in brainstem coordinate autonomic outflow with higher mental functions.

1928. Preganglionic neurons of parasympathetic nervous system leave the central nervous system in all except?
Harrison's 20th Ed. Chapter 432, Page 3158
- A. Third cranial nerve
- B. Sixth cranial nerve
- C. Seventh cranial nerve
- D. Tenth cranial nerve

1929. Preganglionic neurons of parasympathetic nervous system leave the central nervous system in all except?
Harrison's 20th Ed. Chapter 432, Page 3158
- A. Tenth cranial nerve
- B. Eleventh cranial nerve
- C. Second sacral nerve
- D. Third sacral nerve

Preganglionic neurons of PNS leave CNS in third, seventh, ninth & tenth cranial nerves as well as the second & third sacral nerves.

1930. Preganglionic neurons of sympathetic nervous system exit the spinal cord between?
Harrison's 20th Ed. Chapter 432, Page 3158
- A. T1 and L1 segments
- B. T1 and L2 segments
- C. T1 and L3 segments
- D. T1 and L4 segments

Preganglionic neurons of sympathetic nervous system exit spinal cord between first thoracic and the second lumbar segments.

1931. Acetylcholine is the neurotransmitter for all except?
Harrison's 20th Ed. Chapter 432, Page 3158
- A. Preganglionic parasympathetic ANS
- B. Preganglionic sympathetic ANS
- C. Postganglionic parasympathetic ANS
- D. Postganglionic sympathetic ANS

1932. Norepinephrine (NE) is the neurotransmitter for?
Harrison's 20th Ed. Chapter 432, Page 3158
- A. Preganglionic parasympathetic ANS
- B. Preganglionic sympathetic ANS
- C. Postganglionic parasympathetic ANS
- D. Postganglionic sympathetic ANS

Acetylcholine (ACh) is the preganglionic neurotransmitter for both divisions of ANS as well as postganglionic neurotransmitter of parasympathetic neurons. Norepinephrine (NE) is the neurotransmitter of postganglionic sympathetic neurons, except for cholinergic neurons innervating eccrine sweat glands.

1933. Which of the following statements is false?
Harrison's 20th Ed. Chapter 432, Page 3158
- A. Autonomic preganglionic fibers are thinly myelinated
- B. Postganglionic neurons (outside CNS) give rise to postganglionic unmyelinated autonomic nerves
- C. Responses to sympathetic & parasympathetic stimulation are antagonistic
- D. None of the above

1934. With sympathetic activation, which of the following does not occur?
Harrison's 20th Ed. Chapter 432, Page 3159 Table 432-1
- A. Increased bowel motility
- B. Increased bladder sphincter tone
- C. Sweating
- D. Ejaculation, orgasm

1935. With parasympathetic activation, which of the following does not occur?
Harrison's 20th Ed. Chapter 432, Page 3159 Table 432-1
- A. Increased bowel motility
- B. Penile erection
- C. Tearing
- D. Sweating

1936. Which of the following is regulated by autonomic circuits?
Harrison's 20th Ed. Chapter 432, Page 3158
- A. Sleep
- B. Pupils
- C. Bowel & bladder function
- D. All of the above

1937. Which of the following is part of enteric nervous system?
Harrison's 20th Ed. Chapter 432, Page 3159
- A. Meissner's plexus
- B. Auerbach's plexus
- C. Cajal's plexus
- D. All of the above

1938. Which of the following about enteric nervous system is false?
Harrison's 20th Ed. Chapter 432, Page 3159

A. Parasympathetic control of GI system is by craniospinal nerves
B. Sympathetic control of GI system is by thoracolumbar region
C. Number of enteric nervous system cells almost equal number of cells in spinal cord
D. None of the above

Parasympathetic control of GI system is by craniospinal nerves (vagus & S2-S4 nerves). Sympathetic control is by thoracolumbar region. Enteric nervous system comprises of Meissner's (submucosal), Auerbach's (myenteric), Cajal's (deep muscular), mucosal & submucosal plexuses.

1939. Most consistent & severe orthostatic hypotension (OH) is caused by lesion in?
Harrison's 20th Ed. Chapter 432, Page 3159

A. Lesions of the afferent limb of baroreflex arc
B. Lesions of the CNS processing centers
C. Lesions of the efferent limb of reflex arcs
D. All of the above

1940. OH is defined as, within 3 minutes of standing up, a sustained drop in SBP and DBP of?
Harrison's 20th Ed. Chapter 432, Page 3159

A. ≥ 20 and ≥ 20 mm Hg respectively
B. ≥ 20 and ≥ 10 mm Hg respectively
C. ≥ 10 and ≥ 10 mm Hg respectively
D. ≥ 10 and ≥ 5 mm Hg respectively

OH is defined as a sustained drop in systolic (≥20 mm Hg) or diastolic (≥10 mm Hg) BP within three minutes of standing.

1941. Which of the following statements about autonomic control of urinary bladder is false?
Harrison's 20th Ed. Chapter 432, Page 3159

A. Upper motor neuron lesion leads to spastic bladder
B. Lower motor neuron lesion leads to flaccid bladder
C. Bladder volume is a useful test for distinguishing between UMN and LMN bladder dysfunction
D. None of the above

Brain & spinal cord disease above lumbar level results in UMN or spastic bladder. PNS disease results in LMN flaccid bladder (large volumes, urinary frequency & overflow incontinence). Measurement of post-void residual bladder volume is useful test to distinguish between UMN & LMN bladder dysfunction.

1942. Most disabling feature of autonomic dysfunction is?
Harrison's 20th Ed. Chapter 432, Page 3160

A. Orthostatic or postural hypotension
B. Progressively severe constipation
C. Loss of sweat function
D. Impotence

When orthostatic or postural hypotension (OH) is specifically due to dysfunction of ANS, it is referred to as neurogenic OH.

1943. OH can cause which of the following symptom?
Harrison's 20th Ed. Chapter 432, Page 3160

A. Diaphoresis
B. Diminished hearing
C. Shortness of breath
D. All of the above

Symptom spectrum of OH is wide. It includes dimming or loss of vision, light headedness, diaphoresis, diminished hearing, pallor, weakness and shortness of breath.

1944. OH can cause which of the following?
Harrison's 20th Ed. Chapter 432, Page 3160

A. Heart rate that is fixed regardless of posture
B. Postprandial hypotension
C. Excessively high nocturnal BP
D. All of the above

Manifestations of impaired baroreflexes are supine hypertension, a heart rate that is fixed regardless of posture, postprandial hypotension, and an excessively high nocturnal BP.

1945. Which of the following statements about OH is false?
Harrison's 20th Ed. Chapter 432, Page 3161

A. Most common causes of OH are not neurologic in origin
B. Neurogenic OH is aggravated/precipitated by autonomic stressors
C. In non-neurogenic OH, BP drop is leads to a compensatory increase in heart rate of >15 beats/minute.
D. None of the above

1946. Which of the following is an autonomic stressor?
Harrison's 20th Ed. Chapter 432, Page 3161

A. Meal
B. Hot bath
C. Exercise
D. All of the above

Autonomic stressors are a meal, hot bath or exercise. Lack of sweating after a hot bath, during exercise, or on a hot day can suggest sudomotor failure.

1947. Drugs that can cause Orthostatic hypotension (OH) include all except?
Harrison's 20th Ed. Chapter 432, Page 3161

A. Diuretics
B. Phenothiazines
C. Beta adrenergic blockers
D. Calcium channel blockers

1948. Drugs that can cause Orthostatic hypotension (OH) include all except?
Harrison's 20th Ed. Chapter 432, Page 3161

A. Insulin
B. Glucagon
C. Barbiturates
D. Ethanol

Drugs that may cause OH are diuretics, antihypertensives, antidepressants, phenothiazines, ethanol, narcotics, insulin, dopamine agonists, barbiturates & calcium channel blocking agents.

1949. Disorders of autonomic function should be considered in patients with which of the following symptom?
Harrison's 20th Ed. Chapter 432, Page 3161

A. Altered sweating
B. Gastroparesis
C. Impotence
D. All of the above

Disorders of autonomic function should be considered in patients with altered sweating (hyperhidrosis or hypohidrosis), gastroparesis (bloating, nausea, vomiting of old food), impotence, constipation or bladder disturbances (urinary frequency, hesitancy or incontinence).

1950. Which of the following is a non-neurogenic cause of OH?
Harrison's 20th Ed. Chapter 432, Page 3161

- A. Constipation
- B. Hypovolemia
- C. Urinary incontinence
- D. All of the above

Hypovolemia is a non-neurogenic cause of OH.

1951. Heart rate variation with deep breathing (respiratory sinus arrhythmia) is abolished by administration of?
Harrison's 20th Ed. Chapter 432, Page 3162

- A. Atropine
- B. Digoxin
- C. Beta blockers
- D. All of the above

HRDB or Heart rate variation with deep breathing (respiratory sinus arrhythmia) is abolished by atropine but is unaffected by sympathetic blockade (propranolol).

1952. Valsalva response is tested in which position?
Harrison's 20th Ed. Chapter 432, Page 3162

- A. Supine
- B. Sitting
- C. Standing
- D. Any of the above

Valsalva response is tested in the supine position.

1953. In Valsalva maneuver, a constant expiratory pressure of how much is maintained for 15 seconds?
Harrison's 20th Ed. Chapter 432, Page 3162

- A. 10 mm Hg
- B. 20 mm Hg
- C. 30 mm Hg
- D. 40 mm Hg

Valsalva maneuver assesses the integrity of baroreflex control of heart rate (parasympathetic) & BP (adrenergic). With subject supine, a constant expiratory pressure of 40 mmHg is maintained for 15 seconds while measuring changes in heart rate and beat-to-beat BP.

1954. Fall in BP occurs in which phase of Valsalva maneuver?
Harrison's 20th Ed. Chapter 432, Page 3162

- A. Phase I
- B. Early phase II
- C. Late phase II
- D. All of the above

Out of four phases of Valsalva maneuver response, phases I & III are mechanical & related to changes in intrathoracic & intraabdominal pressure. In early phase II, reduced venous return results in a fall in stroke volume and BP, counteracted by a combination of reflex tachycardia and increased total peripheral resistance. Increased total peripheral resistance arrests the BP drop ~5–8 seconds after the onset of maneuver. Late phase II begins with a progressive rise in BP towards or above baseline. Venous return and cardiac output return to normal in phase IV. Persistent peripheral arteriolar vasoconstriction and increased cardiac adrenergic tone results in a temporary BP overshoot and phase IV bradycardia (mediated by baroreceptor reflex).

1955. The 'Valsalva ratio' is defined as?
Harrison's 20th Ed. Chapter 432, Page 3162

- A. Maximum phase 1 tachycardia divided by minimum phase 4 bradycardia
- B. Maximum phase 2 tachycardia divided by minimum phase 4 bradycardia
- C. Maximum phase 3 tachycardia divided by minimum phase 4 bradycardia
- D. Maximum phase 4 tachycardia divided by minimum phase 4 bradycardia

Autonomic function during the Valsalva maneuver can be measured using beat-to-beat blood pressure or heart rate changes. Valsalva ratio is defined as the maximum phase II tachycardia divided by minimum phase IV bradycardia. The ratio reflects cardiovagal function.

1956. Sweating is induced by release of acetylcholine from?
Harrison's 20th Ed. Chapter 432, Page 3162

- A. Preganglionic parasympathetic ANS
- B. Preganglionic sympathetic ANS
- C. Postganglionic parasympathetic ANS
- D. Postganglionic sympathetic ANS

Sweating is induced by release of acetylcholine (ACh) from sympathetic postganglionic fibers.

1957. Which of the following is a test for sweating?
Harrison's 20th Ed. Chapter 432, Page 3162

- A. Quantitative sudomotor axon reflex test (QSART)
- B. Thermoregulatory sweat test (TST)
- C. Measurement of galvanic skin responses
- D. All of the above

1958. A reduced or absent response in 'Quantitative sudomotor axon reflex test (QSART)' indicates?
Harrison's 20th Ed. Chapter 432, Page 3162

- A. Lesion of preganglionic sudomotor axon
- B. Lesion of postganglionic sudomotor axon
- C. Lesion of pre & postganglionic sudomotor axon
- D. None of the above

A reduced or absent response indicates a lesion of the postganglionic sudomotor axon.

1959. If both QSART and TST are absent, the lesion is in?
Harrison's 20th Ed. Chapter 432, Page 3162

- A. Preganglionic sudomotor axon
- B. Postganglionic sudomotor axon
- C. Pre & postganglionic sudomotor axon
- D. None of the above

A postganglionic lesion is present if both QSART and TST show absent sweating.

1960. If QSART is intact but TST shows anhidrosis, lesion is in?
Harrison's 20th Ed. Chapter 432, Page 3162

- A. Preganglionic sudomotor axon
- B. Postganglionic sudomotor axon
- C. Pre & postganglionic sudomotor axon
- D. None of the above

In a preganglionic lesion, QSART is intact but TST shows anhidrosis.

1961. Which of the following is a primary autonomic degenerative disorder?
Harrison's 20th Ed. Chapter 432, Page 126

- A. Multiple system atrophy
- B. Parkinson's disease
- C. Dementia with Lewy bodies
- D. All of the above

Primary autonomic degenerative disorders are multiple system atrophy (Shy-Drager syndrome), Parkinson's disease, dementia with Lewy bodies and pure autonomic failure. These are grouped together as "synucleinopathies" due to the presence of alpha-synuclein, a small protein that precipitates predominantly in the cytoplasm of neurons in the Lewy body disorders (Parkinson's disease, dementia with Lewy bodies and pure autonomic failure) and in the glia in multiple system atrophy.

1962. Which of the following is a small-fiber peripheral neuropathy?
Harrison's 20th Ed. Chapter 432, Page 126

A. Diabetes mellitus
B. Amyloid
C. Hereditary sensory and autonomic neuropathies (HSAN)
D. All of the above

Small-fiber peripheral neuropathies are those seen in diabetes mellitus, amyloid, immune-mediated neuropathies, hereditary sensory and autonomic neuropathies (HSAN; particularly HSAN type III, familial dysautonomia).

1963. Multiple system atrophy (MSA) relates best to which of the following?
Harrison's 20th Ed. Chapter 432, Page 3162

A. Horner's syndrome
B. Wernicke-Korsakoff syndrome
C. Shy-Drager syndrome
D. Shapiro's syndrome

Multiple system atrophy (MSA) comprises of autonomic failure (OH and/or a neurogenic bladder) combined with either striatonigral degeneration (Shy-Drager syndrome) or sporadic olivopontocerebellar atrophy.

1964. Parkinsonism seen in multiple system atrophy features which of the following?
Harrison's 20th Ed. Chapter 432, Page 3163

A. No rest tremor
B. Not responsive to levodopa
C. Levodopa-induced dyskinesia uncommon
D. All of the above

1965. Autonomic dysfunction is a common feature in?
Harrison's 20th Ed. Chapter 432, Page 3163

A. Dementia with Lewy bodies (DLB)
B. Multiple system atrophy (MSA)
C. Parkinson's disease
D. All of the above

Autonomic dysfunction is a feature in dementia with Lewy bodies, MSA & Parkinson's disease.

1966. Autonomic dysreflexia is common in patients with traumatic spinal cord lesion above which level?
Harrison's 20th Ed. Chapter 432, Page 3163

A. T3
B. T6
C. T12
D. L2

Markedly increased autonomic discharge or autonomic dysreflexia is common in patients with traumatic spinal cord lesion above the T6 level.

1967. Neuromuscular junction disorders accompanied by autonomic involvement include?
Harrison's 20th Ed. Chapter 432, Page 3163

A. Porphyria
B. Botulism
C. Chronic alcoholism
D. Guillain-Barré syndrome

Peripheral neuropathies as in diabetes mellitus, amyloidosis, chronic alcoholism, porphyria, and Guillain-Barré syndrome lead to chronic autonomic insufficiency. Neuromuscular junction disorders with autonomic involvement include botulism and Lambert-Eaton syndrome.

1968. Autonomic neuropathy typically begins how many years after the onset of diabetes mellitus?
Harrison's 20th Ed. Chapter 432, Page 3163

A. ~5
B. ~7
C. ~10
D. ~14

Autonomic neuropathy typically begins ~10 years after the onset of DM.

1969. Autonomic dysfunction occurs in which of the following porphyria?
Harrison's 20th Ed. Chapter 432, Page 3163

A. Acute intermittent porphyria
B. Variegate porphyria
C. Hereditary coproporphyria
D. All of the above

Autonomic dysfunction is most extensively documented in acute intermittent porphyria but can also occur with variegate porphyria and hereditary coproporphyria.

1970. Autoantibodies against which of the following is present in autoimmune autonomic ganglionopathy (AAG)?
Harrison's 20th Ed. Chapter 432, Page 3164

A. A_3 AChR
B. B_3 AChR
C. C_3 AChR
D. D_3 AChR

Autoantibodies against ganglionic ACh receptor (A_3 AChR) are present in the serum of patients of autoimmune autonomic ganglionopathy (AAG).

1971. Paraneoplastic AAG is associated with?
Harrison's 20th Ed. Chapter 432, Page 3164

A. Adenocarcinoma or small-cell carcinoma of lung
B. Lymphoma
C. Thymoma
D. All of the above

1972. Botulinum toxin blocks release of which of the following?
Harrison's 20th Ed. Chapter 432, Page 3164

A. Norepinephrine
B. Acetylcholine
C. Serotonin
D. All of the above

Botulinum toxin binds presynaptically to cholinergic nerve terminals and after uptake into cytosol blocks ACh release.

1973. Pure Autonomic Failure (PAF) consists of?
Harrison's 20th Ed. Chapter 432, Page 3164

A. Postural hypotension
B. Impotence & bladder dysfunction
C. Impaired sweating
D. All of the above

1974. Which of the following statements about Pure Autonomic Failure (PAF) is false?
Harrison's 20th Ed. Chapter 432, Page 3164

A. Involvement of postganglionic sympathetic neurons
B. Low supine plasma NE levels
C. Noradrenergic supersensitivity
D. None of the above

In Pure Autonomic Failure (PAF) there is primary involvement of postganglionic sympathetic neurons that results in low supine plasma NE levels & noradrenergic supersensitivity.

1975. **Which of the following is false about Postural Orthostatic Tachycardia Syndrome (POTS)?**
   Harrison's 20th Ed. Chapter 432, Page 3164
   A. Symptomatic orthostatic hypotension
   B. Increase in heart rate of > 30 beats/min with standing
   C. Women affected five times more often than men
   D. Occurs between 15 and 50 years of age

   POTS is characterized by symptomatic orthostatic intolerance (not OH) and by either an increase in heart rate to >120 beats/minute or an increase of 30 beats/minute with standing that subsides on sitting or lying down. Women are affected approximately five times more often than men, and most develop the syndrome between the ages of 15 and 50.

1976. **Which of the following is a presyncopal symptom?**
   Harrison's 20th Ed. Chapter 432, Page 3164
   A. Lightheadedness
   B. Weakness
   C. Blurred vision
   D. All of the above

1977. **Which of the following is a symptom of autonomic overactivity?**
   Harrison's 20th Ed. Chapter 432, Page 3164
   A. Palpitations
   B. Tremulousness
   C. Nausea
   D. All of the above

1978. **Hereditary sensory and autonomic neuropathy I (HSAN I) is best related to which of the following?**
   Harrison's 20th Ed. Chapter 432, Page 3164
   A. Dermatan sulfate
   B. Sphingomyelin
   C. Glucosyl ceramide
   D. Heparan sulfate

   SPTLC is an enzyme in the regulation of ceramide. Cells from HSAN I patients affected by mutation of SPTLC1 gene produce higher-than-normal levels of glucosyl ceramide triggering apoptosis.

1979. **The defective gene in HSAN I is?**
   Harrison's 20th Ed. Chapter 432, Page 3164
   A. SPTLC1
   B. SPTLC2
   C. SPTLC3
   D. SPTLC4

   SPTLC is a key enzyme in the regulation of ceramide. Most common responsible gene for HSAN I is SPTLC1 on chromosome 9q.

1980. **The defective gene in HSAN III is?**
   Harrison's 20th Ed. Chapter 432, Page 3164
   A. IKBKAP
   B. SPTLC2
   C. SPTLC3
   D. SPTLC4

   The defective gene in HSAN III (Riley-Day syndrome or familial dysautonomia) is IKBKAP.

1981. **Cause of autonomic storm is?**
   Harrison's 20th Ed. Chapter 432, Page 3165
   A. Brain and spinal cord injury
   B. Autonomic neuropathy
   C. Pheochromocytoma
   D. All of the above

   Acute autonomic syndrome may be either acute autonomic failure (acute AAN syndrome) or a state of sympathetic overactivity. Autonomic storm is an acute state of sustained sympathetic surge. Causes are brain & spinal cord injury, toxins & drugs, autonomic neuropathy, and pheochromocytoma.

1982. **Which of the following is the most common cause of autonomic storm?**
   Harrison's 20th Ed. Chapter 432, Page 3165
   A. Brain injury
   B. Pheochromocytoma
   C. Cocaine
   D. Tetanus

   Brain injury is the most common cause of autonomic storm and typically follows severe head trauma and postresuscitation encephalopathy anoxic-ischemic brain injury.

1983. **Massive catecholaminergic surge in autonomic storm can cause which of the following?**
   Harrison's 20th Ed. Chapter 432, Page 3165
   A. Seizures
   B. Neurogenic pulmonary edema
   C. Myocardial injury
   D. All of the above

   Massive catecholaminergic surge in autonomic storm can cause seizures, neurogenic pulmonary edema and myocardial injury.

1984. **Drug that can produce autonomic storm is?**
   Harrison's 20th Ed. Chapter 432, Page 3165
   A. Phenylpropanolamine
   B. Cocaine
   C. Amphetamine
   D. All of the above

   Drugs and toxins that can produce autonomic storm include phenylpropanolamine, cocaine, amphetamine & tricyclic antidepressants, tetanus and botulinum.

1985. **Neuroleptic malignant syndrome is seen in psychotic patients treated with?**
   Harrison's 20th Ed. Chapter 432, Page 3165
   A. Amphetamine
   B. Phenylpropanolamine
   C. Phenothiazine
   D. Any of the above

1986. **Which of the following is a feature of neuroleptic malignant syndrome?**
   Harrison's 20th Ed. Chapter 432, Page 3165
   A. Muscle rigidity
   B. Hyperthermia
   C. Hypertension
   D. All of the above

   Neuroleptic malignant syndrome features muscle rigidity, hyperthermia & hypertension in psychotic patients treated with phenothiazines.

1987. **Which of the following drug is effective in chronic and milder autonomic storm?**
   Harrison's 20th Ed. Chapter 432, Page 3165
   A. Morphine sulphate
   B. Labetalol
   C. Clonidine
   D. All of the above

   For chronic and milder autonomic storm, propranolol and/or clonidine can be effective.

1988. Allodynia refers to?
Harrison's 20th Ed. Chapter 432, Page 3165

A. Perception of nonpainful stimulus as painful
B. Exaggerated pain response to a painful stimulus
C. Spontaneous pain
D. All of the above

Allodynia refers to the perception of a nonpainful stimulus as painful while hyperpathia refers to an exaggerated pain response to a painful stimulus.

1989. Which of the following must be present for the diagnosis of complex regional pain syndrome (CRPS)?
Harrison's 20th Ed. Chapter 432, Page 3165

A. Vasomotor dysfunction
B. Sudomotor abnormalities
C. Focal edema
D. Any of the above

Pain is the primary clinical feature of CRPS. Vasomotor dysfunction, sudomotor abnormalities, or focal edema may occur alone or in combination but must be present for diagnosis.

1990. CRPS type II develops after?
Harrison's 20th Ed. Chapter 432, Page 3165

A. Injury to a specific peripheral nerve
B. Myocardial infarction
C. Stroke
D. Limb injury

CRPS type I is a regional pain syndrome that usually develops after tissue trauma (myocardial infarction, minor shoulder or limb injury, stroke). CRPS type II is a regional pain syndrome that develops after injury to a specific peripheral nerve, usually a major nerve trunk.

1991. In the treatment of orthostatic hypotension, enough intake of salt & fluids should produce a urine voiding volume between?
Harrison's 20th Ed. Chapter 432, Page 3165

A. 0.5 & 1.0 Liters
B. 1.0 & 1.5 Liters
C. 1.5 & 2.5 Liters
D. 2.5 & 3.5 Liters

In the treatment of orthostatic hypotension, aim is to consume salt & fluids to produce a voiding volume between 1.5 and 2.5 liters of urine (containing > 170 meq/L of Na+) per day.

1992. Which of the following best relates to treatment of orthostatic hypotension?
Harrison's 20th Ed. Chapter 432, Page 3165

A. Modena treatment
B. Bouillon treatment
C. Mercuro treatment
D. Mancini treatment

Bouillon treatment refers to increasing intake of salt and fluids for transient worsening of OH.

1993. Which of the following drugs is useful in the treatment of orthostatic hypotension?
Harrison's 20th Ed. Chapter 432, Page 3165

A. Midodrine
B. Droxidopa
C. Pyridostigmine
D. All of the above

1994. Which of the following drugs is useful in the treatment of orthostatic hypotension?
Harrison's 20th Ed. Chapter 432, Page 3165

A. Fludrocortisone
B. Atomoxetine and yohimbine
C. Octreotide
D. All of the above

Atomoxetine blocks NE reuptake transporter and yohimbine blocks α2 receptors that mediate the sympathetic feedback loop for downregulation of BP in response to atomoxetine.

Trigeminal Neuralgia, Bell's Palsy, and Other Cranial Nerve Disorders

1995. Trigeminal neuralgia (TN) is also called?
Asian Pac. J. Health Sci., 2015;2(1):108-118

A. Prosopalgia
B. Fothergill's disease
C. Tic-douloureux
D. All of the above

Trigeminal neuralgia (TN) is also known as Tic Douloureux, Fothergill's Disease, Suicide Disease or Prosopalgia. John Fothergill (1712-1780) gave the first full & accurate description of trigeminal neuralgia in 1773. Early descriptions of trigeminal neuralgia (Fothergill's disease) can be found in the writings of Galen, Aretaeus of Cappadocia (born circa AD 81), and in the 11th century by Avicenna ("tortura oris").

1996. Which of the following about Trigeminal nerve is false?
Harrison's 20th Ed. Chapter 433, Page 3166

A. Trigeminal nerve is the largest of the cranial nerves.
B. Trigeminal nerve is predominantly sensory
C. Its motor innervation is exclusively in mandibular V3 division
D. None of the above

1997. Which of the following is best related to trigeminal ganglion?
DeJong's The Neurologic Examination, 7th Ed. Page 132

A. Uhthoff's phenomenon
B. Möbius' syndrome
C. Meckel's cave
D. Cave of septum pellucidum

Trigeminal ganglion lies just beside pons in a depression in the petrous ridge, called Meckel's cave. A large sensory and a smaller motor root join the ganglion to the pons.

1998. Which of the following is false about trigeminal ganglion?
DeJong's The Neurologic Examination, 7th Ed. Page 228

A. Largest ganglion in the peripheral nervous system
B. Named after JL Gasser, also called semilunar ganglion
C. Analogous to a dorsal root ganglion
D. None of the above

Trigeminal or gasserian ganglion is crescent shaped, convex anterolaterally, and is also known as semilunar ganglion. It lies just lateral to internal carotid artery and posterior part of the cavernous sinus. It is analogous to a dorsal root ganglion and contains unipolar sensory neurons, whose central processes enter lateral pons through large sensory root that pass beneath tentorium to connect concave side of ganglion to the brainstem.

1999. Which of the following is related to trigeminal motor dysfunction?
DeJong's The Neurologic Examination, 7th Ed. Page 42

A. Nystagmus
B. Hearing loss
C. Tongue for atrophy/fasciculations
D. Jaw drop

Trigeminal motor function is ascertained by the patient's jaw drop prior to examining mouth and throat. When pterygoids are unilaterally weak, the jaw invariably deviates toward the weak side on opening. It is a sensitive indicator of trigeminal motor root pathology.

2000. Trigeminal motor fibers innervate which of the following muscles?
DeJong's The Neurologic Examination, 7th Ed. Page 135

A. Masseter
B. Temporalis
C. Pterygoids
D. All of the above

Trigeminal motor fibers innervate the masseter, temporalis, and pterygoids (medial & lateral).

2001. Which of the following muscles originate from the skull base?
DeJong's The Neurologic Examination, 7th Ed. Page 227

A. Masseter
B. Temporalis
C. Pterygoids
D. All of the above

2002. Trigeminal nerve supplies which of the following muscles?
DeJong's The Neurologic Examination, 7th Ed. Page 227

A. Anterior belly of digastric
B. Tensor veli palatini
C. Tensor tympani
D. All of the above

Trigeminal (fifth cranial) nerve supplies the mylohyoid, anterior belly of the digastric, tensor veli palatini, and tensor tympani muscles.

2003. Motor part of trigeminal (fifth cranial) nerve innervates which of the following muscle?
Harrison's 20th Ed. Chapter 433, Page 3166

A. Orbicularis oculi
B. Posterior auricular
C. Pterygoid
D. Sternocleidomastoid

The trigeminal (fifth cranial) nerve supplies sensation to the skin of face and anterior half of the head. Its motor part innervates the masseter & pterygoid masticatory muscles as well as the tensor tympani of the middle ear.

2004. Mandibular sensory fibers of trigeminal nerve enter the skull through?
DeJong's The Neurologic Examination, 7th Ed. Page 135

A. Superior orbital fissure
B. Foramen ovale
C. Foramen rotundum
D. Meckel's cave

Ophthalmic division of trigeminal nerve fibers enter skull via superior orbital fissure, and maxillary fibers enter through the foramen rotundum. Both pass through cavernous sinus before joining the gasserian ganglion. Mandibular fibers enter through ovale. Sensory fibers terminate in the principal sensory nucleus in the pons and in the nucleus of the spinal tract, which extends from pons to upper cervical spinal cord.

2005. Motor and principal sensory nuclei of trigeminal nerve are located in?
DeJong's The Neurologic Examination, 7th Ed. Page 227

A. Upper pons
B. Mid pons
C. Lower pons
D. Midbrain

Motor and principal sensory nuclei of trigeminal nerve are located in midpons. The spinal tract & nucleus extend from pons down into upper cervical spinal cord. Trigeminal nuclear structures thus extend from rostral midbrain to rostral spinal cord.

2006. Sensory portion of trigeminal nerve innervates which of the following?
DeJong's The Neurologic Examination, 7th Ed. Page 227

A. Nasal cavities
B. Intracranial dura
C. Cerebral vasculature
D. All of the above

Sensory portion of trigeminal nerve innervates face, teeth, oral & nasal cavities, scalp back to the vertex, intracranial dura & cerebral vasculature, It provides proprioceptive information for muscles of mastication.

2007. Trigeminal neuralgia is rare in which distribution of fifth nerve?
Harrison's 20th Ed. Chapter 433, Page 3166

A. Ophthalmic division
B. Maxillary division
C. Mandibular division
D. None of the above

Trigeminal neuralgia is characterized by excruciating paroxysms of pain in lips, gums, cheek, or chin and, very rarely, in the distribution of the ophthalmic division of the fifth nerve.

2008. Which of the following is the largest of the cranial nerves?
Harrison's 20th Ed. Chapter 433, Page 3166

A. Optic nerve
B. Trigeminal nerve
C. Facial nerve
D. Vestibulocochlear nerve

Trigeminal nerve is the largest of the cranial nerves. Ophthalmic is the smallest of the three divisions while mandibular division is the largest.

2009. Which of the following division of the fifth cranial nerve exits through foramen ovale?
Harrison's 20th Ed. Chapter 433, Page 3166

A. Ophthalmic division
B. Maxillary division
C. Mandibular division
D. None of the above

V1 & V2 traverse the cavernous sinus to exit in the superior orbital fissure and foramen rotundum, located above and below the eye socket respectively. V3 exits through foramen ovale.

2010. Motor innervation of trigeminal nerve is exclusively carried in which division?
Harrison's 20th Ed. Chapter 433, Page 3166

A. Ophthalmic division
B. Maxillary division
C. Mandibular division
D. None of the above

The trigeminal nerve is predominantly sensory and motor innervation is exclusively carried in V3.

2011. Angle of the jaw is innervated by?
DeJong's The Neurologic Examination, 7th Ed. Page 232

A. Greater auricular nerve
B. Auriculotemporal nerve
C. Buccal nerve
D. Lingual nerve

Angle of the jaw is innervated by the greater auricular nerve (C2-3). The three divisions of trigeminal nerve arise from trigeminal ganglion. Each division has a meningeal branch. Terminal branches of V1 are frontal, lacrimal, and nasociliary nerves. Terminal branches of maxillary division are infraorbital, zygomatic, superior alveolar, and pterygopalatine. Terminal branches of mandibular division are buccal, lingual, inferior alveolar, and auriculotemporal.

2012. Trigeminal nerve supplies filaments to which of the ganglia in head?
DeJong's The Neurologic Examination, 7th Ed. Page 232

A. Ciliary
B. Otic
C. Submaxillary
D. All of the above

Trigeminal nerve supplies filaments to 4 ganglia in head—ciliary, sphenopalatine, otic & submaxillary.

2013. Trigeminal nerve is ensheathed by oligodendrocyte-derived myelin for how many millimeters after exit from brainstem?
Harrison's 20th Ed. Chapter 433, Page 3167

A. 2 mm
B. 5 mm
C. 7 mm
D. 11 mm

Trigeminal nerve is ensheathed by oligodendrocyte-derived, rather than Schwann cell-derived, myelin for up to 7 mm after it leaves the brainstem. This may explain high frequency of trigeminal neuralgia in multiple sclerosis which is a disorder of oligodendrocyte myelin.

2014. "Inverse masticatory muscle activity" has been reported in?
DeJong's The Neurologic Examination, 7th Ed. Page 227

A. Syringomyelia
B. Syringobulbia
C. Herpes zoster
D. Encephalitis

"Inverse masticatory muscle activity" has been reported in syringobulbia.

2015. Which cranial nerve carries the efferent limb of jaw jerk reflex?
DeJong's The Neurologic Examination, 7th Ed. Page 235

A. Oculomotor
B. Trigeminal
C. Trochlear
D. Facial

Efferent limb of the jaw jerk is also trigeminal.

2016. Which of the following is a test for trigeminal nerve?
DeJong's The Neurologic Examination, 7th Ed. Page 235, 238

A. Sternutatory reflex
B. Corneal reflex
C. Jaw reflex
D. All of the above

Sternutatory reflex refers to stimulation of nasal mucous membrane with cotton or similar objects. Normally, it causes wrinkling of nose, eye closure & often a forceful exhalation resembling a feeble sneeze, as the nose tries to rid itself of the foreign object. The afferent limb of reflex arc is carried through CN V1, the efferent limb over CNs V, VII, IX, X, and the motor nerves of the cervical and thoracic spinal cord.

2017. Which of the following is a cause of jaw drop?
DeJong's The Neurologic Examination, 7th Ed. Page 238

A. Myasthenia gravis
B. ALS
C. Kennedy's disease
D. All of the above

2018. Which of the following is a cause of trismus?
DeJong's The Neurologic Examination, 7th Ed. Page 239

A. Tetanus
B. Foix-Chavany-Marie syndrome
C. Tetany
D. All of the above

Trismus is marked spasm of the muscles of mastication. It is a classical manifestation of tetanus. It can also occur in encephalitis, rabies, acute dystonic reactions due to neuroleptic medications, tetany, Foix-Chavany-Marie syndrome, polymyositis. Trismus may be psychogenic.

2019. In trigeminal neuralgia, pain lasts for about?
Harrison's 20th Ed. Chapter 433, Page 3167

A. Few seconds to a minute or two
B. Five to ten minutes
C. Half an hour to six hours
D. Twenty four to forty eight hours

In trigeminal neuralgia, pain seldom lasts more than a few seconds or a minute or two. Onset is typically sudden, and bouts tend to persist for weeks or months before remitting spontaneously. Remissions may be long-lasting, but in most patients the disorder ultimately recurs.

2020. Which of the following is related to trigeminal nerve?
DeJong's The Neurologic Examination, 7th Ed. Page 230

A. Balaclava helmet distribution
B. "Onion skin" somatotopic organization
C. Numb chin syndrome
D. All of the above

"Onion skin" somatotopic organization refers to the face being represented as concentric rings from perioral region to preauricular region. Because of "onion skin" somatotopic organization, there is occasionally sparing, less frequently selective involvement of the perioral region compared to the posterior face (balaclava helmet distribution).

2021. In trigeminal neuralgia, trigger zones are least frequent in?
Harrison's 20th Ed. Chapter 433, Page 3167

A. Face
B. Forehead
C. Lips
D. Tongue

Characteristic feature of Trigeminal neuralgia is the presence of trigger zones, typically on the face, lips, or tongue.

2022. In trigeminal neuralgia, objective signs of sensory loss are found in?
Harrison's 20th Ed. Chapter 433, Page 3167

A. Ophthalmic division
B. Maxillary division
C. Mandibular division
D. None of the above

An essential feature of trigeminal neuralgia is that objective signs of sensory loss cannot be demonstrated on examination.

2023. Which of the following artery causes compression of the trigeminal nerve root to cause trigeminal neuralgia?
Harrison's 20th Ed. Chapter 433, Page 3167

A. Superior cerebellar artery
B. Middle cerebral artery
C. Anterior choroidal artery
D. Posterior cerebral artery

Compression of trigeminal nerve root by superior cerebellar artery, anterior inferior cerebellar artery or a tortuous vein causes trigeminal neuralgia in most patients.

2024. Reason of prevalence of trigeminal neuralgia in later life is?
Harrison's 20th Ed. Chapter 433, Page 3167

A. Age-related brain sagging
B. Increased vascular thickness
C. Increased vascular tortuosity
D. All of the above

Age-related brain sagging, increased vascular thickness and tortuosity lead to increased propensity of vascular compression, and this explains the prevalence of trigeminal neuralgia in later life.

2025. Mass lesion that can cause trigeminal neuralgia is?
Harrison's 20th Ed. Chapter 433, Page 3167

A. Aneurysms
B. Neurofibromas & meningiomas
C. Acoustic schwannomas
D. All of the above

2026. Which of the following is characteristic of pain of trigeminal neuralgia?
Harrison's 20th Ed. Chapter 433, Page 3167

A. Superficial stabbing quality
B. Paroxysmal & lancinating
C. Occurs both day and night
D. All of the above

2027. When cluster headache is associated with trigeminal neuralgia, the syndrome is known as?
Harrison's 20th Ed. Chapter 433, Page 3168

A. Glossopharyngeal neuralgia
B. Tic Douloureux
C. Cluster-tic
D. PH-tic syndrome

When cluster headache is associated with trigeminal neuralgia, syndrome is known as cluster-tic.

2028. Which of the following point towards trigeminal neuralgia being related to multiple sclerosis?
Harrison's 20th Ed. Chapter 433, Page 3168, 3189

A. Onset in a young adult
B. Bilateral symptoms
C. Objective sensory loss
D. All of the above

Most cases of trigeminal neuralgia are not MS-related. Atypical features such as onset in a young adult, bilateral symptoms, objective sensory loss, or nonparoxysmal pain should raise concerns that MS could be responsible.

2029. Which of the following about Acute herpes zoster of the trigeminal nerve is false?
DeJong's The Neurologic Examination, 7th Ed. Page 241

A. Affects ophthalmic division (V1) in 80% of cases
B. Cutaneous scarring is common
C. Pain without a cutaneous eruption is called zoster sine zoster
D. None of the above

Acute herpes zoster of trigeminal nerve is extremely painful. It is usually seen in elderly or immunocompromised patients, and affects ophthalmic division (V1) in 80% of cases, causing pain & vesicles over forehead, eyelid & cornea (herpes ophthalmicus). Cutaneous scarring is common. Ophthalmic involvement may lead to keratitis, corneal ulcerations, residual corneal scarring, and sometimes blindness. Zoster may affect any of the trigeminal divisions, and there may be motor involvement. Rarely, trigeminal HZ may be complicated by encephalitis or a syndrome of delayed contralateral hemiparesis due to arteritis. Pain without a cutaneous eruption is referred to as zoster sine zoster or zoster sine herpete.

2030. Pain persisting for how many months after acute HZ eruption is labeled as postherpetic neuralgia (PHN)?
DeJong's The Neurologic Examination, 7th Ed. Page 241

A. 1 month
B. 3 months
C. 6 months
D. 12 months

Pain persisting for more than 3 months after acute HZ eruption is labeled as postherpetic neuralgia (PHN). It is typically dysesthetic with a burning component, constant but with superimposed paroxysms of lacinating pain that may be provoked by touching certain spots within the affected area. It develops in only 10% of those <60, but in 40% of those >60 years.

2031. Roger's sign best relates to?
DeJong's The Neurologic Examination, 7th Ed. Page 241

A. Numb cheek syndrome
B. Numb chin syndrome
C. Trigeminal sensory neuropathy (TSN)
D. Trumpet player's neuropathy

The numb chin syndrome refers to hypesthesia/paresthesias involving lower lip & chin, in the distribution of mental nerve (chin neuropathy, Roger's sign). The numb chin or cheek syndrome can be the presenting manifestation of cancer.

2032. Which of the following drugs are used in cases of trigeminal neuralgia?
Harrison's 20th Ed. Chapter 433, Page 3168

A. Carbamazepine
B. Phenytoin
C. Baclofen
D. All of the above

Drug therapy for trigeminal neuralgia include carbamazepine, oxcarbazepine, lamotrigine, phenytoin and baclofen.

2033. Which of the following is the most important side effect of carbamazepine?
Harrison's 20th Ed. Chapter 433, Page 3168

A. Alopecia
B. Tremor
C. Agranulocytosis
D. Neutrophilia

Therapeutic blood level for carbamazepine is 4 - 12 µg/mL. Carbamazepine, but not oxcarbazepine, induces hepatic metabolism of other medications. Other rare side effects of Carbamazepine are hyponatremia, agranulocytosis, Stevens-Johnson syndrome.

2034. Which of the following is the most widely used procedure in treating trigeminal neuralgia?
Harrison's 20th Ed. Chapter 433, Page 3168

A. Radiofrequency thermal rhizotomy
B. Injection of glycerol in Meckel's cave
C. Microvascular decompression
D. Gamma knife radiosurgery

If drug treatment fails, in surgical therapy, the most widely used method is currently microvascular decompression to relieve pressure on the trigeminal nerve as it exits the pons. This procedure requires a suboccipital craniotomy.

2035. Gasserian ganglion lesions causing trigeminal nerve disorders include all except?
Harrison's 20th Ed. Chapter 433, Page 3168 Table 433-1

A. Trigeminal neuroma
B. Herpes zoster
C. Sarcoidosis
D. Infection

2036. Peripheral trigeminal nerve lesion can be due to?
Harrison's 20th Ed. Chapter 433, Page 3168 Table 433-1

A. Guillain-Barré syndrome
B. Sjögren's syndrome
C. Collagen-vascular diseases
D. All of the above

2037. Which of the following can cause trismus?
Harrison's 20th Ed. Chapter 433, Page 3169

A. Ludwig's angina
B. Phenothiazine
C. Tetanus
D. All of the above

2038. Mental neuropathy is best related to?
Harrison's 20th Ed. Chapter 433, Page 3169

A. Multiple sclerosis
B. Herpes zoster
C. Leprosy
D. Systemic malignancy

Mental neuropathy refers to an isolated sensory loss over chin. It can be the only manifestation of systemic malignancy.

2039. Which of the following about seventh cranial nerve is false?
Harrison's 20th Ed. Chapter 433, Page 3169

A. Supplies all the muscles concerned with facial expression
B. Sensory component is called nervus intermedius
C. Conveys taste sensation from posterior 1/3 of tongue
D. Conveys sensations from anterior wall of external auditory canal

2040. Who's name is best related to phenomenon of neurobiotaxis?
J Anat. 1929;63(Pt 3):396

A. Kappers
B. Marsot
C. Rorick
D. Sumner

CU Ariens Kappers name is closely associated with the phenomenon of neurobiotaxis.

2041. The facial nerve innervates which of the following muscles?
DeJong's The Neurologic Examination, 7th Ed. Page 247

A. Buccinator
B. Platysma
C. Posterior belly of the digastric
D. All of the above

Predominantly motor, the facial nerve innervates muscles of facial expression and muscles of scalp, ear, and buccinator, platysma, stapedius, stylohyoid, and posterior belly of the digastric.

2042. Which of the following is not a component of facial nerve?
DeJong's The Neurologic Examination, 7th Ed. Page 247

A. Motor
B. Sensory
C. Sympathetic
D. Parasympathetic

2043. Facial nerve carries parasympathetic secretory fibers to?
DeJong's The Neurologic Examination, 7th Ed. Page 247

A. Submandibular salivary glands
B. Sublingual salivary glands
C. Lacrimal gland
D. All of the above

Facial nerve carries parasympathetic secretory fibers to submandibular & sublingual salivary glands, lacrimal gland and to mucous membranes of oral & nasal cavities.

2044. Sensory functions of facial nerve include?
DeJong's The Neurologic Examination, 7th Ed. Page 247

A. Taste from anterior two-thirds of tongue
B. Exteroceptive sensation from eardrum
C. Exteroceptive sensation from external auditory canal
D. All of the above

Sensory functions of facial nerve include taste from anterior two-thirds of tongue, exteroceptive sensation from eardrum & external auditory canal.

2045. After its exit from pons, the first branch of facial nerve is?
DeJong's The Neurologic Examination, 7th Ed. Page 247

A. Greater (superficial) petrosal nerve
B. Nerve to the stapedius
C. Chorda tympani
D. Posterior auricular nerve

2046. After its exit from pons, the second branch of facial nerve is?
DeJong's The Neurologic Examination, 7th Ed. Page 256

A. Greater (superficial) petrosal nerve
B. Nerve to the stapedius
C. Chorda tympani
D. Posterior auricular nerve

Facial nerve, from its exit from pons gives branches in the following order : greater (superficial) petrosal nerve, nerve to the stapedius, & chorda tympani, after which facial nerve continues to facial muscles. The mnemonic tear-hear-taste-face helps to recall the sequence.

2047. Which of the following best relates to facial nerve?
DeJong's The Neurologic Examination, 7th Ed. Page 247

A. Pes equinus
B. Pes anserinus
C. Pes cavus
D. Pes planus

2048. Which of the following is related to peripheral facial paralysis?
Harrison's 20th Ed. Chapter 433, Page 3169, DeJong's The Neurologic Examination, 7th Ed. Page 261

A. Marin Amat sign
B. Jaw-winking
C. Facial spasms
D. All of the above

Aberrant regeneration is common after Bell's palsy and after traumatic nerve injury. Axons destined for one muscle regrow to innervate another, so that there is abnormal twitching of face outside the area of intended movement. On blinking or winking, corner of the mouth may twitch. Automatic closure of one eye on opening the mouth is termed as Marin Amat sign, or inverted or reversed Gunn phenomenon (inverse jaw winking). It is a trigeminofacial associated movement.

2049. Which of the following is related to the aberrant regeneration of injured facial nerve?
DeJong's The Neurologic Examination, 7th Ed. Page 261

A. Syndrome of crocodile tears
B. Frey auriculotemporal syndrome
C. Chorda tympani syndrome
D. All of the above

Aberrant regeneration may involve autonomic and taste fibers. Syndrome of crocodile tears is a gustatory-lacrimal reflex, characterized by tearing when eating due to misdirection of salivary axons to lacrimal gland. Frey auriculotemporal syndrome is similar, but with sweating & flushing over cheek rather than lacrimation. In chorda tympani syndrome, there is unilateral swelling & flushing of submental region after eating.

2050. Which of the following is a risk factor for Bell's palsy?
Harrison's 20th Ed. Chapter 433, Page 3169

A. Hypertension
B. Diabetes
C. Migraine
D. All of the above

Most common form of facial paralysis is Bell's palsy & its risk factors are pregnancy & diabetes mellitus.

2051. The annual incidence of Bell's palsy is?
Harrison's 20th Ed. Chapter 433, Page 3169

A. 1 in 60 persons in a lifetime
B. 1 in 600 persons in a lifetime
C. 1 in 6000 persons in a lifetime
D. 1 in 60000 persons in a lifetime

The annual incidence of Bell's palsy is ~25 per 100,000 annually, or about 1 in 60 persons in a lifetime.

2052. In Bell's palsy, maximal weakness is attained by?
Harrison's 20th Ed. Chapter 433, Page 3169

A. 6 hours
B. 12 hours
C. 24 hours
D. 48 hours

The onset of Bell's palsy is abrupt and maximal weakness occurs by 48 hours as a general rule.

2053. Which of the following may precede Bell's palsy for a day or two?
Harrison's 20th Ed. Chapter 433, Page 3169

A. Excessive lacrimations
B. Facial muscle twitching
C. Pain behind the ear
D. Transient blindness

Pain behind the ear may precede Bell's palsy for a day or two.

2054. Which of the following may be present in Bell's palsy?
Harrison's 20th Ed. Chapter 433, Page 3169

A. Loss of taste sensation unilaterally
B. Hyperacusis
C. Mild cerebrospinal fluid lymphocytosis
D. All of the above

2055. Tear production may be quantitated with?
DeJong's The Neurologic Examination, 7th Ed. Page 256, 656

A. Dix-Hallpike test
B. Unterberger-Fukuda stepping test
C. Schwabach test
D. Schirmer test

Tear production may be quantitated with the Schirmer test. Schirmer test, done by placing a strip of sterile filter paper in the lower conjunctival sac and measuring the degree of wetting over 5 minutes.

2056. Which of the following best relates to peripheral facial palsy?
DeJong's The Neurologic Examination, 7th Ed. Page 256

A. Misoplegia
B. Iridoplegia
C. Prosopoplegia
D. Diplegia

With peripheral facial palsy, there is flaccid weakness of all the muscles of facial expression on the involved side, both upper & lower face. This is called prosopoplegia.

2057. Which of the following best relates to peripheral facial palsy?
DeJong's The Neurologic Examination, 7th Ed. Page 257

A. Levator sign of Dutemps and Céstan
B. Bell's phenomenon
C. Negro's sign
D. All of the above

To elicit the levator sign of Dutemps and Céstan, patient is asked to look down, then close the eyes slowly. Because the function of levator palpebrae superioris is no longer counteracted by orbicularis oculi, the upper lid on paralyzed side moves upward slightly. Negro's sign refers to the eyeball on the paralyzed side that deviates outward & elevates more than the normal one when the patient raises the eyes.

2058. Which of the following best relates to peripheral facial palsy?
DeJong's The Neurologic Examination, 7th Ed. Page 257

A. Battle's sign
B. Bergara-Wartenberg sign
C. Marin Amat sign
D. Bon-bon sign

Bergara-Wartenberg sign is a sensitive sign of upper facial weakness. It is loss of the fine vibrations palpable with thumbs or fingertips resting lightly on eyelids as the patient tries to close the eyes as tightly as possible.

2059. Which of the following best relates to peripheral facial palsy?
DeJong's The Neurologic Examination, 7th Ed. Page 260

A. Mona Lisa syndrome
B. Pierre Robin syndrome
C. Löfgren syndrome
D. Wildervanck syndrome

Mona Lisa was pregnant shortly before the famous painting of Leonardo da Vinci was created (1503-1506). It is speculated that Mona Lisa's famous smile is caused by facial muscle contracture and/or synkinesis after Bell's palsy with incomplete nerve regeneration. The risk of facial palsy is three times greater during pregnancy, especially in the third trimester or in the first postpartum week.

2060. Which of the following symptom accompanies Bell's palsy commonly?
DeJong's The Neurologic Examination, 7th Ed. Page 260

A. Increased tearing
B. Pain in or around the ear
C. Taste abnormalities
D. All of the above

The most common symptoms accompanying Bell's palsy are increased tearing, pain in or around the ear, and taste abnormalities.

2061. What percentage of patients of Bell's palsy recover within a few weeks or months?
Harrison's 20th Ed. Chapter 433, Page 3169

A. ~40%
B. ~60%
C. ~80%
D. ~100%

~80% of patients of Bell's palsy recover within a few weeks or months.

2062. Electromyography (EMG) evidence of denervation after how many days indicates axonal degeneration in Bell's palsy?
Harrison's 20th Ed. Chapter 433, Page 3169

A. 7 days
B. 10 days
C. 14 days
D. 21 days

In Bell's palsy, EMG evidence of denervation after 10 days indicates that axonal degeneration has taken place and there will be a long delay (3 months) before regeneration occurs, and that it may be incomplete.

2063. In Bell's palsy, recurrences are reported in what percentage of cases?
Harrison's 20th Ed. Chapter 433, Page 3169

A. ~2%
B. ~5%
C. ~7%
D. ~9%

In Bell's palsy, recurrences are reported in ~7% of cases.

2064. Which of the following statements about causation of Bell's palsy is false?
Harrison's 20th Ed. Chapter 433, Page 3169, N Engl J Med. 2004;351:1323-31

A. HSV-1 is the cause of most cases of Bell's palsy
B. HSV-1 DNA appear to be specific to Bell's palsy
C. Disease probably reflects virus reactivation from latency in geniculate ganglion, rather than primary infection
D. None of the above

2065. Which of the following is implicated in the causation of Bell's palsy?
Harrison's 20th Ed. Chapter 433, Page 3169

A. Herpes simplex virus type 1
B. Varicella-zoster virus
C. Borrelia burgdorferi
D. All of the above

2066. Which of the following is implicated in Bell's palsy among recipients of inactivated intranasal influenza vaccine?
Harrison's 20th Ed. Chapter 433, Page 3169

A. Reactivation of HSV-1
B. Trauma
C. Escherichia coli enterotoxin
D. All of the above

An increased incidence of Bell's palsy among recipients of inactivated intranasal influenza vaccine resulted from the Escherichia coli enterotoxin used as adjuvant or reactivation of latent virus.

2067. Poor prognostic factors in a case of Bell's palsy are all except?
N Engl J Med. 2004;351:1323-31

A. Older age
B. Hypertension
C. Diabetes mellitus
D. Impairment of taste

2068. Poor prognostic factors in a case of Bell's palsy are all except?
N Engl J Med. 2004;351:1323-31

A. Hypertension
B. Pain other than in the ear
C. Anemia
D. Complete facial weakness

2069. For how many days, electrical studies reveal no changes in involved facial muscles in Bell's palsy?
N Engl J Med. 2004;351:1323-31

A. 1 day
B. 2 days
C. 3 days
D. 4 days

2070. Which of the following is a cause of peripheral facial palsy?
DeJong's The Neurologic Examination, 7th Ed. Page 262

A. Möbius' syndrome
B. Kennedy's syndrome
C. Acute attack of paralytic poliomyelitis
D. All of the above

2071. Causes of acquired peripheral facial weakness include all except?
N Engl J Med. 2004;351:1323-31

A. Diabetes mellitus
B. Hypothyroidism
C. Hypertension
D. HIV infection

2072. Causes of acquired peripheral facial weakness include all except?
N Engl J Med. 2004;351:1323-31

A. Lyme disease
B. Ramsay Hunt syndrome
C. Sarcoidosis
D. Rheumatoid arthritis

2073. Causes of acquired peripheral facial weakness include all except?
N Engl J Med. 2004;351:1323-31

A. Sjögren's syndrome
B. Parotid-nerve tumors
C. Eclampsia
D. Dental trauma

2074. Causes of acquired peripheral facial weakness include?
N Engl J Med. 2004;351:1323-31

A. Amyloidosis
B. Recipients of inactivated intranasal influenza vaccine
C. Eclampsia
D. All of the above

2075. Recurrent or bilateral facial palsy is found in?
N Engl J Med. 2004;351:1323-31

A. Lymphoma
B. Sarcoidosis
C. Lyme disease
D. All of the above

2076. Recurrent or bilateral facial palsy is found in all except?
N Engl J Med. 2004;351:1323-31

A. Myasthenia gravis
B. Lesions at base of brain
C. Guillain-Barré syndrome
D. Ramsay Hunt syndrome in immunocompetent people

Facial palsy is often bilateral in sarcoidosis and in Guillain-Barre syndrome.

2077. Ramsay Hunt syndrome best relates to?
Harrison's 20th Ed. Chapter 433, Page 3169

A. Escherichia coli enterotoxin
B. Herpes zoster
C. Borrelia burgdorferi
D. Leprosy

Ramsay Hunt syndrome is caused by reactivation of herpes zoster in the geniculate ganglion, consists of a severe facial palsy associated with a vesicular eruption in the external auditory canal and sometimes in pharynx and other parts of the cranial integument. Often eighth cranial nerve is affected as well.

2078. The Melkersson-Rosenthal syndrome consists of?
Harrison's 20th Ed. Chapter 433, Page 3170

A. Recurrent facial paralysis
B. Facial (labial) edema
C. Plication of tongue
D. All of the above

Melkersson-Rosenthal syndrome is characterized by recurrent attacks of facial palsy, nonpitting facial and lip edema, and a congenitally furrowed and fissured tongue (lingua plicata, scrotal tongue).

2079. Which of the following is the cause of Melkersson-Rosenthal syndrome?
Harrison's 20th Ed. Chapter 433, Page 3170

A. Leprosy
B. Herpes zoster
C. Borrelia burgdorferi
D. None of the above

Melkersson-Rosenthal syndrome consists of recurrent facial paralysis. Recurrent and eventually permanent facial (labial) edema and plication of the tongue. Its cause is unknown.

2080. Parry-Romberg syndrome best relates to?
DeJong's The Neurologic Examination, 7th Ed. Page 265

A. Facial myokymia
B. Blepharospasm
C. Facial hemiatrophy
D. Bilateral facial weakness

In facial hemiatrophy (progressive facial hemiatrophy, Parry-Romberg syndrome, Wartenberg syndrome), there is either congenital failure of development or a progressive atrophy of skin, subcutaneous fat & musculature of one half of face. It may be a form of localized scleroderma.

2081. Which of the following is false about supranuclear facial palsy?
Harrison's 20th Ed. Chapter 433, Page 3170

A. Lower facial muscles involved more than upper facial muscles
B. Dissociation of emotional & voluntary facial movements
C. Paralysis of arm & leg or aphasia may be present
D. None of the above

In supranuclear facial palsy, frontalis & orbicularis oculi muscles of forehead are involved less than those of the lower part of face, because upper facial muscles are innervated by corticobulbar pathways from both motor cortices, whereas the lower facial muscles are innervated only by the opposite hemisphere.

2082. Which of the following is false about Millard-Gubler syndrome?
DeJong's The Neurologic Examination, 7th Ed. Page 262

A. Ipsilateral peripheral facial palsy (PFP)
B. Contralateral hemiparesis
C. Lesion is in pons
D. None of the above

Millard-Gubler syndrome is ipsilateral PFP and contralateral hemiparesis, which may be due to pontine stroke, hemorrhage, or tumor.

2083. Foville syndrome consists of?
DeJong's The Neurologic Examination, 7th Ed. Page 262

A. Ipsilateral peripheral facial palsy (PFP)
B. Horizontal gaze palsy
C. Contralateral hemiparesis
D. All of the above

Foville syndrome is ipsilateral PFP and horizontal gaze palsy with contralateral hemiparesis.

2084. Eight-and-a-Half syndrome is the combination of?
DeJong's The Neurologic Examination, 7th Ed. Page 262

A. Ipsilateral lower motor neuron VIth and VIIth nerve palsy
B. Inter-nuclear ophthalmoplegia
C. Ipsilateral gaze paralysis
D. All of the above

Eight-and-a-half syndrome is characterized by internuclear ophthalmoplegia, horizontal gaze paresis and ipsilateral lower motor neuron seventh cranial nerve palsy, a combination of one-and-a-half syndrome with lower motor neuron seventh cranial nerve palsy. Eight-and-a-Half syndrome is caused by a lesion (vascular or demyelinating) in the dorsal tegmentum of the caudal pons involving ipsilateral paramedian pontine reticular formation (PPRF) or abducens nucleus and medial longitudinal fasciculus (MLF), as well as the nucleus and fasciculus of the facial nerve.

2085. Which of the following is a common site for hemorrhagic stroke?
DeJong's The Neurologic Examination, 7th Ed. Page 262

A. Pons
B. Putamen & thalamus
C. Cerebellum
D. All of the above

Pons is one of the most common sites for hemorrhagic stroke apart from putamen, thalamus and cerebellum.

2086. In MRI, diffuse smooth linear enhancement of facial nerve can be seen in?
Harrison's 20th Ed. Chapter 433, Page 3170 Figure 433-3

A. Lyme disease
B. Sarcoidosis
C. Perineural malignant spread
D. All of the above

2087. Which of the following statements about central weakness of the unilateral lower facial area is false?
N Engl J Med. 2004;351:1323-31

A. Lesion above level of contralateral facial nucleus
B. Facial nucleus innervating lower face receives fibers from ipsilateral cerebral hemisphere
C. Facial nucleus innervating upper face receives fibers from both cerebral hemispheres
D. Unilateral lesion in cortex produces contralateral voluntary central-type facial paralysis and contralateral hemiplegia

2088. Which of the following about facial palsy is false?
N Engl J Med. 2004;351:1323-31

A. Hyperacusis results from paralysis of stapedius muscle
B. Lesions proximal to geniculate ganglion have permanent loss of taste and are unable to produce tears
C. Aberrant regeneration of nerve fibres is the cause of syndrome of crocodile tears
D. None of the above

2089. Which of the following about facial nerve is false?
N Engl J Med. 2004;351:1323-31

A. Facial nerve is predominantly motor
B. Facial nucleus is located in caudal pons
C. Facial nerve encircles nucleus of sixth cranial nerve
D. Facial nerve exits in midpons

2090. Which of the following about facial nerve is false?
N Engl J Med. 2004;351:1323-31

A. 8th nerve, motor root of 7th nerve, and nervus intermedius enter internal auditory meatus
B. Sensory cells located in geniculate ganglion continue distally as chorda tympani nerve
C. Peripheral fibers of nervus intermedius portion of facial nerve initiate salivary, lacrimal, and mucous secretion
D. None of the above

2091. Locate the lesion if there is contralateral central facial weakness, lacrimation, salivation, and taste are intact, contralateral hemiparesis and spasticity?
N Engl J Med. 2004;351:1323-31

A. Cortex, subcortical region
B. Pons
C. Cerebellopontine angle
D. All of the above

2092. Locate the lesion if there is ipsilateral peripheral facial weakness; lacrimation, salivation, and taste intact; contralateral hemiparesis, sensory loss, ataxia, nystagmus, ipsilateral abducens palsy, ophthalmoparesis?
N Engl J Med. 2004;351:1323-31

A. Cortex, subcortical region
B. Pons
C. Cerebellopontine angle
D. All of the above

2093. Locate the lesion if there is ipsilateral peripheral facial weakness; lacrimation, salivation, and taste intact; tinnitus, facial numbness, ataxia, nystagmus?
N Engl J Med. 2004;351:1323-31

A. Cortex, subcortical region
B. Pons
C. Cerebellopontine angle
D. All of the above

2094. Locate the lesion if there is ipsilateral peripheral facial weakness; lacrimation, salivation, and taste likely to be involved; tinnitus, nystagmus, hearing loss?
N Engl J Med. 2004;351:1323-31

A. Cortex, subcortical region
B. Pons
C. Cerebellopontine angle
D. Facial nerve in internal auditory canal proximal to or involving geniculate ganglion

2095. Locate the lesion if there is ipsilateral peripheral facial weakness; lacrimation intact but salivation and taste impaired; tinnitus, nystagmus, hearing loss?
N Engl J Med. 2004;351:1323-31

A. Pons
B. Facial nerve in stylomastoid foramen
C. Facial nerve in internal auditory canal proximal to or involving geniculate ganglion
D. Facial nerve distal to internal auditory canal and geniculate ganglion

2096. Locate the lesion if there is ipsilateral peripheral facial weakness; lacrimation, salivation, and taste intact?
N Engl J Med. 2004;351:1323-31

A. Cerebellopontine angle
B. Facial nerve in internal auditory canal proximal to or involving geniculate ganglion
C. Facial nerve distal to internal auditory canal & geniculate ganglion
D. Facial nerve in stylomastoid foramen

2097. House Brackmann grading system is used for assessing?
N Engl J Med. 2004;351:1323-31

A. Facial muscle function
B. Parotid function
C. Hearing function
D. Salivary function

The House-Brackmann scale, Burres-Fisch index and facial nerve function index may be useful to try to quantitate the degree of weakness.

2098. Facial nerve is compressed at its narrowest point, which is?
N Engl J Med. 2004;351:1323-31

A. Entrance to meatal foramen
B. Middle of internal auditory canal
C. Exit point of internal auditory canal
D. Exit point of facial nerve from pons

2099. Which of the following is useful in treatment of Bell's palsy?
Harrison's 20th Ed. Chapter 433, Page 3170

A. Glucocorticoids
B. IV Ig
C. Plasmapharesis
D. All of the above

Antiviral agents valacyclovir (1000 mg daily for 5-7 days) or acyclovir (400 mg five times daily for 10 days) with glucocorticoids (prednisone 60-80 mg daily for first 5 days, then tapered over next 5 days) might be marginally better than prednisolone alone especially in patients with severe clinical presentations.

2100. Decompression surgery should not be performed?
N Engl J Med. 2004;351:1323-31

A. 7 days after the onset of paralysis
B. 14 days after the onset of paralysis
C. 21 days after the onset of paralysis
D. 28 days after the onset of paralysis

2101. Which of the following may be caused by multiple sclerosis or follow Guillain-Barré syndrome?
Harrison's 20th Ed. Chapter 433, Page 3170

A. Blepharospasm
B. Facial myokymia
C. Hemifacial spasm
D. Facial hemiatrophy

Facial myokymia may be caused by MS, MJD, EA1, neuromyotonia (Isaacs' syndrome) or follow GBS. Facial myokymia consists of either persistent rapid flickering contractions of the facial musculature (especially the lower portion of the orbicularis oculus) or a contraction that slowly spreads across the face. It results from lesions of the corticobulbar tracts or brainstem course of the facial nerve.

2102. Which of the following disorders is associated with pregnancy?
Harrison's 20th Ed. Chapter 433, Page 3444

A. Bell's palsy
B. Carpal tunnel syndrome
C. Meralgia paresthetica
D. All of the above

Bell's palsy (idiopathic facial paralysis) is about three fold more likely to occur during the third trimester and immediate postpartum period than in the general population.

2103. Glossopharyngeal Neuralgia may be due to involvement of which of the following cranial nerves?
Harrison's 20th Ed. Chapter 433, Page 3170

A. X
B. XI
C. XII
D. All of the above

2104. Which of the following is false about Glossopharyngeal Neuralgia?
Harrison's 20th Ed. Chapter 433, Page 3170

A. Involves IX & portions of X cranial nerves
B. Pain may radiate from throat to ear
C. Spasms of pain may be initiated by swallowing or coughing
D. None of the above

Glossopharyngeal neuralgia though uncommon resembles trigeminal neuralgia & involves IX & sometimes portions of vagus cranial nerves. Pain is intense & paroxysmal, originates on one side of throat (tonsillar fossa) and may radiate to the ear (tympanic branch of IX). Spasms of pain may be initiated by swallowing or coughing. There is no motor or sensory deficit.

2105. Which of the following cranial nerves is not involved in pontocerebellar angle syndrome?
Harrison's 20th Ed. Chapter 433, Page 3171 Table 433-2

A. V
B. VII
C. VIII
D. XII

V, VII, VIII and sometimes IX are involved in pontocerebellar angle syndrome.

2106. Which of the following cranial nerves is not involved in jugular foramen syndrome?
Harrison's 20th Ed. Chapter 433, Page 3171 Table 433-2

A. IX
B. X
C. XI
D. XII

IX, X XI cranial nerves are involved in jugular foramen syndrome. Hoarseness due to vocal cord paralysis, difficulty in swallowing, deviation of the soft palate to the intact side, anesthesia of posterior wall of pharynx, and weakness of upper part of trapezius & sternocleidomastoid muscles make up jugular foramen syndrome.

2107. Multiple cranial neuropathy can be caused by?
Harrison's 20th Ed. Chapter 433, Page 3171

A. Wegener's granulomatosis
B. Behcet's disease
C. Sarcoidosis
D. All of the above

2108. Multiple cranial neuropathy can be caused by?
Harrison's 20th Ed. Chapter 433, Page 3171

A. Diabetes mellitus
B. Meningitis
C. Enlarging saccular aneurysms
D. All of the above

2109. Which of the following is true for Tolosa-Hunt syndrome?
Harrison's 20th Ed. Chapter 433, Page 3172

A. Aneurysm of carotid artery
B. Carotid-cavernous fistula
C. Idiopathic granulomatous disorder
D. Meningioma

Tolosa-Hunt syndrome is an idiopathic granulomatous disorder that responds to glucocorticoids.

Diseases of the Spinal Cord

2110. What is the length of adult spinal cord?
Harrison's 20th Ed. Chapter 434, Page 3173
A. ~ 34 cm
B. ~ 40 cm
C. ~ 46 cm
D. ~ 52 cm

Adult spinal cord is ~46 cm (18 inches) long, oval in shape and enlarged in cervical & lumbar regions, where neurons that innervate upper & lower extremities, respectively, are located.

2111. The spinal cord has how many segments?
Harrison's 20th Ed. Chapter 434, Page 3173
A. 30
B. 31
C. 32
D. 33

Spinal cord has 31 segments, each defined by exiting ventral motor root & entering dorsal sensory root.

2112. Lumbar spinal cord segments correspond to which vertebral body?
Harrison's 20th Ed. Chapter 434, Page 3173 Table 434-2
A. T8-T10
B. T10 - T12
C. T12 - L1
D. L1

2113. Sacral spinal cord segments correspond to which vertebral body?
Harrison's 20th Ed. Chapter 434, Page 3173 Table 434-2
A. T11
B. T12
C. T12 - L1
D. L1

Upper cervical - same as cord level, lower cervical - 1 level higher, upper thoracic - 2 levels higher, lower thoracic - 2 to 3 levels higher, lumbar - T10 to T12 and sacral - T12 to L1.

2114. Uppermost level of a spinal cord lesion can be localized by?
Harrison's 20th Ed. Chapter 434, Page 3173
A. Sensory level
B. Segmental signs
C. Band of altered sensation
D. All of the above

2115. Intervertebral disks are responsible for what percentage of spinal column length?
Harrison's 20th Ed. Chapter 14, Page 89
A. 10%
B. 15%
C. 20%
D. 25%

Intervertebral disks are composed of a central gelatinous nucleus pulposus surrounded by a tough cartilaginous ring, the annulus fibrosis. Disks are responsible for 25% of spinal column length.

2116. Intervertebral disks are largest in?
Harrison's 20th Ed. Chapter 14, Page 89
A. Cervical region
B. Thoracic region
C. Sacral region
D. None of the above

Intervertebral disks are largest in cervical & lumbar regions where movements of spine are greatest.

2117. Each vertebral arch gives rise to how many processes?
Harrison's 20th Ed. Chapter 14, Page 89
A. 3
B. 5
C. 7
D. 9

Seven processes arise from each vertebral arch—paired pedicles, paired laminae, paired transverse processes and one spinous process.

2118. Uncinate process is best related to?
Harrison's 20th Ed. Chapter 14, Page 89
A. Cervical vertebral body
B. Thoracic vertebral body
C. Lumbar vertebral body
D. Sacral vertebral body

Beginning at C3 level, each cervical (and first thoracic) vertebral body projects a lateral bony process upward called the uncinate process which articulates with the cervical vertebral body above via uncovertebral joint.

2119. Pain-sensitive structures in spine include all except?
Harrison's 20th Ed. Chapter 14, Page 89
A. Periosteum of vertebrae
B. Nucleus pulposus of intervertebral disk
C. Annulus fibrosus of intervertebral disk
D. Dura

Pain-sensitive structures in the spine include the periosteum of the vertebrae, dura, facet joints, annulus fibrosus of the intervertebral disk, epidural veins, and longitudinal ligaments. The nucleus pulposus of the intervertebral disk is not pain-sensitive.

2120. Activation of agonist muscle is accompanied by inhibition of antagonist muscle refers to?
DeJong's The Neurologic Examination, 7th Ed. Page 559
A. Sherrington's law
B. Pitres' law
C. Alexander's law
D. Hering's law

Sherrington's law of reciprocal innervation describes the balance between the contraction of the agonist and the inhibition of the antagonist. When extensors of a limb are contracted, the flexors are relaxed.

2121. Patrick's test is used to demonstrate pain due to?
Anesth Analg 2005;101:1440-53
A. Lumbar spine disease
B. Hip disease
C. Knee disease
D. Ankle disease

Patrick's test or FABER test (Flexion, ABduction and External Rotation) refers to elicitation of hip pain by internal and external rotation at the hip with the knee and hip in flexion.

2122. Gaenslen's test is used to demonstrate pain due to?
Anesth Analg 2005;101:1440-53

   A. Lumbar spine disease
   B. Hip disease
   C. Knee disease
   D. Ankle disease

2123. Yeoman's test is used to demonstrate pain due to?
Anesth Analg 2005;101:1440-53

   A. Lumbar spine disease
   B. Hip disease
   C. Knee disease
   D. Sacroiliitis

2124. Gillett test is used to demonstrate pain due to?
Anesth Analg 2005;101:1440-53

   A. Lumbar spine disease
   B. Hip disease
   C. Knee disease
   D. Sacroiliitis

2125. Pain is referred to which of the following in diseases affecting upper lumbar spine?
Harrison's 20th Ed. Chapter 14, Page 90

   A. Lumbar region
   B. Groin
   C. Anterior thighs
   D. All of the above

2126. Pain is referred to which of the following in diseases affecting lower lumbar spine?
Harrison's 20th Ed. Chapter 14, Page 90

   A. Buttocks
   B. Posterior thighs
   C. Calves
   D. All of the above

Diseases affecting upper lumbar spine refer pain to lumbar region, groin, or anterior thighs. Diseases affecting lower lumbar spine produce pain referred to buttocks, posterior thighs, calves, or feet.

2127. Which of the following may elicit or worsen radiating pain?
Harrison's 20th Ed. Chapter 14, Page 90

   A. Coughing
   B. Sneezing
   C. Voluntary contraction of abdominal muscles
   D. All of the above

Coughing, sneezing or voluntary contraction of abdominal muscles like lifting heavy objects or straining at stool may elicit or worsen the radiating pain.

2128. Characteristic of pain that favors the diagnosis of radiculopathy is?
Harrison's 20th Ed. Chapter 14, Page 90

   A. Gnawing
   B. Burning
   C. Compressing
   D. Tearing

Burning or electric quality of pain favors radiculopathy rather than referred pain.

2129. In supine position, passive flexion of extended leg at the hip stretches which of the following?
Harrison's 20th Ed. Chapter 14, Page 90

   A. L5 nerve root
   B. S1 nerve root
   C. Sciatic nerve
   D. All of the above

With the patient lying flat, passive flexion of the extended leg at the hip stretches the L5 and S1 nerve roots and the sciatic nerve.

2130. Reverse SLR sign stretches which of the following?
Harrison's 20th Ed. Chapter 14, Page 90

   A. L2-L4 nerve roots
   B. Lumbosacral plexus
   C. Femoral nerve
   D. All of the above

Reverse SLR stretches L2-L4 nerve roots, lumbosacral plexus and femoral nerve.

2131. Ely test refers to?
DeJong's The Neurologic Examination, 7th Ed. Page 698

   A. SLR
   B. Reverse SLR
   C. Crossed SLR
   D. All of the above

Femoral stretch or Ely test refers to reverse SLR. It is a root stretch test and is useful in evaluation of high lumbar radiculopathy.

2132. Ely test is performed with patient in which position?
DeJong's The Neurologic Examination, 7th Ed. Page 698

   A. Supine
   B. Prone
   C. Sitting
   D. Standing

2133. Lasègue test refers to?
DeJong's The Neurologic Examination, 7th Ed. Page 697

   A. SLR
   B. Reverse SLR
   C. Crossed SLR
   D. All of the above

SLR or Lasègue test is performed by slowly raising the symptomatic leg with the knee extended. Nerve roots get tense between ~30° and 70°, and pain increases. Pain at <30° raises the question of nonorganicity, and some discomfort & tightness beyond 70° is routine and insignificant.

2134. Fajersztajn's sign refers to?
DeJong's The Neurologic Examination, 7th Ed. Page 697

   A. SLR
   B. Reverse SLR
   C. Crossed SLR
   D. All of the above

In crossed SLR, raising the good leg produces pain in the symptomatic leg (Fajersztajn's sign). If positive, the likelihood of a root lesion is very high.

2135. Which of the following is related to accentuation of Lasègue's sign (SLR)?
DeJong's The Neurologic Examination, 7th Ed. Page 697

A. Bonnet phenomenon
B. Bragard's sign
C. Sicard's sign
D. All of the above

In SLR, pain may be more severe, or elicited sooner, if test is carried out with thigh & leg in a position of adduction & internal rotation (Bonnet phenomenon). SLR can be enhanced by passively dorsiflexing the patient's foot (Bragard's sign) or great toe (Sicard's sign) at the elevation angle at which the increased root tension begins to produce pain.

2136. O'Connell's test is performed with patient in which position?
DeJong's The Neurologic Examination, 7th Ed. Page 698

A. Supine
B. Prone
C. Sitting
D. Standing

In O'Connell's test, SLR is first done on the sound limb, and angle of flexion & site of pain are recorded. Then, SLR is done on affected limb, and angle & site of pain again noted. Then, both thighs are flexed simultaneously, with knees extended. Angle of flexion permitted may be greater than that allowed when either the affected limb or the sound limb is flexed alone. If at this point, lowering of the sound limb may result in a marked exacerbation of pain in the affected limb.

2137. Bechterew's test is performed with patient in which position?
DeJong's The Neurologic Examination, 7th Ed. Page 698

A. Supine
B. Prone
C. Sitting
D. Standing

Bechterew's test refers to the observation that in sitting position, patient may be able to extend leg alone without pain, but extending both together causes radicular pain.

2138. Which of the following is typical of herniation of the nucleus pulposus (HNP)?
DeJong's The Neurologic Examination, 7th Ed. Page 700

A. Pain worse on sitting
B. Pain lessened with standing
C. Positive SLR
D. All of the above

In HNP, pain may worsen with cough, sneeze, or Valsalva.

2139. Most common lumbosacral radiculopathy (LSR) involve?
DeJong's The Neurologic Examination, 7th Ed. Page 700

A. L2
B. L3
C. L4
D. L5

Most commonly, LSRs involve either L5 or S1. Upper lumbar radiculopathies are rare.

2140. Involvement of which of the following is critical in distinguishing between L5 radiculopathy & peroneal nerve palsy?
DeJong's The Neurologic Examination, 7th Ed. Page 700

A. Tibialis anterior
B. Tibialis posterior
C. Extensor hallucis longus
D. Extensor digitorum longus

Involvement of tibialis posterior is critical in distinguishing between L5 radiculopathy & peroneal nerve palsy.

2141. In S1 lesions, weakness manifests primarily in the?
DeJong's The Neurologic Examination, 7th Ed. Page 700

A. Gastrosoleus
B. Extensor hallucis longus
C. Extensor digitorum longus
D. Gluteus maximus

In S1 lesions, weakness manifests primarily in the gastrosoleus.

2142. Breakaway weakness refers to?
Harrison's 20th Ed. Chapter 14, Page 92

A. Inability to generate maximum power in other half of body
B. Inability to generate maximum power similar to examiner
C. Fluctuations in maximum power during muscle testing
D. None of the above

Breakaway weakness is defined as fluctuations in maximum power generated during muscle testing.

2143. Lumbar spinal stenosis can be caused by?
Harrison's 20th Ed. Chapter 14, Page 94

A. Acromegaly
B. Renal osteodystrophy
C. Hypoparathyroidism
D. All of the above

Lumbar spinal stenosis can be caused by epidural lipomatosis, osteoporosis, acromegaly, renal osteodystrophy, hypoparathyroidism, and Paget's disease.

2144. Which of the following is false about Tethered cord syndrome?
Harrison's 20th Ed. Chapter 14, Page 96

A. Presents as progressive cauda equina disorder
B. Perineal or perianal pain
C. Low-lying conus (below L1-L2)
D. Long and thickened filum terminale

Tethered cord syndrome presents as a progressive cauda equina disorder or myelopathy in a young adult who complains of perineal or perianal pain. Neuroimaging studies show a low-lying conus (below L1-L2) and a short & thickened filum terminale.

2145. Which of the following spinal root value innervates axilla?
Harrison's 20th Ed. Chapter 14, Page 100 Table 14-4

A. C8
B. T1
C. T2
D. T3

2146. Spurling's sign relates to?
Harrison's 20th Ed. Chapter 14, Page 100

A. Extension & lateral rotation of neck
B. Flexion & lateral rotation of neck
C. Extreme extension of neck
D. Extreme flexion of neck

Extension & lateral rotation of neck narrows ipsilateral intervertebral foramen resulting in radicular symptoms (Spurling's sign).

2147. Cervical angina syndrome relates best with?
Harrison's 20th Ed. Chapter 14, Page 100

A. Vertebrobasilar syndrome
B. Coronary artery ischemia
C. Subclavian steal syndrome
D. All of the above

Cervical angina syndrome refers to pain in neck that is due to coronary artery ischemia.

2148. Horner's syndrome accompanies cervical cord lesion at?
Harrison's 20th Ed. Chapter 434, Page 3173

A. C5
B. C6
C. C7
D. Any cervical level

Horner's syndrome (miosis, ptosis & facial hypohidrosis) may accompany cervical cord lesion at any level.

2149. Which cervical root lesion is most common?
DeJong's The Neurologic Examination, 7th Ed. Page 695

A. C5
B. C6
C. C7
D. C8

In the cervical spine, C7 root lesions are the most common, followed by C6, C5 and C8 lesions. Involvement of the upper cervical roots is rare.

2150. Weakness of triceps & pronator teres is pathognomonic of lesion at?
DeJong's The Neurologic Examination, 7th Ed. Page 696

A. C5
B. C6
C. C7
D. C8

Weakness of triceps & pronator teres is pathognomonic of C7 lesions, since C7 is their only common innervation.

2151. Lesions at C7 produce all except?
Harrison's 20th Ed. Chapter 434, Page 3173

A. Weakness in finger extensors
B. Weakness in wrist extensors
C. Weakness in brachioradialis
D. Weakness in triceps

At C7 lesion, weakness is found only in finger and wrist extensors and triceps.

2152. Lesions at C8 produces?
Harrison's 20th Ed. Chapter 434, Page 3173

A. Weakness in finger and wrist flexors
B. Weakness in finger extensors
C. Weakness in wrist extensors
D. Weakness in supination

At C8, finger and wrist flexion are impaired.

2153. Sensory dermatome at the level of nipples is?
Harrison's 20th Ed. Chapter 434, Page 3173

A. T2
B. T3
C. T4
D. T5

Dermatome at nipples is T4 and at umbilicus is T10.

2154. Beevor's sign is positive in spinal cord lesion at?
Harrison's 20th Ed. Chapter 434, Page 3173

A. T7 - T8
B. T8 - T9
C. T9 - T10
D. T11 - T12

Lesions at T9-T10 paralyze the lower, but not the upper abdominal muscles, resulting in upward movement of the umbilicus when the abdominal wall contracts (Beevor's sign).

2155. Lesions at L2 - L4 cause all except?
Harrison's 20th Ed. Chapter 434, Page 3173

A. Weakness of flexion of thigh
B. Weakness of abduction of thigh
C. Weakness of leg extension at knee
D. Absent patellar reflex

Lesions at L2 - L4 spinal cord levels paralyze flexion & adduction of thigh, weaken leg extension at knee and abolish the patellar reflex.

2156. Lesions at L5-S1 cause all except?
Harrison's 20th Ed. Chapter 434, Page 3173

A. Paralyze movements of foot and ankle
B. Weakness of flexion at knee
C. Weakness of flexion of thigh
D. Absent ankle jerk

Lesions at L5 - S1 paralyse movements of the foot & ankle, flexion at knee, and extension of thigh and abolish the ankle jerks (S1).

2157. Conus medullaris comprises of?
Harrison's 20th Ed. Chapter 434, Page 3173

A. Lower lumbar + sacral + coccygeal segments
B. Sacral + coccygeal segments
C. Lower sacral + coccygeal segments
D. None of the above

Conus medullaris is the tapered caudal termination of the spinal cord, comprising of the lower sacral and single coccygeal segments.

2158. The conus syndrome is characterized by all except?
Harrison's 20th Ed. Chapter 434, Page 3173

A. Bilateral saddle anesthesia
B. Asymmetric leg weakness
C. Bladder and bowel dysfunction
D. Impotence

2159. The conus syndrome is characterized by all except?
Harrison's 20th Ed. Chapter 434, Page 3173

A. Absent bulbocavernosus reflex
B. Absent anal reflex
C. Asymmetric sensory loss in leg
D. Bilateral saddle anesthesia

2160. The root value of bulbocavernosus reflex is?
Harrison's 20th Ed. Chapter 434, Page 3173

A. S1 - S2
B. S2 - S4
C. S3 - S5
D. S4 - S5

2161. The root value of anal reflex is?
Harrison's 20th Ed. Chapter 434, Page 3173

A. S1 - S2
B. S2 - S4
C. S3 - S5
D. S4 - S5

Conus syndrome consists of bilateral saddle anesthesia (S3-S5), prominent bladder & bowel dysfunction (urinary retention & incontinence with lax anal tone), and impotence. Bulbocavernosus (S2-S4) & anal (S4-S5) reflexes are absent. Muscle strength is largely preserved.

2162. Cauda equina lesion is characterized by all except?
Harrison's 20th Ed. Chapter 434, Page 3173

A. Radicular pain
B. Asymmetric leg weakness
C. Variable areflexia in lower extremities
D. Bladder and bowel dysfunction

Lesions of cauda equina are characterized by low back & radicular pain, asymmetric leg weakness & sensory loss, variable areflexia in the lower extremities & relative sparing of bowel & bladder function.

2163. Which of the following is false about cauda equina syndrome?
Harrison's 20th Ed. Chapter 434, Page 3173

A. Sphincters are affected
B. Hip flexion is spared
C. Sensation over anterolateral thighs is spared
D. None of the above

2164. In spinal cord, sacral fibres are placed laterally in all except?
Harrison's 20th Ed. Chapter 434, Page 3174 Figure 434-1

A. Ventral spinothalamic tract
B. Lateral spinothalamic tract
C. Lateral corticospinal tract
D. Posterior column

2165. In spinal posterior columns, fibres from which part of the body are nearest midline?
Harrison's 20th Ed. Chapter 434, Page 3174 Figure 434-1

A. Cervical
B. Thoracic
C. Lumbar
D. Sacral

2166. In lateral spinothalamic tracts, fibres from which part of the body are nearest midline?
Harrison's 20th Ed. Chapter 434, Page 3174 Figure 434-1

A. Cervical
B. Thoracic
C. Lumbar
D. Sacral

2167. In lateral corticospinal tracts, fibres from which part of the body are nearest midline?
Harrison's 20th Ed. Chapter 434, Page 3174 Figure 434-1

A. Cervical
B. Thoracic
C. Lumbar
D. Sacral

2168. Which of the following motor neurons in anterior horn of spinal cord are placed anteriorly?
Harrison's 20th Ed. Chapter 434, Page 3174 Figure 434-1

A. Proximal
B. Distal
C. Flexors
D. Extensors

2169. Brown-Sequard hemicord syndrome features all except?
Harrison's 20th Ed. Chapter 434, Page 3173

A. Ipsilateral weakness
B. Ipsilateral loss of joint position & vibratory sensation
C. Contralateral loss of pain & temperature sensation
D. Bilateral segmental signs

2170. Brown-Sequard syndrome is characterized by?
Harrison's 20th Ed. Chapter 434, Page 3174

A. Absence of cranial nerve signs
B. Ipsilateral loss of propioception
C. Contralateral loss pain & temperature
D. All of the above

Brown-Sequard hemicord syndrome consists of ipsilateral weakness (corticospinal tract) and loss of joint position and vibratory sense (posterior column), with contralateral loss of pain and temperature sense (spinothalamic tract) one or two levels below the lesion. Segmental signs, such as radicular pain, muscle atrophy, or loss of a deep tendon reflex, are unilateral.

2171. Central cord syndrome results from all except?
Harrison's 20th Ed. Chapter 434, Page 3174

A. Spinal trauma
B. Infection
C. Syringomyelia
D. Intrinsic cord tumors

Central cord syndrome is due to damage to gray matter nerve cells & crossing spinothalamic tracts near the central spinal canal. Trauma, syringomyelia, tumors & intrinsic cord tumors cause central cord syndrome.

2172. Dissociated sensory loss in central cord syndrome means?
Harrison's 20th Ed. Chapter 434, Page 3174

A. Loss of JPS & vibration sense with preservation of pain & temperature sense
B. Loss of pain & temperature sense with preservation of JPS & vibration sense
C. Loss of pain sense with preservation of temperature sense
D. Loss of temperature sense with preservation of pain sense

In cervical cord, central cord syndrome produces arm weakness out of proportion to leg weakness and "dissociated" sensory loss (loss of pain & temperature sense with preservation of light touch, joint position, and vibration sense over shoulders, lower neck & upper trunk.

2173. Which of the following is false about anterior spinal artery syndrome?
Harrison's 20th Ed. Chapter 434, Page 3174

A. Due to occlusion of anterior spinal artery
B. Motor, sensory & autonomic functions are lost below the level of lesion
C. Preserved vibration & position sensation
D. None of the above

Anterior spinal artery syndrome is due to infarction of spinal cord due to its occlusion or diminished flow. Destruction spares posterior columns. Motor, sensory and autonomic functions are lost below the level of lesion, Vibration and position sensation are retained.

2174. "Around the clock" pattern of weakness is seen in?
Harrison's 20th Ed. Chapter 434, Page 3174

- A. Central cord syndrome
- B. Anterior spinal artery syndrome
- C. Foramen magnum syndrome
- D. All of the above

Compressive lesions near foramen magnum produce weakness of ipsilateral shoulder & arm followed by weakness of ipsilateral leg, then contralateral leg, & finally contralateral arm, an "around the clock" pattern that may begin in any of four limbs. Typical sub-occipital pain spreading to neck & shoulders is present.

2175. Which of the following features does not favour the diagnosis of extramedullary lesions?
Harrison's 20th Ed. Chapter 434, Page 3174

- A. Radicular pain
- B. Early sacral sensory loss
- C. Sparing of sensation in perineal & sacral areas
- D. Spastic weakness in legs

Prominent radicular pain with early sacral sensory loss (lateral spinothalamic tract) & spastic weakness in legs (corticospinal tract) with incontinence indicate extramedullary lesions. Extradural masses are generally malignant while intradural masses are generally benign. Therefore, a long duration of symptoms favors an intradural origin.

2176. Which of the following features favours the diagnosis of intramedullary lesions?
Harrison's 20th Ed. Chapter 434, Page 3174

- A. Radicular pain
- B. Early corticospinal tract signs
- C. Sparing of sensation in perineal & sacral areas
- D. Spastic weakness in legs

Intramedullary lesions produce poorly localized burning pain & spare sensation in perineal and sacral areas ("sacral sparing"), due to laminated configuration of spinothalamic tract with sacral fibers outermost. Corticospinal tract signs appear later.

2177. Which of the following features favours noncompressive myelopathy?
Harrison's 20th Ed. Chapter 434, Page 3175

- A. Neck or back pain preceding paralysis
- B. Bladder disturbances preceding paralysis
- C. Sensory symptoms preceding paralysis
- D. Myelopathy without antecedent symptoms

Epidural compression causes warning signs of neck or back pain, bladder disturbances and sensory symptoms that precede development of paralysis. Noncompressive etiologies produce myelopathy without antecedent symptoms.

2178. Which of the following malignant tumors usually do not metastasize to "thoracic" spinal cord?
Harrison's 20th Ed. Chapter 434, Page 3175

- A. Breast
- B. Kidney
- C. Ovary
- D. Lymphoma

Almost any malignant tumor can metastasize to spinal column with breast, lung, prostate, kidney, lymphoma & myeloma being frequent because of high proportion of bone marrow in axial skeleton. Thoracic cord is most commonly involved. Metastases from prostate & ovarian cancer occur disproportionately in sacral & lumbar vertebrae.

2179. Batson's plexus is composed of?
Harrison's 20th Ed. Chapter 434, Page 3175

- A. Nerves
- B. Arteries
- C. Veins
- D. Capillaries

Batson's plexus is a network of veins along the anterior epidural space.

2180. Pain in neoplastic epidural compressive myelopathy worsens with?
Harrison's 20th Ed. Chapter 434, Page 3175

- A. Movement
- B. Coughing
- C. Sneezing
- D. All of the above

Pain in neoplastic epidural compressive myelopathy typically worsens with movement, coughing or sneezing & awakens patients at night.

2181. Which of the following segment of spine is uncommonly involved by spondylosis?
Harrison's 20th Ed. Chapter 434, Page 3175

- A. Cervical spine
- B. Thoracic spine
- C. Lumbar spine
- D. Sacral spine

2182. Which of the following is false about intradural mass lesions?
Harrison's 20th Ed. Chapter 434, Page 3175

- A. Slow-growing & benign
- B. Initial symptom is radicular pain
- C. Asymmetric, progressive spinal cord syndrome
- D. None of the above

Most intradural mass lesions are slow-growing & benign. Symptoms usually begin with radicular sensory symptoms followed by an asymmetric, progressive spinal cord syndrome.

2183. Intradural neurofibromas typically arise near?
Harrison's 20th Ed. Chapter 434, Page 3176

- A. Anterior root
- B. Posterior root
- C. Radicle
- D. Any of the above

Intradural neurofibromas typically arise near the posterior root.

2184. Which of the following is a primary intramedullary tumor?
Harrison's 20th Ed. Chapter 434, Page 3176

- A. Ependymomas
- B. Hemangioblastomas
- C. Low-grade astrocytoma
- D. All of the above

Primary intramedullary tumors of spinal cord include ependymomas, hemangioblastomas, or low-grade astrocytomas in adults. They present as central cord or hemicord syndromes, mostly in cervical region.

2185. Clinical triad of spinal epidural abscess consists of all except?
Harrison's 20th Ed. Chapter 434, Page 3176

- A. Midline dorsal pain
- B. Fever
- C. Progressive limb weakness
- D. Sensory loss

Clinical triad of spinal epidural abscess consists of midline dorsal pain, fever & progressive limb weakness.

2186. Which of the following about spinal epidural abscess is false?
Harrison's 20th Ed. Chapter 434, Page 3176

A. Infections of skin is a risk factor
B. Commonly due to hematogenous spread
C. *Streptococcus* aureus most common causative bacteria
D. Lumbar puncture is not recommended

Most cases of spinal epidural abscess are due to Staphylococcus aureus. Gram-negative bacilli, streptococcus, anaerobes, fungi and tuberculosis are other important causes.

2187. The spinal cord is supplied by how many arteries?
Harrison's 20th Ed. Chapter 434, Page 3177

A. 1
B. 2
C. 3
D. 4

Spinal cord is supplied by 3 arteries—single anterior spinal artery & paired posterior spinal arteries.

2188. Which of the following about blood supply of spinal cord is false?
Harrison's 20th Ed. Chapter 434, Page 3177

A. Anterior spinal artery originates in paired branches of vertebral arteries at cranciocervical junction
B. Anterior spinal artery is fed by additional radicular vessels C6, upper thoracic and at T11-L2 level
C. Anterior spinal artery supplies anterior three-fourths of cord
D. Posterior spinal arteries supply the posterior columns

Anterior spinal artery supplies the anterior two-thirds of cord.

2189. Anterior spinal artery feeder - Artery of Adamkiewicz arises at?
Harrison's 20th Ed. Chapter 434, Page 3177

A. C6
B. T4 - T5
C. T11 - L2
D. L4 - L5

Anterior spinal artery is fed by radicular vessels that arise at C6, at an upper thoracic level, and most consistently, at T11 - L2 (artery of Adamkiewicz).

2190. Posterior spinal arteries become less distinct below?
Harrison's 20th Ed. Chapter 434, Page 3177

A. Midcervical level
B. Midthoracic level
C. Midlumbar level
D. Midsacral level

Posterior spinal arteries supply posterior columns & become less distinct below midthoracic level.

2191. With systemic hypotension, greatest ischemic risk of cord infarction is at the level of?
Harrison's 20th Ed. Chapter 434, Page 3177

A. C6
B. T3 - T4
C. T11 - L2
D. L5 - S1

With systemic hypotension, greatest ischemic risk is at T3-T4 and also at boundary zones between anterior & posterior spinal artery territories.

2192. Which of the following is not a feature of anterior cord syndrome?
Harrison's 20th Ed. Chapter 434, Page 3177

A. Paraplegia or quadriplegia
B. Loss of pain & temperature sense
C. Sparing of vibration & position sense
D. Preservation of sphincter control

Anterior cord syndrome is due to acute infarction in the territory of anterior spinal artery that presents as paraplegia or quadriplegia, dissociated sensory loss affecting pain & temperature sense but sparing vibration & position sense, and loss of sphincter control. Sharp midline or radiating back pain localized to the area of ischemia is frequent.

2193. Spinal cord infarction is associated with?
Harrison's 20th Ed. Chapter 434, Page 3177

A. Aortic atherosclerosis
B. Dissecting aortic aneurysm
C. Hypotension from any cause
D. All of the above

Spinal cord infarction results from aortic atherosclerosis, dissecting aortic aneurysm, vertebral artery occlusion or dissection in neck, profound hypotension from any cause, cardiogenic emboli, vasculitis related to collagen vascular disease, and surgical interruption of aortic aneurysms.

2194. Presentation of surfer's myelopathy resembles which of the following?
Harrison's 20th Ed. Chapter 434, Page 3177

A. Anterior cord syndrome
B. Brown-Sequard hemicord syndrome
C. Central cord syndrome
D. Foramen magnum syndrome

A surfer's myelopathy usually occurs in thoracic region. It is caused by prolonged back extension due to lifting upper body off the board while waiting for waves. It typically manifests as anterior cord syndrome.

2195. Recurrent episodes of myelitis are usually due to?
Harrison's 20th Ed. Chapter 434, Page 3177

A. SLE
B. Sarcoid
C. Infection with HSV- 2
D. All of the above

Recurrent episodes of myelitis are due to immune-mediated disease like SLE and sarcoid or to infection with HSV type 2.

2196. Which of the following is a demyelinating condition?
Harrison's 20th Ed. Chapter 434, Page 3177

A. Multiple sclerosis (MS)
B. Neuromyelitis optica (NMO)
C. Postinfectious myelitis
D. All of the above

2197. Acute myelitis in multiple sclerosis presents most commonly as?
Harrison's 20th Ed. Chapter 434, Page 3178

A. Transverse myelopathy
B. Partial cord syndrome
C. Anterior cord syndrome
D. Central cord syndrome

MS may present with acute myelitis and is among the most common causes of partial cord syndrome. MS attacks rarely cause a transverse myelopathy.

2198. Which of the following about neuromyelitis optica (NMO) is false?
Harrison's 20th Ed. Chapter 434, Page 3178

A. Immune-mediated demyelinating disorder
B. Longitudinally extensive severe myelopathy
C. Associated with optic neuritis
D. None of the above

NMO is an immune-mediated demyelinating disorder associated with a severe myelopathy that is typically longitudinally extensive (lesion spans ≥3 vertebral segments) and optic neuritis (often bilateral & may precede or follow myelitis). Brainstem, hypothalamic or focal cerebral white matter involvement may occur. Recurrent myelitis without optic nerve involvement can also occur in NMO.

2199. Neuromyelitis optica (NMO) is associated with?
Harrison's 20th Ed. Chapter 434, Page 3178

A. Antiphospholipid antibodies
B. SLE
C. Connective tissue diseases
D. All of the above

NMO is also associated with SLE, antiphospholipid antibodies and with other connective tissue diseases.

2200. Which of the laboratory findings are observed in NMO?
Harrison's 20th Ed. Chapter 434, Page 3178

A. Oligoclonal bands in CSF absent
B. Serum autoantibodies against aquaporin-4 present
C. Autoantibodies against myelin oligodendrocyte glycoprotein (MOG) may be found
D. All of the above

2201. Which of the following about neuromyelitis optica is false?
European Journal of Neurology 2010,17:1019–1032

A. Also called Devic's disease
B. Idiopathic immune-mediated inflammatory demyelinating disease
C. Predominantly involves spinal cord and optic nerves
D. None of the above

Association between optic neuritis (ON) & spinal cord impairment was first described by Sir Clifford Albutt in 1870. In 1894, Eugene Devic and his student Fernand Gault proposed the nature of the pathological process and named the syndrome as neuromyelitis optica.

2202. Endocrinopathies associated with NMO include?
European Journal of Neurology 2010,17:1019–1032

A. Amenorrhea, galactorrhea
B. Diabetes insipidus
C. Hypothyroidism, hyperphagia (class IV)
D. All of the above

Endocrinopathies associated with NMO include amenorrhea, galactorrhea, diabetes insipidus, hypothyroidism or hyperphagia (class IV).

2203. Cardinal clinical feature of neuromyelitis optica is?
Harrison's 20th Ed. Chapter 434, Page 3178

A. Longitudinally extensive transverse myelitis
B. Optic neuritis—unilateral or bilateral
C. Repeated relapses
D. All of the above

Complete transverse myelitis is typical of NMO & partial transverse myelitis syndromes is indicative of MS.

2204. Which of the following is false about NMO-IgG autoantibody?
Harrison's 20th Ed. Chapter 434, Page 3178

A. Target antigen is AQP4 water-pump channel
B. AQP4 is an integral protein of astrocytic plasma membranes
C. AQP4 is highly concentrated in astrocyte foot processes
D. None of the above

2205. Immune-mediated disorders causing acute transverse myelopathies (ATM) include?
Harrison's 20th Ed. Chapter 434, Page 3178

A. SLE
B. Sjogren's syndrome
C. Behcet's syndrome
D. All of the above

Immune-mediated myelitides include SLE, Sjögren's syndrome, antiphospholipid antibody syndrome, mixed connective tissue disease, Behçet's syndrome and vasculitis related to polyarteritis nodosa, perinuclear antineutrophilic cytoplasmic (p-ANCA) antibodies, primary central nervous system vasculitis and sarcoidosis.

2206. Antiphospholipid antibodies are found in which of the following immune-mediated disorders?
Harrison's 20th Ed. Chapter 434, Page 3178

A. SLE
B. Sjogren's syndrome
C. Behcet's syndrome
D. RA

Myelitis occurs in SLE associated with antiphospholipid antibodies.

2207. In which of the following myelopathies, a large edematous swelling of spinal cord mimicing tumor is observed?
Harrison's 20th Ed. Chapter 434, Page 3178

A. SLE
B. Sarcoidosis
C. Sjogren's syndrome
D. Behcet's syndrome

In sarcoid myelopathy, an edematous swelling of spinal cord may mimic tumor.

2208. Typical neurologic manifestation of sarcoidosis is?
Harrison's 20th Ed. Chapter 434, Page 3178

A. Cranial neuropathy
B. Hypothalamic involvement
C. Meningeal enhancement visualized by MRI
D. All of the above

Typical neurologic manifestation of sarcoidos are cranial neuropathy, hypothalamic involvement or meningeal enhancement visualized by MRI.

2209. Recurrent sacral myelitis which mimic multiple sclerosis is due to?
Harrison's 20th Ed. Chapter 434, Page 3178

A. HSV - 2
B. Herpes zoster
C. Epstein-Barr virus (EBV)
D. Cytomegalovirus (CMV)

HSV-2 causes recurrent sacral myelitis along with outbreaks of genital herpes mimicking MS.

2210. Which of the following about Elsberg's syndrome is false?
Harrison's 20th Ed. Chapter 434, Page 3179

- A. HSV-2
- B. Recurrent sacral cauda equina neuritis
- C. Genital herpes
- D. None of the above

HSV-2 produces a syndrome of recurrent sacral cauda equina neuritis in association with outbreaks of genital herpes (Elsberg's syndrome).

2211. A polio-like syndrome can also be caused by which of the following?
Harrison's 20th Ed. Chapter 434, Page 3179

- A. Enterovirus 71 & coxsackie
- B. Japanese encephalitis virus
- C. West Nile virus
- D. All of the above

Prototype of viral myelitis is poliomyelitis. A polio-like syndrome can also be caused by enteroviruses (enterovirus 71 & coxsackie), Japanese encephalitis virus and flaviviruses like West Nile virus.

2212. Which of the following can cause myelitis?
Harrison's 20th Ed. Chapter 434, Page 3179

- A. Treponema pallidum
- B. Borrelia burgdorferi
- C. Listeria monocytogenes
- D. All of the above

Borrelia burgdorferi (Lyme disease), Listeria monocytogenes, Mycobacterium tuberculosis, and Treponema pallidum (syphilis) can cause myelitis.

2213. Which of the following can cause myelitis?
Harrison's 20th Ed. Chapter 434, Page 3179

- A. Schistosomiasis
- B. Toxoplasmosis
- C. Cysticercosis
- D. All of the above

2214. Acyclovir is useful in treatment of myelitis caused by which of the following viruses?
Harrison's 20th Ed. Chapter 434, Page 3179

- A. Herpes zoster
- B. HSV
- C. EBV
- D. All of the above

Herpes zoster, HSV & EBV myelitis are treated with IV acyclovir or oral valacyclovir for 10 - 14 days.

2215. Ganciclovir plus foscarnet is indicated for the treatment of?
Harrison's 20th Ed. Chapter 434, Page 3179

- A. Herpes zoster
- B. HSV
- C. EBV
- D. CMV

CMV myelitis is treated with ganciclovir plus foscarnet or cidofovir.

2216. Which of the following is not a type of chronic myelopathy?
Harrison's 20th Ed. Chapter 434, Page 3179

- A. Syringomyelia
- B. Tabes dorsalis
- C. HSV myelitis
- D. Subacute combined degeneration of cord

2217. Foix-Alajouanine syndrome best relates with?
Harrison's 20th Ed. Chapter 434, Page 3179

- A. Dural arteriovenous malformations
- B. Progressive thoracic myelopathy
- C. Paraparesis
- D. All of the above

Foix-Alajouanine syndrome or subacute necrotic myelopathy refers to a progressive thoracic myelopathy with paraparesis developing over weeks or months, characterized by dural arteriovenous malformation (dAVF) of spinal cord, mostly lower thoracic & lumbar in location.

2218. Which of the following about Klippel-Trenaunay-Weber syndrome (KTWS) is false?
Journal of Vascular Surgery: Venous and Lymphatic Disorders 2017;5(4):587

- A. Port-wine stain ((nevus flammeus)
- B. Varicose veins
- C. Bony & soft tissue hypertrophy involving an extremity
- D. None of the above

Klippel-Trenaunay-Weber syndrome (KTWS) is characterized by a triad of cutaneous capillary malformations (port-wine stain), varicose veins, and bony and soft tissue hypertrophy involving an extremity.

2219. Differential diagnosis of Klippel-Trenaunay-Weber syndrome include?
Journal of Vascular Surgery: Venous and Lymphatic Disorders 2017;5(4):587

- A. Sturge-Weber syndrome
- B. Triploid syndrome
- C. Proteus syndrome
- D. All of the above

Differential diagnosis for patients being considered for KTS includes Sturge-Weber syndrome, Parkes Weber syndrome, lymphatic filariasis, Beckwith Wiedemann syndrome, Russell-Silver syndrome, congenital hemidysplasia with ichthyosiform erythroderma and limb defects (CHILD) syndrome, neurofibromatosis 1, triploid syndrome and Proteus syndrome.

2220. Which of the following disorders is associated with lymphedema?
Harrison's 20th Ed. Chapter 276, Page 1934

- A. Neurofibromatosis type 1
- B. Noonan's syndrome
- C. Yellow nail syndrome
- D. All of the above

Disorders associated with lymphedema include Klippel-Trénaunay syndrome, Parkes-Weber syndrome, Noonan's syndrome, yellow nail syndrome, intestinal lymphangiectasia syndrome, lymphangiomyomatosis, and neurofibromatosis type 1.

2221. Tropical spastic paraparesis best relates to?
Harrison's 20th Ed. Chapter 434, Page 3179

- A. Human T cell lymphotropic virus-1 (HTLV-1)
- B. Epstein-Barr Virus (EBV)
- C. *Helicobacter pylori*
- D. *Campylobacter jejuni*

2222. Syrinx cavities are caused by all except?
Harrison's 20th Ed. Chapter 434, Page 3180

A. Syringomyelia
B. Trauma
C. Myelitis
D. Chronic arachnoiditis due to tuberculosis

Syringomyelia is a developmental cavity of the cervical cord. Syrinx cavities are acquired cavitations of spinal cord in areas of necrosis. They may be due trauma, myelitis, necrotic spinal cord tumors and chronic arachnoiditis due to tuberculosis.

2223. Which of the following is false about syringomyelia?
Harrison's 20th Ed. Chapter 434, Page 3180

A. Acquired or developmental
B. Symptoms begin in adolescence or early adulthood
C. Associated with Chiari type 1 malformations
D. None of the above

2224. Which of the following is false about syringomyelia?
Harrison's 20th Ed. Chapter 434, Page 3180

A. Dissociated sensory loss in upper limbs
B. Areflexic weakness in upper limbs
C. Spasticity and weakness of the legs
D. None of the above

Dissociated sensory loss can reflect spinothalamic tract involvement in spinal cord (bilateral spinothalamic tract involvement occurs in syringomyelia). There occurs impairment of pinprick & temperature appreciation but relative preservation of light touch, position sense & vibration appreciation.

2225. Which of the following is related to the sensory deficit in syringomyelia?
Harrison's 20th Ed. Chapter 434, Page 3180

A. Poisson distribution
B. Limb-girdle distribution
C. Cape distribution
D. Tibial distribution

In syringomyelia, cape distribution refers to the sensory deficit has a distribution that is "suspended" over nape of the neck, shoulders and upper arms or in the hands. This central cord syndrome initially produces signs & symptoms caused by dysfunction of crossing spinothalamic tract fibers that pass through anterior white commissure at that level. As the lesion expands to anterior gray matter of spinal cord, it may destroy anterior horn cells, causing weakness & wasting of muscles (LMN signs) at the involved levels.

2226. Which of the following is related to the sensory deficit in syringomyelia?
Harrison's 20th Ed. Chapter 434, Page 3180

A. Sparing the face
B. Sacral sparing
C. Pupil-sparing oculomotor palsy
D. Bladder-sparing

In syringomyelia, further enlargement of central lesion leads to involvement of spinothalamic tracts. As spinothalamic tract fibers from sacral areas are most distant from the center of spinal cord, the saddle area is spared ("sacral sparing").

2227. Syringobulbia causes which of the following?
Harrison's 20th Ed. Chapter 434, Page 3180

A. Horizontal or vertical nystagmus
B. Palatal or vocal cord paralysis
C. Tongue weakness with atrophy
D. All of the above

Syringobulbia causes palatal or vocal cord paralysis, dysarthria, horizontal or vertical nystagmus, episodic dizziness or vertigo, and tongue weakness with atrophy.

2228. Which of the following is false about chronic myelopathy of multiple sclerosis?
Harrison's 20th Ed. Chapter 434, Page 3181

A. Bilateral
B. Asymmetric
C. Motor, sensory, and bladder/bowel disturbances
D. None of the above

In chronic progressive myelopathy of MS, involvement is typically bilateral but asymmetric & produces motor, sensory & bladder/bowel disturbances.

2229. Which of the following drugs is effective in patients with primary progressive MS?
Harrison's 20th Ed. Chapter 434, Page 3181

A. Natalizumab
B. Alemtuzumab
C. Ocrelizumab
D. All of the above

Treatment with ocrelizumab, an anti-CD20 B-cell monoclonal antibody, is effective in patients with primary progressive MS.

2230. Which of the following is false about subacute combined degeneration of cord?
Harrison's 20th Ed. Chapter 434, Page 3181

A. Loss of deep tendon reflexes
B. Babinski sign
C. Romberg's sign
D. None of the above

2231. Which of the following is false about subacute combined degeneration of cord?
Harrison's 20th Ed. Chapter 434, Page 3181

A. Macrocytic red blood cells
B. Elevated serum levels of homocysteine
C. Elevated serum levels of methylmalonic acid
D. None of the above

2232. Which of the following condition is virtually identical to subacute combined degeneration?
Harrison's 20th Ed. Chapter 434, Page 3181

A. Adrenomyeloneuropathy
B. Tabes dorsalis
C. Familial spastic paraplegia
D. Hypocupric myelopathy

Hypocupric myelopathy is virtually identical to subacute combined degeneration except there is no neuropathy. Serum levels of B12 are normal, serum copper & ceruloplasmin levels are low.

2233. Which of the following is a copper-binding protein?
Harrison's 20th Ed. Chapter 434, Page 3181

A. Rubinstein
B. Lectin
C. Metallothionein
D. Haptocorrin

Metallothionein is a copper-binding protein.

2234. Which of the following condition producing myelopathy identical to subacute combined degeneration?
Harrison's 20th Ed. Chapter 434, Page 3181

A. Adrenomyeloneuropathy
B. Tabes dorsalis
C. Familial spastic paraplegia
D. Nitrous oxide inhalation

Nitrous oxide inhalation producing a myelopathy identical to subacute combined degeneration.

2235. Which of the following is false about tabes dorsalis?
Harrison's 20th Ed. Chapter 434, Page 3181

A. Fleeting & repetitive lancinating pains in legs
B. Ataxia
C. Acute abdominal pain with vomiting
D. None of the above

2236. Which of the following is false about tabes dorsalis?
Harrison's 20th Ed. Chapter 434, Page 3181

A. Loss of deep tenson reflexes in legs
B. Impaired position & vibratory sense
C. Romberg's sign
D. None of the above

2237. Which of the following polyradiculopathy may simulate tabes dorsalis?
Harrison's 20th Ed. Chapter 434, Page 3181

A. Non-Hodgkin's lymphoma
B. EBV polyradiculopathy
C. CMV polyradiculopathy
D. Diabetic polyradiculopathy

2238. Which of the following is false about adrenomyeloneuropathy?
Harrison's 20th Ed. Chapter 434, Page 3181

A. Mixed motor & sensory neuropathy
B. Flaccid paraplegia
C. Elevated levels of very long chain fatty acids
D. Adrenal insufficiency

Adrenomyeloneuropathy is associated with a mixed motor & sensory neuropathy with spastic paraplegia in adults associated with elevated circulating levels of very long chain fatty acids and adrenal insufficiency. The responsible gene encodes ADLP.

2239. Which of the following is false about Tethered cord syndrome?
Harrison's 20th Ed. Chapter 434, Page 3181

A. Developmental disorder of lower spinal cord & nerve roots
B. A dimple, hair patch, or sinus tract on skin overlying lower back
C. Diastematomyelia
D. None of the above

2240. Lathyrism is due to ingestion of faulty?
Harrison's 20th Ed. Chapter 434, Page 3181

A. Peas
B. Chick peas
C. Soyabean
D. Barley

Lathyrism due to ingestion of chick peas containing the excitotoxin β-N-oxylylaminoalanine (BOAA).

2241. The prospects for recovery from an acute destructive spinal cord lesion fade after?
Harrison's 20th Ed. Chapter 434, Page 3182

A. ~ 1 month
B. ~ 3 months
C. ~ 6 months
D. ~ 12 months

The prospects for recovery from an acute destructive spinal cord lesion fade after ~6 months.

2242. Which of the following is a feature of quadriplegic fever?
Harrison's 20th Ed. Chapter 434, Page 3182

A. Loss of normal thermoregulation
B. Inability to maintain normal body temperature
C. Recurrent fever
D. None of the above

2243. Which of the following is an α2 adrenergic agonist?
Harrison's 20th Ed. Chapter 434, Page 3182

A. Dantrolene
B. Tizanidine
C. Terazosin hydrochloride
D. Oxybutynin

Tizanidine is an α2 adrenergic agonist that increases presynaptic inhibition of motor neurons.

2244. In cervical radiculopathy, weakness of deltoid, supraspinatus & infraspinatus muscles signify lesion in which root?
N Engl J Med. 2005;353:392-9

A. C5
B. C6
C. C7
D. C8

2245. In cervical radiculopathy, weakness of biceps, brachioradialis, wrist extensor muscles signify lesion in the root?
N Engl J Med. 2005;353:392-9

A. C5
B. C6
C. C7
D. C8

2246. In cervical radiculopathy, weakness of triceps, wrist flexor, finger extensor muscles signify lesion in the root?
N Engl J Med. 2005;353:392-9

A. C5
B. C6
C. C7
D. C8

2247. In cervical radiculopathy, weakness of thumb flexors, abductors, intrinsic hand muscles signify lesion in the root?
N Engl J Med. 2005;353:392-9

A. C5
B. C6
C. C7
D. C8

2248. In cervical radiculopathy, sensory loss over lateral upper arm signifies lesion in the root?
   N Engl J Med. 2005;353:392-9
   A. C5
   B. C6
   C. C7
   D. C8

2249. In cervical radiculopathy, sensory loss over thumb and index finger signifies lesion in the root?
   N Engl J Med. 2005;353:392-9
   A. C5
   B. C6
   C. C7
   D. C8

2250. In cervical radiculopathy, sensory loss over posterior forearm and third finger signifies lesion in the root?
   N Engl J Med. 2005;353:392-9
   A. C5
   B. C6
   C. C7
   D. C8

2251. In cervical radiculopathy, sensory loss over fifth finger signifies lesion in the root?
   N Engl J Med. 2005;353:392-9
   A. C5
   B. C6
   C. C7
   D. C8

2252. In cervical radiculopathy, loss of supinator reflex signifies lesion in the root?
   N Engl J Med. 2005;353:392-9
   A. C5
   B. C6
   C. C7
   D. C8

2253. In cervical radiculopathy, loss of biceps reflex signifies lesion in the root?
   N Engl J Med. 2005;353:392-9
   A. C5
   B. C6
   C. C7
   D. C8

2254. In cervical radiculopathy, loss of triceps reflex signifies lesion in the root?
   N Engl J Med. 2005;353:392-9
   A. C5
   B. C6
   C. C7
   D. C8

2255. In cervical radiculopathy, pain in the region of medial scapular border, lateral upper arm to elbow signifies lesion in the root?
   N Engl J Med. 2005;353:392-9
   A. C5
   B. C6
   C. C7
   D. C8

2256. In cervical radiculopathy, pain in the region of lateral forearm, thumb and index finger signifies lesion in the root?
   N Engl J Med. 2005;353:392-9
   A. C5
   B. C6
   C. C7
   D. C8

2257. In cervical radiculopathy, pain in the region of medial scapula, posterior arm, dorsum of forearm & third finger signifies lesion in the root?
   N Engl J Med. 2005;353:392-9
   A. C5
   B. C6
   C. C7
   D. C8

2258. In cervical radiculopathy, pain in the region of shoulder, ulnar side of forearm, fifth finger signifies lesion in the root?
   N Engl J Med. 2005;353:392-9
   A. C5
   B. C6
   C. C7
   D. C8

2259. Spurling maneuver is?
   N Engl J Med. 2005;353:392-9
   A. Foraminal compression test in cervical radiculopathy
   B. Opposite of Valsalva maneuver
   C. Other name of hyperventilation
   D. Breath holding test

2260. Parsonage-Turner syndrome refers to?
   N Engl J Med. 2005;353:392-9
   A. Acute brachial-plexus neuritis
   B. Peripheral entrapment neuropathies
   C. Disorders of the rotator cuff and shoulder
   D. Referred somatic pain from the neck

2261. Differential diagnosis of cervical radiculopathy include?
   N Engl J Med. 2005;353:392-9
   A. Peripheral entrapment neuropathies
   B. Disorders of rotator cuff & shoulder
   C. Acute brachial-plexus neuritis
   D. All of the above

2262. Differential diagnosis of cervical radiculopathy include?
N Engl J Med. 2005;353:392-9

A. Thoracic outlet syndrome
B. Herpes zoster
C. Pancoast syndrome
D. All of the above

2263. Tinel's sign and Phalen's maneuver best relate to?
N Engl J Med. 2005;353:392-9

A. Thoracic outlet syndrome
B. Acute brachial-plexus neuritis
C. Carpal tunnel syndrome
D. Pancoast syndrome

2264. Hypoesthesia and weakness in medial three digits and opponens pollicis occurs in?
N Engl J Med. 2005;353:392-9

A. Median nerve entrapment
B. Ulnar nerve entrapment
C. Thoracic outlet syndrome
D. Pancoast syndrome

2265. Hypoesthesia and weakness in the fourth and fifth digits and thumb adductor occurs in?
N Engl J Med. 2005;353:392-9

A. Median nerve entrapment
B. Ulnar nerve entrapment
C. Thoracic outlet syndrome
D. Pancoast syndrome

2266. Which of the following statements about Roo's test is false?
N Engl J Med. 2005;353:392-9

A. It is a kind of provocation test
B. Used for diagnosis of thoracic outlet syndrome
C. Done by rapid flexion and extension of fingers while the arms are abducted at 90° and externally rotated 90°
D. Intermittent paresthesia, most commonly in C5 region

2267. Which of the following is false about paraplegia in extension?
Proc. Rom. Acad., Series B, 2013;15(3):197-215

A. Cause is lesion in pyramidal tracts
B. Clonus present
C. Mass reflex present
D. Position of lower limbs is extended

Paraplegia in extension has following feature : cause is lesion in pyramidal tracts, hypertonia is more in extensors, position of lower limbs is extended, deep reflexes are exaggerated, clonus is present, mass reflex is absent and bladder precipitancy is apparent.

2268. Which of the following is false about paraplegia in flexion?
Proc. Rom. Acad., Series B, 2013;15(3):197-215

A. Cause is lesion in pyramidal tracts and extrapyramidal
B. Clonus present
C. Mass reflex may be present
D. Position of lower limbs is in flexion

Paraplegia in flexion has following feature : cause is lesion in pyramidal and extrapyramidal tracts, hypertonia is more in flexors, position of lower limbs is flexed, deep reflexes are less exaggerated, clonus is absent, mass reflex may be present and automatic bladder is apparent.

2269. Which of the following about central cord syndrome is false?
Proc. Rom. Acad., Series B, 2013;15(3):197-215

A. Occurs almost exclusively in cervical region
B. Due to hyperextension pathogenic mechanism
C. Also known as "inverse paraplegia"
D. None of the above

Central cord syndrome occurs almost exclusively in the cervical region, usually by a hyperextension pathogenic mechanism. It produces localized sensitivity alteration for pain and temperature, with tendon reflex weakness. If the lesion enlarges - greater motor loss in the upper limbs than in lower ones occurs. It is therefore also known as "inverse paraplegia". Sacral sparing is noted.

2270. Which of the following about lateral (Brown-Sequard) syndrome is false?
Proc. Rom. Acad., Series B, 2013;15(3):197-215

A. Ipsilateral proprioceptive loss
B. Ipsilateral motor weakness
C. Controlateral loss of touch, pain and temperature
D. None of the above

In lateral (Brown-Sequard) syndrome, the lesion (e.g. stab wound - injury on a lateral side/hemi-section) produces greater ipsilateral proprioceptive, vibration, light touch sensitivity (posterior column impairment), paresthesias and motor weakness, possible reflex changes, and controlateral loss of sensitivity to touch, pain and temperature.

2271. Which of the following about anterior (ventral) cord syndrome is false?
Proc. Rom. Acad., Series B, 2013;15(3):197-215

A. Frequently occurs after a hyperflexion injury
B. Preserved proprioception
C. Variable loss of motor function, urinary continence
D. None of the above

In anterior (ventral) cord syndrome, the lesion, frequently occurs after a hyperflexion injury. It produces a variable loss of motor function, urinary continence, sensitivity to pain and temperature perception with preserved proprioception.

2272. Which of the following about posterior (dorsal) cord syndrome is false?
Proc. Rom. Acad., Series B, 2013;15(3):197-215

A. Lesion is often nontraumatic
B. Loss of two points discrimination
C. Ataxia
D. None of the above

In posterior (dorsal) cord syndrome, the lesion is more often nontraumatic. It produces loss of two points discrimination (epicritic sensitivity) and of proprioception, associated with ataxia, paresthesias and possibly urinary incontinece. Sensitivity for pain, and light touch, as well as motor function, remain intact.

2273. Which of the following about transverse/transsection (total) cord syndrome is false?
Proc. Rom. Acad., Series B, 2013;15(3):197-215

A. Complete loss of sensory modalities
B. Complete loss of motor functions
C. Complete loss of autonomic modalities
D. None of the above

In transverse/transsection (total) cord syndrome, the lesion results from a crush, and also possibly secondary to hemorrhagic or infectious, insults. It produces complete interruption/loss of any spinal cord control (sensory, motor, also autonomic) in terms of efficient functionality below the lesion level.

2274. "Osinski reflex" is best related to?

A. Anal reflex
B. Bulbo-cavernosus reflex
C. Cremasteric reflex
D. Anterior abdominal reflex

2275. Which of the following about conus medullaris syndrome is false?

A. Injury occurs between T11 and L2
B. Results in neurological impairments of bladder & bowel
C. Results in sexual impairment
D. None of the above

In conus medullaris syndrome, the lesion is due to injury of the distal cord (conus), typically between T11 and L2. It results in neurological impairments of bladder, bowel, sexual and lower limbs functionality (mild/symmetrical). The affected segments may occasionally show preserved reflexes (e.g. bulbo-cavernosus or "Osinski reflex", perianal wink/ano-cutaneous reflex related to micturition). If still absent after the spinal shock has passed, this proves the irreversibility of damage to such neural structures.

2276. Which of the following about cauda equina syndrome is false?

A. Injury occurs to lumbar-sacral nerve roots
B. Results in neurological impairments of bladder & bowel
C. Results in sexual impairment
D. None of the above

In cauda equina syndrome, injury to the lumbar-sacral (2 or more of its 18) nerve roots within the spinal canal, result in neurological impairments of bladder, bowel, sexual function and/or lower limbs. If there are affected mainly high and/or medium levels (L1-S1), the main symptoms consist in low back pain and somatic sensitive, motor, reflex and/or trophic deficits, whereas insults in the lowest ones (S2-S4) affect the sacral and perineum dermatomes, including with sphincters and/or sexual functions. The prognostic is better.

2277. Which dermatome is represented in apex of the axilla?

A. T1
B. T2
C. T3
D. T4

Root value at various locations on the body are : C2 – Occipital protuberance, C3 – Supraclavicular fossa, C4 – Top of the acromioclavicular joint, C5 – Lateral side of the antecubital fossa, C6 – Thumb, C7 – Middle finger, C8 – Little finger, T1 – Medial (ulnar) side of the antecubital fossa, T2 – Apex of the axilla, T3 – Third intercostal space, T4 – Fourth ICS (nipple line), T5 – Fifth ICS (midway between T4 and T6), T6 – Sixth IS (level of xiphisternum), T7 – Seventh IS (midway between T6 and T8), T8 – Eighth ICS (midway between T6 and T10), T9 – Ninth IS (midway between T8 and T10), T10 – Tenth ICS (umbilicus), T11 – Eleventh IS (midway between T10 and T12), T12 – Inguinal ligament at mid-point, L1 – Half the distance between T12 and L2, L2 – Mid-anterior thigh, L3 – Medial femoral condyle, L4 – Medial malleolus, L5 – Dorsum of the foot at the third metatarsal phalangeal joint, S1 – Lateral heel, S2 – Popliteal fossa in the mid-line, S3 – Ischial tuberosity, S4 – 5 Perianal area.

2278. Which of the following is a cause of pure motor paraplegia without sensory loss?

A. Hereditary spastic paraplegia
B. Lathyrism
C. Amyotrophic lateral sclerosis
D. All of the above

Causes of pure motor paraplegia without sensory loss are Hereditary spastic paraplegia, Lathyrism, Amyotrophic lateral sclerosis, Fluorosis, Guillain-Barre syndrome.

2279. Which of the following is a cause of cord compression at multiple levels?

A. Arachnoiditis
B. Neurofibromatosis
C. Spondylosis—cervical and lumbar level
D. All of the above

Causes of cord compression at multiple levels are Arachnoiditis, Multiple secondaries, Multiple sclerosis, Neurofibromatosis, Spondylosis—cervical and lumbar level.

2280. Which of the following is false about mass reflex?

A. Stimulation below level of lesion produces flexion reflexes of the lower limb
B. Evacuation of bowel & bladder
C. Sweating of skin below the level of lesion
D. None of the above

In mass reflex occurs in severe injury of spinal cord wherein stimulation below the level of lesion produces flexion reflexes of the lower limbs, evacuation of bowel & bladder and sweating of the skin below the level of lesion.

2281. Which of the following mediates reflex head & neck movements in response to visual & vestibular stimuli?

A. Corticobulbar tract
B. Rubrospinal tract
C. Medical longitudinal fasciculus
D. All of the above

Descending Medical longitudinal fasciculus (MLF) contains vestibulospinal and reticulospinal fibers, mediates reflex head and neck movements in response to visual and vestibular stimuli.

2282. Which of the following is a trigeminal mediated reflex?

A. Zygomatic reflex
B. Head retraction
C. Nasal reflex of Bechterew
D. All of the above

Various trigeminal mediated reflexes are : Head retraction (A sharp tap with the reflex hammer just below the nose with the head bent slightly forward produces a quick, involuntary backward jerk of the head. Present in bilateral corticospinal lesions rostral to the cervical spine, e.g. amyotrophic lateral sclerosis (ALS). Not present in normals.), Zygomatic reflex (A modification of the jaw jerk. Percussion over the zygoma produces ipsilateral deviation of the mandible. Seen only with supranuclear lesions.), Oculosensory or oculopupillary reflex (Constriction of the pupil, or dilation followed by constriction, in response to a painful stimulus directed toward the eye or its adnexa.), Corneo-oculogyric reflex (Contralateral or upward deviation of the eyes in response to stimulation of the conjunctive or cornea, with associated contraction of the orbicularis.), Corneomandibular reflex (Stimulation of cornea causes contralateral movement of the mandible. May be an associated movement rather than a true reflex. Indicates supranuclear interruption of the ipsilateral corticotrigeminal tract. Said to be the only eye sign in ALS.), Nasal reflex of Bechterew (Similar to sternutatory reflex. Tickling of the nasal mucosa causes contraction of the ipsilateral facial muscles.), Trigeminobrachial reflex (Contralateral flexion and supination of the forearm after stimulation in the distribution of CN V), Trigeminocervical reflex (Contralateral head turn after stimulation in the distribution of CN V).

2283. Which of the following is a facial reflex?

A. McCarthy's reflex
B. Myerson's sign
C. Chvostek's sign
D. All of the above

Transverse Myelitis

2284. Which of the following does not relate well with transverse myelitis?
N Engl J Med. 2010;363:564-72

A. Inflammatory disorder
B. Acute
C. Subacute
D. Chronic

Transverse myelitis is a heterogeneous group of acute or subacute inflammatory disorders with motor, sensory and autonomic (bladder, bowel, and sexual) spinal cord dysfunction.

2285. Transverse myelitis syndrome "most often" occurs due to?
N Engl J Med. 2010;363:564-72

A. Autoimmune phenomenon after infection or vaccination
B. Direct infection
C. Underlying systemic autoimmune disease
D. Acquired demyelinating disease

Transverse myelitis syndrome most often occurs as an autoimmune phenomenon after an infection or vaccination or as a result of a direct infection, an underlying systemic autoimmune disease, acquired demyelinating disease (multiple sclerosis) or idiopathic (15–30%).

2286. In transverse myelitis, most of the recovery occurs over?
N Engl J Med. 2010;363:564-72

A. First 3 months after the event
B. First 6 months after the event
C. First 12 months after the event
D. First 18 months after the event

Most of the recovery in transverse myelitis cases occurs in the first 3 months after the event. Although, improvement may continue for a year or longer.

2287. Pathological hallmark of transverse myelitis within the spinal cord is?
N Engl J Med. 2010;363:564-72

A. Focal collections of neutrophils
B. Focal collections of lymphocytes & monocytes
C. Focal collections of eosinophils
D. Focal collections of basophils

In spinal cord, pathological hallmark of transverse myelitis is the presence of focal collections of lymphocytes and monocytes, with varying degrees of demyelination, axonal injury and astroglial and microglial activation.

2288. Prognosis in transverse myelitis associated with multiple sclerosis is?
N Engl J Med. 2010;363:564-72

A. Good
B. Bad
C. Worse
D. Worst

Transverse myelitis associated with multiple sclerosis may have a substantial or even complete recovery. Transverse myelitis or neuromyelitis optica associated with other diseases usually have clinically significant residual neurologic deficits.

2289. "Spinal shock" consists of all except?
N Engl J Med. 2010;363:564-72

A. Areflexia
B. Sensory loss
C. Severe weakness
D. Hypotonia

"Spinal shock" refers to a combination of severe weakness, hypotonia and areflexia. It is the only recognized predictor of a poor outcome in transverse myelitis.

2290. Which of the following best distinguishes myelopathy from cerebral lesions and peripheral neuropathies?
N Engl J Med. 2010;363:564-72

A. Seizure
B. Sensory level
C. Babinski signs
D. Course of illness

A well-defined truncal sensory level, below which the sensation of pain & temperature is altered or lost, distinguishes myelopathy from cerebral lesions & peripheral neuropathies.

2291. Which of the following is responsible for the Lhermitte's sign in transverse myelitis?
N Engl J Med. 2010;363:564-72

A. Demyelination
B. Axonal injury
C. Astroglial activation
D. Microglial activation

Demyelination is responsible for the Lhermitte's sign that refers to the paresthesias that radiate down the spine or limbs with neck flexion. Demyelination is responsible for the paroxysmal tonic spasms i.e. involuntary dystonic contractions of limb or trunk muscles.

2292. Which of the following is false about idiopathic transverse myelitis?
N Engl J Med. 2010;363:564-72

A. No cerebrospinal fluid abnormalities
B. No MRI abnormalities
C. No identifiable underlying cause
D. None of the above

Patients with possible idiopathic transverse myelitis have clinical events consistent with transverse myelitis but that are not associated with cerebrospinal fluid abnormalities or abnormalities detected on MRI and that have no identifiable underlying cause.

2293. Presentation in transverse myelitis include?
N Engl J Med. 2010;363:564-72

A. Sensory spinal cord dysfunction
B. Motor spinal cord dysfunction
C. Autonomic spinal cord dysfunction
D. All of the above

Diagnostic criteria for transverse myelitis include bilateral (not necessarily symmetric) sensorimotor and autonomic spinal cord dysfunction.

2294. In transverse myelitis, clinical deficits progress to nadir between?
N Engl J Med. 2010;363:564-72

A. 4 hours and 7 days after symptom onset
B. 4 hours and 14 days after symptom onset
C. 4 hours and 21 days after symptom onset
D. 4 hours and 28 days after symptom onset

Progression to nadir of clinical deficits between 4 hours and 21 days after symptom onset is characteristic of transverse myelitis.

2295. Which of the following is true for MRI findings characteristic of myelitis?
N Engl J Med. 2010;363:564-72

A. More than one intrinsic cord lesions
B. Intrinsic cord lesions span at least two vertebral segments
C. Lesions enhance with intravenous gadolinium
D. All of the above

MRI finding of more than one intrinsic cord lesion is characteristic of myelitis. In acute phase, lesions enhance with intravenous gadolinium administration. Lesions in idiopathic transverse myelitis usually span at least two vertebral segments. Normal MRI should prompt a reconsideration of the diagnosis of myelopathy in favor of other disorders of the central or peripheral nervous system.

2296. Serum autoantibodies like antinuclear antibody or extractable nuclear antigen are present in?
N Engl J Med. 2010;363:564-72

A. Multiple sclerosis
B. Neuromyelitis optica
C. Systemic lupus erythematosus
D. All of the above

Serum autoantibodies like antinuclear antibody or extractable nuclear antigen may be present in patients with multiple sclerosis or neuromyelitis optica, systemic lupus erythematosus.

2297. MRI findings in multiple sclerosis include?
N Engl J Med. 2010;363:564-72

A. Short lesions spanning less than two vertebral segments
B. Lesions located in the periphery of the cord
C. Concomitant MRI evidence of demyelinating brain lesions
D. All of the above

Multiple sclerosis is associated with short lesions, spanning fewer than two vertebral segments, located in the periphery of the cord, affecting mainly white matter ("partial" transverse myelitis), and concomitant MRI evidence of demyelinating brain lesions.

2298. MRI findings in Neuromyelitis optica include?
N Engl J Med. 2010;363:564-72

A. Longitudinally extensive lesions spanning three or more vertebral segments
B. Symmetric lesions
C. Lesions situated centrally within the cord
D. All of the above

Neuromyelitis optica is strongly associated with longitudinally extensive transverse myelitis, defined by a lesion that spans three or more vertebral segments on MRI. Such lesions tend to be symmetric and situated centrally within the cord (involving both gray and white matter) and may extend into the brain stem, causing nausea, vomiting, and hiccups.

2299. Serum autoantibody marker NMO-IgG targets?
N Engl J Med. 2010;363:564-72

A. Beta2GPI
B. aCL
C. Astrocytic water channel, aquaporin-4
D. Anti-LKM3

Neuromyelitis optica is specifically associated with the serum autoantibody marker NMO-IgG, which targets the astrocytic water channel, aquaporin-4.

2300. Which of the following is not a monophasic syndrome?
N Engl J Med. 2010;363:564-72

A. Postinfectious transverse myelitis
B. Postvaccination transverse myelitis
C. Idiopathic transverse myelitis
D. Multiple sclerosis

Postinfectious, postvaccination and idiopathic forms of transverse myelitis are usually monophasic syndromes, whereas multiple sclerosis and neuromyelitis optica.spectrum disorders are relapsing diseases that are associated with a high risk of future attacks of transverse myelitis and other neurologic events.

2301. What happens to the IgG index in transverse myelitis?
N Engl J Med. 2010;363:564-72

A. Normal
B. Decreased
C. Increased
D. Any of the above

IgG index is a measure of intrathecal synthesis of immunoglobulin and is calculated by the following formula - (CSF IgG ÷ serum IgG) ÷ (CSF albumin ÷ serum albumin).

Multiple Sclerosis

2302. Which of the following is false about demyelinating disorders?
Harrison's 20th Ed. Chapter 436, Page 3188

A. Immune-mediated preferential destruction of CNS myelin
B. Peripheral nervous system (PNS) is spared
C. No evidence of associated systemic illness
D. None of the above

Demyelinating disorders are immune-mediated conditions characterized by preferential destruction of central nervous system (CNS) myelin. The peripheral nervous system (PNS) is spared, and most patients have no evidence of an associated systemic illness.

2303. Which about Multiple sclerosis (MS) is false?
Harrison's 20th Ed. Chapter 436, Page 3188

A. Onset of MS may be abrupt or insidious
B. Symptoms may be severe or trivial
C. Course can be relapsing or progressive
D. None of the above

2304. Triad in multiple sclerosis (MS) includes all except?
Harrison's 20th Ed. Chapter 436, Page 3188

A. Chronic inflammation
B. Demyelination
C. Remyelination
D. Gliosis

Multiple sclerosis is characterized by a triad of chronic inflammation, demyelination, and gliosis (scarring) with neuronal loss specially in advanced cases. Demyelination is the pathological hallmark. Relative sparing of axons is typical of MS. Lesions of MS typically occur at different times and in different CNS locations (i.e., disseminated in time and space).

2305. Which out of the following is the most common initial symptoms of MS?
Harrison's 20th Ed. Chapter 436, Page 3188 Table 436-1

A. Paresthesias
B. Diplopia
C. Ataxia
D. Vertigo

2306. Which out of the following is the most common initial symptoms of MS?
Harrison's 20th Ed. Chapter 436, Page 3188 Table 436-1

A. Sensory loss
B. Diplopia
C. Optic neuritis
D. Bladder dysfunction

2307. Which of the following about sensory symptoms in MS is false?
Harrison's 20th Ed. Chapter 436, Page 3188

A. Paresthesias
B. Hypesthesia
C. Sensory level
D. None of the above

Sensory symptoms in MS include paresthesias, hypesthesia, unpleasant sensations, bandlike sensation of tightness around torso.

2308. In MS, optic neuritis (ON) is least likely to present as?
Harrison's 20th Ed. Chapter 436, Page 3188

A. Diminished visual acuity
B. Dimness
C. Decreased color perception
D. Complete loss of light perception

Optic neuritis (ON) presents as diminished visual acuity, dimness, or decreased color perception (desaturation) in the central field of vision. Rarely, there is complete loss of light perception.

2309. In MS, which of the following statements is false?
Harrison's 20th Ed. Chapter 436, Page 3188

A. Visual symptoms are generally bilateral
B. Periorbital pain precedes or accompanies visual loss
C. Afferent pupillary defect is usually present
D. Uveitis is uncommon

Visual symptoms are generally monocular but may be bilateral. Periorbital pain often precedes or accompanies visual loss. Afferent pupillary defect is usually present. Funduscopic examination may be normal or reveal optic disc swelling (papillitis). Pallor of optic disc (optic atrophy) commonly follows ON. Uveitis is uncommon.

2310. Which of the following is uncommon in MS?
Harrison's 20th Ed. Chapter 436, Page 3188

A. Hearing loss
B. Uveitis
C. Complete loss of light perception
D. All of the above

2311. Which of the following is characteristic of MS?
Harrison's 20th Ed. Chapter 436, Page 3188

A. Movement-induced muscle spasms
B. Exercise-induced weakness of limbs
C. Monocular visual loss
D. Acquired pendular nystagmus

Exercise-induced weakness of limbs is characteristic of MS. Weakness is of UMN type accompanied by spasticity, hyperreflexia & Babinski signs.

2312. In MS, facial weakness is characterised by?
Harrison's 20th Ed. Chapter 436, Page 3188

A. Resembles idiopathic Bell's palsy
B. Not associated with ipsilateral loss of taste sensation
C. Not associated with retroauricular pain
D. All of the above

Facial weakness due to a MS lesion in pons resembles idiopathic Bell's palsy but is not associated with ipsilateral loss of taste or retroauricular pain.

2313. Which of the following is strongly suggestive of MS?
Harrison's 20th Ed. Chapter 436, Page 3188

A. Horizontal gaze palsy
B. Bilateral internuclear ophthalmoplegia (INO)
C. "One and a half" syndrome
D. Acquired pendular nystagmus

Bilateral internuclear ophthalmoplegia (INO) is particularly suggestive of MS. Other gaze disturbances include horizontal gaze palsy, "one and a half" syndrome (horizontal gaze palsy + an INO) & acquired pendular nystagmus.

2314. Visual blurring in MS may result from?
Harrison's 20th Ed. Chapter 436, Page 3188

A. Keratitis
B. Diplopia
C. Uveitis
D. Retinitis

Visual blurring in MS may result from optic neuritis (ON) or diplopia (double vision).

2315. Ataxia in MS usually manifests as?
Harrison's 20th Ed. Chapter 436, Page 3188

A. Cerebellar tremors
B. Hyperthyroid tremors
C. Episodic ataxia
D. Gait apraxia

Ataxia usually manifests as cerebellar tremors. It involves head and trunk or voice, producing a characteristic cerebellar dysarthria (scanning speech).

2316. In MS, paroxysmal symptoms are due to?
Harrison's 20th Ed. Chapter 436, Page 3188

A. Plaque rupture
B. Spontaneous discharges
C. Neovascularization
D. Disruption in blood-brain barrier

In MS, paroxysmal symptoms are due to spontaneous discharges arising at the edges of demyelinated plaques & spreading to adjacent white matter tracts.

2317. In MS, which of the following is false about paroxysmal symptoms?
Harrison's 20th Ed. Chapter 436, Page 3188

A. Brief duration (10 secopnds to 2 minutes), self-limited
B. High frequency (5–40 episodes per day)
C. No change in consciousness or background EEG
D. None of the above

2318. In MS, paroxysmal symptoms may be precipitated by?
Harrison's 20th Ed. Chapter 436, Page 3188

A. Sleep
B. Anxiety
C. Hyperventilation
D. Hunger

In MS, paroxysmal symptoms may be precipitated by hyperventilation or movement.

2319. Which of the following is false about Lhermitte's symptom?
Harrison's 20th Ed. Chapter 436, Page 3189

A. Electric shock-like sensation
B. Evoked by neck flexion
C. Radiates down the back into legs
D. None of the above

Lhermitte's symptom is an electric shock like sensation, typically induced by flexion of neck, that radiates down the back into legs. Lhermitte's symptom can also occur with compression of cervical spinal cord (cervical spondylosis), radiation-associated myelopathy (6 - 12 weeks after treatment) & Vitamin B12 deficiency syndrome.

2320. In MS, 'Uhthoff's symptom' is related to?
Harrison's 20th Ed. Chapter 436, Page 3189

A. Facial myokymia
B. Visual symptoms
C. Heat sensitivity
D. Movement

Heat sensitivity refers to neurologic symptoms produced by elevation of body's core temperature. Unilateral visual blurring may occur during a hot shower or with physical exercise (Uhthoff's symptom).

2321. Symptoms of bladder dysfunction are present in what percentage of MS patients?
Harrison's 20th Ed. Chapter 436, Page 3189

A. 50%
B. 65%
C. 75%
D. 90%

Bladder dysfunction is present in >90% of MS patients.

2322. Which of the following was once thought to be characteristic of MS?
Harrison's 20th Ed. Chapter 436, Page 3189

A. Euphoria
B. Impaired attention
C. Memory loss
D. Slowed information processing

Euphoria (elevated mood) was once thought to be characteristic of MS but is actually uncommon, occurring in <20% of patients.

2323. In MS, fatigue can be exacerbated by?
Harrison's 20th Ed. Chapter 436, Page 3189

A. Elevated temperatures
B. Depression
C. Sleep disturbances
D. All of the above

90% of patients of MS experience fatigue which is exacerbated by elevated temperatures, depression, or sleep disturbances.

2324. At onset, which of the following is the commonest clinical type of MS?
Harrison's 20th Ed. Chapter 436, Page 3189

A. Relapsing MS (RMS)
B. Secondary progressive MS (SPMS)
C. Primary progressive MS (PPMS)
D. All of the above

Relapsing or bout onset MS (RMS) accounts for 90% of MS cases.

2325. Secondary progressive MS (SPMS) always begins as?
Harrison's 20th Ed. Chapter 436, Page 3189

A. Relapsing MS (RMS)
B. Secondary progressive MS (SPMS)
C. Primary progressive MS (PPMS)
D. Any of the above

Secondary progressive MS (SPMS) always begins as RRMS.

2326. For a patient with RMS, the risk of developing SPMS is?
Harrison's 20th Ed. Chapter 436, Page 3189

A. ~1% each year
B. ~2% each year
C. ~3% each year
D. ~4% each year

For a patient with RMS, the risk of developing SPMS is ~2% each year, meaning thereby that great majority of RMS ultimately evolves into SPMS.

2327. Which of the following clinical type of MS experience relapses more?
Harrison's 20th Ed. Chapter 436, Page 3189

A. Relapsing MS (RMS)
B. Secondary progressive MS (SPMS)
C. Primary progressive MS (PPMS)
D. All of the above

Patients with SPMS or PPMS will occasionally experience relapses, far less often than in RMS though.

2328. Which of the following clinical type of MS has a more favorable prognosis?
Harrison's 20th Ed. Chapter 436, Page 3189

A. Relapsing MS (RMS)
B. Secondary progressive MS (SPMS)
C. Primary progressive MS (PPMS)
D. All of the above

Relapsing MS (RMS) is characterized by discrete attacks that evolve over days to weeks with complete recovery over weeks to months. Between attacks, patients are neurologically stable.

2329. Which of the following is false about multiple sclerosis?
Harrison's 20th Ed. Chapter 436, Page 3189

A. Thrice more common in women than men
B. Age of onset is between 20 and 40 years
C. Prevalence decreases at higher latitudes
D. ~10% cases begin <18 years of age

Prevalence rates of MS increase at higher latitudes.

2330. Highest known prevalence for MS is in?
Harrison's 20th Ed. Chapter 436, Page 3189

A. Middle east
B. Orkney Islands
C. Tasmania
D. Fiji

Highest known prevalence for MS is in Orkney Islands (Scotland) (250 per 100,000).

2331. Deficiency of which of the following vitamins is associated with an increase in MS risk?
Harrison's 20th Ed. Chapter 436, Page 3190

A. A
B. D
C. E
D. C

Vitamin D deficiency is associated with an increase in MS risk. Ongoing deficiency may increase the relapse rate in established MS.

2332. Well-established risk factor for MS is?
Harrison's 20th Ed. Chapter 436, Page 3190

A. Vitamin D deficiency
B. Exposure to Epstein-Barr virus (EBV) after early childhood
C. Cigarette smoking
D. All of the above

Well-established risk factors for MS include vitamin D deficiency, exposure to Epstein-Barr virus (EBV) after early childhood and cigarette smoking.

2333. Which of the following races are inherently at higher risk for MS?
Harrison's 20th Ed. Chapter 436, Page 3190

A. Whites
B. Africans
C. Asians
D. All of the above

Whites are inherently at higher risk for MS than Africans or Asians.

2334. Risk of developing MS is highest?
Harrison's 20th Ed. Chapter 436, Page 3190 Table 436-2

A. If an identical twin has MS
B. If a sibling has MS
C. If a parent has MS
D. If a spouse has MS

Risk of developing MS is highest if an identical twin has MS (1 in 3).

2335. If no one in the family has MS, what is the risk of developing MS?
Harrison's 20th Ed. Chapter 436, Page 3190 Table 436-2

A. 1 in 1000
B. 1 in 5000
C. 1 in 10000
D. 1 in 100000

2336. Which of the following is the strongest MS susceptibility region in the genome?
Harrison's 20th Ed. Chapter 436, Page 3190

A. HLA-DRB1 gene in class II region of MHC
B. HLA-DRB2 gene in class II region of MHC
C. HLA-DRB3 gene in class II region of MHC
D. HLA-DRB4 gene in class II region of MHC

The strongest susceptibility signal in genome-wide studies maps to HLA-DRB1 gene in the class II region of the major histocompatibility complex (MHC).

2337. Genes for which of the following have a role in adaptive immune system?
Harrison's 20th Ed. Chapter 436, Page 3190

A. Interleukin (IL) 7 receptor (CD127)
B. IL-2 receptor (CD25)
C. T cell costimulatory molecule LFA-3 (CD58)
D. All of the above

2338. New MS lesions begin with?
Harrison's 20th Ed. Chapter 436, Page 3190

A. Astrocytic proliferation
B. Disruption of blood-brain barrier (BBB)
C. Perivenular cuffing by inflammatory mononuclear cells
D. Infiltration of nervous system by B lymphocytes

New MS lesions begin with perivenular cuffing by inflammatory mononuclear cells, predominantly T cells and macrophages.

2339. Which of the following about MS is false?
Harrison's 20th Ed. Chapter 436, Page 3190

A. Susceptibility to MS is polygenic
B. Proinflammatory autoimmune response against a component of CNS myelin
C. No disruption of the BBB
D. Demyelination

At sites of inflammation in MS lesions, blood-brain barrier (BBB) is disrupted, but unlike vasculitis, the vessel wall is preserved.

2340. "Shadow plaques" refer to?
Harrison's 20th Ed. Chapter 436, Page 3190

A. Astrocytic proliferation (gliotic areas)
B. Remyelination of surviving naked axons
C. Aggregates of T and B cells
D. Any of the above

Surviving oligodendrocytes partially remyelinate surviving naked axons, producing "shadow plaques".

2341. 'Sclerosis' in MS best relates to?
Harrison's 20th Ed. Chapter 436, Page 3190

A. Axonal destruction
B. Astrocytic proliferation (gliosis)
C. Demyelination
D. All of the above

In MS, term sclerosis refers to the prominent astrocytic proliferation leading to gliotic plaques that have a rubbery or hardened texture at autopsy.

2342. In MS, "dirty white matter" refers to?
Harrison's 20th Ed. Chapter 436, Page 3190

A. Prominent astrocytic proliferation
B. Subpial cortical demyelination and neurodegeneration
C. Diffuse low-grade inflammation with microglial proliferation
D. Ectopic clusters of lymphocytic aggregates in white matter

In MS, "dirty white matter" refers to a diffuse low-grade inflammation with microglial proliferation seen across large areas of white matter, associated with reduced myelin staining & axonal injury.

2343. Nerve conduction in myelinated axons occurs in a saltatory manner at a velocity of?
Harrison's 20th Ed. Chapter 436, Page 3190

A. ~ 50 meters / second
B. ~ 70 meters / second
C. ~ 90 meters / second
D. ~ 110 meters / second

Nerve conduction in myelinated axons occurs in saltatory manner at a velocity of ~70 meter per second. In unmyelinated nerves, continuous propagation occurs at ~1 meter per second.

2344. Which of the following is best related to pathophysiology of MS?
Harrison's 20th Ed. Chapter 436, Page 3190

A. Redistribution of potassium channels along naked axon
B. Redistribution of sodium channels along naked axon
C. Redistribution of calcium channels along naked axon
D. Redistribution of chloride channels along naked axon

In MS, due to demyelination, conduction blocks occur. Axons that are normally buried underneath the myelin sheath are exposed. Thereafter, resting axon membrane becomes hyperpolarized due to exposure of voltage-dependent potassium channels. Sodium channels are concentrated at the nodes of Ranvier. With demyelination sodium channels redistribute along the naked axon allowing slow, rather than saltatory, continuous propagation of nerve action potentials through the demyelinated segment.

2345. In northern hemisphere, babies born in which month are significantly more likely to develop MS?
Eur Neurol 2016;76:202-209

A. February
B. May
C. September
D. December

In northern hemisphere, babies born in May are significantly more likely to develop MS than those born in November. This is called "month-of-birth effect". Opposite is true for southern hemisphere.

2346. For diagnosis of MS, symptoms must last for?
Harrison's 20th Ed. Chapter 436, Page 3191

A. 1 day
B. 3 days
C. 5 days
D. 7 days

2347. For diagnosis of MS, symptom episodes must be separated by?
Harrison's 20th Ed. Chapter 436, Page 3191

A. 1 week
B. 2 weeks
C. 3 weeks
D. 4 weeks

Diagnostic criteria for clinically definite MS require documentation of ≥2 episodes of symptoms and ≥2 signs that relate to pathology in anatomically noncontiguous white matter tracts of CNS. Also, symptoms must last for >24 hours and occur as distinct episodes that are separated by a month or more. Abnormal MRI or evoked potentials (EPs) could be considered as a sign.

2348. MS-typical region of CNS involvement is?
Harrison's 20th Ed. Chapter 436, Page 3192 Table 436-3

A. Periventricular
B. Juxtacortical, infratentorial
C. Spinal cord
D. All of the above

As MRI evidence for diagnosis of MS, ≥1 T2 lesion in at least 2 out of 4 MS-typical regions of the CNS, i.e. periventricular, juxtacortical, infratentorial, or spinal cord. Also, simultaneous presence of asymptomatic gadolinium-enhancing and nonenhancing lesions at any time or a new T2 and/or gadolinium-enhancing lesion(s) on follow-up MRI, irrespective of its timing with reference to a baseline scan.

2349. On MRI in MS, characteristic abnormalities are found in what percentage of patients?
Harrison's 20th Ed. Chapter 436, Page 3191

A. > 65%
B. > 75%
C. > 85%
D. > 95%

On MRI in MS, characteristic abnormalities are found in >95% of patients, although >90% of lesions visualized by MRI are asymptomatic.

2350. On MRI in MS, which of the following is the characteristic abnormality?
Harrison's 20th Ed. Chapter 436, Page 3191

A. Posterior brain edema
B. Dawson's fingers
C. Spot sign
D. Mammillary body atrophy

2351. Which of the following statements about MS is false?
Harrison's 20th Ed. Chapter 436, Page 3191

A. Early in MS, most disease activity is clinically silent
B. >90% of lesions visualized by MRI are asymptomatic
C. Patients with benign MS, 15 years after onset are likely to maintain their benign course
D. None of the above

2352. Which of the following does not favour the diagnosis of MS?
Harrison's 20th Ed. Chapter 436, Page 3192

A. Mild CSF pleocytosis (> 5 cells/µL)
B. CSF protein concentration of > 100 mg/dL
C. Lesions in the anterior corpus callosum
D. Dawson's fingers

Pleocytosis of >75 cells/µL, presence of polymorphonuclear leukocytes, or a protein concentration of >100 mg/dL in CSF should raise doubts about MS. Lesions in the anterior corpus callosum are frequent in MS and rare in vascular disease. Dawson's fingers refers to lesions as seen in MRI that are oriented perpendicular to ventricular surface, and corresponding to pathologic pattern of perivenous demyelination.

2353. Which of the following ratio is used to calculate CSF IgG index?
Harrison's 20th Ed. Chapter 436, Page 3192

A. IgG to albumin in CSF divided by IgG to albumin in serum
B. IgG to albumin in serum divided by IgG to albumin in CSF
C. IgG to globulin in CSF divided by IgG to globulin in serum
D. IgG to globulin in serum divided by IgG to globulin in CSF

CSF IgG index is the ratio of IgG to albumin in CSF divided by IgG to albumin in serum. Also calculated as CSF IgG index = (CSF IgG x serum albumin) / (CSF albumin x serum IgG).

2354. Which of the following is a marker of axonal integrity?
Harrison's 19th Ed. 2665

A. Propionyl-CoA carboxylase
B. Argininosuccinate lyase
C. N-acetyl aspartate
D. N-Acetylglutamate synthase

N-acetyl aspartate, which is a marker of axonal integrity. Proton magnetic resonance spectroscopic imaging (MRSI) can quantitate it.

2355. Which of the following is uncommon in MS?
Harrison's 20th Ed. Chapter 436, Page 3192

A. Aphasia
B. Seizures
C. Chorea
D. All of the above

Uncommon or rare symptoms in MS are aphasia, parkinsonism, chorea, isolated dementia, severe muscular atrophy, peripheral neuropathy, episodic loss of consciousness, fever, headache, seizures, or coma.

2356. Disorders that can mimic multiple sclerosis are all except?
Harrison's 20th Ed. Chapter 436, Page 3194 Table 436-4

A. Vitamin B12 deficiency
B. Syphilis
C. Sarcoid
D. HSV-1 encephalitis

Disorders that can mimic multiple sclerosis are acute disseminated encephalomyelitis (ADEM), Antiphospholipid antibody syndrome (APLA), Behçet's disease, Cerebral autosomal dominant arteriopathy, subcortical infarcts, and leukoencephalopathy (CADASIL), Congenital leukodystrophies (adrenoleukodystrophy, metachromatic leukodystrophy), HIV infection, Ischemic optic neuropathy, Lyme disease, Mitochondrial encephalopathy with lactic acidosis and stroke (MELAS), Neoplasms (lymphoma, glioma, meningioma), Sarcoid, Sjögren's syndrome, Stroke & ischemic cerebrovascular disease, Syphilis, Systemic lupus erythematosus, Tropical spastic paraparesis (HTLV I/II infection), Vascular malformations, Vasculitis, Vitamin B12 deficiency.

2357. Clinical features that have a more favorable prognosis in MS include all except?
Harrison's 20th Ed. Chapter 436, Page 3194

A. Optic neuritis or sensory symptoms at onset
B. Pyramidal symptoms
C. Women
D. Age < 40 years at onset

Clinical features that point towards favorable prognosis in MS are ON or sensory symptoms at onset, <2 relapses in 1st year of illness & minimal impairment after 5 years. Those with truncal ataxia, action tremor, pyramidal symptoms or progressive disease are likely to be disabled.

2358. Likelihood of having benign MS is about?
Harrison's 20th Ed. Chapter 436, Page 3193

A. 2%
B. 5%
C. 10%
D. 20%

In benign variant of MS, patients never develop neurologic disability & maintain a benign course. Likelihood of having benign MS is <10%.

2359. Pregnant MS patients experience fewer attacks than expected during?
Harrison's 20th Ed. Chapter 436, Page 3193

A. First trimester
B. Second trimester
C. Third trimester
D. First 3 months postpartum

Pregnant MS patients experience fewer attacks than expected during gestation especially in the last trimester but more attacks than expected in the first 3 months postpartum.

2360. Kurtzke Expanded Disability Status Score (EDSS) is used for?
Harrison's 20th Ed. Chapter 436, Page 3194

A. Parkinson disease
B. Multiple sclerosis
C. Alzheimer's disease
D. Creutzfeldt-Jakob disease

2361. Most patients with Kurtzke Expanded Disability Status Score (EDSS) scores < 3.5 have?
Harrison's 20th Ed. Chapter 436, Page 3194

A. Relapsing/remitting MS (RRMS)
B. Secondary progressive MS (SPMS)
C. Primary progressive MS (PPMS)
D. Progressive/relapsing MS (PRMS)

Kurtzke Expanded Disability Status Score (EDSS) is a measure of neurologic impairment in MS. Most patients with EDSS scores <3.5 have RRMS and are generally not disabled. Patients with EDSS scores >5.5 have progressive MS (SPMS or PPMS), are gait-impaired and occupationally disabled.

2362. Which of the following is used to manage first attacks or acute exacerbations of MS?
Harrison's 20th Ed. Chapter 436, Page 3194

A. Glucocorticoids
B. Mitoxantrone
C. Glatiramer acetate
D. All of the above

Glucocorticoids are used to manage first attacks or acute exacerbations of MS. A 2-3 week course provides short-term clinical benefit. Mild attacks are managed with physical & occupational therapy. Plasma exchange may benefit patients with fulminant attacks of demyelination that are unresponsive to glucocorticoids.

2363. Disease modifying therapies for RMS include?
Harrison's 20th Ed. Chapter 436, Page 3194

A. IFN β1a
B. Mitoxantrone (MTX)
C. Glatiramer acetate (GA)
D. All of the above

Disease-Modifying Therapies for Relapsing Forms of MS (RMS, SPMS with Exacerbations) include IFN-β-1a, IFN-β-1b, glatiramer acetate, natalizumab, ocrelizumab, fingolimod, dimethylfumarate, teriflunomide, mitoxantrone and alemtuzumab.

2364. Which of the following is the mode of action of Interferon β?
Harrison's 20th Ed. Chapter 436, Page 3194

A. Downregulating expression of MHC molecules on APCs
B. Reducing proinflammatory & raising regulatory cytokine levels
C. Inhibiting T-cell proliferation
D. All of the above

Interferon β (IFN-β) is a class I interferon with antiviral properties. Efficacy in MS results from immunomodulatory properties i.e. downregulating expression of MHC molecules on antigen-presenting cells, reducing proinflammatory & increasing regulatory cytokine levels, inhibiting T-cell proliferation and limiting trafficking of inflammatory cells in CNS.

2365. Glatiramer acetate is composed of which of the following amino acids?
Harrison's 20th Ed. Chapter 436, Page 3194

A. L-glutamic acid
B. L-lysine
C. L-tyrosine
D. All of the above

2366. Which of the following is the mechanism of action of Glatiramer acetate?
Harrison's 20th Ed. Chapter 436, Page 3195

A. Induction of antigen-specific suppressor T cells
B. Binding to MHC molecules and displacing bound MBP
C. Altering balance between proinflammatory & regulatory cytokines
D. All of the above

Glatiramer acetate is a synthetic polypeptide composed of four amino acids (L-glutamic acid, L-lysine, L-alanine and L-tyrosine). It acts by induction of antigen-specific suppressor T cells, binding to MHC molecules thereby displacing bound MBP or altering balance between proinflammatory & regulatory cytokines.

2367. Which of the following is a side effect of Fingolimod?
Harrison's 20th Ed. Chapter 436, Page 3196

A. 1° & 2° heart block, bradycardia & QT prolongation
B. Macular edema
C. Disseminated varicella-zoster virus & cryptococcal infections
D. All of the above

2368. Risk of progressive multifocal leukoencephalopathy (PML) is associated with?
Harrison's 20th Ed. Chapter 436, Page 3196

A. Mitoxantrone
B. Fingolimod
C. Dimethyl Fumarate (DMF)
D. Glatiramer acetate

Dimethyl Fumarate (DMF) is a small molecule and a Krebs cycle metabolite. Its use carries a risk of developing progressive multifocal leukoencephalopathy (PML).

2369. Which of the following about Natalizumab is false?
Harrison's 20th Ed. Chapter 436, Page 3197

A. Monoclonal antibody against α4 subunit of α4β1 integrin
B. Its use carries a risk of progressive multifocal leukoencephalopathy (PML)
C. Recommended only for JC antibody—negative patients
D. None of the above

2370. Which of the following about Ocrelizumab is false?
Harrison's 20th Ed. Chapter 436, Page 3197

A. Monoclonal antibody against CD20 on surface of mature B cell
B. IV methylprednisolone is given prior to each infusion
C. Carries a nonzero risk of PML
D. None of the above

2371. Which of the following about Teriflunomide is false?
Harrison's 20th Ed. Chapter 436, Page 3197

A. Cytostatic rather than cytotoxic
B. Can remain in the bloodstream for 2 years
C. Active metabolite of leflunomide
D. None of the above

2372. Which of the following drugs used in MS can cause malignancies?
Harrison's 20th Ed. Chapter 436, Page 3197

A. Mitoxantrone Hydrochloride
B. Teriflunomide
C. Ocrelizumab
D. Natalizumab

Mitoxantrone Hydrochloride use carries a risk of acute leukemia.

2373. Which of the following drugs used in MS can cause malignancies?
Harrison's 20th Ed. Chapter 436, Page 3197

A. Alemtuzumab
B. Teriflunomide
C. Ocrelizumab
D. Natalizumab

2374. Which of the following drugs used in MS can cause cardiomyopathy & irreversible congestive heart failure?
Harrison's 20th Ed. Chapter 436, Page 3197

A. Mitoxantrone Hydrochloride
B. Teriflunomide
C. Ocrelizumab
D. Natalizumab

2375. Which of the following drugs used in MS can cause toxic epidermal necrolysis or Stevens-Johnson syndrome?
Harrison's 20th Ed. Chapter 436, Page 3197

A. Mitoxantrone Hydrochloride
B. Teriflunomide
C. Ocrelizumab
D. Natalizumab

2376. Worsening RMS is defined as?
Harrison's 20th Ed. Chapter 436, Page 3197

A. Neurologic status abnormal between MS attacks
B. Worsening CSF IgG index
C. MRI lesions >3 mm in diameter
D. Involvement of more sites of CNS

Rapidly worsening MS is defined as patients whose neurologic status remains significantly abnormal between MS attacks.

2377. Which of the following drugs is used for patients with progressive disability in MS?
Harrison's 20th Ed. Chapter 436, Page 3194

A. Glucocorticoid
B. Plasma exchange
C. Mitoxantrone
D. Glatiramer acetate

Mitoxantrone is an immune suppressant generally reserved for patients with progressive disability who have failed other treatments. Mitoxantrone should not be used as a first-line agent in either RRMS or relapsing SPMS.

2378. Untreated patients of MS should be followed with?
Harrison's 20th Ed. Chapter 436, Page 3199

A. Objective clinical CNS examination
B. Evoked potential testing
C. Kurtzke expanded disability status score (EDSS)
D. Periodic brain MRI scans

Untreated patients are followed closely with periodic brain MRI scans.

2379. In MS, initiating treatment can be delayed if?
Harrison's 20th Ed. Chapter 436, Page 3194

A. Neurologic examinations are normal
B. Single attack or a low attack frequency
C. Low burden of disease as assessed by brain MRI
D. All of the above

In MS, initial treatment may be delayed in patients with normal neurologic examinations, a single attack or a low attack frequency and (3) a low burden of disease as assessed by brain MRI.

2380. Which of the following is the first-line therapy for RMS?
Harrison's 20th Ed. Chapter 436, Page 3194

A. IFN β
B. IV Ig
C. Mitoxantrone
D. Natalizumab

Relapsing forms of MS are treated with IFN-β or glatiramer acetate as first-line therapy.

2381. Which of the following is administered by IV infusion?
Harrison's 20th Ed. Chapter 436, Page 3194

A. IFN-β-1a
B. IFN-β-1b
C. Glatiramer acetate
D. Natalizumab

IFN-β-1a (IM), IFN-β-1b (SC), Glatiramer acetate (SC), Natalizumab (IV infusion).

2382. Which of the following is administered orally?
Harrison's 20th Ed. Chapter 436, Page 3194

A. IFN-β-1a
B. Mitoxantrone
C. Glatiramer acetate
D. Fingolimod

Fingolimod and Dimethyl Fumarate (DMF) are administered orally.

2383. Mitoxantrone is indicated for use in?
Harrison's 20th Ed. Chapter 436, Page 3198

A. SPMS
B. PRMS
C. Worsening RRMS
D. All of the above

Mitoxantrone is indicated in SPMS, PRMS, and worsening RRMS.

2384. Which of the following therapies is effective in treating PPMS?
Harrison's 20th Ed. Chapter 436, Page 3198

A. Glucocorticoids
B. IFN β1a
C. Glatiramer acetate
D. None of the above

No currently available therapies have shown any promise for treating PPMS at this time.

2385. In Marburg's variant of multiple sclerosis, the course of disease is?
Harrison's 20th Ed. Chapter 436, Page 3200

A. Hyperacute
B. Subacute
C. Fulminant
D. Chronic

Acute MS (Marburg's variant) is a fulminant demyelinating process that in some cases progresses inexorably to death within 1-2 years.

2386. Which of the following about Marburg's variant of multiple sclerosis is false?
Harrison's 20th Ed. Chapter 436, Page 3200

A. There are no remissions
B. Does not follow infection or vaccination
C. Death occurs within 1-2 years
D. None of the above

2387. Which of the following is a fulminant demyelinating syndrome?
Harrison's 20th Ed. Chapter 436, Page 3200

A. Weston-Hurst syndrome
B. Balo's concentric sclerosis
C. Acute hemorrhagic leukoencephalitis
D. All of the above

Balo's concentric sclerosis is a fulminant demyelinating syndrome characterized by concentric brain or spinal cord lesions with alternating spheres of demyelination and remyelination.

2388. Which of the following about multiple sclerosis is false?
N Engl J Med. 2006;354:942-55

A. Plaque is a chronic inflammatory, demyelinating lesion
B. Plaque lesions develop in white matter
C. Primary targets are myelin sheath & oligodendrocyte
D. Gray matter lesions are known to occur

2389. Which of the following about acute lesions of multiple sclerosis is false?

N Engl J Med. 2006;354:942-55

A. Indistinct margin, hypercellularity, intense perivascular infiltration, loss of myelin and oligodendrocytes
B. Widespread axonal damage, plasma cells, myelin-laden macrophages
C. Hypertrophic astrocytes
D. Astroglial scarring

2390. Most explosive form of acute disseminated encephalomyelitis (ADEM) is called?

Harrison's 20th Ed. Chapter 436, Page 3200

A. Mitochondrial encephalopathy
B. Acute hemorrhagic leukoencephalitis
C. Tropical spastic paraparesis
D. Metachromatic leukodystrophy

Acute hemorrhagic leukoencephalitis is the most explosive form of ADEM. Lesions are vasculitic & hemorrhagic & the clinical course is devastating.

2391. Which of the following is false about acute disseminated encephalomyelitis (ADEM)?

Harrison's 20th Ed. Chapter 436, Page 3200

A. Polyphasic course
B. Postvaccinal encephalomyelitis
C. Postinfectious encephalomyelitis
D. Perivenular inflammation & demyelination

ADEM has a monophasic course & is associated with antecedent immunization (postvaccinal encephalomyelitis) or infection (postinfectious encephalomyelitis). Hallmark of ADEM is presence of widely scattered small foci of perivenular inflammation & demyelination.

2392. ADEM can follow infections with all except?

Harrison's 20th Ed. Chapter 436, Page 3200

A. Measles
B. Varicella
C. Mycoplasma
D. Legionella

2393. ADEM can follow infections with all except?

Harrison's 20th Ed. Chapter 436, Page 3200

A. Rubella
B. Hepatitis B
C. Mumps
D. Infectious mononucleosis virus

Postvaccinal encephalomyelitis may follow administration of smallpox vaccine & rabies vaccine. Postinfectious encephalomyelitis is associated with infection with measles virus, varicella (chickenpox), rubella, mumps, influenza, parainfluenza, infectious mononucleosis viruses and Mycoplasma.

2394. Which CNS antigens correlates with development of ADEM?

Harrison's 20th Ed. Chapter 436, Page 3200

A. Vascular cell adhesion molecule (VCAM)
B. Myelin basic protein (MBP)
C. Bruton's tyrosine kinase (BTK)
D. Stromal-cell derived factor (SDF)

All forms of ADEM result from a cross-reactive immune response to infectious agent or vaccine that triggers an inflammatory demyelinating response. Autoantibodies to MBP and to other myelin antigens have been detected in the CSF from many patients with ADEM.

2395. Cerebellar involvement in ADEM is common in infections due to?

Harrison's 20th Ed. Chapter 436, Page 3200

A. Measles
B. Varicella
C. Mycoplasma
D. Mumps

In ADEM due to chickenpox, cerebellar involvement is often conspicuous.

2396. ADEM is differentiated from MS by?

Harrison's 20th Ed. Chapter 436, Page 3200

A. Simultaneous onset of disseminated symptoms & signs
B. Drowsiness or coma
C. Seizures
D. All of the above

2397. ADEM is differentiated from MS by?

Harrison's 20th Ed. Chapter 436, Page 3200

A. Bilateral involvement of optic nerve
B. Complete transverse myelopathy
C. Monophasic course
D. All of the above

Features that suggest ADEM rather than MS are monophasic course, simultaneous onset of disseminated symptoms & signs, meningismus, drowsiness, coma, seizures, bilateral optic nerve involvement, complete transverse myelopathy.

Neuromyelitis Optica

2398. Devic's disease refers to which of the following?
Harrison's 20th Ed. Chapter 437, Page 3202

- A. Acute disseminated encephalomyelitis (ADEM)
- B. Isolated dementia
- C. Neuromyelitis optica (NMO)
- D. Mitochondrial encephalopathy

Neuromyelitis optica (NMO) is also called Devic's disease. Eugène Devic (1858-1930) was a French physician who described clinical pathological features of "acute neuromyelitis optica" (NMO) in 1894.

2399. Which of the following is a limited form of NMO?
Neurology 2015;85:177–189

- A. Bilateral recurrent optic neuritis (BRON)
- B. Opticospinal MS
- C. ON or LETM associated with systemic autoimmune disease
- D. All of the above

2400. Which of the following about NMO Spectrum Disorder (NMOSD) is false?
Harrison's 20th Ed. Chapter 437, Page 3202, Neurology 2015;85:177–189

- A. Term NMO spectrum disorders (NMOSD) introduced in 2007
- B. Incorporates NMO individuals with partial forms
- C. Incorporates NMO individuals with involvement of additional structures in CNS
- D. None of the above

2401. Which of the following about NMO is false?
Harrison's 20th Ed. Chapter 437, Page 3202

- A. More frequent in women than men (>3:1)
- B. ON can be bilateral & produces severe visual loss
- C. Myelitis can be severe, transverse & typically longitudinally extensive involving ≥3 contiguous vertebral segments
- D. None of the above

2402. Which of the following about NMO is false?
Harrison's 20th Ed. Chapter 437, Page 3202

- A. Typically progressive symptoms do not occur
- B. Astrocytopathy with inflammation
- C. Absence of staining of AQP4 by immunohistochemistry
- D. None of the above

2403. In neuromyelitis optica, which of the following is involved?
Harrison's 20th Ed. Chapter 437, Page 3202

- A. Brainstem
- B. Cerebellum
- C. Cognitive functions
- D. None of the above

In contrast to MS, patients with NMO do not experience brainstem, cerebellar & cognitive involvement, & the brain MRI is typically normal. Over three or more spinal cord segments are involved.

2404. Which is the best available detection method for AQP4-IgG?
Harrison's 20th Ed. Chapter 437, Page 3202 Table 437-1

- A. Direct assay
- B. Cell-based assay
- C. Hybridization assay
- D. Heterophile agglutination assay

2405. Which of the following is a chemosensitive vomiting center in brain?
Harrison's 20th Ed. Chapter 437, Page 3202 Table 437-1

- A. Habenular trigone
- B. Pretectal area
- C. Arcuate nucleus
- D. Area postrema

Area postrema (AP), located in dorsal medulla, is the chemosensitive vomiting center and has high AQP-4 expression. AP is highly vascularized and lacks blood-brain-barrier, potentially increasing its exposure to blood-borne AQP-4 IgG. AP syndrome with unexplained hiccups, nausea & vomiting is clinical characteristic for NMOSDs and may occur concurrently with a myelitis episode.

2406. Which of the following about longitudinal extensive transverse myelitis (LETM) is false?
Harrison's 20th Ed. Chapter 437, Page 3202

- A. LETM is defined as a spinal cord lesion that extends ≥3 contiguous vertebral segments as seen on MRI of spine
- B. LETM is a characteristic feature of neuromyelitis optica
- C. LETM can also occur in multiple sclerosis, sarcoidosis or Sjögren syndrome
- D. None of the above

2407. Autoantibody against which of the following is seen in neuromyelitis optica?
Harrison's 20th Ed. Chapter 437, Page 3202

- A. Aquaporin-1
- B. Aquaporin-2
- C. Aquaporin-3
- D. Aquaporin-4

A highly specific autoantibody directed against water channel protein aquaporin-4 is seen in >70% patients of NMO. Aquaporin-4 (AQP4) is localized to foot processes of astrocytes in close apposition to endothelial surfaces, as well as at paranodal regions near nodes of Ranvier.

2408. Levels of which of the following is elevated during acute attacks of myelitis in NMO?
Harrison's 20th Ed. Chapter 437, Page 3203

- A. CSF levels of interleukin-6
- B. CSF levels of Glial fibrillary acidic protein (GFAP)
- C. Levels of AQP4 antibodies
- D. All of the above

During acute attacks of myelitis in NMO, CSF levels of interleukin-6 (IL-6) and glial fibrillary acidic protein (GFAP) levels are markedly elevated. Proinflammatory T-lymphocytes of Th17 type recognize an immunodominant epitope of AQP4 and may contribute to its pathogenesis.

2409. The course of NMO is monophasic in what percentage of patients?
Harrison's 20th Ed. Chapter 437, Page 3203

A. 10%
B. 20%
C. 40%
D. 50%

NMO is typically a recurrent disease. Its course is monophasic in <10% of patients. AQP-4 antibodies negative patients are more likely to have a monophasic course.

2410. The highest reported prevalence of NMO is from?
Harrison's 20th Ed. Chapter 437, Page 3203, Multiple Sclerosis Journal 2017;18:1-8

A. Rio de Janeiro
B. Martinique
C. Buenos Aires
D. Caracas

The highest reported prevalence is from Martinique, a region in Latin America (LATAM).

2411. What percentage of NMO patients have a systemic autoimmune disorder?
Harrison's 20th Ed. Chapter 437, Page 3204

A. ~ 10%
B. ~ 20%
C. ~ 30%
D. ~ 40%

Up to 40% of NMO patients have a systemic autoimmune disorder, such as SLE, Sjögren's syndrome, perinuclear antineutrophil cytoplasmic antibody (p-ANCA)-associated vasculitis, myasthenia gravis, Hashimoto's thyroiditis, or mixed connective tissue disease.

2412. Onset of NMO may be associated with acute infection with?
Harrison's 20th Ed. Chapter 437, Page 3204

A. Varicella zoster virus
B. Epstein-Barr virus
C. HIV
D. Any of the above

Onset of NMO may be associated with acute infection with varicella zoster virus, Epstein-Barr virus, HIV, or tuberculosis. Rare cases appear to be paraneoplastic & associated with breast, lung, or other cancers.

2413. In NMO, prophylaxis against relapses is done with which of the following medicines?
Harrison's 20th Ed. Chapter 437, Page 3204

A. Mycophenolate mofetil
B. Rituximab
C. Glucocorticoids plus azathioprine
D. Any of the above

2414. Which is the first line of treatment for acute attacks of NMO?
Harrison's 20th Ed. Chapter 437, Page 3204

A. Plasma exchange
B. High-dose glucocorticoids
C. Interferon beta
D. Alemtuzumab

2415. Which of the following drugs is ineffective & paradoxically increases the risk of NMO relapses?
Harrison's 20th Ed. Chapter 437, Page 3204

A. Interferon beta
B. Glatiramer acetate
C. Fingolimod
D. Natalizumab

Interferon beta is ineffective and paradoxically increases the risk of NMO relapses. Glatiramer acetate, fingolimod, natalizumab & alemtuzumab are ineffective.

2416. Clinical feature that distinguishes ON associated with anti-MOG antibodies from NMO or MS is?
Harrison's 20th Ed. Chapter 437, Page 3204

A. Cerebrospinal fluid (CSF) pleocytosis
B. Papillitis
C. Hiccups
D. Nausea or vomiting

Clinical feature that distinguishes ON associated with anti-MOG antibodies from NMO or MS is the presence of papillitis seen by funduscopy or orbital MRI.

Peripheral Neuropathy

2417. Peripheral nerves are composed of which of the following elements?
Harrison's 20th Ed. Chapter 438, Page 3204

A. Sensory
B. Motor
C. Autonomic
D. All of the above

Peripheral nerves are composed of sensory, motor and autonomic elements.

2418. Which of the following is not a major class of nerves?
Harrison's 20th Ed. Chapter 438, Page 3204

A. Large myelinated
B. Large unmyelinated
C. Small myelinated
D. Small unmyelinated

Nerves can be subdivided into three major classes: large myelinated (6 to 12 μm), small myelinated (2 to 6 μm), and small unmyelinated (0.2 to 2.0 μm). Small myelinated fibers are about three times more numerous than large myelinated axons.

2419. Motor axons conduct impulses at the speed of about?
Harrison's 20th Ed. Chapter 438, Page 3204

A. 25 m/sec
B. 50 m/sec
C. 75 m/sec
D. 100 m/sec

Motor axons are usually large myelinated fibers & conduct impulses at ~ 50 m/sec. Conduction is most efficient when the ratio of axon diameter to total fiber diameter is 0.5 to 0.7.

2420. Sensory fibers are of which type?
Harrison's 20th Ed. Chapter 438, Page 3204

A. Large-diameter myelinated
B. Small-diameter myelinated
C. Small-diameter unmyelinated
D. Any of the above

Sensory fibers may be any of the three types namely, large myelinated, small myelinated or small unmyelinated.

2421. Remak cell best relates to?
DeJong's The Neurologic Examination, 7th Ed. Page 369

A. Schwann cell
B. Neurofilaments
C. Neurotubules
D. All of the above

In unmyelinated axons, a single Schwann cell, sometimes called Remak cell, sends out processes to support several adjacent axons, providing a cytoplasmic coat with minimal myelin.

2422. Large fiber neuropathies spare which of the following?
DeJong's The Neurologic Examination, 7th Ed. Page 369

A. Pain and temperature sensation
B. Proprioception
C. Strength
D. Reflexes

2423. Small fiber neuropathies affect which of the following?
DeJong's The Neurologic Examination, 7th Ed. Page 369

A. Pain
B. Temperature
C. Autonomic function
D. All of the above

Large fiber neuropathies affect strength, reflexes, and proprioception with relative sparing of pain & temperature sensation. Small fiber neuropathies primarily affect pain, temperature & autonomic function.

2424. Proprioception & vibratory sensation are conducted to the brain by?
Harrison's 20th Ed. Chapter 438, Page 3204

A. Large-diameter sensory fibers
B. Smaller-diameter myelinated fibers
C. Smaller-diameter unmyelinated fibers
D. All of the above

Large-diameter sensory fibers conduct proprioception and vibratory sensation to the brain, while the smaller-diameter myelinated and unmyelinated fibers transmit pain and temperature sensation.

2425. Which of the following is a peripheral neuropathy?
Harrison's 20th Ed. Chapter 438, Page 3204

A. Neuronopathy or ganglionopathy
B. Myelinopathy
C. Axonopathy
D. All of the above

Peripheral neuropathies are classified into those that primarily affect the cell body (neuronopathy or ganglionopathy), myelin (myelinopathy) and the axon (axonopathy).

2426. Which of the following is a possibility in symmetric proximal and distal weakness with sensory loss?
Harrison's 20th Ed. Chapter 438, Page 3206 Table 438-2

A. Chronic inflammatory demyelinating polyneuropathy (CIDP)
B. Charcot-Marie-Tooth disease
C. Spinal muscular atrophy (SMA)
D. Diabetes mellitus

In the scenario of symmetric proximal and distal weakness with sensory loss, inflammatory demyelinating polyneuropathy (GBS and CIDP) are a possibility.

2427. Which of the following is a possibility in symmetric distal sensory loss with or without distal weakness?
Harrison's 20th Ed. Chapter 438, Page 3206 Table 438-2

A. Chronic inflammatory demyelinating polyneuropathy (CIDP)
B. Guillain-Barré syndrome
C. Spinal muscular atrophy (SMA)
D. Diabetes mellitus

In the scenario of symmetric distal sensory loss with or without distal weakness, cryptogenic or idiopathic sensory polyneuropathy (CSPN), diabetes mellitus and other metabolic disorders, drugs, toxins, familial (HSAN), CMT, amyloidosis and others are a possibility.

2428. Which of the following is a possibility in asymmetric distal weakness with sensory loss with involvement of multiple nerves?
Harrison's 20th Ed. Chapter 438, Page 3206 Table 438-2

- A. Multifocal CIDP
- B. Sarcoidosis
- C. Hereditary neuropathy with liability to pressure palsies
- D. All of the above

Asymmetric distal weakness with sensory loss with involvement of multiple nerves may occur in multifocal CIDP, vasculitis, cryoglobulinemia, amyloidosis, sarcoid, infectious (leprosy, Lyme, hepatitis B, C or E, HIV, CMV), hereditary neuropathy with liability to pressure palsies (HNPP), tumor infiltration

2429. Which of the following is a possibility in asymmetric proximal and distal weakness with sensory loss?
Harrison's 20th Ed. Chapter 438, Page 3206 Table 438-2

- A. Diabetes mellitus
- B. Meningeal carcinomatosis
- C. Hereditary neuropathy with liability to pressure palsies
- D. All of the above

Asymmetric proximal and distal weakness with sensory loss can be seen in polyradiculopathy or plexopathy due to diabetes mellitus, meningeal carcinomatosis or lymphomatosis, hereditary plexopathy (HNPP, HNA), idiopathic.

2430. Which of the following is a possibility in asymmetric distal weakness (UMN) without sensory loss?
Harrison's 20th Ed. Chapter 438, Page 3206 Table 438-2

- A. Diabetes mellitus
- B. Multifocal motor neuropathy
- C. Motor neuron disease
- D. Progressive muscular atrophy

Asymmetric distal weakness without sensory loss with upper motor neuron findings is seen in motor neuron disease. Those without upper motor neuron findings is seen in progressive muscular atrophy, juvenile monomelic amyotrophy (Hirayama disease), multifocal motor neuropathy, multifocal acquired motor axonopathy.

2431. Which of the following is a possibility in symmetric sensory loss and distal areflexia with upper motor neuron findings?
Harrison's 20th Ed. Chapter 438, Page 3206 Table 438-2

- A. Vitamin B12 deficiency
- B. Vitamin E deficiency
- C. Copper deficiency
- D. All of the above

Symmetric sensory loss and distal areflexia with upper motor neuron findings is seen in Vitamin B12, vitamin E, and copper deficiency with combined system degeneration with peripheral neuropathy, hereditary leukodystrophies (adrenomyeloneuropathy).

2432. Which of the following is a possibility in symmetric weakness without sensory loss?
Harrison's 20th Ed. Chapter 438, Page 3206 Table 438-2

- A. Guillain-Barré syndrome
- B. Spinal muscular atrophy
- C. Diabetes mellitus
- D. Chronic inflammatory demyelinating polyneuropathy (CIDP)

Symmetric weakness without sensory loss with proximal and distal weakness is seen in spinal muscular atrophy and with distal weakness seen in hereditary motor neuropathy ("distal" SMA) or atypical CMT.

2433. If the patient has only weakness without any evidence of sensory or autonomic dysfunction, the diagnosis can be?
Harrison's 20th Ed. Chapter 438, Page 3204

- A. Motor neuropathy
- B. Neuromuscular junction abnormality
- C. Myopathy
- D. Any of the above

If the patient has only weakness without any evidence of sensory or autonomic dysfunction, a motor neuropathy, neuromuscular junction abnormality, or myopathy can be the cause.

2434. Heat intolerance is a symptom due to which of the following abnormalities?
Harrison's 20th Ed. Chapter 438, Page 3205

- A. Motor
- B. Sensory
- C. Autonomic
- D. All of the above

Symptoms of autonomic neuropathy are fainting spells or orthostatic lightheadedness (orthostatic fall in blood pressure without an appropriate increase in heart rate), heat intolerance or any bowel, bladder, or sexual dysfunction.

2435. Majority of neuropathies are predominantly?
Harrison's 20th Ed. Chapter 438, Page 3205

- A. Motor
- B. Sensory
- C. Autonomic
- D. Combined

Majority of neuropathies are predominantly sensory in nature.

2436. Symmetric proximal and distal weakness is the hallmark of?
Harrison's 20th Ed. Chapter 438, Page 3205

- A. Charcot-Marie-Tooth disease
- B. Guillain-Barré syndrome (GBS)
- C. Motor neuron disease
- D. Diabetes mellitus

Symmetric proximal & distal weakness is the hallmark of acquired immune demyelinating polyneuropathies, both acute form (AIDP) also known as Guillain-Barré syndrome (GBS) and the chronic inflammatory demyelinating polyneuropathy (CIDP).

2437. Sharp and lancinating (epicritic pain), relayed by?
Harrison's 20th Ed. Chapter 438, Page 3206

- A. A-delta fibers
- B. B-delta fibers
- C. C-delta fibers
- D. D-delta fibers

Neuropathic pain can be burning, dull and poorly localized (protopathic pain, presumably transmitted by polymodal C nociceptor fibers or sharp and lancinating (epicritic pain), relayed by A-delta fibers.

2438. Most likely cause of small-fiber neuropathies is?
Harrison's 20th Ed. Chapter 438, Page 3206

- A. Hepatitis B
- B. Motor neuron disease
- C. Sjogren's syndrome
- D. Diabetes mellitus

Most likely cause of small-fiber neuropathies is diabetes mellitus or glucose intolerance.

2439. Which of the following is the cause of combined system degeneration with neuropathy?
Harrison's 20th Ed. Chapter 438, Page 3206

A. Vitamin B12 deficiency
B. Copper deficiency
C. HIV infection
D. All of the above

Symmetric distal sensory neuropathy, with symmetric upper motor neuron involvement, suggests combined system degeneration with neuropathy as seen in vitamin B12 deficiency, copper deficiency, HIV infection, severe hepatic disease & adrenomyeloneuropathy.

2440. Which of the following neuropathies does not present acutely or subacutely?
Harrison's 20th Ed. Chapter 438, Page 3206

A. GBS
B. Diabetes
C. Lyme disease
D. Porphyria

Neuropathies with acute and subacute presentations include GBS, vasculitis, and radiculopathies related to diabetes or Lyme disease. A relapsing course is seen in CIDP and porphyria.

2441. Fixatives containing which element can lead to copper deficiency?
Harrison's 20th Ed. Chapter 438, Page 3206

A. Aluminium
B. Lead
C. Zinc
D. Nickel

Fixatives that contain zinc that can lead to copper deficiency.

2442. Which of the following is not a EDx finding in axonal neuropathy?
Harrison's 20th Ed. Chapter 438, Page 3207

A. Low-amplitude potentials
B. Absence of fibrillations
C. Relatively preserved distal latencies
D. Relatively preserved conduction velocities

Nerve conduction studies (NCS) are helpful in differentiating between axonal degeneration or segmental demyelination. Low-amplitude potentials with relatively preserved distal latencies, conduction velocities, and late potentials, along with fibrillations suggest an axonal neuropathy. Relatively preserved amplitudes, slow conduction velocities, prolonged distal latencies and late potentials, and absence of fibrillations imply a primary demyelinating neuropathy.

2443. Laboratory workup in a suspected case of vasculitis includes?
Harrison's 20th Ed. Chapter 438, Page 3208

A. Cryoglobulins
B. Western blot for Lyme disease
C. Cytomegalovirus (CMV) titer
D. All of the above

Laboratory workup in a suspected case of vasculitis includes antineutrophil cytoplasmic antibodies (ANCA), cryoglobulins, hepatitis serology, Western blot for Lyme disease, HIV, and cytomegalovirus (CMV) titer.

2444. Which of the following tests is done to detect a monoclonal gammopathy?
Harrison's 20th Ed. Chapter 438, Page 3208

A. Serum protein electrophoresis (SPEP)
B. Serum-free light chains
C. Serum kappa / lambda ratio
D. All of the above

2445. Severe painful sensorimotor & autonomic neuropathy and alopecia point towards?
Harrison's 20th Ed. Chapter 438, Page 3207

A. Arsenic toxicity
B. Thallium toxicity
C. Lead toxicity
D. Zinc toxicity

2446. Severe painful sensorimotor neuropathy with or without gastrointestinal disturbance & Mee's lines point towards?
Harrison's 20th Ed. Chapter 438, Page 3207

A. Arsenic toxicity
B. Thallium toxicity
C. Lead toxicity
D. Zinc toxicity

2447. Wrist or finger extensor weakness and anemia with basophilic stippling of blood cells point towards?
Harrison's 20th Ed. Chapter 438, Page 3207

A. Arsenic toxicity
B. Thallium toxicity
C. Lead toxicity
D. Zinc toxicity

Severe painful sensorimotor and autonomic neuropathy and alopecia—thallium toxicity. Severe painful sensorimotor neuropathy with or without gastrointestinal disturbance and Mee's lines—arsenic toxicity and wrist or finger extensor weakness and anemia with basophilic stippling of blood cells—lead toxicity.

2448. Most common cause of sensory ganglionopathies is?
Harrison's 20th Ed. Chapter 438, Page 3207

A. Porphyria
B. Diabetes mellitus
C. Vitamin B12 deficiency
D. Sjögren syndrome

Most common causes of sensory ganglionopathies presenting as severe sensory ataxia are Sjögren syndrome and paraneoplastic neuropathy.

2449. Which of the following investigation is done in patients with neuropathy due to Sjögren's syndrome?
Harrison's 20th Ed. Chapter 438, Page 3207

A. ANA
B. SS-A/Ro antibodies in serum
C. SS-B/La antibodies in serum
D. All of the above

Patients with neuropathy due to Sjögren's syndrome may have ANAs, SS-A/Ro, and SS-B/La antibodies in the serum, but most do not.

2450. Anti-Hu antibodies are 'most commonly' seen in patients with?
Harrison's 20th Ed. Chapter 438, Page 3207

A. Breast cancer
B. Ovarian cancer
C. Lymphoma
D. Small-cell carcinoma of the lung

Antineuronal nuclear antibodies—anti-Hu antibodies are most commonly seen in patients with small-cell carcinoma of the lung but are seen also in breast, ovarian, lymphoma, and other cancers.

2451. Which of the following is an onconeuronal antibody?
Harrison's 20th Ed. Chapter 90, Page 994, 669 Table 90-3

A. Anti-Hu
B. Anti-Amphiphysin
C. Anti-CRMP5
D. All of the above

Onconeuronal antibodies are anti-Hu, anti-Yo, anti-Ma2, anti-amphiphysin, anti-CRMP5, anti-CV2.

2452. Most commonly biopsied nerve is?
Harrison's 20th Ed. Chapter 438, Page 3208

A. Superficial peroneal nerve
B. Common peroneal nerve
C. Sural nerve
D. Superficial lateral cuteneous nerve

Nerve biopsies should be done only if NCS studies are abnormal. Sural nerve is most commonly biopsied because it is a pure sensory nerve and biopsy will not result in loss of motor function.

2453. Which of the following about skin biopsies in a case of neutopathy is false?
Harrison's 20th Ed. Chapter 438, Page 3208

A. Used to diagnose a small-fiber neuropathy
B. Useful when NCS is normal
C. Useful when routine nerve biopsies are normal
D. None of the above

2454. In mnemonic DANG THERAPIST, which is helpful in recalling common causes of peripheral neuropathy, "S" stands for?

A. Syphilis
B. Sepsis
C. Sarcoid
D. Secondaries

The mnemonic DANG THERAPIST for common causes of peripheral neuropathy Diabetes mellitus, Alcohol, Nutritional (B12 deficiency), Guillain-Barre syndrome, Toxins (Pb, As, Zn, Hg), Hematologic (paraproteins), Endocrine (hypothyroid), Rheumatologic (SLE, rheumatoid arthritis, vasculitis), Amyloid, Porphyria, Infectious (syphilis, HIV), Sarcoid, Tumor (paraneoplastic neuropathy).

2455. Which of the following is the most common type of hereditary neuropathy?
Harrison's 20th Ed. Chapter 438, Page 3208

A. Charcot-Marie-Tooth (CMT) disease
B. Hereditary neuropathy with liability to pressure palsies
C. Hereditary neuralgic amyotrophy
D. Hereditary sensory and autonomic neuropathy

Charcot-Marie-Tooth (CMT) disease is the most common type of hereditary neuropathy. CMT used to be called peroneal muscular atrophy. It was also referred to as hereditary motor/sensory neuropathy (HMSN).

2456. Various subtypes of CMT are classified according to?
Harrison's 20th Ed. Chapter 438, Page 3208

A. Predominant pathology
B. Nerve conduction velocities
C. Inheritance pattern
D. All of the above

Various subtypes of CMT are classified according to the nerve conduction velocities and predominant pathology (demyelination or axonal degeneration), inheritance pattern (autosomal dominant, recessive, or X-linked), and the specific mutated genes.

2457. In CMT1, motor conduction velocities in the arms are slowed to?
Harrison's 20th Ed. Chapter 438, Page 3208

A. < 38 m/sec
B. < 48 m/sec
C. < 58 m/sec
D. < 68 m/sec

By definition, motor conduction velocities in the arms are slowed to < 38 m/sec in CMT1 and are greater than 38 m/sec in CMT2.

2458. Transmission of Charcot-Marie-Tooth (CMT) neuropathy diseases is?
Harrison's 20th Ed. Chapter 438, Page 3208

A. Autosomal dominant
B. Autosomal recessive
C. X-linked
D. All of the above

CMT is usually transmitted as autosomal dominant trait, as X-linked-dominant CMT in ~10%. Rare autosomal recessive forms (CMT4) have an early onset & are more severe than dominant types.

2459. Inheritance of CMT1 is?
Harrison's 20th Ed. Chapter 438, Page 3208

A. Autosomal dominant
B. Autosomal recessive
C. X-linked
D. Any of the above

Inheritance of CMT1 is autosomal dominant.

2460. Which of the following is false about Charcot-Marie-Tooth Disease (CMT)?
Harrison's 20th Ed. Chapter 438, Page 3208

A. Heritable neuromuscular disorder
B. Chronic distal sensory and motor neuropathy
C. CMT does not reduce the life span
D. None of the above

CMT is the most common heritable neuromuscular disorder. It is a chronic distal sensory & motor neuropathy. Pes cavus & hammer toes indicate that neuropathy dates from early life. CMT does not reduce life span & rarely involves respiratory muscles.

2461. Which of the following about Charcot–Marie–Tooth disease is false?
Harrison's 20th Ed. Chapter 438, Page 3208

A. CMT1 and 2 are autosomal dominant
B. CMT1 is a demyelinating polyneuropathy
C. CMT2 is an axonal polyneuropathy
D. None of the above

Charcot–Marie–Tooth disease type 1 is most common inherited demyelinating sensorimotor neuropathy, followed by type 2. Both are autosomal dominant. Type 1 is a demyelinating polyneuropathy, whereas type 2 is an axonal sensory polyneuropathy.

2462. Which of the following is an autosomal recessive neuropathy?
Harrison's 20th Ed. Chapter 438, Page 3208

A. CMT1
B. CMT2
C. CMT3
D. CMT4

CMT1, CMT2 and CMT3 have autosomal dominant inheritance (with a few exceptions). CMT4 (genetically heterogenic) is an autosomal recessive neuropathy.

2463. The ratio of occurrence of CMT1:CMT2 is approximately?
Harrison's 20th Ed. Chapter 438, Page 3208

A. 1:1
B. 2:1
C. 3:1
D. 4:1

CMT1 is the most common form of hereditary neuropathy. The ratio of CMT1:CMT2 is ~2:1.

2464. CMT1 is which form of CMT?
Harrison's 20th Ed. Chapter 438, Page 3208

A. Demyelinating
B. Axonal
C. Intermediate
D. Any of the above

2465. CMT2 is which form of CMT?
Harrison's 20th Ed. Chapter 438, Page 3208

A. Demyelinating
B. Axonal
C. Intermediate
D. Any of the above

Demyelinating forms of CMT are classified as CMT1, and axonal forms as CMT2. Nerve conduction velocities (NCVs) intermediate between CMT1 & CMT2 are classified as "intermediate CMT" and most of these are X-linked.

2466. Which of the following physical finding favours diagnosis of CMT?
Harrison's 20th Ed. Chapter 438, Page 3208

A. Inverted champagne bottle appearance of legs
B. Hammer toes
C. High arched feet (pes cavus)
D. All of the above

Wasting & weakness of distal muscles of legs lead to inverted champagne bottle like appearance. Hammer toes & pes cavus are common & indicate onset of CMT in early life.

2467. Which of the following manifestation prompts suspicion of CMT1?
Harrison's 20th Ed. Chapter 438, Page 3208

A. Bed sore
B. Numbness or tingling
C. Footdrop
D. Frequent falls

CMT1 usually present in the first to third decade of life with distal leg weakness (footdrop). People with CMT generally do not complain of numbness or tingling, which helps in distinguishing CMT from acquired forms of neuropathy in which sensory symptoms usually predominate.

2468. Which of the following manifestation prompts suspicion of CMT1?
Harrison's 20th Ed. Chapter 438, Page 3208

A. Reduced sensation to all modalities
B. Reduced muscle stretch reflexes
C. Atrophy of muscles below knee
D. All of the above

In CMT1, reduced sensation to all modalities is apparent on examination. Muscle stretch reflexes are absent or reduced. Atrophy of muscles below knee (particularly anterior compartment), leads to inverted champagne bottle legs.

2469. In CMT1, characteristic nerve biopsy appearance is?
Harrison's 20th Ed. Chapter 438, Page 3208

A. Mulberry appearance
B. Cabbage appearance
C. Potato peel appearance
D. Onion bulb appearance

Nerve biopsies show evidence of repeated demyelination & remyelination. Supernumerary, concentrically arranged, Schwann cells attempting to remyelinate axons give a characteristic "onion bulb" appearance.

2470. The most common form of CMT1 is?
Harrison's 20th Ed. Chapter 438, Page 3208

A. 1A subtype
B. 2A subtype
C. 2B subtype
D. 2C subtype

CMT1A is the most common subtype of CMT1, representing 70% of cases.

2471. CMT 1A subtype is caused by?
Harrison's 20th Ed. Chapter 438, Page 3208

A. Duplication of PMP22 gene
B. Deletion in PMP22
C. Translocation in PMP22
D. All of the above

CMT1A is caused by a 1.5-megabase (Mb) duplication within peripheral myelin protein-22 (PMP-22) gene containing chromosome 17p11.2-12 resulting in patients having three copies of the PMP-22 gene rather than two.

2472. Charcot-Marie-Tooth disease (CMT) type 1B is caused by mutations in gene for?
Harrison's 20th Ed. Chapter 438, Page 3208

A. Proteolipid protein (PLP)
B. MPZ
C. Myelin oligodendrocyte glycoprotein (MOG)
D. Myelin basic protein (MBP)

CMT1B is due to a mutation in the myelin protein zero (MPZ, or P0) gene.

2473. CMT2 is caused by mutations for which gene?
Harrison's 20th Ed. Chapter 438, Page 3208

A. Alpha-galactosidase gene
B. ATP-binding cassette transporter 1 (ABC1) gene
C. Mitofusin 2 (MFN2) gene
D. Transthyretin (TTR) gene

Most common cause of CMT2 is a mutation in the gene for mitofusin 2 (MFN2) which is localized to the outer mitochondrial membrane, where it regulates the mitochondrial network architecture by fusion of mitochondria.

2474. Diagnosis of CMT is favoured by which of the following observation?
Harrison's 20th Ed. Chapter 438, Page 3208

A. Early age of onset
B. Positive family history
C. Long standing symptoms
D. All of the above

Diagnosis of CMT is favoured by an early age of onset, positive family history, and long standing symptoms. If EDx findings indicate a demyelinating process, diagnosis of CMT can be made with confidence.

2475. Which of the following is associated with pes cavus?
Harrison's 20th Ed. Chapter 438, Page 3208, 2975, 3157

A. CMT1x
B. Friedreich's ataxia
C. Plantar fasciitis
D. All of the above

Pes cavus is associated with CMT1x, Friedreich's ataxia, Nemaline myopathy, Central core disease and Plantar fasciitis.

2476. Which of the following is false about Schmidt-Lanterman incisures?
The Journal of Neuroscience. 2005;25(13):3259-3269

A. Noncompacted regions of myelin
B. Contains cytoplasm
C. Transport metabolic substances across myelin sheath
D. None of the above

Schwann cells form myelin sheath around peripheral nerve axons as either highly compacted membrane or noncompacted cytoplasmic regions (Schmidt-Lanterman incisures or SLI). SLI are important for transport of metabolic substances across myelin sheath and for metabolic maintenance & longitudinal growth of sheath.

2477. When NCV is faster than seen in CMT1 but slower than in CMT2, the condition is termed as?
Harrison's 20th Ed. Chapter 438, Page 3208

A. CMT3
B. CMT4
C. Intermediate CMT (iCMT)
D. Dominant-intermediate CMT (CMTDI)

In dominant-intermediate CMTs (CMTDIs), NCVs are faster than seen in CMT1 (>38 m/s) but slower than in CMT2.

2478. Palpably thickened nerves in CMT1 is due to increase in?
Harrison's 20th Ed. Chapter 438, Page 3208

A. Hyaline
B. Mucopolysaccharides
C. Collagen
D. Glycogen

In CMT1, increased collagen between layers of supernumerary Schwann cells leads to palpably thickened nerves.

2479. Which of the following appears in infancy & is associated with severe demyelination or hypomyelination?
Harrison's 20th Ed. Chapter 438, Page 3208

A. CMT1
B. CMT2
C. CMT3
D. CMT4

CMT3 is an autosomal dominant neuropathy that appears in infancy and is associated with severe demyelination or hypomyelination.

2480. Which of the following type of CMT have an onset later in life?
Harrison's 20th Ed. Chapter 438, Page 3208

A. CMT1
B. CMT2
C. CMT3
D. CMT4

2481. Which of the following is false about myelin?
Harrison's 20th Ed. Chapter 417 Page 3039

A. It speeds impulse conduction
B. Single oligodendrocyte ensheaths multiple CNS axons
C. Each Schwann cell myelinates a single PNS axon
D. It is a protein-rich material

Myelin is a lipid-rich material formed by a spiraling process of the membrane of myelinating cell around the axon.

2482. Pelizaeus Merzbacher disease is caused by mutations in gene for?
Harrison's 20th Ed. Chapter 429 Page 3148

A. Proteolipid protein (PLP)
B. P0 protein
C. Myelin oligodendrocyte glycoprotein (MOG)
D. Myelin basic protein (MBP)

Pelizaeus-Merzbacher syndrome is a dysmyelinating X-linked allelic disorder of CNS, caused by mutations in gene for proteolipid protein (PLP) that promotes extracellular compaction between adjacent myelin lamellae.

2483. Protein restricted to CNS myelin is which of the following?
Harrison's 19th Ed. 444e-4

A. Proteolipid protein (PLP)
B. P_0
C. PMP_{22}
D. GM_1

2484. Protein restricted to PNS myelin is which of the following?
Harrison's 19th Ed. 444e-4

A. Proteolipid protein (PLP)
B. P_0
C. Myelin oligodendrocyte glycoprotein (MOG)
D. GM_1

2485. Protein in both CNS & PNS myelin is?
Harrison's 19th Ed. 444e-4

A. Proteolipid protein (PLP)
B. P_0
C. Myelin oligodendrocyte glycoprotein (MOG)
D. GM_1

2486. DéJerine-Sottas disease is also called?
Harrison's 20th Ed. Chapter 438, Page 3208

A. CMT Type 1
B. CMT Type 2
C. CMT Type 3
D. CMT Type 4

CMT3 was originally described by Deéjerine and Sottas as a hereditary demyelinating sensorimotor polyneuropathy presenting in infancy or early childhood.

2487. DéJerine-Sottas syndrome is similar to?
Harrison's 20th Ed. Chapter 438, Page 3209 Table 438-4

A. CMT2A
B. CMT2B
C. Congenital hypomyelinating neuropathy (CHN)
D. Roussy-Levy Syndrome

DéJerine-Sottas syndrome & congenital hypomyelinating neuropathy are indistinguishable. Nerve biopsy can distinguish them.

2488. DéJerine-Sottas syndrome is caused by mutations of?
Harrison's 20th Ed. Chapter 438, Page 3208

A. PMP22
B. Myelin protein zero (MPZ)
C. Early growth response gene (ERG2)
D. All of the above

Most cases of CMT3 are caused by point mutations in the genes for PMP-22, MPZ, or ERG-2, which are also the genes responsible for CMT1.

2489. Which of the following CMT is extremely rare?
Harrison's 20th Ed. Chapter 438, Page 3208

A. CMT1
B. CMT2
C. CMT3
D. CMT4

CMT4 is extremely rare & is characterized by a severe, childhood-onset sensorimotor polyneuropathy.

2490. Gap junctions consist of membrane-spanning proteins called?
Harrison's 20th Ed. Chapter 438, Page 3210

A. Spannins
B. Membranins
C. Connexins
D. All of the above

Connexins are gap junction structural proteins that are important in cell-to-cell communication. Gap junctions provide direct neuron-neuron electrical conduction and also create openings for the diffusion of ions and metabolites between cells. Gap junctions membrane-spanning proteins, expressed by Schwann cells are connexins, that pair across adjacent cells.

2491. Mutation of which gene of gap junction protein is responsible for X-linked Charcot-Marie-Tooth disease?
Harrison's 20th Ed. Chapter 438, Page 3208

A. Connexin 26
B. Connexin 32
C. Connexin 42
D. Connexin 48

Mutations in connexin 32 are responsible for X-linked form of CMT disease (CMT1X). Mutated gene is GJB1. Connexin 32 is found in both central and peripheral nervous systems.

2492. Connexins have a role in which of the following conditions?
Harrison's 20th Ed. Chapter 438, Page 3208

A. Hereditary hearing impairment (HHI)
B. Angiogenic endothelium
C. Re-entrant cardiac arrhythmias
D. All of the above

2493. Which of the following is false about CMT1X?
Harrison's 20th Ed. Chapter 438, Page 3208, Eur J Neurol. 2015;22:406–9

A. Severe in males than in females
B. NCS shows both demyelination & axonal degeneration
C. Caused by mutations in connexin 32 gene (GJB1)
D. None of the above

Molecular genetic testing of GJB1 (Cx32) detects ~90% of cases of X-linked CMTX1. Affected males pass the abnormal gene to all of their daughters & none of their sons i.e. no male-to-male inheritance. Penetrance is complete in males with GJB1 pathogenic variants. Females who are carriers are at a 50% risk of passing the pathogenic gene to each offspring.

2494. Clinical presentation of CMTX1 can overlap with?
Harrison's 20th Ed. Chapter 438, Page 3208

A. CMT1
B. CMT2
C. Hereditary neuropathy with liability to pressure palsies
D. All of the above

2495. Which of the following is a clinical feature of CMTX1?
Harrison's 20th Ed. Chapter 438, Page 3208

A. Bilateral foot drop
B. Symmetrical atrophy of muscles below knee (stork leg appearance)
C. Absent tendon reflexes in both upper & lower extremities
D. All of the above

The typical CMTX1 affected adult has bilateral foot drop, symmetrical atrophy of muscles below knee (stork leg appearance), pes cavus, atrophy of intrinsic hand muscles, especially thenar muscles of thumb, & absent tendon reflexes in both upper & lower extremities. Proximal muscles usually remain strong. Mild to moderate sensory deficits of position, vibration & pain/temperature occur in feet.

2496. Which of the following is an X-linked disorder?
Harrison's 20th Ed. Chapter 438, Page 3210

A. CMT1X
B. Adrenomyeloneuropathy
C. Pelizeaus-Merzbacher disease
D. All of the above

2497. Cowchock syndrome relates best with?
Eur J Neurol. 2015;22:406–9

A. CMTX1
B. CMTX2
C. CMTX3
D. CMTX4

CMTX4 is also called Cowchock syndrome. It presents as peripheral neuropathy with deafness and intellectual disability.

2498. Which of the following is called tomaculous neuropathy?
J Neurol Sci 1975;25:415-418

A. DéJerine-Sottas Syndrome (DSS)
B. Hereditary neuropathy with liability to pressure palsies
C. Roussy-Levy syndrome
D. Congenital hypomyelinating neuropathy (CHN)

Autosomal dominant disorder hereditary neuropathy with liability to pressure palsies (HNPP) is also called tomaculous neuropathy. Tomaculae are sausage-shaped bodies that indicate segmental demyelination. The first published description of HNPP was in 1947 by De Jong.

2499. HNPP is an autosomal dominant disorder related to?
Harrison's 20th Ed. Chapter 438, Page 3210

A. CMT1A
B. CMT1B
C. CMT1X
D. DéJerine-Sottas Syndrome (DSS)

Hereditary neuropathy with liability to pressure palsies (HNPP) is an autosomal dominant disorder related to CMT1A.

2500. Which of the following about HNPP is false?
Harrison's 20th Ed. Chapter 438, Page 3210

A. Affected individuals have only one copy of PMP-22 gene
B. Weakness in distribution of single peripheral nerves
C. Symptoms precipitated by trivial compression of nerve
D. None of the above

CMT1A is associated with duplication in chromosome 17p11.2 resulting in an extra copy of PMP-22 gene, whereas in HNPP, affected individuals have only one copy of the PMP-22 gene.

2501. Which of the following about HNPP is false?
Harrison's 20th Ed. Chapter 438, Page 3210

A. Painless motor weakness that recovers early
B. Presence of familiar history facilitates early diagnosis
C. Molecular studies are decisive
D. None of the above

Painless acute or subacute mononeuropathy is the classical phenotype of HNPP. It presents as a focal sensory & motor neuropathy in the territory of a single nerve or brachial plexus.

2502. Which of the following have overlapping clinical features?
Harrison's 20th Ed. Chapter 438, Page 3210

A. CMT1A
B. Hereditary neuralgic amyotrophy (HNA)
C. Hereditary neuropathy with liability to pressure palsies
D. All of the above

2503. Most commonly involved nerve in HNPP is?
Harrison's 20th Ed. Chapter 438, Page 3210, Case Rep Neurol 2014;6:281–286

A. Peroneal
B. Ulnar
C. Radial
D. Median

HNPP presents as recurrent focal entrapment neuropathy (numbness & weakness) most frequently is peroneal then ulnar, radial & median nerves.

2504. Electrodiagnostic findings in HNPP include?
Harrison's 20th Ed. Chapter 438, Page 3210

A. Prolongation of distal latencies
B. Conduction block / slowing at entrapment sites
C. Short terminal latency index (TLI)
D. All of the above

2505. Hereditary neuralgic amyotrophy (HNA) is caused by mutations in?
Harrison's 20th Ed. Chapter 438, Page 3210

A. Septin 9 (SEPT9)
B. ATP-binding cassette transporter 1 (ABC1) gene
C. Mitofusin 2 (MFN2) gene
D. Transthyretin (TTR) gene

HNA is caused by mutations in septin 9 (SEPT9). Septins may be important in formation of the neuronal cytoskeleton and have a role in cell division (cytokinesis). It is also called hereditary brachial plexus neuropathy.

2506. Which of the following is best related to hereditary neuralgic amyotrophy (HNA)?
Harrison's 20th Ed. Chapter 438, Page 3210

A. Lumbosacral plexus
B. Brachial plexus
C. Charcot joints
D. Deep dermal ulcerations

HNA is an autosomal dominant disorder characterized by recurrent attacks of pain, weakness, and sensory loss in the distribution of brachial plexus. The lumbosacral plexus, lower cranial nerves, phrenic nerve, autonomic nervous system or a combination of these may also be involved. Attacks may occur in postpartum period, following surgery or at other times of stress.

2507. Symptoms of which of the following disorders can be similar to those of HNA?
Harrison's 20th Ed. Chapter 438, Page 3210

A. Congenital hypomyelinating neuropathy (CHN)
B. Parsonage-Turner syndrome (PTS)
C. Roussy-Levy syndrome
D. Fabry's disease

Parsonage-Turner syndrome (PTS) is also known as idiopathic neuralgic amyotrophy. as with HNA, PTS mainly involves the brachial plexus. Unlike HNA, PTS usually occurs in a older age group (~40 years). The distinctive facial features found in some individuals with HNA do not occur in PTS.

2508. Apart from demyelinating CMT, what else characterizes Roussy-Levy syndrome?
Harrison's 20th Ed. Chapter 438, Page 3210

A. Action tremor
B. Deafness
C. Blindness
D. Spina bifida

Roussy-Levy syndrome is a combination of demyelinating CMT with postural and action tremor.

2509. SPTLC is a key enzyme in the regulation of?
Harrison's 20th Ed. Chapter 438, Page 3164

A. Salicylamide
B. Globotriaosylceramide
C. Ceramide
D. Pyroglutamyl histidylprolinamide

Five hereditary sensory and autonomic neuropathies (HSANs) exist, designated HSAN I–V. The most important autonomic variants are HSAN I and HSAN III. HSAN I is dominantly inherited and manifests as a distal small-fiber neuropathy (burning feet syndrome) associated with sensory loss & foot ulcers. The responsible gene on chromosome 9q, is SPTLC1. SPTLC is a key enzyme in the regulation of ceramide. Cells from HSAN I patients with the mutation produce higher-than-normal levels of glucosyl ceramide. HSAN III (Riley-Day syndrome; familial dysautonomia) is an autosomal recessive disorder and is less prevalent than HSAN I. Decreased tearing, hyperhidrosis, reduced sensitivity to pain, areflexia, absent fungiform papillae on tongue, and labile BP may be present. Individuals with HSAN III have afferent baroreflex failure that causes the classic episodic abdominal crises and blood pressure surges in response to emotional stimuli. Pathologic examination of nerves reveals a loss of sympathetic, parasympathetic, and sensory neurons. The defective gene, IKBKAP, prevents normal transcription of important molecules in neural development.

2510. Riley-Day syndrome is also called?
Harrison's 20th Ed. Chapter 438, Page 3164

A. HSAN 1
B. HSAN 2
C. HSAN 3
D. HSAN 4

Hereditary sensory neuropathies (HSN) are also called hereditary sensory & autonomic neuropathies (HSANs). Out of five subtypes, HSAN 1 is most common. HSAN 3 is also called Riley-Day syndrome. Both are autonomic variants of HSAN.

2511. Hereditary sensory and autonomic neuropathy 1A (HSAN1A) is caused by mutations in?
Harrison's 20th Ed. Chapter 438, Page 3210

A. Septin 9 (SEPT9)
B. Serine palmitoyltransferase long-chain base 1 (SPTLC1)
C. Mitofusin 2 (MFN2)
D. Transthyretin (TTR)

HSAN1A is caused by mutations in serine palmitoyltransferase long-chain base 1 (SPTLC1) gene on chromosome 9q.

2512. Hereditary sensory and autonomic neuropathy III (HSAN III) is caused by mutations in?
Harrison's 20th Ed. Chapter 438, Page 3164

A. Septin 9 (SEPT9)
B. IKBKAP
C. Mitofusin 2 (MFN2)
D. Transthyretin (TTR)

The defective gene in HSAN III is IKBKAP. It prevents normal transcription of important molecules in neural development.

2513. Which of the following is a feature of HSAN1?
Harrison's 20th Ed. Chapter 438, Page 3210

A. Deep dermal ulcerations
B. Recurrent osteomyelitis
C. Gross foot and hand deformities
D. All of the above

HSAN1 is associated with degeneration of small myelinated & unmyelinated nerve fibers leading to severe loss of pain & temperature sensation, deep dermal ulcerations, recurrent osteomyelitis, Charcot joints, bone loss, gross foot and hand deformities, and amputated digits. Autonomic neuropathy is not a prominent feature.

2514. Fabry's disease is also called?
Harrison's 20th Ed. Chapter 438, Page 3210

A. Globoid cell leukodystrophy
B. Pediculus humanus corporis
C. Angiokeratoma corporis diffusum
D. Cerebrotendinous xanthomatosis

2515. Which of the following about Fabry disease is false?
Harrison's 20th Ed. Chapter 438, Page 3210

A. X-linked dominant disorder
B. Reddish-purple maculopapular lesions (Angiokeratomas)
C. Premature atherosclerosis
D. None of the above

Premature atherosclerosis (hypertension, renal failure, cardiac disease & stroke) lead to death by fifth decade of life and overshadow the neuropathy manifesting as burning or lancinating pain in hands & feet.

2516. Affected organs in Fabry disease include which of the following?
Harrison's 20th Ed. Chapter 308, Page 2146

A. Endothelium
B. Heart
C. Brain
D. All of the above

Affected organs include the vascular endothelium, heart, brain and kidneys.

2517. Classically, Fabry's disease presents in childhood in males with?
Harrison's 20th Ed. Chapter 308, Page 2146

A. Acroparesthesias
B. Angiokeratoma
C. Hypohidrosis
D. All of the above

Classically, Fabry's disease presents in childhood in males with acroparesthesias, angiokeratoma and hypohidrosis.

2518. Which of the following is related to Fabry's disease?
Harrison's 20th Ed. Chapter 308, Page 2146

A. Zebra bodies
B. Maltese cross
C. Cornea verticillata
D. All of the above

Renal biopsy reveals small clear vacuoles containing globotriaosylceramide in glomeruli, parietal and tubular epithelia. These vacuoles of electron-dense materials in parallel arrays (zebra bodies) are easily seen on electron microscopy. Urinalysis in Fabry's disease may reveal oval fat bodies and birefringent glycolipid globules under polarized light called Maltese cross.

2519. Manifestations of Fabry disease include all except?
Harrison's 20th Ed. Chapter 411, Page 3007

A. Angiokeratomas (telangiectatic skin lesions)
B. Hyperhidrosis
C. Corneal and lenticular opacities
D. Acroparesthesia

Fabry's disease manifests with angiokeratomas (telangiectatic skin lesions), hypohidrosis, corneal and lenticular opacities, acroparesthesia and small-vessel disease of kidney, heart, and brain.

2520. Angiokeratomas in Fabry's disease are best seen in?
Harrison's 20th Ed. Chapter 438, Page 3210, 3007

A. Between umbilicus and knees
B. Nape of the neck
C. Fingers of hand
D. Nose

Angiokeratomas in Fabry's disease are punctate, dark red to blue-black, flat or slightly raised, and usually symmetric. They do not blanch with pressure. They are most dense between umbilicus and knees "bathing suit area" (umbilicus, scrotum, inguinal region and perineum).

2521. Red papules like those seen in angiokeratomas of Fabry disease are seen in?
Harrison's 20th Ed. Chapter 54, Page 350, Table 54-15

A. Cutaneous polyarteritis nodosa
B. Bacillary angiomatosis
C. Lupus pernio
D. Urticaria pigmentosa

2522. Which of the following is related to Fabry disease?
Harrison's 20th Ed. Chapter 54, Page 351

A. Lattice corneal dystrophy
B. Keratoconus
C. Cornea verticillata
D. Corneal beading

Associated findings in Fabry disease include chronic renal disease, peripheral neuropathy & corneal opacities (cornea verticillata).

2523. Which of the following best relates to Fabry disease?
Harrison's 20th Ed. Chapter 411, Page 3007

A. GALA mutations
B. GBA1 mutations
C. LIPA mutations
D. GUSB mutations

Fabry disease results from mutations in GALA (cytogenetic location: Xq22.1) which encodes α-galactosidase A. The GLA gene provides instructions for making an enzyme called alpha-galactosidase A which is active in lysosomes. Alpha-galactosidase A breaks down globotriaosylceramide. Alterations in GLA gene produce an abnormal version of enzyme that is unable to break down globotriaosylceramide effectively. As a result, globotriaosylceramide builds up in body's cells, particularly cells lining blood vessels in the skin and cells in the kidneys, heart & nervous system, damaging the cells. Other names of GALA are AGAL_HUMAN, Agalsidase alfa, Alpha-D-galactosidase A, alpha-D-galactoside galactohydrolase, Alpha-galactosidase, alpha-Galactosidase A, ceramidetrihexosidase, GALA, galactosidase alpha, Melibiase.

2524. Which of the following about angiokeratomas in Fabry disease is false?
Harrison's 20th Ed. Chapter 411, Page 3007

A. Punctate, dark red to blue-black
B. Symmetric
C. Do not blanch with pressure
D. None of the above

Angiokeratomas are punctate, dark red to blue-black, flat or slightly raised, and usually symmetric; they do not blanch with pressure.

2525. Which of the following may occur in Fabry disease?
Harrison's 20th Ed. Chapter 411, Page 3007

A. Isosthenuria
B. Idiopathic hypertrophic myocardiopathy
C. Leg lymphedema without hypoproteinemia
D. All of the above

2526. Fabry disease is caused by mutations in?
Harrison's 20th Ed. Chapter 308, Page 2146

A. Alpha-galactosidase A gene
B. ATP-binding cassette transporter 1 (ABC1) gene
C. Mitofusin 2 (MFN2) gene
D. Transthyretin (TTR) gene

Fabry's disease is an X-linked inborn error of globotriaosylceramide metabolism secondary to deficient lysosomal α-galactosidase A activity, resulting in excessive intracellular storage of globotriaosylceramide.

2527. Accumulation in nerves and blood vessels of which of the following occurs Fabry disease?
Harrison's 20th Ed. Chapter 411, Page 3007

A. Aspartyl glucosamine
B. Galactosylsphingosine
C. Ceramide trihexoside (Globotriaosylceramide)
D. Glycogen

Fabry disease is caused by mutations in alpha-galactosidase A gene that leads to accumulation of ceramide trihexoside in nerves and blood vessels. Fabry's disease is an X-linked inborn error of globotriaosylceramide metabolism secondary to deficient lysosomal α-galactosidase A activity resulting in excessive intracellular storage of globotriaosylceramide.

2528. Accessory pathways (APs) are associated with which of the following?
Harrison's 20th Ed. Chapter 244, Page 1739

A. Ebstein's anomaly
B. Danon's disease
C. Fabry's disease
D. All of the above

Accessory pathways (APs) are associated with Ebstein's anomaly of tricuspid valve & forms of hypertrophic cardiomyopathy including PRKAG2 mutations, Danon's disease and Fabry's disease. APs are associated with various arrhythmias including narrow-complex PSVT, wide-complex tachycardias & sudden death.

2529. Which of the following is a heritable form of CKD?
Harrison's 20th Ed. Chapter 305, Page 2119

A. Alport disease
B. Fabry disease
C. Cystinosis
D. All of the above

Heritable form of CKD are Alport or Fabry disease, cystinosis.

2530. Which of the following is a lysosomal storage disease?
Harrison's 20th Ed. Chapter 411, Page 3003

A. Tay-Sachs disease
B. Pompe disease
C. Fabry disease
D. All of the above

There are more than 50 different lysosomal storage diseases (LSDs), classified according to the nature of the stored material. These include Tay-Sachs disease, Fabry disease, Gaucher disease, Niemann-Pick disease, lysosomal acid lipase deficiencies, the mucopolysaccharidoses and Pompe disease.

2531. Which of the following lysosomal storage diseases is X-linked?
Harrison's 20th Ed. Chapter 411, Page 3004 Table 411-1

A. Hunter (mucopolysaccharidosis type II) disease
B. Danon disease
C. Fabry disease
D. All of the above

All LSDs are inherited as autosomal recessive disorders except for Hunter (mucopolysaccharidosis type II), Danon and Fabry diseases, which are X-linked.

2532. Footdrop is a prominent feature of?
Harrison's 20th Ed. Chapter 438, Page 3210

A. Facioscapulohumeral muscular dystrophy (FSH)
B. Peroneal neuropathy
C. CMT1
D. All of the above

Footdrop is a prominent feature of Refsum disease, myotonic dystrophy type 1 (DM1), Facioscapulohumeral muscular dystrophy (FSH), Type 1 lepra reaction, Udd, and Markesbery-Griggs type distal myopathies.

2533. Adrenoleukodystrophy (ALD) & adrenomyeloneuropathy (AMN) are caused by mutations in?
Harrison's 20th Ed. Chapter 438, Page 3211

A. Alpha-galactosidase A gene
B. ATP-binding cassette transporter 1 (ABC1) gene
C. Mitofusin 2 (MFN2) gene
D. Transthyretin (TTR) gene

2534. Level in urine of very long chain fatty acid (VLCFA) is increased in which of the following?
Harrison's 20th Ed. Chapter 438, Page 3211

A. Fabry's disease
B. Refsum disease
C. Adrenoleukodystrophy & adrenomyeloneuropathy
D. All of the above

Very long chain fatty acid (VLCFA) levels (C24, C25 and C26) are increased in the urine of patients of Adrenoleukodystrophy (ALD) & adrenomyeloneuropathy (AMN). Demonstration of increased plasma VLCFA such as hexacosanoic acid (C26:0) levels is the most frequently used diagnostic assay.

2535. Which of the following is a major phenotype of adrenoleukodystrophy (ALD)?
Arch Neurol. 2005;62(7):1073-1080

A. Rapidly progressive cerebral ALD (CERALD)
B. Adrenomyeloneuropathy (AMN)
C. Addison-only phenotype
D. All of the above

There are 4 major phenotypes of ALD: (1) rapidly progressive cerebral ALD (CERALD) phenotypes, which are most common in childhood and are associated with inflammatory demyelination; (2) adrenomyeloneuropathy (AMN), a slowly progressive noninflammatory distal axonopathy that involves the spinal cord long tracts; (3) Addison-only phenotype of primary adrenocortical insufficiency without demonstrable neurological deficit; and (4) asymptomatic status without clinically evident neurological or endocrine abnormality.

2536. Which of the following represents Lorenzo's oil (LO)?
Arch Neurol. 2005;62(7):1073-1080

- A. 1-O-alkyl-2-acyl-sn-glyceryl-3-phosphorylcholine
- B. 4:1 glyceryl trioleate - glyceryl trierucate
- C. Acyl-monoserine lactone
- D. None of the above

2537. Lorenzo's Oil contains?
N Engl J Med. 1993;328:1126-1127

- A. 20% erucic acid and 80% oleic acid
- B. 40% erucic acid and 60% oleic acid
- C. 50% erucic acid and 50% oleic acid
- D. 80% erucic acid and 20% oleic acid

Lorenzo's Oil contains 20 percent erucic acid (22:1) and 80 percent oleic acid (18:1).

2538. VLCFA levels are increased in?
Ann Neurol. 1999;45:100-110

- A. Zellweger syndrome (cerebrohepatorenal syndrome)
- B. Neonatal adrenoleukodystrophy
- C. Infantile Refsum's disease
- D. All of the above

VLCFA levels are increased in patients homozygous for Zellweger syndrome (cerebrohepatorenal syndrome), neonatal adrenoleukodystrophy, infantile Refsum's disease, and in patients with deficiencies of peroxisomal acyl-coenzyme A oxidase, bifunctional enzyme, and 3-oxoacyl-coenzyme A thiolase.

2539. Diets supplemented with Lorenzo's oil is of use in which of the following?
Harrison's 20th Ed. Chapter 438, Page 3211

- A. Fabry's disease
- B. Refsum disease
- C. Adrenoleukodystrophy & adrenomyeloneuropathy
- D. All of the above

Diets low in VLCFAs and supplemented with Lorenzo's oil (erucic & oleic acids) reduce levels of VLCFAs and increase the levels of C22 in serum, fibroblasts and liver.

2540. Refsum disease is caused by accumulation of which of the following in the central & peripheral nervous systems?
Harrison's 20th Ed. Chapter 438, Page 3211

- A. Formic acid
- B. Glycolic acid
- C. Oxalic acid
- D. Phytanic acid

Refsum disease (autosomal recessive) is caused by mutations in the gene that encodes for phytanoyl-CoA alpha-hydroxylase (PAHX). This mutations lead to elevation of serum phytanic acid levels and accumulation of phytanic acid in central and peripheral nervous systems. Refsum disease is treated by removing phytanic precursors (phytols: fish oils, dairy products, and ruminant fats) from diet.

2541. The classic tetrad of Refsum disease include all except?
Harrison's 20th Ed. Chapter 438, Page 3211

- A. Peripheral neuropathy
- B. Retinitis pigmentosa
- C. Cerebellar ataxia
- D. Normal CSF protein concentration

The classic tetrad of Refsum disease include peripheral neuropathy, retinitis pigmentosa, cerebellar ataxia, and elevated CSF protein concentration.

2542. Presentation of Refsum disease include?
Harrison's 20th Ed. Chapter 438, Page 3211

- A. Anosmia
- B. Sensorineural deafness
- C. Ichthyosis
- D. All of the above

Features of Refsum disease include sensorimotor demyelinating neuropathy, sensorineural deafness, cerebellar ataxia, anosmia, retinitis pigmentosa, ichthyosis, syndactyly, shortening of the fourth toe, cardiac conduction abnormalities, cardiomyopathy and cataracts.

2543. Retinitis pigmentosa occurs in association with which of the following diseases?
Harrison's 20th Ed. Chapter 28, Page 188

- A. Olivopontocerebellar degeneration
- B. Bassen-Kornzweig disease
- C. Bardet-Biedl syndrome
- D. All of the above

Retinitis pigmentosa occur in association with rare hereditary systemic diseases like olivopontocerebellar degeneration, Bassen-Kornzweig disease, Kearns-Sayre syndrome, Bardet-Biedl syndrome, Refsum's disease, Cranioectodermal dysplasia (Sensenbrenner syndrome), Senior-Loken syndrome, Leigh disease, NARP (neuropathy, ataxia, and retinitis pigmentosa), Usher's syndrome (retinitis pigmentosa and hearing loss), abetalipoproteinemia.

2544. Severe deficiency of which of the following occurs in Tangier Disease (TD)?
Harrison's 20th Ed. Chapter 438, Page 3211

- A. High-density lipoproteins (HDL)
- B. Low-density lipoproteins (HDL)
- C. Very low-density lipoproteins (HDL)
- D. Triglycerides

Tangier disease is caused by mutations in the ATP-binding cassette transporter 1 (ABC1) gene, which leads to markedly reduced levels of high-density lipoprotein (HDL) cholesterol levels while triacylglycerol levels are increased.

2545. Presentation of Tangier disease resembles those of?
Harrison's 20th Ed. Chapter 438, Page 3211

- A. Guillain-Barré syndrome
- B. Syringomyelia
- C. Multiple sclerosis
- D. Amyotrophic lateral sclerosis

Tangier disease is a rare autosomal recessive disorder that can present as asymmetric multiple mononeuropathies, slowly progressive symmetric polyneuropathy predominantly in legs, and a pseudo-syringomyelia pattern with dissociated sensory loss (i.e. abnormal pain/temperature perception but preserved position/vibration in the arms.

2546. Which of the following is characteristic of Tangier disease?
Harrison's 20th Ed. Chapter 234, Page 1667, 2899

- A. Orange tonsils
- B. Howship's lacunae
- C. Lenticonus
- D. Strawberry gums

2547. Which of the following about Tangier disease is false?
Harrison's 20th Ed. Chapter 400, Page 2899

- A. Very low levels of HDL-C
- B. Low plasma levels of LDL-C
- C. Low plasma levels of apoA-I
- D. All of the above

2548. Which of the following forms of porphyria are associated with peripheral neuropathy?
Harrison's 20th Ed. Chapter 438, Page 3211

A. Acute intermittent porphyria (AIP)
B. Hereditary coproporphyria (HCP)
C. Variegate porphyria (VP)
D. All of the above

Three forms of porphyria are associated with peripheral neuropathy - acute intermittent porphyria (AIP), hereditary coproporphyria (HCP), and variegate porphyria (VP).

2549. Photosensitive rash is not seen with which of the following porphyrias?
Harrison's 20th Ed. Chapter 438, Page 3211

A. Acute intermittent porphyria (AIP)
B. Hereditary coproporphyria (HCP)
C. Variegate porphyria (VP)
D. All of the above

A photosensitive rash is seen with HCP and VP but not in AIP.

2550. Which of the following tests is useful in porphyria?
Harrison's 20th Ed. Chapter 438, Page 3211

A. Increased urinary excretion of aminolevulinic acid
B. Increased urinary excretion of porphobilinogen
C. Increased urinary excretion of coproporphyrinogen
D. All of the above

Accumulation of intermediary precursors of heme like d-aminolevulinic acid, porphobilinogen, uroporphobilinogen, coproporphyrinogen and protoporphyrinogen is found in urine of patients of porphyria.

2551. Which of the following is decreased in axonal degeneration in motor nerve conduction studies?
Harrison's 20th Ed. Chapter 438, Page 3211

A. F wave
B. Conduction velocity
C. CMAP amplitude
D. Distal latency

The primary abnormalities on EDx are marked reductions in compound motor action potential (CMAP) amplitudes and signs of active axonal degeneration on needle EMG.

2552. Mutations in which of the following genes is responsible for familial amyloid neuropathy?
Harrison's 20th Ed. Chapter 438, Page 3212

A. Transthyretin (FAP 1 & 2)
B. Apolipoprotein A1 (FAP 3)
C. Gelsolin
D. All of the above

Familial amyloid polyneuropathy (FAP) is phenotypically and genetically heterogeneous and is caused by mutations in the genes for transthyretin (TTR), apolipoprotein A1, or gelsolin. The majority of patients with FAP have mutations in the TTR gene.

2553. Which of the following modalities halts disease progression in familial amyloid neuropathy (FAP)?
Harrison's 20th Ed. Chapter 438, Page 3212

A. Plasmapheresis
B. Liver transplantation
C. Kidney transplantation
D. IVIg

Because the liver produces much of the body's TTR, liver transplantation has been used to treat FAP related to TTR mutations. Liver transplantation halts disease progression of FAP.

2554. Which of the following about TTR-related FAP is false?
Harrison's 20th Ed. Chapter 438, Page 3212

A. Carpal tunnel syndrome (CTS) is common
B. Autonomic involvement can be severe
C. Liver transplantation beneficial
D. None of the above

2555. Which of the following about Gelsolin-related amyloidosis (Finnish type) is false?
Harrison's 20th Ed. Chapter 438, Page 3212

A. Lattice corneal dystrophy
B. Multiple cranial neuropathies
C. Autonomic dysfunction does not occur
D. None of the above

2556. Which of the following drugs is beneficial in familial amyloid neuropathy (FAP)?
Harrison's 20th Ed. Chapter 438, Page 3212

A. Paroxetine
B. Nacetyl cysteine
C. Epigallocatechin gallate
D. Tafamidis meglumine

Tafamidis meglumine & diflunisal which prevent misfolding & deposition of mutated TTR, appear to slow the rate of deterioration patients with TTR-related FAP.

2557. AL amyloidosis occurs in?
Harrison's 20th Ed. Chapter 438, Page 3212

A. Multiple myeloma (MM)
B. Waldenström's macroglobulinemia
C. Lymphoma
D. All of the above

AL amyloidosis occurs with multiple myeloma (MM), Waldenström's macroglobulinemia, lymphoma, other plasmacytomas, or lymphoproliferative disorders, or idiopathic.

2558. Presence of which of the following is a risk factors for diabetic neuropathy?
Harrison's 20th Ed. Chapter 438, Page 3212

A. Long-standing, poorly controlled DM
B. Presence of retinopathy
C. Presence of nephropathy
D. All of the above

Risk factors for the development of diabetic neuropathy include long-standing, poorly controlled DM and presence of retinopathy & nephropathy.

2559. Which of the following is the most common form of diabetic neuropathy?
Harrison's 20th Ed. Chapter 438, Page 3212

A. Diabetic truncal radiculoneuropathy (DTRN)
B. Diabetic lumbosacral radiculoplexus neuropathy
C. Oculomotor (III or VI nerve) neuropathy
D. Diabetic sensorimotor polyneuropathy (DSPN)

Diabetic Distal Symmetric Sensory and Sensorimotor Polyneuropathy (DSPN) is the most common form of diabetic neuropathy. Other types of polyneuropathy include autonomic neuropathy, diabetic neuropathic cachexia, polyradiculoneuropathies, cranial neuropathies & other mononeuropathies.

2560. Sensory loss in DSPN begins in?
Harrison's 20th Ed. Chapter 438, Page 3212

A. Nose
B. Fingers
C. Toes
D. Buttocks

DSPN manifests as sensory loss beginning in the toes that gradually progresses over time up the legs and into the fingers and arms.

2561. Which of the following nerves are involved in diabetic sensorimotor polyneuropathy (DSPN)?
Harrison's 20th Ed. Chapter 438, Page 3212

A. Small- and large-fiber sensory
B. Autonomic
C. Motor
D. All of the above

DSPN is a mixed neuropathy with small- & large-fiber sensory, autonomic, & motor nerve involvement in various combinations. Sensory & autonomic symptoms are more prominent than motor.

2562. Which of the following has relevance in the pathogenesis of diabetic sensorimotor polyneuropathy (DSPN)?
Diabetes. 1983;32(11):988-992

A. Myo-inositol
B. Betaine
C. Glutamine
D. All of the above

DSPN could be caused by an increased neuronal glucose conversion to sorbitol by aldose reductase using NADPH as a coenzyme. Sorbitol decreases levels of myo-inositol and phosphoinositides, leading to a decrease in diacylglycerol, protein kinase C, and Na+, K+, ATPase activity. This sequence of events leads to axonal loss & demyelination.

2563. Diabetic autonomic neuropathy is typically seen in combination with?
Harrison's 20th Ed. Chapter 438, Page 3212

A. DSPN
B. Diabetic neuropathic cachexia
C. Polyradiculoneuropathies
D. Cranial neuropathies

Autonomic neuropathy is typically seen in combination with DSPN.

2564. Initial presentation in diabetic amyotrophy or Bruns-Garland Syndrome is?
Harrison's 20th Ed. Chapter 438, Page 3212

A. Pain
B. Sensory loss
C. Muscle weakness
D. Diplopia

Typically, patients of diabetic radiculoplexus neuropathy present with severe pain in low back, hip, and thigh in one leg. Atrophy & weakness of proximal & distal muscles in the affected leg become apparent within a few days or weeks. Neuropathy is often accompanied by severe weight loss.

2565. Asymmetric abrupt-onset diabetic neuropathy is?
Harrison's 20th Ed. Chapter 438, Page 3212

A. Diabetic truncal radiculoneuropathy (DTRN)
B. Diabetic lumbosacral radiculoplexus neuropathy
C. Cranial neuropathy
D. All of the above

Asymmetric abrupt-onset diabetic neuropathies include diabetic truncal radiculoneuropathy (DTRN), diabetic lumbosacral radiculoplexus neuropathy (DLSRPN) & oculomotor (III or VI nerve) neuropathy.

2566. Which is the most frequently involved cranial nerve in diabetes?
Harrison's 20th Ed. Chapter 438, Page 3212

A. III
B. IV
C. VI
D. VII

In regard to cranial mononeuropathies, a seventh nerve palsy is most common, followed by third nerve, sixth nerve, and, less frequently, fourth nerve palsies.

2567. Which of the following is not a feature of diabetic third nerve palsy?
Harrison's 20th Ed. Chapter 438, Page 3212

A. Abrupt in onset
B. Intense retro-orbital pain
C. Bilateral ptosis
D. Restriction of medial gaze & upgaze

Diabetic III nerve palsy is abrupt in onset, heralded by intense retro-orbital pain, double vision, unilateral ptosis & restriction of medial gaze & upgaze.

2568. Which of the following is not a feature of diabetic third nerve palsy?
Harrison's 20th Ed. Chapter 438, Page 3212

A. Abrupt in onset
B. Intense retro-orbital pain
C. Dilated pupil
D. Improve spontaneously in 3–6 months

Pupil is nearly always spared in diabetic III nerve palsy as pupillomotor fibers are present on the outer layers of III nerve fascicle, and an ischemic lesion tends to involve the center of the fascicle. Thus, diabetic third nerve palsies are characteristically pupil-sparing.

2569. Trigeminal neuropathy occurs in which of the following illnesses?
Harrison's 20th Ed. Chapter 433, Page 2556, 3168

A. Systemic sclerosis (Scleroderma)
B. Sjögren syndrome
C. Leprosy
D. All of the above

In Systemic sclerosis (SSc), the central nervous system is generally spared, sensory trigeminal neuropathy due to fibrosis or vasculopathy can occur. Other causes include Sjögren syndrome, systemic lupus erythematosus, mixed connective tissue disease, herpes zoster (acute or postherpetic) and leprosy.

2570. Which of the following is related to insulin treatment for diabetes?
Curr Diabetes Rev. 2013 9(3):267-74

A. Diabetic truncal radiculoneuropathy
B. Diabetic amyotrophy
C. Insulin neuritis
D. All of the above

Insulin neuritis or "treatment induced neuropathy" is a reversible painful neuropathy seen with initiation of insulin treatment for diabetes.

2571. Which of the following about diabetic neuropathic cachexia is false?
Curr Diabetes Rev. 2013 9(3):267-74

A. Unintentional weight loss
B. Acute symmetrical painful peripheral neuropathy, no weakness
C. Burning pain in lower limbs & allodynia
D. None of the above

"Diabetic neuropathic cachexia" is a rare disorder associated with poor diabetic control that presents with large amounts of unintentional weight loss associated with an acute symmetrical painful peripheral neuropathy without weakness. Pain is characteristically burning in nature with predominant lower limb involvement and allodynia.

2572. Which of the following is a finding in Sjögren's syndrome?
Harrison's 20th Ed. Chapter 438, Page 3213

A. Sicca complex of xerophthalmia & xerostomia
B. Length-dependent axonal sensorimotor neuropathy
C. Trigeminal neuropathy
D. All of the above

Sjögren's syndrome is characterized by sicca complex of xerophthalmia, xerostomia & dryness of other mucous membranes, length-dependent axonal sensorimotor neuropathy, small-fiber neuropathy, trigeminal neuropathy, or sensory neuronopathy/ganglionopathy.

2573. Which of the following causes vasculitic neuropathy?
Harrison's 20th Ed. Chapter 438, Page 3213

A. Polyarteritis nodosa (PAN)
B. Churg-Strauss syndrome (CSS)
C. Rheumatoid arthritis
D. All of the above

Diagnosis of suspected vasculitic neuropathy is made by a combined nerve & muscle biopsy, with serial section or skip-serial techniques.

2574. Which of the following causes necrotizing vasculitis?
Harrison's 20th Ed. Chapter 438, Page 3213

A. Extrapulmonary pneumocystosis
B. Eosinophilic granulomatosis with polyangiitis (EGPA)
C. Malignant hypertension
D. All of the above

2575. Which of the following causes small-vessel venulitis isolated to the skin?
Harrison's 20th Ed. Chapter 456, Page 2589

A. Systemic lupus erythematosus
B. Rheumatoid arthritis
C. Sjögren's syndrome
D. All of the above

Systemic lupus erythematosus, rheumatoid arthritis, inflammatory myositis, relapsing polychondritis, and Sjögren's syndrome cause small-vessel venulitis isolated to the skin.

2576. In sarcoidosis, most common cranial nerve involved is?
Harrison's 20th Ed. Chapter 438, Page 3214

A. Third nerve
B. Fifth nerve
C. Seventh nerve
D. Twelfth nerve

In sarcoidosis, most common cranial nerve involved is seventh nerve, which can be affected bilaterally.

2577. In celiac disease, which of the neurologic finding may be present?
Harrison's 20th Ed. Chapter 438, Page 3214

A. Ataxia
B. Peripheral neuropathy
C. Neuromyotonia
D. All of the above

In celiac disease, various neurologic complications including ataxia, generalized sensorimotor polyneuropathy, pure motor neuropathy, multiple mononeuropathies, autonomic neuropathy, small-fiber neuropathy, and neuromyotonia have been reported.

2578. Which of the following drugs can cause peripheral neuropathy?
Harrison's 20th Ed. Chapter 438, Page 3214

A. Tumor necrosis blockers
B. Leflunomide
C. Metronidazole
D. All of the above

2579. Which of the following can complicate arteriovenous shunts created in arm for dialysis?
Harrison's 20th Ed. Chapter 438, Page 3214

A. Lymphedema
B. Ischemic monomelic neuropathy
C. Steal syndrome
D. All of the above

The most important complications of fistulae for HD are lymphedema, infection, aneurysm, stenosis, congestive heart failure, steal syndrome, ischemic neuropathy and thrombosis.

2580. Weakness developing in critically ill patients while in ICU is caused by?
Harrison's 20th Ed. Chapter 438, Page 3214

A. Critical illness polyneuropathy (CIP)
B. Critical illness myopathy (CIM)
C. Prolonged neuromuscular blockade
D. Any of the above

Most common causes of acute generalized weakness leading to admission to medical ICU are GBS & myasthenia gravis. Weakness that develops in critically ill patients while in ICU is caused by critical illness polyneuropathy (CIP) or critical illness myopathy (CIM) or by prolonged neuromuscular blockade.

2581. Neurologic finding in a case of critical illness polyneuropathy (CIP) include?
Harrison's 20th Ed. Chapter 301, Page 2083

A. Diffuse weakness, decreased reflexes
B. Distal sensory loss
C. Electrophysiologic studies show axonal degeneration
D. All of the above

2582. Carpal tunnel syndrome can be a presentation of which of the following illnesses?
Harrison's 20th Ed. Chapter 438, Page 3214

A. Familial amyloid polyneuropathy (FAP)
B. Hypothyroidism
C. Uremic neuropathy
D. All of the above

2583. Clinical presentation can mimic Guillain-Barré syndrome in?
N Engl J Med. 2012;366:2294-304

A. Porphyria
B. Sarcoidosis
C. Arsenic neuropathy
D. All of the above

2584. Acute, severe sensorimotor polyneuropathy can resemble Guillain-Barré syndrome in?
N Engl J Med. 2012;366:2294-304

A. Nitrofurantoin
B. Inflammatory bowel disease
C. Uremic neuropathy
D. All of the above

2585. Mycobacterium leprae causes?
Harrison's 20th Ed. Chapter 438, Page 3214

A. Mononeuropathy
B. Mononeuropathy multiplex
C. Polyneuropathy
D. Plexopathy

M. leprae causes mononeuropathy multiplex affecting peripheral nerves in cooler regions of body.

2586. Peripheral nerves are affected in which type of leprosy?
Harrison's 20th Ed. Chapter 438, Page 3214

A. Tuberculoid
B. Lepromatous
C. Borderline
D. All of the above

Peripheral nerves may be affected in all three types of leprosy. Neuropathies are most common in patients with borderline leprosy.

2587. In leprosy, sensory loss does not occur in all except?
Harrison's 20th Ed. Chapter 116, Page 869

A. Groin
B. Axilla
C. Pinnae of ears
D. Scalp

In leprosy, sensory loss spares midline of trunk anteriorly, groin, axilla & scalp - the warmer regions of the body.

2588. Which of the following cranial nerves is involved in leprosy?
Harrison's 20th Ed. Chapter 438, Page 3214

A. III
B. V
C. VI
D. XI

V & VII cranial nerves, greater auricular nerve in neck, median & ulnar nerves, and peroneal nerves are involved in leprosy.

2589. Lyme disease is caused by?
Harrison's 20th Ed. Chapter 438, Page 3215

A. Borrelia recurrentis
B. Borrelia burgdorferi
C. Borrelia hermsii
D. Borrelia turicatae

Lyme disease is caused by infection with Borrelia burgdorferi, a spirochete usually transmitted by the deer tick Ixodes dammini.

2590. Which of the following about Lyme disease is false?
Harrison's 20th Ed. Chapter 438, Page 3215

A. Facial neuropathy is common
B. Asymmetric polyradiculoneuropathy or multiple mononeuropathies
C. EDx is suggestive of a primary axonopathy
D. None of the above

2591. Diphtheritic neuropathy develops how many months after the initial infection?
Harrison's 20th Ed. Chapter 438, Page 3215

A. 1 or 2 months
B. 2 or 3 months
C. 3 or 4 months
D. 4 or 5 months

A generalized polyneuropathy may manifest 2 or 3 months following the initial diphtheritic infection. Early treatment with antitoxin and antibiotics does not alter natural history of associated peripheral neuropathy which resolves after several months.

2592. HIV-infected individuals develop a neuropathy due to?
Harrison's 20th Ed. Chapter 438, Page 3215

A. Direct result of the virus itself
B. Other associated viral infections (CMV)
C. Neurotoxicity secondary to antiviral medications
D. All of the above

2593. Which of the following is the presentation of nerve involvement in HIV infection?
Harrison's 20th Ed. Chapter 438, Page 3215

A. Polyradiculopathy
B. Distal symmetric polyneuropathy (DSP)
C. Inflammatory demyelinating polyneuropathy
D. Any of the above

Major presentations of peripheral neuropathy associated with HIV infection include distal symmetric polyneuropathy (DSP), inflammatory demyelinating polyneuropathy (GBS & CIDP), multiple mononeuropathies (vasculitis, CMV-related), polyradiculopathy (CMV-related), autonomic neuropathy, and sensory ganglionitis.

2594. Most common form of peripheral neuropathy associated with HIV infection is?
Harrison's 20th Ed. Chapter 438, Page 3215

A. Distal symmetric polyneuropathy (DSP)
B. Inflammatory demyelinating polyneuropathy
C. Autonomic neuropathy
D. Sensory ganglionitis

DSP is the most common form of peripheral neuropathy associated with HIV infection and usually is seen in patients with AIDS.

2595. Which of the following Anti-HIV drug is neurotoxic & causes a painful sensory neuropathy?
Harrison's 20th Ed. Chapter 438, Page 3215

A. Dideoxycytidine
B. Dideoxyinosine
C. Stavudine
D. All of the above

2596. Anti-HIV drug not associated with neuropathy is?
Harrison's 20th Ed. Chapter 438, Page 3215

A. Zidovudine
B. Lamivudine
C. Abacavir
D. All of the above

Zidovudine, lamivudine and abacavir are not associated with neuropathy. Dideoxycytidine, dideoxyinosine & stavudine are neurotoxic and can cause a painful sensory neuropathy.

2597. Which of the following neuropathy usually develops at the time of seroconversion in HIV infection?
Harrison's 20th Ed. Chapter 438, Page 3215

A. HIV-associated polyradiculoneuropathy
B. Acute inflammatory demyelinating polyneuropathy (AIDP)
C. Chronic inflammatory demyelinating polyneuropathy (CIDP)
D. HIV-related multiple mononeuropathies

Acute inflammatory demyelinating polyneuropathy (AIDP) usually develops at the time of seroconversion, whereas CIDP can occur any time in the course of the HIV infection.

2598. Lumbosacral polyradiculopathy in patients with AIDS is due to?
Harrison's 20th Ed. Chapter 438, Page 3215

A. Herpes zoster
B. CMV infection
C. Tuberculosis
D. Lymphoma

Lumbosacral polyradiculopathies are usually due to CMV infection in patients with AIDS.

2599. Which of the following can be caused by HIV infection?
Harrison's 20th Ed. Chapter 438, Page 3215

A. Distal symmetric polyneuropathy (DSP)
B. Inflammatory demyelinating polyradiculoneuropathy
C. Progressive polyradiculopathy
D. All of the above

2600. Which of the following can be caused by HIV infection?
Harrison's 20th Ed. Chapter 438, Page 3215

A. Multiple mononeuropathies
B. Inflammatory demyelinating polyradiculoneuropathy
C. Sensory neuronopathy/ganglionopathy
D. All of the above

2601. Which of the following about peripheral neuropathy due to herpes varicella-zoster (HVZ) infection is false?
Harrison's 20th Ed. Chapter 438, Page 3215

A. Due to reactivation of latent virus
B. Due to a primary infection
C. 25% of affected patients have postherpetic neuralgia (PHN)
D. HVZ vaccine recipients has no effect on PHN

Postherpetic neuralgia (PHN) is reduced by 67% in those who have received HVZ vaccine.

2602. Most common malignancy causing neuropathies is?
Harrison's 20th Ed. Chapter 438, Page 3215

A. Lung cancer
B. Carcinoma breast
C. Carcinoma ovary
D. Carcinoma stomach

Most common malignancy causing neuropathy is lung cancer. Neuropathies also complicate carcinoma of breast, ovaries, stomach, colon, rectum.

2603. Paraneoplastic encephalomyelitis/sensory neuronopathy (PEM/SN) usually complicates which of the following malignancies?
Harrison's 20th Ed. Chapter 438, Page 3216

A. Small cell lung carcinoma
B. Carcinoma breast
C. Carcinoma ovary
D. Carcinoma stomach

Paraneoplastic encephalomyelitis/sensory neuronopathy (PEM/SN) usually complicates small cell lung carcinoma.

2604. Autoantigen found in sera / CSF of patients with paraneoplastic PEM/SN is?
Harrison's 20th Ed. Chapter 438, Page 3216

A. Amphiphysin
B. Hu protein
C. Gephyrin
D. Cyclin B1

Polyclonal antineuronal antibodies (IgG) directed against Hu antigen are found in sera or CSF in the majority of patients with paraneoplastic PEM/SN.

2605. Which of the following is beneficial in PEM/SN?
Harrison's 20th Ed. Chapter 438, Page 3216

A. Plasmapheresis
B. Intravenous immunoglobulin
C. Immunosuppressive agents
D. None of the above

Treatment of the underlying cancer generally does not affect the course of PEM/SN. However, occasional patients may improve following treatment of the tumor.

2606. Which of the following is a potentially neurotoxic drug?
Harrison's 20th Ed. Chapter 438, Page 3216

A. Isoniazid
B. Disulfiram
C. Pyridoxine
D. All of the above

Nitrofurantoin, isoniazid, disulfiram and pyridoxine are potentially neurotoxic drugs. They cause a sensory greater than motor length-dependent axonal neuropathy or neuronopathy/ganglionopathy.

2607. What dose of Chloroquine causes neuromyopathy?
Harrison's 20th Ed. Chapter 438, Page 3216

A. 500 mg/day for one year
B. 1000 mg/day for one year
C. 500 mg/day for two years
D. 1000 mg/day for two years

Signs & symptoms of chloroquine neuropathy & myopathy are reversible with its discontinuation.

2608. Which of the following can cause neuromyopathy similar to chloroquine & hydroxychloroquine?
Harrison's 20th Ed. Chapter 438, Page 3216

A. Amiodarone
B. Thalidomide
C. Colchicine
D. All of the above

Amiodarone neuromyopathy, similar to chloroquine & hydroxychloroquine neuromyopathy, typically appears after patients have taken Amiodarone for 2–3 years. Inclusions in muscle & nerve biopsies may persist for ~2 years following discontinuation of Amiodarone.

2609. Thalidomide is used to treat?
Harrison's 20th Ed. Chapter 438, Page 3217

- A. Multiple myeloma (MM)
- B. GVHD
- C. Leprosy
- D. All of the above

Thalidomide is an immunomodulating agent used to treat MM, GVHD & leprosy.

2610. What dose of Pyridoxine (Vitamin B6) can cause toxicity?
Harrison's 20th Ed. Chapter 438, Page 3217

- A. 100 mg/day
- B. 106 mg/day
- C. 110 mg/day
- D. 116 mg/day

At high doses of Pyridoxine (116 mg/day), patients can develop a severe sensory neuropathy with dysesthesias and sensory ataxia.

2611. Toxic effects of which of the following drugs continue even after stopping the drug?
Harrison's 20th Ed. Chapter 438, Page 3217

- A. Chloroquine
- B. Hydroxychloroquine
- C. Thalidomide
- D. All of the above

Even after stopping Thalidomide for 4–6 years, ~50% patients continue to have significant symptoms.

2612. Which of the following is inhibited by isoniazid (INH) resulting in pyridoxine deficiency and neuropathy?
Harrison's 20th Ed. Chapter 438, Page 3217

- A. Pyridoxal phosphate
- B. Pyridoxal 5'-phosphate
- C. Pyridoxal kinase
- D. Pyridoxal phosphokinase

INH inhibits pyridoxal phosphokinase, resulting in pyridoxine deficiency and consequent neuropathy. Prophylactic administration of pyridoxine 100 mg/day can prevent this neuropathy. Pyridoxine (Vitamin B6) refers to a family of compounds that include pyridoxine, pyridoxal, pyridoxamine, and their 5'-phosphate derivatives.

2613. Coasting effect refers to?
Harrison's 20th Ed. Chapter 438, Page 3219

- A. Response to drug varies is same patient
- B. Drug effect amplified by addition of another drug
- C. Drug effect reduced by addition of another drug
- D. Adverse effects of drug continue even after stopping medication

Severity of neuropathy increases with duration of treatment & progression stops once drug treatment is completed. Platinum compounds are an exception where sensory loss may progress for several months after cessation of treatment - The coasting effect.

2614. Which of the following about hexacarbons is false?
Harrison's 20th Ed. Chapter 438, Page 3219

- A. n-Hexane and methyl n-butyl ketone
- B. Water-insoluble industrial organic solvent
- C. Leads to covalent cross-linking between axonal neurofilaments
- D. None of the above

2615. Most common presentation of lead poisoning is?
Harrison's 20th Ed. Chapter 438, Page 3219

- A. Sensory neuropathy
- B. Motor neuropathy
- C. Autonomic neuropathy
- D. Encephalopathy

Most common presentation of lead poisoning is an encephalopathy. Motor neuropathy can also occur. Sensation is generally preserved. Autonomic nervous system can be affected.

2616. In lead poisoning, serum levels of which of the following is elevated?
Harrison's 20th Ed. Chapter 438, Page 3219

- A. Alpha fetoprotein
- B. Ceruloplasmin
- C. Coproporphyrin
- D. Prolactin

Serum coproporphyrin level is elevated in lead poisoning.

2617. In lead poisoning, chelation therapy with which of the following is beneficial?
Harrison's 20th Ed. Chapter 438, Page 3220

- A. Calcium disodium ethylene-diaminetetraacetic acid (EDTA)
- B. British anti-Lewisite (BAL)
- C. Penicillamine
- D. All of the above

2618. In mercury toxicity, the primary site of neuromuscular pathology is in?
Harrison's 20th Ed. Chapter 438, Page 3220

- A. Motor neurons
- B. Lateral spinothalamic tract
- C. Medical longitudnal fasciculus
- D. Dorsal root ganglia

In mercury toxicity, the primary site of neuromuscular pathology is in the dorsal root ganglia.

2619. Potassium ferric ferrocyanide II is useful in intoxication with which of the following?
Harrison's 20th Ed. Chapter 438, Page 3220

- A. Mercury
- B. Arsenic
- C. Lead
- D. Thallium

With acute intoxication, potassium ferric ferrocyanide II may be effective in preventing absorption of thallium from the gut.

2620. Which of the following is not helpful in Thallium toxicity?
Harrison's 20th Ed. Chapter 438, Page 3220

- A. Potassium ferric ferrocyanide II
- B. Adequate diuresis
- C. Chelating agents
- D. All of the above

2621. Mee's lines are related to which of the following?
Harrison's 20th Ed. Chapter 438, Page 3220

- A. Organophosphates
- B. Thallium
- C. Hexacarbons
- D. Lithium

2622. Mee's lines are related to which of the following?
Harrison's 20th Ed. Chapter 438, Page 3220

A. Mercury
B. Arsenic
C. Lead
D. Gold

Mee's lines are transverse lines at the base of fingernails & toenails. Mee's lines are seen in arsenic toxicity and also in thallium poisoning.

2623. Which of the following in arsenic toxicity is not diagnostically helpful?
Harrison's 20th Ed. Chapter 438, Page 3220

A. Arsenic levels in serum
B. Arsenic levels in urine
C. Arsenic levels in hair
D. Arsenic levels in fingernails

Because arsenic is cleared from blood rapidly, serum level of arsenic is not diagnostically helpful.

2624. Diagnosis of vitamin B12 deficiency is made by?
Harrison's 20th Ed. Chapter 438, Page 3220

A. Low serum cobalamin levels
B. Raised levels of methylmalonic acid
C. Raised levels of homocysteine
D. All of the above

Serum methylmalonic acid & homocysteine, the metabolites that accumulate when cobalamin-dependent reactions are blocked, are elevated.

2625. Which of the following anesthetic agent can produce acute cobalamin deficiency neuropathy?
Harrison's 20th Ed. Chapter 438, Page 3220

A. Halothane
B. Nitrous oxide
C. Isoflurane
D. Methoxyflurane

Use of nitrous oxide as an anesthetic agent can produce acute cobalamin deficiency neuropathy and subacute combined degeneration of cord.

2626. Beriberi in Singhalese language means?
Harrison's 20th Ed. Chapter 438, Page 3220

A. I'm sick, I'm sick
B. I can't, I can't
C. I'm tired, I'm tired
D. I want to be alone, I want to be alone

Beriberi means "I can't, I can't" in Singhalese, the language of natives of Sri Lanka. Dry beriberi refers to neuropathic symptoms. The term wet beriberi is used when cardiac manifestations predominate (in reference to edema).

2627. Erythrocyte transketolase activity is reduced in the blood of which nutritional neuropathy?
Harrison's 20th Ed. Chapter 438, Page 3220

A. Thiamine (Vitamin B1)
B. Pyridoxine (Vitamin B6)
C. Cobalamin (Vitamin B12)
D. Riboflavin

Blood & urine assays for thiamine are not reliable for diagnosis of deficiency. Erythrocyte transketolase activity and the percentage increase in activity (in vitro) following the addition of thiamine pyrophosphate (TPP) are more accurate & reliable.

2628. The term vitamin E is usually used for?
Harrison's 20th Ed. Chapter 438, Page 3221

A. α-tocopherol
B. β-tocopherol
C. γ-tocopherol
D. δ-tocopherol

Term vitamin E is usually used for α-tocopherol, most active of the four main types of vitamin E.

2629. Vitamin E deficiency usually occurs secondary to?
Harrison's 20th Ed. Chapter 438, Page 3221

A. Abetalipoproteinemia
B. Short-bowel syndromes
C. Cystic fibrosis
D. All of the above

Vitamin E deficiency usually occurs secondary to lipid malabsorption or in uncommon disorders of vitamin E transport like Abetalipoproteinemia, cystic fibrosis, as a consequence of various cholestatic and hepatobiliary disorders as well as short-bowel syndromes.

2630. Abetalipoproteinemia is characterized by?
Harrison's 20th Ed. Chapter 438, Page 3221

A. Pigmentary retinopathy
B. Acanthocytosis
C. Progressive ataxia
D. All of the above

Abetalipoproteinemia is a rare autosomal dominant disorder characterized by steatorrhea, pigmentary retinopathy, acanthocytosis and progressive ataxia.

2631. The main clinical feature of Vitamin E deficiency is?
Harrison's 20th Ed. Chapter 438, Page 3221

A. Pancytopenia and aplastic anemia
B. Subacute combined degeneration of cord
C. Spinocerebellar ataxia
D. Autonomic instability

2632. Clinical features of vitamin E deficiency resemble those of?
Harrison's 20th Ed. Chapter 438, Page 3221

A. Subacute combined degeneration of spinal cord
B. Friedreich's ataxia
C. Pellagra
D. Tabes dorsalis

The main clinical features of Vitamin E deficiency are spinocerebellar ataxia and polyneuropathy, resembling Friedreich's ataxia or other spinocerebellar ataxias. Patients manifest progressive ataxia & signs of posterior column dysfunction (impaired joint position & vibratory sensation). Because of the polyneuropathy, there is hyporeflexia, but plantar responses may be extensor as a result of the spinal cord involvement. Other neurologic manifestations may include ophthalmoplegia, pigmented retinopathy, night blindness, dysarthria, pseudoathetosis, dystonia and tremor.

2633. Drug that acts as pyridoxine (Vitamin B6) antagonist is?
Harrison's 20th Ed. Chapter 438, Page 3221

A. Isoniazid
B. Cycloserine
C. Penicillamine
D. All of the above

Isoniazid, cycloserine and penicillamine act as pyridoxine antagonists by combining to aldehyde moiety of vitamin B6. Vitamin B6 deficiency is most commonly seen in patients treated with isoniazid or hydralazine.

2634. Measurement of xanthurenic acid after tryptophan loading helps in the diagnosis of?
Molecular Aspects of Medicine (2016), doi: 10.1016/j.mam.2016.08.001

A. Thiamine (Vitamin B1) deficiency
B. Pyridoxine (Vitamin B6) deficiency
C. Cobalamin (Vitamin B12) deficiency
D. Riboflavin deficiency

Measurement of xanthurenic acid after tryptophan loading can help confirm the diagnosis of pyridoxine (Vitamin B6) deficiency.

2635. Strachan's syndrome is characterized by?
Rev Neurol. 1997;25:1950-1956

A. Painful sensory neuropathy
B. Orogenital dermatitis
C. Amblyopia and deafness
D. All of the above

Strachan's syndrome is characterized by a painful sensory neuropathy associated with orogenital dermatitis, amblyopia and deafness.

2636. Which of the following is a feature of copper deficiency?
Harrison's 20th Ed. Chapter 438, Page 3221

A. Lower limb paresthesias, spasticity and gait difficulties
B. Microcytic anemia
C. Neutropenia, pancytopenia
D. All of the above

2637. Excess of which of the following is an established cause of copper deficiency?
Harrison's 20th Ed. Chapter 438, Page 3221

A. Vitamin E excess
B. Vitamin B6 excess
C. Zinc excess
D. Iron excess

Excess zinc is an established cause of copper deficiency. Zinc upregulates enterocyte production of metallothionine, which results in decreased absorption of copper.

2638. Which of the following damage neurons in dorsal root ganglion?
Harrison's 20th Ed. Chapter 438, Page 3217 Table 438-7

A. Cisplatin
B. Varicella zoster virus (VZV)
C. Vitamin E deficiency
D. All of the above

Others that damage neurons in dorsal root ganglion include Mercury toxicity, Vitamin B6 deficiency, Nitrofurantoin, INH, Etoposide, Cisplatin, Ataxia Telangiectasia, Friedreich's Ataxia.

2639. Which of the following is toxic to dorsal root ganglia neurons?
Harrison's 20th Ed. Chapter 438, Page 3217 Table 438-7

A. Cisplatin
B. Paclitaxel
C. Vincristine
D. Thalidomide

Cisplatin is toxic to dorsal root ganglia neurons, producing a dose-related large-fiber sensory neuropathy (neuronopathy).

2640. Which of the following is not a feature of cisplatin toxicity?
Harrison's 20th Ed. Chapter 438, Page 3217

A. Hearing loss
B. Lhermitte's sign
C. Sensory ataxia
D. Decrease in motor strength

Small-fiber sensation (pain & temperature) and motor strength are spared in cisplatin toxicity (asymmetric proprioceptive sensory loss without weakness).

2641. Which of the following is a median neuropathy?
Harrison's 20th Ed. Chapter 438, Page 3222

A. Pronator teres syndrome
B. Anterior interosseous neuropathy
C. Carpal tunnel syndrome
D. All of the above

2642. The number of tendons in carpal tunnel is?

A. 7
B. 8
C. 9
D. 10

2643. In carpal tunnel syndrome (CTS), nocturnal paresthesia is common in?
Harrison's 19th Ed. 49

A. Thumb
B. Index finger
C. Middle finger
D. All of the above

2644. Systemic diseases associated with carpal tunnel syndrome include?
Harrison's 20th Ed. Chapter 438, Page 3222

A. Hypothyroidism
B. Rheumatoid arthritis
C. Diabetes mellitus
D. All of the above

Other diseases include Uremic neuropathy, AL primary amyloidosis, Familial amyloid polyneuropathy (FAP), Acromegaly, Systemic Sclerosis,

2645. Which of the following signs relate to diagnosis of mononeuropathy of upper limb?
Harrison's 20th Ed. Chapter 438, Page 3222

A. Tinel's sign
B. Phalen's sign
C. Froment sign
D. All of the above

In carpal tunnel syndrome (CTS), sensation of tingling can be reproduced when a percussion hammer is tapped over wrist (Tinel's sign) or wrist is flexed for 30–60 sec. (Phalen's sign). Froment sign indicates thumb adductor weakness and consists of flexion of thumb at the interphalangeal joint when attempting to oppose the thumb against lateral border of the second digit. This is seen in cubital tunnel syndrome.

2646. The root value of median nerve is?
Harrison's 20th Ed. Chapter 22, Page 141

A. C5 - T1
B. C6 - T1
C. C7 - T1
D. C8 - T1

2647. The root value of ulnar nerve is?
Harrison's 20th Ed. Chapter 22, Page 141

A. C5 - T1
B. C6 - T1
C. C7 - T1
D. C8 - T1

2648. The root value of radial nerve is?
Harrison's 20th Ed. Chapter 22, Page 141

A. C5 - T1
B. C6 - T1
C. C7 - T1
D. C8 - T1

2649. Which of the following nerve is involved if the site of lesion is 'Cubital tunnel'?
Harrison's 20th Ed. Chapter 438, Page 3222

A. Radial nerve
B. Ulnar nerve
C. Median nerve
D. All of the above

Ulnar nerve passes through the condylar groove between the medial epicondyle and the olecranon. Ulnar neuropathy at the elbow is called "Cubital Tunnel Syndrome" (tardy ulnar palsy).

2650. Which of the following nerve is involved in Saturday night palsy?
Harrison's 20th Ed. Chapter 438, Page 3222

A. Radial nerve
B. Ulnar nerve
C. Median nerve
D. All of the above

2651. Meralgia paresthetica relates best to?
Harrison's 20th Ed. Chapter 438, Page 3222

A. Radial neuropathy
B. Lateral femoral cutaneous neuropathy
C. Ulnar neuropathy at the elbow
D. Peroneal neuropathy

The neuropathy affecting lateral femoral cutaneous nerve is also known as meralgia paresthetica.

2652. Which of the following neuropathies occur during pregnancy?
Harrison's 20th Ed. Chapter 438, Page 3222

A. Peroneal neuropathy
B. Meralgia paresthetica
C. Carpal tunnel syndrome
D. All of the above

Compressive mononeuropathies during pregnancy and delivery are peroneal neuropathy, meralgia paresthetica, carpal tunnel syndrome, femoral neuropathy, isolated obturator neuropathy. There is a clear association between pregnancy and an increased frequency of idiopathic facial palsy (Bell's palsy). Restless leg syndrome is the most common peripheral nerve and movement disorder in pregnancy.

2653. Peroneal neuropathy needs to be distinguished from?
Harrison's 20th Ed. Chapter 438, Page 3222

A. L5 radiculopathy
B. Pott's disease
C. Diabetic radiculopathy
D. Sciatic neuropathy

Peroneal neuropathy needs to be distinguished from L5 radiculopathy. In L5 radiculopathy, ankle invertors and evertors are weak and needle EMG reveals denervation.

2654. Which of the following is false for Brachial Plexus?
Harrison's 20th Ed. Chapter 438, Page 3223

A. Four roots
B. Three trunks
C. Two divisions per trunk
D. Three cords

Brachial plexus is composed of five roots, three trunks (upper, middle, & lower), with two divisions (anterior & posterior) per trunk. Trunks divide into three cords (medial, lateral, & posterior).

2655. Parsonage-Turner syndrome relates best with?
Harrison's 20th Ed. Chapter 438, Page 3223

A. Brachial plexus
B. Lumbosacral plexus
C. Radiation-Induced plexopathy
D. Peroneal neuropathy

Immune-mediated brachial plexus neuropathy (IBPN) is also called acute brachial plexitis, neuralgic amyotrophy and Parsonage - Turner syndrome.

2656. Pain in immune-mediated brachial plexus neuropathy (IBPN) is at?
Harrison's 20th Ed. Chapter 438, Page 3223

A. Neck
B. Shoulder
C. Arm
D. Hand

IBPN usually presents with an acute onset of severe pain in the shoulder region.

2657. Out of the following, which is most commonly involved in IBPN?
Harrison's 20th Ed. Chapter 438, Page 3223

A. Root
B. Trunk
C. Division
D. Cord

Most common pattern of IBPN involves the upper trunk or a single or multiple mononeuropathies primarily involving the suprascapular, long thoracic, or axillary nerves.

2658. Which of the following surgical procedures is the most common cause of brachial plexopathy?
Harrison's 20th Ed. Chapter 438, Page 3223

A. Reduction of subluxated shoulder
B. Repair of fracture of neck of humerus
C. Median sternotomy
D. Repair of fracture of clavicle

Most common surgical procedures associated with brachial plexopathy as a complication are those that involve median sternotomies.

2659. Which of the following is false about electrodiagnostic features of demyelination?
Harrison's 20th Ed. Chapter 438, Page 3207

A. Slowing of nerve conduction velocity (NCV)
B. Dispersion of evoked compound action potentials
C. Conduction block & prolongation of distal latencies
D. None of the above

2660. Electrodiagnostic studies (EDx) help to diagnose which of the following neuropathies?
Harrison's 20th Ed. Chapter 438, Page 3207

A. Axonal
B. Demyelinating
C. Neuronal
D. All of the above

Electrodiagnostic studies help to classify neuropathy into either axonal, demyelinating or neuronal.

2661. Mononeuropathy multiplex syndrome may be a manifestation of all except?
Harrison's 20th Ed. Chapter 438, Page 3214

A. Leprosy
B. Sarcoidosis
C. Syphilis
D. NeuroAIDS

2662. Mononeuropathy multiplex syndrome may be a manifestation of?
Harrison's 20th Ed. Chapter 438, Page 3214

A. Eosinophilic granulomatosis with polyangiitis
B. Rheumatoid vasculitis
C. Tangier disease (ABCA I deficiency)
D. All of the above

2663. Sensory neuronopathy (or ganglionopathy) is best related to?
Harrison's 20th Ed. Chapter 22, Page 142

A. Amyloidosis
B. Sarcoidosis
C. Sjogren's syndrome
D. Gaucher disease Type 1

2664. Example of motor neuronopathies include?
Harrison's 20th Ed. Chapter 90, Page 673

A. Lower-motor form of amyotrophic lateral sclerosis
B. Poliomyelitis
C. Hereditary spinal muscular atrophies
D. All of the above

2665. Which of the following is a motor-predominant neuropathy?
Am Fam Physician. 2010;81(7):887-892

A. Acute intermittent porphyria
B. Diphtheritic neuropathy
C. Lead neuropathy
D. All of the above

2666. Which of the following is a neuronal neuropathy?
Am Fam Physician. 2010;81(7):887-892

A. Sjögren's syndrome
B. Cisplatin toxicity
C. Pyridoxine toxicity
D. All of the above

2667. Which of the following is not a demyelinating neuropathy?
Am Fam Physician. 2010;81(7):887-892

A. Guillain-Barré syndrome
B. Multifocal motor neuropathy (MMN)
C. HIV neuropathy
D. Diphtheria neuropathy

2668. Which of the following is not a axonal neuropathy?
Am Fam Physician. 2010;81(7):887-892

A. Toxic
B. HIV
C. Charcot-Marie-Tooth 2 (CMT2)
D. All of the above

Most toxic neuropathies are distal axonal degenerations. In HIV, length-dependent axonal degeneration of sensory fibers without nerve-fiber regeneration occurs.

2669. Which of the following is a acute onset neuropathy?
Am Fam Physician. 2010;81(7):887-892

A. Porphyria
B. Diphtheria
C. Guillain-Barré syndrome
D. All of the above

2670. Which of the following is a recurrent neuropathy?
Am Fam Physician. 2010;81(7):887-892

A. Porphyria
B. Refsum's disease
C. Hereditary neuropathy with pressure palsies (HNPP)
D. All of the above

2671. Example of motor neuronopathies include?
Harrison's 20th Ed. Chapter 90, Page 673

A. Lead intoxication
B. Dapsone intoxication
C. Porphyria
D. All of the above

2672. Peripheral neuropathy includes disorders of?
Am Fam Physician. 2010;81(7):887-892

A. Peripheral nerves
B. Dorsal or ventral nerve roots
C. Dorsal root ganglia
D. All of the above

Peripheral neuropathy includes disorders of peripheral nerves, dorsal or ventral nerve roots, dorsal root ganglia, brachial or lumbosacral plexus, cranial nerves (except I & II) & other sensory, motor, autonomic or mixed nerves.

2673. Which of the following is false about peripheral neuropathy?
Am Fam Physician. 2010;81(7):887-892

A. Sensory symptoms precede motor symptoms
B. Small-fiber neuropathies present with paresthesias
C. Large-fiber neuropathies present as gait disturbance
D. None of the above

2674. Term ataxic-neuropathy is used for?
Am Fam Physician. 2010;81(7):887-892

A. Small-fiber sensory neuropathies
B. Large-fiber sensory neuropathies
C. Motor-predominant neuropathies
D. Autonomic neuropathies

2675. Which of the following is not a small-fiber sensory neuropathy?
Ann Indian Acad Neurol. 2008;11(2):89–97

A. Amyloidosis
B. Sjogren's syndrome
C. Hereditary sensory and autonomic neuropathy
D. Friedreich's ataxia

Causes of small fiber neuropathy include Diabetes, Amyloidosis, Fabry's disease, Tangier's disease, Hereditary sensory and autonomic neuropathy, Sjogren's syndrome & Chronic idiopathic small fiber sensory neuropathy.

2676. Which of the following is not a large-fiber sensory neuropathy?
Ann Indian Acad Neurol. 2008;11(2):89–97

A. Sjögren's syndrome
B. Fabry's disease
C. Cisplatin neuropathy
D. Pyridoxine toxicity

Guillain-Barré Syndrome and Other Immune-Mediated Neuropathies

2677. Guillain-Barré syndrome was first described in which year?
N Engl J Med. 2012;366:2294-304

- A. 1869
- B. 1898
- C. 1916
- D. 1934

Guillain–Barré syndrome, characterized by acute areflexic paralysis with albuminocytologic dissociation (elevated protein in CSF and normal cell counts), was described in 1916.

2678. Miller Fisher syndrome was first reported in which year?
N Engl J Med. 2012;366:2294-304

- A. 1923
- B. 1943
- C. 1956
- D. 1966

Miller Fisher syndrome, characterized by ophthalmoplegia, ataxia & areflexia, was reported in 1956 as a likely variant of Guillain–Barré syndrome, because the CSF of affected patients showed albuminocytologic dissociation.

2679. Feature not typical of Guillain-Barre syndrome is?
Harrison's 20th Ed. Chapter 439, Page 3225

- A. Acute onset
- B. Males & females are at equal risk
- C. Autoimmune
- D. Polyradiculoneuropathy

Males are at 1.5-fold higher risk for GBS than females. Adults are more frequently affected than children.

2680. Facial diparesis is present in what proportion of GBS patients?
Harrison's 20th Ed. Chapter 439, Page 3225

- A. 10%
- B. 20%
- C. 50%
- D. 80%

Facial diparesis is present in 50% of GBS patients.

2681. Bilateral facial nerve palsy occurs in which of the following?
Harrison's 20th Ed. Chapter 439, Page 3214

- A. Leprosy
- B. Sarcoidosis
- C. Sjogren's syndrome
- D. All of the above

Facial palsy that is often bilateral occurs in sarcoidosis and in Guillain-Barre syndrome.

2682. GBS manifests as?
Harrison's 20th Ed. Chapter 439, Page 3225

- A. Rapidly evolving areflexic ascending motor paralysis
- B. With or without sensory disturbance
- C. Autonomic involvement is common
- D. All of the above

2683. Which of the following about GBS is false?
Lancet. 2016;388:717-27

- A. Annual incidence rate of GBS increases with age
- B. Estimated lifetime risk of developing GBS <1 in 1000
- C. Post-infectious, rapidly progressive, monophasic disorder
- D. None of the above

2684. Which of the following is not typical of Guillain-Barre syndrome?
Harrison's 20th Ed. Chapter 439, Page 3225

- A. Fever & constitutional symptoms are absent at onset
- B. Lower cranial nerves are frequently involved
- C. DTRs disappear within first few days of onset
- D. Bladder dysfunction is a prominent feature

Presence of fever & constitutional symptoms at onset cast doubt on the diagnosis of GBS. Transient bladder dysfunction may occur in severe GBS. If bladder dysfunction is a prominent & early in the course, GBS is unlikely.

2685. In GBS, clinical worsening reaches a plateau in how many weeks of onset?
Harrison's 20th Ed. Chapter 439, Page 3225

- A. 1 week
- B. 4 weeks
- C. 8 weeks
- D. 12 weeks

Clinical worsening stops and GBS patient reaches a plateau almost always within 4 weeks of onset.

2686. Limited or regional GBS syndromes include?
Harrison's 20th Ed. Chapter 439, Page 3225

- A. Acute motor axonal neuropathy (AMAN)
- B. Acute motor sensory axonal neuropathy (AMSAN)
- C. Miller Fisher syndrome (MFS)
- D. All of the above

Limited or regional GBS syndromes are Miller Fisher syndrome, pure sensory forms, ophthalmoplegia with anti-GQ1b antibodies (severe motor-sensory GBS), GBS with severe bulbar & facial paralysis associated with cytomegalovirus (CMV) infection & anti-GM2 antibodies & acute pandysautonomia.

2687. Which of the following is the most common form of GBS?
Harrison's 20th Ed. Chapter 439, Page 3225

- A. Acute inflammatory demyelinating polyradiculoneuropathy
- B. Acute axonal motor disorder
- C. Acute sensory & motor axonal neuropathy
- D. Miller Fisher syndrome (MFS)

In Europe & North America ~95% of GBS are acute inflammatory demyelinating polyradiculoneuropathy. ~5% are AMAN & AMSAN.

2688. Nationality of Charles Miller Fisher was?

- A. Canadian
- B. American
- C. British
- D. Brazilian

Charles Miller Fisher was a Canadian stroke specialist.

2689. Which of the following is a demyelinating disorder?
Harrison's 20th Ed. Chapter 439, Page 3226 Table 439-1

- A. Acute motor axonal neuropathy (AMAN)
- B. Acute motor sensory axonal neuropathy (AMSAN)
- C. Miller Fisher syndrome (MFS)
- D. All of the above

Acute motor axonal neuropathy (AMAN) and acute motor sensory axonal neuropathy (AMSAN) subtypes are axonal variants of Guillain-Barré syndrome (GBS).

2690. Which of the following is a regional variant of GBS?
Harrison's 20th Ed. Chapter 439, Page 3225

- A. Pure sensory form
- B. GBS with severe bulbar & facial paralysis
- C. Acute pandysautonomia
- D. All of the above

Regional variants of GBS include pure sensory forms, ophthalmoplegia with anti-GQ1b antibodies as part of severe motor-sensory GBS, GBS with severe bulbar & facial paralysis, sometimes associated with antecedent cytomegalovirus (CMV) infection and anti-GM2 antibodies and acute pandysautonomia.

2691. Organisms involved in antecedent infections in Guillain-Barre syndrome include?
Harrison's 20th Ed. Chapter 439, Page 3225, N Engl J Med. 2012;366:2294-304

- A. Campylobacter jejuni
- B. Human herpes virus
- C. Cytomegalovirus
- D. All of the above

~70% of GBS occur 1–3 weeks after an acute infectious process (respiratory or gastrointestinal). Antecedent infection or reinfection with Campylobacter jejuni, human herpes virus infection, CMV, Epstein-Barr virus, HIV, hepatitis E, Zika, chikungunya, Mycoplasma pneumoniae & swine influenza vaccine have been identified. Case clusters are rare. Presence of sialylated lipopolysaccharides on C. jejuni strains is a form of molecular mimicry that promotes autoimmune recognition of sialylated cell surface molecules on axons. Asymptomatic Campylobacter infection also may trigger Guillain-Barre syndrome.

2692. Which of the following is false if preceding infection in GBS case is C. jejuni?
Lancet. 2016;388:717–27

- A. A pure motor axonal form of GBS occurs
- B. Seropositivity against GM1 & GD1a gangliosides
- C. Poorer outcome
- D. None of the above

2693. Which of the following vaccinations could predispose to Guillain-Barre syndrome?
Harrison's 20th Ed. Chapter 439, Page 3225

- A. Swine influenza vaccine
- B. Influenza A vaccine
- C. Older type rabies vaccine
- D. All of the above

Immunizations with swine influenza vaccine, influenza A vaccines and older-type (Semple) rabies vaccine are implicated as a trigger of GBS. There is no increased risk of GBS with meningococcal vaccinations.

2694. Guillain-Barre syndrome occurs more frequently in patients with following diseases except?
Harrison's 20th Ed. Chapter 439, Page 3225

- A. Hodgkin's disease
- B. Chronic myeloid leukemia
- C. HIV-seropositive individuals
- D. Systemic lupus erythematosus

GBS also occurs more frequently in patients with lymphoma (Hodgkin's disease), HIV-seropositive individuals and in patients with SLE.

2695. Which of the following statements is false about GBS?
Harrison's 20th Ed. Chapter 439, Page 3226

- A. Both cellular & humoral immune mechanisms involved
- B. Analogous to experimental allergic neuritis (EAN)
- C. Molecular mimicry mechanism
- D. None of the above

2696. Which of the following is the critical event in the development of GBS?
N Engl J Med. 2012;366:2294-304

- A. B cells recognize glycoconjugates on C. jejuni
- B. Activation of B cells T cell
- C. Escape of activated B cells from Peyer's patches into regional lymph nodes
- D. All of the above

In the immunopathogenesis of GBS, a critical event in the development of GBS is the escape of activated B cells from Peyer's patches into regional lymph nodes.

2697. Which of the following is a functional region of myelinated axons?
Harrison's 20th Ed. Chapter 439, Page 3226 Figure 439-1

- A. Internodes
- B. Paranode
- C. Juxtaparanodes
- D. All of the above

Myelinated axons are divided into four functional regions. They are the nodes of Ranvier, paranodes, juxtaparanodes & internodes.

2698. Which of the following antiganglioside antibody is common in GBS?
Harrison's 20th Ed. Chapter 439, Page 3228 Table 439-2

- A. Anti GM1
- B. Anti GM2
- C. Anti GM3
- D. Anti GM4

Anti GM1, an antiganglioside antibody is common in GBS (20–50%), particularly in those preceded by C. jejuni infection.

2699. Which of the following is most relevant to Gangliosides?
N Engl J Med. 2012;366:2294-304

- A. Lectin
- B. Heparan
- C. Ceramide
- D. Mannose

Gangliosides are composed of a ceramide attached to one or more sugars (hexoses) and contain sialic acid (N-acetylneuraminic acid) linked to an oligosaccharide core. Gangliosides are important components of the peripheral nerves.

2700. Which of the following is a Ganglioside?
N Engl J Med. 2012;366:2294-304

- A. GM1
- B. GD1a
- C. GT1a
- D. All of the above

GM1, GD1a, GT1a, and GQ1b are gangliosides.

2701. Which of the following gangliosides is strongly expressed at the nodes of Ranvier?

Harrison's 20th Ed. Chapter 439, Page 3228 Table 439-2, N Engl J Med. 2012;366: 2294-304

- A. GM1
- B. GT1a
- C. GQ1b
- D. All of the above

Gangliosides GM1 and GD1a are strongly expressed at the nodes of Ranvier, where voltage-gated sodium (Nav) channels are localized. Contactin associated protein (Caspr) & voltage-gated potassium (Kv) channels are present at paranodes and juxtaparanodes respectively. IgG anti-GM1 or anti-GD1a autoantibodies bind to the nodal axolemma, leading to membrane-attack complex (MAC) formation. This results in disappearance of Nav clusters and detachment of paranodal myelin, which can lead to nerve-conduction failure and muscle weakness.

2702. IgG autoantibodies to GQ1b cross-react with which of the following?

N Engl J Med. 2012;366:2294-304

- A. GM1
- B. GD1a
- C. GT1a
- D. All of the above

IgG autoantibodies to GQ1b, which cross-react with GT1a, are strongly associated with the Miller Fisher syndrome, its incomplete forms (acute ophthalmoparesis and acute ataxic neuropathy), and its CNS variant, Bickerstaff's brainstem encephalitis (acute ophthalmoplegia, ataxia, and impaired consciousness after an infectious episode).

2703. The anti-GQ1b antibody syndrome includes which of the following?

N Engl J Med. 2012;366:2294-304

- A. Bickerstaff's brainstem encephalitis
- B. Miller Fisher syndrome
- C. Pharyngeal-cervical-brachial weakness
- D. All of the above

The anti-GQ1b antibody syndrome includes the Miller Fisher syndrome, acute ophthalmoparesis, acute ataxic neuropathy, Bickerstaff's brainstem encephalitis, and pharyngeal–cervical–brachial weakness.

2704. GQ1b is strongly expressed in which of the following cranial nerves?

N Engl J Med. 2012;366:2294-304

- A. Oculomotor nerve
- B. Trochlear nerve
- C. Abducens nerve
- D. All of the above

GQ1b is strongly expressed in the oculomotor, trochlear, and abducens nerves, as well as muscle spindles in the limbs. Glossopharyngeal and vagus nerves strongly express GT1a and GQ1b, possibly accounting for dysphagia.

2705. Which of the following is false about Miller Fisher syndrome?

N Engl J Med. 2012;366:2294-304

- A. Anti-GQ1b antibodies are found in > 90% patients
- B. IgG titers are highest early in the course
- C. Areflexia of limbs without weakness
- D. None of the above

Anti-GQ1b IgG antibodies are found in >90% of patients with MFS, and titers of IgG are highest early in the course. Anti-GQ1b antibodies are not found in other forms of GBS unless there is extraocular motor nerve involvement.

2706. Which of the following is not found in Miller Fisher syndrome?

N Engl J Med. 2012;366:2294-304

- A. Ataxia
- B. Areflexia of limbs
- C. Weakness of limbs
- D. Ophthalmoplegia

Miller Fisher's syndrome is an ocular variant of Guillain-Barre syndrome. It produces ophthalmoplegia with areflexia and mild ataxia, reflexes are normal. Antiganglioside antibodies (GQIb) can be detected in about 50% of cases.

2707. Which of the following is false about Miller Fisher syndrome?

N Engl J Med. 2012;366:2294-304

- A. Rapidly evolving ataxia
- B. Areflexia of limbs without weakness
- C. Ophthalmoplegia often with pupillary paralysis
- D. None of the above

2708. MFS is strongly associated with which of the following antibodies?

N Engl J Med. 2012;366:2294-304

- A. GQ1a
- B. GQ1b
- C. GQ1c
- D. GQ1d

Miller Fisher syndrome (MFS) presents as rapidly evolving ataxia & areflexia of limbs without weakness, and ophthalmoplegia, often with pupillary paralysis. MFS is strongly associated with antibodies to ganglioside GQ1b.

2709. Which of the following is a central nervous system variant of Miller Fisher syndrome?

N Engl J Med. 2012;366:2294-304

- A. Anti-Hu–associated paraneoplastic encephalitis (PEM)
- B. Bickerstaff's brainstem encephalitis
- C. Post–infectious brainstem encephalitis
- D. All of the above

Antibodies against ganglioside GQ1b have also been detected in patients with Bickerstaff's brainstem encephalitis. Bickerstaff's encephalitis is characterized by ophthalmoplegia and ataxia but is also accompanied by pyramidal and sensory tract findings and cerebrospinal fluid pleocytosis.

2710. In demyelinating GBS, basis for flaccid paralysis & sensory disturbance is?

Harrison's 20th Ed. Chapter 439, Page 3227

- A. Conduction block
- B. Neurodegeneration
- C. Apoptosis
- D. All of the above

In demyelinating forms of GBS, basis for flaccid paralysis & sensory disturbance is conduction block. Secondary axonal degeneration usually occurs in severe cases.

2711. CSF findings in Guillain-Barre syndrome include all except?

Harrison's 20th Ed. Chapter 439, Page 3227

- A. Elevated CSF proteins
- B. CSF protein elevated by end of first week
- C. No pleocytosis
- D. CSF is normal when symptoms are present for < 6 hours

CSF is often normal when symptoms have been present for 48 hours. By the end of first week the level of protein is usually elevated without accompanying pleocytosis. Sustained CSF pleocytosis suggests an alternative diagnosis (viral myelitis, unrecognized HIV infection, leukemia or lymphoma with infiltration of nerves or neurosarcoidosis.

2712. Cytoalbuminologic dissociation best relates to?
Lancet. 2016;388:717–27

A. Normal CSF protein level & CSF TLC > 5 cells/μL
B. Raised CSF protein level & CSF TLC < 5 cells/μL
C. Normal CSF protein level & CSF TLC > 50 cells/μL
D. Raised CSF protein level & CSF TLC < 50 cells/μL

Cytoalbuminologic dissociation implies elevation of CSF protein level above laboratory normal value and CSF total white cell count <50 cells/μL).

2713. Electrodiagnostic feature of GBS is?
Harrison's 20th Ed. Chapter 439, Page 3227

A. Prolonged F-wave latencies
B. Prolonged distal latencies
C. Reduced amplitudes of compound muscle action potentials
D. All of the above

Edx features are mild or absent in the early stages of GBS and lag behind the clinical evolution. In AIDP, the earliest features are prolonged F-wave latencies, prolonged distal latencies and reduced amplitudes of compound muscle action potentials (CMAPs).

2714. Which of the following criteria is used for the diagnosis of Guillain-Barre syndrome?
Harrison's 20th Ed. Chapter 439, Page 3227

A. Amsel criteria
B. CASPAR criteria
C. Research Domain Criteria (RDoCs)
D. Brighton Criteria

Brighton criteria. Brain 137:33,2014.

2715. In CSF of GBS patient, increase in which of the following reflects axonal damage & predicts a residual deficit?
Harrison's 20th Ed. Chapter 439, Page 3227

A. Tau
B. Amyloid precursor protein (APP)
C. Chymotrypsin
D. Apolipoprotein E

Tau & 14-3-3 protein levels are elevated early in some cases of GBS. Tau increases in CSF may reflect axonal damage & predict a residual deficit.

2716. Which of the following can cause ptosis?
Harrison's 20th Ed. Chapter 28, Page 190

A. Guillain-Barre syndrome
B. Miller Fisher syndrome
C. Lambert-Eaton syndrome
D. All of the above

2717. Which of the following can cause ptosis without ophthalmoparesis?
Harrison's 20th Ed. Chapter 441, Page 3240 Table 441-1

A. Myotonic dystrophy
B. Congenital myopathies
C. Neuromuscular junction disorders
D. All of the above

2718. Differential diagnosis of Guillain-Barré syndrome includes?
Harrison's 20th Ed. Chapter 439, Page 3228

A. Hypokalemia
B. Polymyositis
C. Porphyria
D. All of the above

Differential diagnosis of Guillain-Barré syndrome include transverse myelitis & neuromyelitis optica, Lyme polyradiculitis, porphyria, vasculitic neuropathy, poliomyelitis, West Nile virus, CMV polyradiculitis, critical illness neuropathy or myopathy, myasthenia gravis, botulism, poisonings with organophosphates, thallium, or arsenic, paralytic shellfish poisoning, severe hypophosphatemia.

2719. Which of the following must be considered in the differential diagnosis of Guillain Barre syndrome?
Harrison's 20th Ed. Chapter 148, Page 1107

A. Adult botulism
B. Tick paralysis
C. Eaton Lambert syndrome
D. All of the above

Adult botulism, myasthenia gravis, stroke syndromes, Eaton Lambert syndrome and tick paralysis must be considered in the differential diagnosis of cases include Guillain Barre syndrome (GBS).

2720. Type of respiratory failure in GBS is?
Harrison's 20th Ed. Chapter 293, Page 2026

A. I
B. II
C. III
D. IV

Type II respiratory failure is a consequence of alveolar hypoventilation and results from the inability to eliminate carbon dioxide effectively due to impaired CNS drive to breathe, impaired strength with failure of neuromuscular function in the respiratory system and increased load(s) on the respiratory system. Reduced strength can be due to impaired neuromuscular transmission as in myasthenia gravis, Guillain-Barre syndrome, amyotrophic lateral sclerosis or respiratory muscle weakness (e.g. myopathy, electrolyte derangements, fatigue).

2721. What length of time after the first motor symptoms in GBS, immunotherapy is no longer effective?
Harrison's 20th Ed. Chapter 439, Page 3229

A. 3 days
B. 14 days
C. 30 days
D. 60 days

Each day counts in the treatment of GBS. ~2 weeks after first motor symptoms, immunotherapy is no longer effective.

2722. What percentage of patients with GBS require ventilatory assistance?
Harrison's 20th Ed. Chapter 439, Page 3229

A. ~10%
B. ~20%
C. ~30%
D. ~40%

~30% of patients with GBS require ventilatory assistance, sometimes for prolonged periods of time.

2723. Which of the following about treatment of GBS is false?
Harrison's 20th Ed. Chapter 439, Page 3229

A. High-dose IVIg & plasmapheresis are equally effective
B. Combination of IVIg & plasmapheresis offers no advantage
C. After successful treatment of GBS, relapse may occur in II or III week
D. None of the above

IVIg is administered as five daily infusions for a total dose of 2 g/kg body weight. A course of plasmapheresis usually consists of 40–50 mL/kg plasma exchange (PE) four to five times over a week. Glucocorticoids have not been found to be effective in GBS.

2724. Guillain-Barre syndrome best relates to which of the following?
Harrison's 20th Ed. Chapter 344, Page 2497

A. Autoimmune lymphoproliferative syndrome (ALPS)
B. Hemophagocytic lymphohistiocytosis (HLH)
C. Hyper-IgM (HIGM) Syndromes
D. Wiskott-Aldrich Syndrome

Autoimmune lymphoproliferative syndrome (ALPS) is characterized by nonmalignant T and B lymphoproliferation causing splenomegaly and enlarged lymph nodes. 70% of patients also display autoimmune manifestations like autoimmune cytopenias, Guillain-Barre syndrome, uveitis & hepatitis.

2725. Which of the following statements about Gullain-Barre syndrome (GBS) is false?
Harrison's 20th Ed. Chapter 439, Page 3229

A. Escape of activated B cells from Peyers patches into regional lymph nodes
B. Anti GQ1b IgG antibodies are found in >90% of patients with Miller Fisher subtype of GBS
C. Glucocorticoids are effective in GBS
D. Severe proximal motor & sensory axonal damage is a poor prognostic sign

Glucocorticoids have not been found to be effective in GBS. CIDP responds to glucocorticoids, whereas GBS does not.

2726. Factor that worsen the outlook for recovery in GBS is?
Harrison's 20th Ed. Chapter 439, Page 3230

A. Severe proximal motor & sensory axonal damage
B. Fulminant or severe attack
C. Delay in the onset of treatment
D. All of the above

2727. Patient characteristic consistently related to poor prognostic outcome in GBS is?
Harrison's 20th Ed. Chapter 439, Page 3230, Lancet. 2016;388:717–27

A. Age > 40 years
B. Preceding diarrhea (or C. jejuni infection in past 4 weeks)
C. High disability at nadir
D. All of the above

Factors that worsen the outlook for recovery in AIDP are patients with severe proximal motor and sensory axonal damage, advanced age, a fulminant or severe attack and a delay in the onset of treatment.

2728. What percentage of patients with GBS achieve a full functional recovery?
Harrison's 20th Ed. Chapter 439, Page 3230

A. ~ 65%
B. ~ 75%
C. ~ 85%
D. ~ 95%

~85% of patients with GBS achieve a full functional recovery within several months to a year.

2729. In optimal settings, mortality rate in patients with GBS is?
Harrison's 20th Ed. Chapter 439, Page 3230

A. <1%
B. <3%
C. <5%
D. <7%

In optimal settings, mortality rate in patients with GBS is <5%. Death usually results from secondary pulmonary complications.

Chronic Inflammatory Demyelinating Polyneuropathy

2730. Which of the following is false about chronic inflammatory demyelinating polyneuropathy (CIDP)?
Harrison's 20th Ed. Chapter 439, Page 3230

A. Initial attack is indistinguishable from that of GBS
B. Acute-onset form of CIDP may mimic GBS
C. CIDP should be considered if it deteriorates >9 weeks after onset or relapses at least three times
D. None of the above

2731. Which of the following is false about chronic inflammatory demyelinating polyneuropathy (CIDP)?
Harrison's 20th Ed. Chapter 439, Page 3230

A. Onset is usually gradual over a few months
B. Motor & sensory symptoms present
C. Death from CIDP is uncommon
D. None of the above

2732. Lewis-Sumner Syndrome is?
Harrison's 20th Ed. Chapter 439, Page 3230, N Engl J Med. 2005;352:1343-56

A. Multifocal acquired demyelinating sensory & motor neuropathy
B. Multifocal motor neuropathy
C. Distal acquired demyelinating symmetric neuropathy
D. Motor neuron disease

Lewis-Sumner syndrome is also called multifocal acquired demyelinating sensory and motor (MADSAM) neuropathy. It is a variant of CIDP in which discrete peripheral nerves are involved.

2733. Lewis-Sumner Syndrome is characterized by all except?
Harrison's 20th Ed. Chapter 439, Page 3230, N Engl J Med. 2005;352:1343-56

A. Motor and sensory deficits
B. Discrete peripheral nerves are involved
C. Asymmetrical presentation of symptoms
D. Poor response to intravenous immune globulin in presence of antibodies to gangliosides

Weakness of the limbs is usually symmetric in CIDP, but can be strikingly asymmetric in Lewis-Sumner syndrome.

2734. Classic chronic inflammatory demyelinating polyneuropathy is characterized by all except?
N Engl J Med. 2005;352:1343-56

A. Symmetrical weakness in proximal muscles
B. Symmetrical weakness in distal muscles
C. Weakness progressively increases for > 2 months
D. Not associated with impaired sensation

2735. Which of the following electrodiagnostic findings is not a feature of classic chronic inflammatory demyelinating polyneuropathy?
N Engl J Med. 2005;352:1343-56

A. Partial motor-nerve conduction block
B. Reduced motor-nerve conduction velocity
C. Prolonged distal motor latencies
D. Absent F-wave latencies

Edx findings in CIDP reveal variable degrees of conduction slowing, prolonged distal latencies, distal and temporal dispersion of CMAPs, and conduction block as the principal features. Presence of conduction block is a certain sign of an acquired demyelinating process. Evidence of axonal loss, presumably secondary to demyelination, is present in >50% of patients.

2736. Chronic inflammatory demyelinating polyneuropathy may be associated with all of the following except?
Harrison's 20th Ed. Chapter 439, Page 3230

A. HIV
B. SLE
C. Diabetes mellitus
D. Hypothyroidism

In all patients with presumptive CIDP, it is also reasonable to exclude vasculitis, collagen vascular disease (SLE), chronic hepatitis, HIV infection, amyloidosis, diabetes mellitus, inflammatory bowel disease and lymphoma.

2737. Which of the following is related to CIDP?
Harrison's 20th Ed. Chapter 439, Page 3230

A. Contactin-1 (CNTN1)
B. Contactin-associated protein-1 (CASPR1)
C. Neurofascin-155 (NF155)
D. All of the above

2738. Presence of IgG4 CNTN1 antibodies in CIDP patients leads to?
Harrison's 20th Ed. Chapter 439, Page 3230

A. Early axonal damage & severe distal motor involvement
B. Sensory ataxia with tremor
C. Poor response to IVIg
D. All of the above

Antibodies of IgG4 isotype directed against contactin-1 (CNTN1) or neurofascin-155 (NF155) are associated with early axonal damage, severe distal motor involvement or sensory ataxia with tremor, and a poor response to IVIg. CNTN1 and its partner contactin-associated protein-1 (CASPR1) interact with NF155 at paranodal axoglial junctions.

2739. Patients with clinical features of CIDP may also have?
Harrison's 20th Ed. Chapter 439, Page 3230

A. Monoclonal gammopathy of undetermined significance
B. POEMS syndrome
C. Churg-Strauss syndrome
D. Sjögren's syndrome

As many as 25% of patients with clinical features of CIDP also have a monoclonal gammopathy of undetermined significance (MGUS).

2740. Which of the following treatments is effective in CIDP?
Harrison's 20th Ed. Chapter 439, Page 3230

A. High-dose IVIg
B. Plasma exchange (PE)
C. Glucocorticoids
D. All of the above

High-dose IVIg, PE & glucocorticoids are all more effective than placebo in CIDP. Patients who fail therapy with IVIg, PE & glucocorticoids may benefit from treatment with azathioprine, methotrexate, cyclosporine, cyclophosphamide, and anti-CD20 (rituximab).

2741. Intravenous immune globulin has been established to be efficacious in?

A. Guillain-Barré syndrome
B. Chronic inflammatory demyelinating polyneuropathy
C. Myasthenia gravis
D. All of the above

2742. Intravenous Immunoglobulin (IVIg) has been used successfully in which of the following diseases?

A. Kawasaki disease
B. Graft-versus-host disease
C. Multiple sclerosis
D. All of the above

Intravenous Immunoglobulin (IVIg) has been used successfully to block reticuloendothelial cell function and immune complex clearance in various immune cytopenias such as immune thrombocytopenia. In addition, IVIg is useful for prevention of tissue damage in certain inflammatory syndromes such as Kawasaki disease and as Ig replacement therapy for certain types of immunoglobulin deficiencies. Use of IVIg in selected patients with graft-versus-host disease, multiple sclerosis, myasthenia gravis, Guillain-Barre syndrome and chronic demyelinating polyneuropathy is established.

2743. Intravenous immune globulin has been established to be efficacious in?

A. Corticosteroid-resistant dermatomyositis
B. Kawasaki's syndrome
C. GVHD prevention in allogeneic BM transplants
D. All of the above

IVIg blocks reticuloendothelial cell function and immune complex clearance in immune thrombocytopenia. In addition, IVIg is useful for prevention of tissue damage in certain inflammatory syndromes such as Kawasaki disease and as Ig replacement therapy for certain types of immunoglobulin deficiencies. IVIg is also useful in selected patients with graft-versus-host disease, multiple sclerosis, myasthenia gravis, Guillain-Barré syndrome, and chronic demyelinating polyneuropathy.

2744. The mode of action of immune globulin involves?

A. Modulation of expression & function of Fc receptors
B. Interference with activation of complement & cytokines
C. Provision of antiidiotypic antibodies
D. All of the above

2745. The half-life of infused immune globulin in immunocompetent persons is?

A. Two weeks
B. Three weeks
C. Four weeks
D. Five weeks

2746. Most natural autoantibodies in adult serum are of?

A. IgG class
B. IgM class
C. IgA class
D. All of the above

2747. Which of the following about total dose of Intravenous immune globulin is true?

A. 1 grams per kilogram over 3 days
B. 1 grams per kilogram over 5 days
C. 2 grams per kilogram over 3 days
D. 2 grams per kilogram over 5 days

Intravenous immune globulin has replaced plasma exchange as the treatment of choice in GBS patients who are not able to walk unaided. Immune globulin is given at a total dose of 2 grams per kilogram of body weight over a period of 5 days.

2748. Which of the following is true regarding definition of partial nerve conduction block?

A. Drop of 20% or more in negative peak area
B. Drop of 20% or more in peak-to-peak amplitude
C. Change of <15% in duration between proximal & distal site stimulation
D. All of the above

2749. Which of the following is false about Multifocal Motor Neuropathy?

A. Symmetric weakness
B. Relative sparing of sensory fibres
C. Starts in distal arm muscles
D. A partial motor-conduction block at multiple sites

Multifocal motor neuropathy (MMN) presents as slowly progressive motor weakness & atrophy evolving over years in the distribution of selected nerve trunks, associated with sites of persistent focal motor conduction block in the same nerve trunks. Sensory fibers are relatively spared. The arms are affected more frequently than the legs, and >75% of all patients are male.

2750. Which of the following is effective in the treatment of Multifocal Motor Neuropathy?

A. Corticosteroids
B. Plasma exchange (PE)
C. Immune globulin therapy
D. Methotrexate

2751. Which of the following is effective in the treatment of Multifocal Motor Neuropathy?

A. Corticosteroids
B. Plasma exchange (PE)
C. Cyclophosphamide
D. Methotrexate

Most patients with Multifocal motor neuropathy (MMN) respond to high-dose IVIg. Refractory patients may respond to rituximab or cyclophosphamide. Glucocorticoids and PE are not effective.

Myasthenia Gravis and Other Diseases of the Neuromuscular Junction

2752. Who was the first person to describe clinical features of MG?

A. Howard Wolfe
B. Amato Beeson
C. Nicolle Gilhus
D. Thomas Willis

A physiologist by the name of Thomas Willis was the first to describe the clinical features of MG in 1672. He wrote of a woman who, when she tried to talk for a prolonged period, "temporarily lost her power of speech and became mute as a fish."

2753. Myasthenia gravis (MG) is a neuromuscular disorder involving?
Harrison's 20th Ed. Chapter 440, Page 3232

A. Skeletal muscle
B. Smooth muscle
C. Cardiac muscle
D. All of the above

MG is a neuromuscular disorder characterized by weakness & fatigability of skeletal muscles.

2754. At neuromuscular junctions in myasthenia gravis, the defect in acetylcholine receptors (AChRs) is?
Harrison's 20th Ed. Chapter 440, Page 3232

A. Decrease in their number
B. Decrease in their size
C. Alteration in their shape
D. All of the above

In MG, underlying pathogenetic defect is decrease in number of available AChRs at neuromuscular junctions due to antibody-mediated autoimmune attack. This was first demonstrated by the use of a radioactively labeled snake toxin, α-bungarotoxin, which binds specifically, quantitatively, and irreversibly to acetylcholine receptors of skeletal muscles.

2755. Which of the following is false about neuromuscular junction in MG?
Harrison's 20th Ed. Chapter 440, Page 3233 Figure 440-1

A. Normal nerve terminal
B. Flattened, simplified postsynaptic folds
C. Widened synaptic space
D. None of the above

In MG, NM junction has a normal nerve terminal, reduced number of AChRs (stippling), flattened, simplified postsynaptic folds, & widened synaptic space.

2756. ACh from how many vesicles is released when action potential reaches nerve terminal?
Harrison's 20th Ed. Chapter 440, Page 3232

A. 5 to 20
B. 50 to 100
C. 150 to 200
D. 500 to 800

When an action potential travels down a motor nerve & reaches nerve terminal, acetylcholine (Ach) from 150 to 200 vesicles is released and combines with AChRs that are densely packed at peaks of postsynaptic folds.

2757. Structure of AChR consists of?
Harrison's 20th Ed. Chapter 440, Page 3232

A. 1-alpha, 2-beta, 1-delta, and 1-gamma or epsilon
B. 1-alpha, 1-beta, 2-delta, and 1-gamma or epsilon
C. 1-alpha, 1-beta, 1-delta, and 2-gamma or epsilon
D. 2-alpha, 1-beta, 1-delta, and 1-gamma or epsilon

Structure of nicotinic AChR consists of five subunits - 2-alpha, 1-beta, 1-delta, and 1-gamma or epsilon arranged around a central pore. Each of the two α subunits has an acetylcholine-binding site that is located extracellularly & centered around amino acids 192 and 193.

2758. Which of the following about Myasthenia gravis is false?
Harrison's 20th Ed. Chapter 440, Page 3232

A. Acetylcholine receptor consists of five subunits - 1-alpha, 2-beta, 1-gamma, 1-delta or 1-epsilon
B. Pathologic antibodies are IgG & are T cell dependent
C. Absence of anti AChR antibodies does not exclude diagnosis
D. Mycophenolate mofetil is useful

2759. SNARE stands for?
Mol Cell Neurosci. 2012 ;50(1):58–69

A. Soluble N-ethylmaleimide-sensitive fusion protein attachment protein receptors
B. Soluble N-ethylmaleimide-sensitive fusion protein adherent protein receptors
C. Soluble N-ethylmaleimide-sensitive fusion protein assembly protein receptors
D. Soluble N-ethylmaleimide-sensitive fusion protein absorbing protein receptors

In exocytosis/neurosecretion, SNAREs (soluble N-ethylmaleimide-sensitive fusion protein attachment protein receptors) play a role in vesicle docking, priming, fusion & synchronization of neurotransmitter release. Neurotransmitter release at neuronal synapses is directed by action potentials, whereas in sensory synapses, release is driven by receptor potentials that direct graded exocytosis. SNARE proteins associated with the vesicles are termed vesicle-SNAREs (v-SNAREs) and those on the presynaptic plasma membrane are called target-SNAREs (t-SNAREs).

2760. Which of the following is the most abundant protein of neuronal synaptic vesicles?
Mol Cell Neurosci. 2012 ;50(1):58–69

A. Synapsin
B. Actin
C. Synaptotagmin 4
D. Synaptobrevin

Synaptobrevin is the most abundant protein of neuronal synaptic vesicles. Others include synapsin, actin, and synaptotagmin 4. Synaptotagmins are the vesicle-bound calcium sensors. Complexins act as calcium-dependent switches.

2761. Which of the following is a criteria that provides supporting evidence for an antibody-mediated process?
N Engl J Med. 1994; 330:1797-1810

A. Presence of antibody
B. Antibody interacts with target antigen

C. Passive transfer reproduces disease features
D. All of the above

Myasthenia gravis is a disease due to an antibody-mediated autoimmune attack directed against acetylcholine receptors at neuromuscular junctions. The supporting evidence satisfies a set of five criteria that define the pathogenesis of autoantibody-mediated disorders. First, antibody is present. Second, antibody interacts with target antigen, acetylcholine receptor. Third, passive transfer reproduces disease features. Fourth, immunization with antigen produces a model disease. Fifth, a reduction of antibody levels ameliorates disease.

2762. Number of available acetylcholine receptors in NMJ is reduced by antibodies through?
N Engl J Med. 1994; 330:1797-1810

A. Accelerated endocytosis & degradation of receptors
B. Functional blockade of acetylcholine-binding sites
C. Complement-mediated damage to acetylcholine receptors
D. All of the above

2763. The first step in vesicle fusion at NMJ is?
Mol Cell Neurosci. 2012 ;50(1):58–69

A. Docking
B. Tethering
C. Priming
D. Fusion

The first step in vesicle fusion is tethering followed by docking, priming and fusion.

2764. Which of the following is a protein in SNARE complex?
Mol Cell Neurosci. 2012 ;50(1):58–69

A. Synaptobrevin
B. Syntaxin
C. SNAP-25/23 (synaptosomal-associated proteins)
D. All of the above

2765. With the opening of the channel in AChR, which of the following cation gains rapid entry?
Harrison's 20th Ed. Chapter 440, Page 3232

A. Sodium
B. Potassium
C. Calcium
D. Magnesium

ACh combines with binding sites on alpha subunits of AChR to open the channel permitting rapid entry of cations, chiefly sodium.

2766. Acetylcholinesterase (AChE) rapidly terminates the action of ACh by?
Harrison's 20th Ed. Chapter 440, Page 3232

A. Oxidation
B. Reduction
C. Hydrolysis
D. Phosphorylation

Acetylcholinesterase (AChE) rapidly terminates the action of acetylcholine (ACh) by hydrolysis.

2767. Which of the following about myasthenia gravis is false?
Harrison's 20th Ed. Chapter 440, Page 3232

A. ACh is released normally
B. Decrease in number of available ACh receptors
C. Increased presynaptic rundown
D. Thymus abnormal in ~ 75% of patients

Amount of ACh released per impulse normally declines on repeated activity (presynaptic rundown). In MG, this "normal" rundown along with decreased efficiency of NM transmission results in weakness or myasthenic fatigue. Thymus is abnormal in ~75% of patients with MG.

2768. In MG, the autoimmune antibody is targeted against?
Harrison's 20th Ed. Chapter 440, Page 3232

A. Acetylcholine
B. Acetylcholine receptor (AChR)
C. Acetylcholinesterase (AChE)
D. All of the above

In MG, specific anti-AChR autoimmune antibody is targeted against Acetylcholine receptor (AChR).

2769. In MG, anti-AChR antibodies reduce the number of available AChRs at NM junctions by which mechanism?
Harrison's 20th Ed. Chapter 440, Page 3232

A. Cross-linking & rapid endocytosis of AChR receptors
B. Blockade of the active site of AChR
C. Damage to postsynaptic muscle membrane
D. All of the above

Anti-AChR antibodies reduce the number of available AChRs at NM junctions by accelerated turnover of AChRs by its rapid endocytosis, blockade of the active binding site of AChR, and damage to postsynaptic muscle membrane by the antibody + complement.

2770. What is the role of protein muscle-specific kinase (MuSK)?
Harrison's 20th Ed. Chapter 440, Page 3232

A. AChR activation at NMJ
B. AChR blocking at NMJ
C. AChR clustering at NMJ
D. All of the above

An immune response to muscle-specific kinase (MuSK), a protein involved in AChR clustering at neuromuscular junctions, can also result in MG, with reduction of AChRs.

2771. Which of the following is involved in the pathogenesis of MG?
Harrison's 20th Ed. Chapter 440, Page 3232, 3233

A. Antibodies against agrin
B. Muscle-specific kinase (MuSK)
C. Antibodies against low-density lipoprotein receptor related protein 4 (LRP4)
D. All of the above

2772. Pathogenic anti-AChR antibody in myasthenia gravis is which immunoglobulin type?
Harrison's 20th Ed. Chapter 440, Page 3232

A. IgA
B. IgG
C. IgM
D. IgE

Anti-MuSK antibody occurs in about 40% of patients without AChR antibody. A small proportion of patients whose sera are negative for both AChR and MuSK antibodies have antibodies to another protein at the neuromuscular junction-low-density lipoprotein receptor related protein 4 (LRP4) - that is important for clustering of AChRs. The pathogenic antibodies are IgG and are T cell dependent. Antibodies against agrin have recently been found in some patients with MG. Agrin is a protein derived from motor nerves that normally binds to LRP4 and thus may also interfere with clustering of AChRs at neuromuscular junctions.

2773. Thymus is abnormal in what proportion of patients with MG?
Harrison's 20th Ed. Chapter 440, Page 3232

A. 25%
B. 50%
C. 75%
D. 100%

Thymus is abnormal in 75% of patients with MG. In 65%, thymus is "hyperplastic" though not necessarily enlarged. 10% of patients have thymic tumors (thymomas). Muscle-like cells within the thymus (myoid cells), which bear AChRs on their surface, may serve as a source of autoantigen & trigger the autoimmune reaction within thymus gland.

2774. Thymoma along with which of the following is called Good's syndrome?
Arch Intern Med. 1985;145:1704–7

A. Pure red cell aplasia
B. Hypogammaglobulinemia
C. Systemic lupus erythematosus
D. Ulcerative colitis

Thymoma with hypogammaglobulinemia also is called Good's syndrome.

2775. Hypogammaglobulinemia is observed in association with?
Harrison's 20th Ed. Chapter 344, Page 2496, 502

A. Thymoma
B. Chronic lymphocytic leukemia (CLL)
C. Myeloma
D. All of the above

2776. Individuals with hypogammaglobulinemia are at particular risk of?
Harrison's 20th Ed. Chapter 117, Page 881

A. C. difficile colitis
B. Giardiasis
C. Septic shock caused by P. aeruginosa
D. All of the above

Individuals with hypogammaglobulinemia are at particular risk of C. difficile colitis and giardiasis.

2777. WHIM syndrome consists of all except?
Harrison's 20th Ed. Chapter 60, Page 398

A. Warts
B. Hypogammaglobulinemia
C. Infections
D. Myelofibrosis

WHIM syndrome consists of warts, hypogammaglobulinemia, infections & myelokathexis (retention of WBCs in marrow). WHIM syndrome is caused by dominant gain-of-function mutation of CXCR4, resulting in cell retention in bone marrow.

2778. Paraneoplastic syndrome associated with thymic tumors presents as?
Harrison's 20th Ed. Chapter 74, Page 553

A. Myasthenia gravis
B. Pure red cell aplasia
C. Hypogammaglobulinemia
D. Any of the above

2779. Staging system for thymomas is named after?
Harrison's 20th Ed. Chapter 74, Page 554 Table 74-14

A. Atkin
B. Falkson
C. Masaoka
D. Tomaszek

The staging system for thymoma was developed by Masaoka and colleagues.

2780. Thymoma and / or myasthenia gravis is associated with which of the following?
Harrison's 20th Ed. Chapter 55, Page 357

A. Pemphigus vulgaris
B. Pemphigus foliaceus
C. Paraneoplastic pemphigus
D. Bullous pemphigoid

2781. Which of the following muscles are typically involved early in the course of MG?
Harrison's 20th Ed. Chapter 440, Page 3233

A. Chewing muscles
B. Facial muscles
C. Lids & extraocular muscles
D. Palate, tongue & pharyngeal muscles

In MG, due to early involvement of lids & extraocular muscles (EOMs), diplopia & fluctuating fatigable ptosis are common initial complaints.

2782. Involvement of extraocular muscles leads to all except?
Harrison's 20th Ed. Chapter 440, Page 3233

A. Diplopia
B. Ophthalmoplegia
C. Ptosis
D. Nystagmus

Most frequently affected muscle in MG is levator palpebrae superioris. Its weakness leads to ptosis, with or without Cogan's lid twitch. Ptosis may first ocur one eye, it almost always becomes bilateral with time.

2783. Which of the following is best related to ptosis?

A. Inverse-care law
B. Hering's law of equal innervation
C. Sutton's law
D. Hy's law

Heing's law, or the law of equal innervation, states that the same amount of innervation goes to an extraocular muscle and to its yoked fellow. The amount of innervation to the yoked pair is always determined by the fixating eye. Hering's law is important in understanding the topic of primary and secondary deviations.

2784. Which of the following about myasthenia gravis is false?
Harrison's 20th Ed. Chapter 440, Page 3233

A. Women more affected than men
B. Lids & extraocular muscles involved early
C. Limb weakness is proximal and asymmetric
D. Deep tendon reflexes diminished

Women are affected more frequently than men, in a ratio of ~3:2. Cranial muscles, particularly lids & extraocular muscles are involved early in MG. Diplopia & ptosis are common initial complaints. Limb weakness is proximal & asymmetric. Deep tendon reflexes are preserved.

2785. Dysarthric "mushy" quality speech in MG is due to?
Harrison's 20th Ed. Chapter 440, Page 3233

A. Weakness of the palate
B. Weakness of the tongue
C. Weakness of the pharynx
D. All of the above

In MG, speech has a nasal timbre caused by weakness of the palate or dysarthric "mushy" quality due to tongue weakness.

2786. In MG, when patient attempts to smile, facial weakness manifests as?
Harrison's 20th Ed. Chapter 440, Page 3233

A. "Elfin" facies
B. "Snarling" expression
C. "Chipmunk" facies
D. Leonine facies

Facial weakness produces a vertical myasthenic "snarling" expression when patient attempts to smile.

2787. Which of the following is related to myasthenia gravis?
DeJong's The Neurologic Examination, 7th Ed. Page 323

A. Dropped Head Syndrome
B. Ectropion
C. Trident tongue
D. All of the above

Causes of dropped head syndrome (head ptosis, floppy head, camptocormia) are inflammatory myopathy, ALS, and myasthenia gravis.

2788. Weakness out of proportion to wasting occurs in?
DeJong's The Neurologic Examination, 7th Ed. Page 479

A. Inflammatory myopathy
B. Myasthenia gravis
C. Periodic paralysis
D. All of the above

Weakness out of proportion to wasting occurs in inflammatory myopathy, myasthenia gravis, and periodic paralysis.

2789. Oculomasticatory myorhythmia is characteristic of which of the following?
Harrison's 20th Ed. Chapter 171, Page 1225

A. Leigh's disease
B. Lambert-Eaton syndrome
C. CNS Whipple's disease
D. Guillain-Barré syndrome

Oculomasticatory myorhythmia refers to pendular vergence movements of eyes synchronous with contractions of masticatory muscles. It is characteristic for CNS Whipple's disease.

2790. Which of the following is not a feature of Rowland Payne syndrome?
DeJong's The Neurologic Examination, 7th Ed. Page 315

A. Unilateral Horner syndrome
B. Ipsilateral vocal cord paralysis
C. Ipsilateral paralysis of hemidiaphragm
D. Ipsilateral deviation of tongue

Rowland Payne syndrome is a triad of unilateral Horner syndrome, ipsilateral vocal cord paralysis, and ipsilateral paralysis of hemidiaphragm. It is due to disruption of the oculosympathetic nerve, vagus nerve, and phrenic nerve in anterior neck (tumour, trauma).

2791. To grade clinical severity of myasthenia gravis, which of the following scale is used?
N Engl J Med. 1994; 330:1797-1810

A. Nicole scale
B. Wolfe scale
C. Gilhus scale
D. Osserman scale

Osserman scale: grade I involves focal disease (restricted to ocular muscles); grade II, generalized disease that is either mild (IIa) or moderate (IIb); grade III, severe generalized disease; and grade IV, a crisis, with life-threatening impairment of respiration. MGFA (Myasthenia Gravis Foundation of America) is also used to classify MG.

2792. Which of the following weakness is prominent in MuSK antibody positive MG?
Harrison's 20th Ed. Chapter 440, Page 3233

A. Facial weakness
B. Bulbar weakness
C. Lids & extraocular muscle weakness
D. Tongue weakness

Bulbar weakness is prominent in MuSK antibody positive MG.

2793. In MG, weakness becomes generalized, affecting limb muscles in what proportion of cases?
Harrison's 20th Ed. Chapter 440, Page 3233

A. ~55%
B. ~65%
C. ~75%
D. ~85%

In ~85% of patients, the weakness becomes generalized, affecting the limb muscles as well.

2794. MG muscle weakness will not become generalized if it remains restricted to extraocular muscles for?
Harrison's 20th Ed. Chapter 440, Page 3233

A. 6 months
B. 1 year
C. 2 years
D. 3 years

In MG, if muscle weakness remains restricted to extraocular muscles for 3 years (ocular MG), it is unlikely to become generalized.

2795. Which of the following is false about MG?
Harrison's 20th Ed. Chapter 440, Page 3233

A. No loss of reflexes
B. No impairment of sensation
C. No HMF neurologic defect
D. None of the above

MG is characterized by typical distribution of skeletal muscle weakness & fatigability, without loss of reflexes or impairment of sensation or other neurologic function.

2796. At which place is an ice-pack applied in ice-pack test (IPT) for NMJ defect?
Harrison's 20th Ed. Chapter 440, Page 3233, N Engl J Med. 2016;375:e39

A. Ear
B. Tongue
C. Eye
D. Any of the above

If ptosis is due to an NMJ defect, application of a pack of ice over the ptotic eye often results in improvement due to less depletion of quanta of AChR in cold & reduced activity of AChE at NMJ. However, IPT is limited by the need for ptosis and is therefore not suitable for all cases of MG. It is useful in cardiac patients and the elderly, where use of anticholinestrase agents is contraindicated.

2797. Ice is applied over the eye for how many minutes in ice pack test?
Neurol India 2016;64:1173-4

A. 1 minute
B. 2 minutes
C. 3 minutes
D. 4 minutes

Ice pack test consists of application of ice to eyes for 2 minutes, ensuring that eyes are covered to prevent burns. Reduction in muscle fiber temperature <22°C reduces the contractile force of muscle leading to a false negative result.

2798. Ice pack test is considered positive when there is an increase in palpebral fissure of?
Neurol India 2016;64:1173-4

A. 1 mm
B. 2 mm
C. 3 mm
D. 4 mm

Ice pack test is considered positive when there is an increase in palpebral fissure of 2 mm or more of the palpebral fissure on removal of the ice pack.

2799. Which of the following is a nonpharmacological test for evaluation of MG?
Neurol India 2016;64:1173-4

A. Ice pack test
B. Rest test
C. Sleep test
D. All of the above

For the rest test, patient is asked to close eyes for 5 minutes, and then improvement in ptosis is measured. For sleep test, patient is asked to lie down with eyes closed for 30 minutes in a quiet, dark room. Improvement in ptosis & ophthalmoparesis is then assessed.

2800. Pain in the head or eye in association with diplopia occurs in?
DeJong's The Neurologic Examination, 7th Ed. Page 204

A. Posterior communicating aneurysm
B. Ophthalmoplegic migraine
C. Tolosa-Hunt syndrome
D. All of the above

Pain in head or eye in association with diplopia occurs in diabetic third nerve palsy, posterior communicating aneurysm, ophthalmoplegic migraine, Tolosa-Hunt syndrome (painful ophthalmoplegia) & giant cell arteritis.

2801. Simpson's test refers to?
Neurol India 2016;64:1173-4

A. Increased ptosis on sustained down gaze
B. Increased ptosis on sustained up gaze
C. Increased ptosis on sustained lateral gaze
D. Any of the above

In Simpson test, the patient is asked to maintain upgaze for 2–3 minutes testing for fatigue induced ptosis.

2802. Which of the following test is used to diagnose MG?
Arch. Ophthalmol. 1979;97:678, Arch. Neurol. 1981;31:531

A. 'Peek' sign
B. Gorelick's test
C. Cogan's lid twitch sign
D. All of the above

The earliest manifestation of ocular MG is slowing of saccadic movement on rapid refixation. The 'peek' sign occurs when palpebral fissure widens after a period of voluntary eyelid closure. Gorelick's test is for bilateral asymmetrical ptosis. Finger elevation of opposite side eyelid while patient looks up, causes decreased ptosis on contralateral side. Cogan's lid twitch sign is characteristic of MG. It consists of a brief overshoot twitch of lid retraction following sudden return of eyes to primary position after a period of downgaze. Curtain sign or seesaw ptosis is elicited by manually raising the more ptotic lid. It causes the eye with less or no ptosis to suddenly crash.

2803. In myasthenia gravis (MG), which of the following about "trident tongue" is false?
DeJong's The Neurologic Examination, 7th Ed. Page 331

A. Occurs in long-standing disease
B. Tongue atrophy
C. Triple furrowed, grooves along median sulcus on each side
D. None of the above

Except for MG, neuromuscular junction disorders & myopathies rarely involve tongue to clinically significant degree. Tongue weakness & fatigability occurs in MG but generally only with severe involvement.

2804. Lingua plicata is characteristic of?
DeJong's The Neurologic Examination, 7th Ed. Page 38

A. Myasthenia gravis
B. Melkersson-Rosenthal syndrome
C. Myxedema
D. Down's syndrome

A triple furrowed tongue is seen in myasthenia gravis. Lingua plicata is seen in Melkersson-Rosenthal syndrome while macroglossia is typical of amyloid, myxedema & Down's syndrome.

2805. Which of the following is a cause of jaw drop?
DeJong's The Neurologic Examination, 7th Ed. Page 238

A. Myasthenia gravis (MG)
B. ALS
C. Kennedy's disease
D. All of the above

2806. Acquired autoimmune channelopathies include?
DeJong's The Neurologic Examination, 7th Ed. Page 791

A. Myasthenia gravis (MG)
B. Lambert-Eaton syndrome
C. Neuromyotonia & paraneoplastic cerebellar degeneration
D. All of the above

2807. Genetic channelopathies include?
DeJong's The Neurologic Examination, 7th Ed. Page 791

A. Periodic paralysis
B. Myotonia congenita, paramyotonia
C. Congenital myasthenia syndromes
D. All of the above

Genetic channelopathies include periodic paralysis, myotonia congenita, paramyotonia, the congenital myasthenia syndromes, malignant hyperthermia (MH), familial hemiplegic migraine, familial episodic ataxia, and the idiopathic generalized epilepsies.

2808. "Look of perpetual surprise" is a characteristic facial expression in?
DeJong's The Neurologic Examination, 7th Ed. Page 37

A. Progressive supranuclear palsy
B. Pseudobulbar palsy
C. Myasthenia gravis
D. Athetosis and dystonia

2809. "Immobile face with precipitate laughter & crying" is a characteristic facial expression in?
DeJong's The Neurologic Examination, 7th Ed. Page 37

  A. Progressive supranuclear palsy
  B. Pseudobulbar palsy
  C. Myasthenia gravis
  D. Athetosis and dystonia

Fixed ("masked") face is typical of parkinsonism. Look of perpetual surprise is seen in progressive supranuclear palsy, immobile face with precipitate laughter & crying is seen in pseudobulbar palsy, grimacing is typical of athetosis & dystonia. Ptosis & weakness of facial muscles is seen in some myopathies & myasthenia gravis.

2810. In seronegative MG, antibodies can be found against?
Harrison's 20th Ed. Chapter 440, Page 3233

  A. Muscle-specific tyrosine kinase
  B. Myasthenia-specific tyrosine kinase
  C. Membrane-specific tyrosine kinase
  D. None of the above

Presence of anti-AChR antibodies is diagnostic of MG, but a negative test does not exclude MG. Antibodies to muscle-specific tyrosine kinase (MuSK) are present in ~40% of AChR antibody-negative patients with generalized MG.

2811. Anti-AChR antibodies are detectable in what percentage of all myasthenic patients?
Harrison's 20th Ed. Chapter 440, Page 3233

  A. ~45%
  B. ~65%
  C. ~85%
  D. ~99%

2812. Anti-AChR antibodies are detectable in what percentage of ocular MG patients?
Harrison's 20th Ed. Chapter 440, Page 3233

  A. ~25%
  B. ~50%
  C. ~75%
  D. ~99%

Anti-AChR antibodies are detectable in ~85% of all MG patients & in only ~50% of ocular MG patients.

2813. Anti-MuSK antibodies are found in what percentage of AChR antibody-negative patients with generalized MG?
Harrison's 20th Ed. Chapter 440, Page 3233

  A. ~10%
  B. ~40%
  C. ~80%
  D. ~100%

~40% of AChR antibody-negative patients with generalized MG have anti-MuSK antibodies.

2814. Anti MuSK antibodies are present in what percentage of AChR antibody-positive MG patients?
Harrison's 20th Ed. Chapter 440, Page 3233

  A. Rare
  B. 25%
  C. 50%
  D. 80%

2815. Anti MuSK antibodies are present in what percentage of patients with MG limited to ocular muscles?
Harrison's 20th Ed. Chapter 440, Page 3233

  A. Rare
  B. 25%
  C. 50%
  D. 80%

MuSK antibodies are rarely present in AChR antibody-positive MG patients or in patients with MG limited to ocular muscles.

2816. Which of the following statements about antibodies to muscle-specific kinase (MuSK) is false?
Harrison's 20th Ed. Chapter 440, Page 3233

  A. Found in ~40% of AChR antibody-negative generalized MG
  B. Not present in AChR antibody-positive patients
  C. Not present in MG limited to ocular muscles
  D. None of the above

2817. It is best to test which of the following muscles in repetitive nerve stimulation for evidence of MG?
Harrison's 20th Ed. Chapter 440, Page 3234

  A. Proximal muscle groups
  B. Distal muscle groups
  C. Interosseous muscles
  D. Any of the above

It is best to test weak muscles or proximal muscle groups in repetitive nerve stimulation for evidence of MG. Anti-AChE medication must be stopped 6–24 hours before testing.

2818. In myasthenic patients, rapid reduction of what proportion in amplitude of evoked responses is noted?
Harrison's 20th Ed. Chapter 440, Page 3234

  A. > 10%
  B. > 20%
  C. > 30%
  D. > 50%

In repetitive nerve stimulation for evidence of MG, electric shocks are delivered at a rate of three per second (3 Hz) to the appropriate nerves, and action potentials are recorded from muscles. In myasthenic patients there is a rapid reduction of > 10% in the amplitude of the evoked responses. (Normal <10%).

2819. In myasthenia gravis, which of the following spirometric statement is false?
Harrison's 20th Ed. Chapter 279, Page 1950

  A. Normal FRC
  B. Low TLC
  C. Elevated RV
  D. Normal FVC

In MG, FRC remains normal, as both lung recoil & passive chest wall recoil are normal. TLC is low and RV is elevated, as respiratory muscle strength is insufficient. Caught between the low TLC and the elevated RV, FVC and FEV1 are reduced as "innocent bystanders." As airway size and the lung vasculature are unaffected, both airways resistance (R_{aw}) and DL_{CO} are normal.

2820. Type of respiratory failure in MG is usually?
Harrison's 20th Ed. Chapter 293, Page 2026

  A. Type I
  B. Type II
  C. Type III
  D. Type IV

In myasthenia gravis, reduced strength due to impaired neuromuscular transmission results in type II respiratory failure i.e. alveolar hypoventilation and inability to eliminate carbon dioxide effectively.

2821. Fluctuating ptosis that worsens late in the day is typical of?
Harrison's 20th Ed. Chapter 28, Page 190

A. Myasthenia gravis
B. Glaucoma
C. Optic nerve glioma
D. Orbital cellulitis

Fluctuating ptosis that worsens late in the day is typical of myasthenia gravis.

2822. Which of the following is a cause of myogenic ptosis?
Harrison's 20th Ed. Chapter 28, Page 190

A. Myasthenia gravis
B. Chronic progressive external ophthalmoplegia
C. Oculopharyngeal dystrophy
D. All of the above

2823. Which of the following muscles open the eyelid?
Harrison's 20th Ed. Chapter 28, Page 190

A. Tenon's muscle
B. Müller's muscle
C. Zinn muscle
D. All of the above

Two muscles that open the eyelid are Müller's muscle & levator palpebrae superioris.

2824. Which of the following is an eye-related finding in myasthenia gravis?
Harrison's 20th Ed. Chapter 28, Page 190

A. Pupils are always normal
B. Diplopia is intermittent & variable
C. Diplopia is not confined to any single ocular motor nerve
D. All of the above

MG is a major cause of painless diplopia which is intermittent, variable, and not confined to any single ocular motor nerve distribution. Pupils are always normal. Fluctuating ptosis may be present.

2825. Cause of episodic generalized weakness is?
Harrison's 20th Ed. Chapter 21, Page 138

A. Myasthenia gravis
B. Lambert-Eaton myasthenic syndrome
C. Multiple sclerosis
D. All of the above

Causes of episodic generalized weakness include electrolyte disturbances (hypokalemia, hyperkalemia, hypercalcemia, hypernatremia, hyponatremia, hypophosphatemia, hypermagnesemia), muscle disorders (periodic paralyses, metabolic defects of muscle), neuromuscular junction disorders (myasthenia gravis, Lambert-Eaton myasthenic syndrome), central nervous system disorders (transient ischemic attacks of brainstem, transient global cerebral ischemia, multiple sclerosis).

2826. The edrophonium test is now used in which of the following patients of suspected MG?
Harrison's 20th Ed. Chapter 440, Page 3235

A. Who have negative antibody
B. Who have negative electrodiagnostic testing
C. Who have negative ice-pack test
D. All of the above

2827. Which of the following drug must be kept at hand while conducting Edrophonium anticholinesterase test?
Harrison's 20th Ed. Chapter 440, Page 3235

A. Atropine
B. Neostigmine
C. Adrenaline
D. All of the above

Atropine (0.6 mg) should be drawn up in a syringe, ready for IV use if nausea, diarrhea, salivation, fasciculations, syncope or bradycardia develop following IV edrophonium.

2828. Apart from Edrophonium which drug can be used for Anticholinesterase Test?
Harrison's 20th Ed. Chapter 440, Page 3235

A. Atropine
B. Neostigmine
C. Adrenaline
D. All of the above

A longer acting drug like neostigmine (orally) may be used for anticholinesterase test, as it permits more time for detailed evaluation of strength.

2829. Which of the following diseases can cause false-positive Edrophonium anticholinesterase test?
Harrison's 20th Ed. Chapter 440, Page 3235

A. Amyotrophic lateral sclerosis
B. Hodgkin lymphoma
C. Charcot-Marie-Tooth disease
D. Creutzfeldt-Jakob disease (CJD)

False-positive Edrophonium anticholinesterase test occur in occasional patients with amyotrophic lateral sclerosis, and in placebo-reactors.

2830. Which of the following is a cause of autoimmune MG?
Harrison's 20th Ed. Chapter 440, Page 3235

A. Congenital myasthenic syndromes (CMS)
B. Treatment with penicillamine
C. Kearns-Sayre syndrome
D. Botulism

Treatment with penicillamine and check point inhibitors for cancer may result in autoimmune MG.

2831. Drugs that can exacerbate weakness in myasthenic patients are all except?
Harrison's 20th Ed. Chapter 440, Page 3235

A. Penicillamine
B. Aminoglycoside antibiotics
C. Procainamide
D. Diazepam

Drugs that may exacerbate MG include aminoglycosides (streptomycin, tobramycin, kanamycin), Quinolones (ciprofloxacin, levofloxacin, ofloxacin, gatifloxacin), macrolides (erythromycin, azithromycin), Nondepolarizing muscle relaxants (D-Tubocurarine, pancuronium, vecuronium, atracurium), Beta-blockers (Propranolol, atenolol, metoprolol), Local anesthetics (Procaine, Xylocaine), Procainamide, Botulinum toxin, Quinine derivatives (Quinine, quinidine, chloroquine, mefloquine), Magnesium, Penicillamine.

2832. Which of the following drugs contain a thiol group in their chemical structure?
Harrison's 20th Ed. Chapter 55, Page 357

A. Penicillamine
B. Captopril
C. Enalapril
D. All of the above

Drugs containing a thiol group in their chemical structure are penicillamine, captopril, enalapril. They are most commonly associated with drug-induced pemphigus.

2833. Which of the following component of the neuromuscular junction may be affected in congenital myasthenic syndromes (CMS)?

Harrison's 20th Ed. Chapter 440, Page 3235

A. Presynaptic nerve terminal
B. Various subunits of AChR
C. Various subunits of AChE
D. All of the above

Congenital myasthenic syndromes (CMS) are disorders of neuromuscular junction that are not autoimmune but are due to genetic mutations in which virtually any component of the neuromuscular junction may be affected. Alterations in function of presynaptic nerve terminal or in various subunits of the AChR or AChE have been identified in different forms of CMS.

2834. Which of the following statements about congenital myasthenic syndromes (CMS) is false?

Harrison's 20th Ed. Chapter 440, Page 3235

A. Due to genetic mutations, not autoimmune
B. Symptoms begin in infancy or childhood
C. AChR antibody tests are consistently negative
D. A subunit of AChR is affected in ~75% of cases

CMS should be suspected when symptoms of myasthenia begin in infancy or childhood & AChR antibody tests are consistently negative. CMS that involve AChR, ε subunit is affected in ~75%.

2835. Double seronegative MG i.e. absence of AChR & MuSK antibodies occurs in what percentage of generalized MG patients?

Harrison's 20th Ed. Chapter 440, Page 3235

A. ~ 2%
B. ~ 5%
C. ~ 8%
D. ~ 10%

Double seronegative MG i.e. absence of AChR & MuSK antibodies occurs in ~10% of generalized MG patients.

2836. Which of the following CMS patients worsen with AChE inhibitors?

Harrison's 20th Ed. Chapter 440, Page 3235

A. Slow channel syndrome
B. AChE deficiency
C. DOK-7 related CMS
D. All of the above

2837. Myasthenia gravis is related to which of the following?

Harrison's 20th Ed. Chapter 440, Page 3235

A. Neuromyelitis optica (NMO)
B. M component on electrophoretic analysis
C. Hyperthyroidism
D. All of the above

2838. Disorders associated with myasthenia gravis include?

Harrison's 20th Ed. Chapter 440, Page 3235

A. Hashimoto's thyroiditis
B. Graves' disease
C. Systemic lupus erythematosus
D. All of the above

Disorders associated with Myasthenia Gravis are thymoma, thymus hyperplasia, Hashimoto's thyroiditis, Graves' disease, rheumatoid arthritis, lupus erythematosus, skin disorders, family history of autoimmune disorder. Hyperthyroidism or hypothyroidism, occult infection, medical treatment for other conditions may exacerbate myasthenia gravis. Tuberculosis, diabetes, peptic ulcer, gastrointestinal bleeding, renal disease, hypertension, asthma, osteoporosis, obesity are disorders that may interfere with therapy.

2839. Which of the following is false about Lambert-Eaton myasthenic syndrome (LEMS)?

Harrison's 20th Ed. Chapter 440, Page 3235

A. Presynaptic disorder of neuromuscular junction
B. Proximal muscles of lower limbs most commonly affected
C. Normal deep tendon reflexes
D. Incremental responses on repetitive nerve stimulation

LEMS is a presynaptic disorder of NM junction. Proximal muscles of lower limbs are most commonly affected. Ptosis & diplopia occur in ~70% of patients. Patients with LEMS have depressed or absent reflexes, experience autonomic changes such as dry mouth and impotence, and have incremental responses on repetitive nerve stimulation.

2840. Which of the following is false about Lambert-Eaton myasthenic syndrome (LEMS)?

Harrison's 20th Ed. Chapter 440, Page 3235

A. Autoantibodies against P/Q type calcium channels
B. Associated small-cell carcinoma of lung
C. Plasmapheresis ineffective
D. 3,4 Diaminopyridine (3,4-DAP) helpful

LEMS is caused by autoantibodies directed against P/Q type calcium channels at the motor nerve terminals impairing release of ACh & are detected in ~85% of LEMS patients. Small cell lung carcinoma is common in LEMS. Treatment of LEMS involves plasmapheresis & immunosuppression, 3,4-Diaminopyridine (3,4-DAP) & pyridostigmine.

2841. Muscle testing reveals "jerky release" or "give-away weakness" in which of the following?

Harrison's 20th Ed. Chapter 440, Page 3235

A. Lambert-Eaton myasthenic syndrome (LEMS)
B. Botulism
C. Hyperthyroidism
D. Neurasthenia

Muscle testing reveals "jerky release" or "give-away weakness" characteristic of non-organic disorders like Neurasthenia - a myasthenia-like fatigue syndrome without an organic basis.

2842. Which of the following cause weakness of somatic musculature due to presynaptic neuromuscular junction abnormality?

Harrison's 20th Ed. Chapter 440, Page 3235

A. Lambert-Eaton myasthenic syndrome (LEMS)
B. Botulism
C. Congenital myasthenic syndromes (CMS)
D. All of the above

CMS are not due to autoimmune but due to genetic mutations presynaptic nerve terminal or in subunits of AChR or AChE. In Botulism, bacterial toxin interferes with release of acetylcholine from presynaptic nerve terminal.

2843. Morvan's syndrome consists of?

Harrison's 20th Ed. Chapter 440, Page 3236

A. Encephalitis
B. Autonomic dysfunction
C. Neuromyotonia
D. All of the above

Morvan's syndrome consists of encephalitis, insomnia, confusion, hallucinations, autonomic dysfunction and neuromyotonia.

2844. Myasthenic patients have an increased incidence of?
Harrison's 20th Ed. Chapter 440, Page 3236

A. Hyperthyroidism
B. Systemic lupus erythematosus
C. Rheumatoid arthritis
D. All of the above

2845. Myasthenic patients have an increased incidence of?
Harrison's 20th Ed. Chapter 440, Page 3236

A. Neuromyelitis optica
B. Rippling muscle disease
C. Chronic inflammatory demyelinating polyneuropathy
D. All of the above

Myasthenic patients have an increased incidence of neuromyelitis optica, neuromyotonia, Morvan's syndrome (encephalitis, insomnia, confusion, hallucinations, autonomic dysfunction, and neuromyotonia), rippling muscle disease, granulomatous myositis/myocarditis & CIDP.

2846. Rippling muscle disease is associated with?
Journal of Clinical Neuroscience 2006;13(5):576-578

A. Caveolin-3
B. Connexin 26
C. MYO7A
D. TMC1

Caveolin-3 protein is expressed exclusively in muscle cells and forms scaffolding on cytoplasmic surface of sarcolemmal membrane. Improper caveolin-3 oligomerization results in skeletal muscle T-tubule system derangement, sarcolemmal membrane alterations, and large subsarcolemmal vesicle formation. Caveolin-3 mutations can result in four muscle disease phenotypes: limb girdle muscular dystrophy, rippling muscle disease, distal myopathy, and hyperCKemia.

2847. Botulinum toxin is produced by?
Harrison's 20th Ed. Chapter 148, Page 1105

A. Clostridium botulinum
B. Clostridium argentinense
C. Clostridium butyricum
D. All of the above

Botulinum toxin is produced by four recognized species of clostridia namely Clostridium botulinum, Clostridium argentinense, Clostridium baratii, and Clostridium butyricum.

2848. Which serotype of botulinum toxin produces the most severe syndrome?
Harrison's 20th Ed. Chapter 148, Page 1106

A. Serotype A
B. Serotype B
C. Serotype E
D. Serotype F

2849. Clinical syndrome of botulism consists of?
Harrison's 20th Ed. Chapter 148, Page 1106

A. Bilateral cranial-nerve palsies
B. Respiratory compromise
C. Bilateral descending flaccid paralysis of voluntary muscles
D. All of the above

Clinical syndrome of botulism consists of bilateral cranial-nerve palsies, respiratory compromise, bilateral descending flaccid paralysis of voluntary muscles and even death.

2850. Which of the following illnesses is considered in the differential diagnosis of adult botulism?
Harrison's 20th Ed. Chapter 148, Page 1107

A. Miller Fisher syndrome
B. Myasthenia gravis
C. Eaton-Lambert syndrome
D. All of the above

2851. The universally accepted method for confirmation of botulism is?
Harrison's 20th Ed. Chapter 148, Page 1108

A. Muscle biopsy
B. Nerve stimulation studies
C. Mouse bioassay
D. HPLC

The universally accepted method for confirmation of botulism is the mouse bioassay.

2852. Muscarinic side effects of anticholinesterase medication include all except?
Harrison's 20th Ed. Chapter 440, Page 3237

A. Diarrhea
B. Abdominal cramps
C. Dry mouth
D. Nausea

Muscarinic side effects of anticholinesterase medication are diarrhea, abdominal cramps, salivation and nausea.

2853. Thymoma is suspected if thymus is enlarged after?
Harrison's 20th Ed. Chapter 440, Page 3237

A. > 10 years
B. > 20 years
C. > 30 years
D. > 40 years

Thymic shadow on CT is normal in young adulthood, but thymus enlargement in a patient >40 years is highly suspicious of thymoma.

2854. By consensus, thymectomy should be done in all patients with generalized MG between?
Harrison's 20th Ed. Chapter 440, Page 3237

A. Puberty and 55 years
B. 30 and 55 years
C. 40 and 65 years
D. 50 and 75 years

It is the consensus that thymectomy should be carried out in all patients with generalized MG who are between puberty and at least 55 years of age.

2855. Which of the following patients may not benefit from thymectomy?
Harrison's 20th Ed. Chapter 440, Page 3237

A. Ocular myasthenia
B. MuSK-positive MG
C. Seronegative MG
D. All of the above

2856. Which of the following statements about MG is false?
Harrison's 20th Ed. Chapter 440, Page 3237

A. Patients with anti-MuSK MG get less benefit from anticholinesterase agents
B. Patients with anti-MuSK - positive MG respond less well to thymectomy
C. Rituximab is effective in MG patients with MuSK antibody
D. None of the above

2857. If immediate improvement is essential, which of the following is used to manage MG?
Harrison's 20th Ed. Chapter 440, Page 3237

A. Thymectomy
B. High-dose cyclophosphamide
C. Glucocorticoids
D. Intravenous immunoglobulin (IVIg)

In MG, if immediate improvement is essential, IVIg is given or plasmapheresis instituted.

2858. Which of the following produce clinical improvement within a period of 1–3 months?
Harrison's 20th Ed. Chapter 440, Page 3237

A. Glucocorticoids
B. Cyclosporine
C. Tacrolimus
D. All of the above

For the intermediate term goal of improvement, glucocorticoids, cyclosporine or tacrolimus produce clinical improvement within a period of 1–3 months.

2859. Which of the following immunosuppressive agents is preferred (toxicity & cost) in treatment of MG?
Harrison's 20th Ed. Chapter 440, Page 3237

A. Azathioprine
B. Cyclosporine
C. Mycophenolate mofetil
D. Cyclophosphamide

2860. Beneficial effect of azathioprine takes how long to appear?
Harrison's 20th Ed. Chapter 440, Page 3237

A. 7 – 21 days
B. 1 – 3 months
C. 3 – 6 months
D. 18 months

Beneficial effects of azathioprine & mycophenolate mofetil begin after many months (up to a year) because mycophenolate mofetil does not kill or eliminate preexisting autoreactive lymphocytes.

2861. Which of the following is used in MG patients refractory to optimal treatment with immunosuppressive agents?
Harrison's 20th Ed. Chapter 440, Page 3237

A. Tacrolimus
B. High-dose cyclophosphamide
C. Mycophenolate mofetil
D. Intravenous immunoglobulin (IVIg)

Patient with MG refractory to optimal treatment with conventional immunosuppressive agents, high-dose cyclophosphamide may induce long-lasting benefit by "rebooting" the immune system.

2862. Drug of choice for long-term treatment of myasthenic patients is?
Harrison's 20th Ed. Chapter 440, Page 3238

A. Azathioprine
B. Mycophenolate mofetil
C. Cyclosporine
D. Tacrolimus

2863. In patients taking azathioprine, which out of the following drugs should not be used?
Harrison's 20th Ed. Chapter 440, Page 3238

A. Paracetamol
B. Allopurinol
C. Cephalosporins
D. Terfenadine

In patients taking azathioprine, allopurinol should never be used to treat hyperuricemia, because due to a common degradation pathway, severe bone marrow depression may occur.

2864. Which of the following may be used as indications of adequacy of azathioprine dosage?
Harrison's 20th Ed. Chapter 440, Page 3238

A. Increase in hemoglobin
B. Decrease in ESR
C. Increase in hematocrit
D. Increase of RBC mean corpuscular volume

Reduction of lymphocytes to <1000/μL and/or an increase of MCV may be used as indications of adequacy of azathioprine dosage.

2865. Which of the following drug is useful in the treatment of anti-MuSK antibody positive MG?
Harrison's 20th Ed. Chapter 440, Page 3238

A. Tacrolimus
B. Rituximab
C. Cyclophosphamide
D. Azathioprine

Rituximab, a monoclonal antibody that depletes CD20 B cells, is useful in the treatment of anti-MuSK antibody positive MG.

2866. Which of the following has been found beneficial in MG patients?
Harrison's 20th Ed. Chapter 440, Page 3238

A. Trastuzumab
B. Eculizumab
C. Tocilizumab
D. Bevacizumab

Eculizumab is an anti-C5 complement inhibitor.

2867. Eculizumab is used in the treatment of?
Harrison's 20th Ed. Chapter 440, Page 3238

A. Paroxysmal nocturnal hemoglobinuria
B. Familial (Atypical) Hemolytic-Uremic Syndrome (aHUS)
C. Acute cellular rejection (ACR)
D. All of the above

2868. Most common cause of myasthenic crisis is?
Harrison's 20th Ed. Chapter 440, Page 3238

A. Hyperthyroidism
B. Hypothyroidism
C. Intercurrent infection
D. Drug underdose

The most common cause of myasthenic crisis is intercurrent infection.

2869. Which of the following is useful to assess MG patient's clinical status?
Cleveland clinic J of Med. 2013;80(11):711-21

A. Forward arm abduction time (5 min)
B. Forced vital capacity
C. Time to development of ptosis on upward gaze
D. All of the above

Most useful clinical tests to assess MG patient's clinical status include forward arm abduction time (up to a full 5 min.), forced vital capacity, range of eye movements, and time to development of ptosis on upward gaze. Patient's AChR antibody level also provides clinically valuable confirmation of the effectiveness of treatment.

2870. Which of the following is false about Myasthenia gravis?
Cleveland clinic J of Med. 2013;80(11):711-21

A. Age of onset has a bimodal distribution
B. Fluctuating muscle weakness with fatigue
C. Generalized fatigue without objective weakness
D. Ptosis alternating from one eye to the other

In MG, age of onset has a bimodal distribution, with an early incidence peak in the second to third decade with a female predominance and a late peak in the 6th to the 8th decade with a male predominance. Generalized fatigue without objective weakness is inconsistent with myasthenia gravis. Ptosis alternating from one eye to the other is fairly characteristic of myasthenia gravis.

2871. Myasthenia gravis is commonly associated with?
Cleveland clinic J of Med. 2013;80(11):711-21

A. Hypothyroidism
B. Hyperthyroidism
C. Rheumatoid arthritis
D. All of the above

Myasthenia gravis is commonly associated with hypothyroidism, hyperthyroidism, systemic lupus erythematosus, rheumatoid arthritis, vitiligo, diabetes and neuromyelitis optica.

2872. Which of the following is an AChR antibody subtype?
Cleveland clinic J of Med. 2013;80(11):711-21

A. Binding
B. Blocking
C. Modulating
D. All of the above

There are three AChR antibody subtypes: binding, blocking, and modulating. Binding antibodies are present in 80% to 90% of patients with generalized myasthenia gravis and 50% of those with ocular myasthenia gravis. Testing for blocking and modulating AChR antibodies increases the sensitivity by less than 5% when added to testing for binding antibodies.

2873. MuSK stands for?
Cleveland clinic J of Med. 2013;80(11):711-21

A. Membrane-specific kinase (MuSK)
B. Muscle-specific kinase (MuSK)
C. Membrane-specific tyrosine kinase (MuSK)
D. Muscle-specific tyrosine kinase (MuSK)

In most cases of myasthenia gravis the patient has autoimmune antibodies against constituents of the neuromuscular junction, specifically acetylcholine receptor (AChR) and muscle-specific tyrosine kinase (MuSK).

2874. Which of the following about MuSK is false?
Cleveland clinic J of Med. 2013;80(11):711-21

A. Transmembrane component of postsynaptic neuromuscular junction
B. Activated through binding of agrin to lipoprotein-related protein 4
C. Antibodies against MuSK activate complement system
D. MG with MuSK antibodies is rarely associated with thymoma

Like AChR, MuSK is a transmembrane component of the postsynaptic neuromuscular junction. During formation of the neuromuscular junction, MuSK is activated through the binding of agrin (a nerve-derived proteoglycan) to lipoprotein-related protein 4 (LRP4, receptor for agrin), after which complicated intracellular signaling promotes the assembly and stabilization of AChR. Unlike AChR antibodies, antibodies against MuSK do not activate the complement system, and complement fixation is not essential for clinical myasthenic symptoms to appear. Also, myasthenia gravis with MuSK antibodies is rarely associated with thymoma. MuSK antibodies block the binding of MuSK to acetylcholinesterase. MuSK antibody-positive myasthenia gravis tend to respond poorly to acetylcholinesterase inhibitors. Most MuSK antibody-positive patients have a favorable response to immunosuppressive therapy.

2875. Decremental response on repetitive nerve stimulation studies can be seen in?
Cleveland clinic J of Med. 2013;80(11):711-21

A. Myasthenia gravis
B. Motor neuron disease
C. Lambert-Eaton myasthenic syndrome
D. All of the above

Repetitive nerve stimulation studies use a slow rate (2 - 5 Hz) of repetitive electrical stimulation. The study is positive if the motor response declines by >10%. Decremental response may be seen in myasthenia gravis, motor neuron disease or Lambert-Eaton myasthenic syndrome.

2876. Medication that can exacerbate weakness in myasthenia gravis is?
Cleveland clinic J of Med. 2013;80(11):711-21

A. Penicillamine
B. Procainamide
C. Aminoglycosides
D. All of the above

Medications that can exacerbate weakness in myasthenia gravis are penicillamine, interferons, procainamide, quinidine, and antibiotics, including quinolones and aminoglycosides.

Muscular Dystrophies and Other Muscle Diseases

2877. Clinical findings of a myopathy include all except?
Harrison's 20th Ed. Chapter 441, Page 3239

A. Proximal limb weakness
B. Symmetric limb weakness
C. Depressed reflexes
D. Preserved sensation

Clinical findings of a myopathy are proximal, symmetric limb weakness (arms or legs) with preserved reflexes and sensation.

2878. Muscular dystrophies are characterized by the progressive loss of muscle in accordance with?
Current Opinion in Genetics and Development. 2003;13(3):231-238

A. Age of onset
B. Severity
C. Group of muscles affected
D. All of the above

2879. Which of the following is not a childhood muscular dystrophy?
doi:10.1155/2012/485376

A. Limb-girdle muscular dystrophy
B. Duchenne muscular dystrophy (DMD)
C. Becker muscular dystrophy (BMD)
D. Emery-Dreifuss muscular dystrophy (EDMD)

Duchenne muscular dystrophy (DMD), Becker muscular dystrophy (BMD) and Emery-Dreifuss muscular dystrophy (EDMD) have their first clinical manifestations during childhood. Laminopathies such as myotonic dystrophy or limb-girdle muscular dystrophy appear during adulthood.

2880. Which of the following is not a cause of intermittent weakness of muscles?
Harrison's 20th Ed. Chapter 441, Page 3240

A. Myasthenia gravis
B. Polymyositis
C. Myophosphorylase deficiency
D. Carnitine palmitoyltransferase deficiency

Disorders causing intermittent muscle weakness include myasthenia gravis, periodic paralyses (hypokalemic, hyperkalemic), and metabolic energy deficiencies of glycolysis (myophosphorylase deficiency), fatty acid utilization (carnitine palmitoyltransferase deficiency), and some mitochondrial myopathies.

2881. Which of the following about limb-girdle weakness is false?
Harrison's 20th Ed. Chapter 441, Page 3240

A. Proximal muscles are weaker than the distal
B. Symmetrically affected
C. Facial muscles are spared
D. None of the above

2882. Which of the following is characteristic of facioscapulohumeral dystrophy (FSHD)?
Harrison's 20th Ed. Chapter 441, Page 3240

A. Difficulty with eye closure
B. Impaired smile
C. Scapular winging
D. All of the above

Facial weakness manifesting as difficulty with eye closure and impaired smile along with scapular winging are characteristic of facioscapulohumeral dystrophy (FSHD).

2883. Which of the following is virtually diagnostic of myotonic dystrophy type 1?
Harrison's 20th Ed. Chapter 441, Page 3240

A. Facial weakness
B. Distal limb weakness
C. Hand grip myotonia
D. All of the above

Facial & distal limb weakness associated with hand grip myotonia is virtually diagnostic of myotonic dystrophy type 1.

2884. Ptosis or extraocular muscle weakness is caused by?
Harrison's 20th Ed. Chapter 441, Page 3240

A. Neuromuscular junction disorders
B. Oculopharyngeal muscular dystrophy
C. Mitochondrial myopathies
D. All of the above

Ptosis or extraocular muscle weakness can be caused by neuromuscular junction disorders, oculopharyngeal muscular dystrophy, mitochondrial myopathies, and some congenital myopathies.

2885. Which of the following is characteristic of inclusion body myositis?
Harrison's 20th Ed. Chapter 441, Page 3240

A. Atrophy and weakness of wrist flexors
B. Atrophy and weakness of finger flexors
C. Atrophy and weakness of quadriceps muscles
D. All of the above

A pathognomonic pattern characteristic of inclusion body myositis (IBM) is atrophy & weakness of wrist flexors, finger flexors and quadriceps muscles, often asymmetric.

2886. Which of the following can have a presentation of "dropped head syndrome"?
Harrison's 20th Ed. Chapter 441, Page 3240

A. Myasthenia gravis
B. Amyotrophic lateral sclerosis
C. Hyperparathyroidism
D. All of the above

Dropped head syndrome indicates selective neck extensor muscle weakness. Neuromuscular diseases associated with this pattern of weakness include myasthenia gravis, amyotrophic lateral sclerosis, late-onset nemaline myopathy, hyperparathyroidism, focal myositis, and some forms of inclusion body myopathy.

2887. Pathologic fatigability occurs in which of the following?
Harrison's 20th Ed. Chapter 441, Page 3241

A. Disorders of neuromuscular transmission
B. Disorders of defects in glycolysis
C. Chronic myopathies
D. All of the above

Pathologic fatigability refers to inability to maintain or sustain a force. It occurs in disorders of neuromuscular transmission and in disorders altering energy production (glycolysis, lipid metabolism, or mitochondrial energy production), chronic myopathies.

2888. Muscle cramps often occur in which of the following neurogenic disorders?
Harrison's 20th Ed. Chapter 441, Page 3241

A. Motor neuron disease
B. Radiculopathies
C. Polyneuropathies
D. All of the above

Muscle cramps often occur in neurogenic disorders, especially motor neuron disease, radiculopathies, and polyneuropathies. They are not a feature of most primary muscle diseases. There are no pathologic reflexes in myopathies.

2889. Which of the following is false in myopathies?
Harrison's 20th Ed. Chapter 441, Page 3241

A. There are no pathologic reflexes
B. There is no sensory loss
C. There is no bowel & bladder dysfunction
D. None of the above

2890. Fixed contracture is a distinctive feature of?
Harrison's 20th Ed. Chapter 441, Page 3242

A. Motor neuron disease
B. Stiff-Person syndrome
C. Emery-Dreifuss muscular dystrophy
D. Paramyotonia congenita (PC)

In Emery-Dreifuss muscular dystrophy and Bethlem myopathy, fixed contractures are an early and distinctive feature.

2891. Which of the following is a chloride channel disorder?
Harrison's 20th Ed. Chapter 441, Page 3242

A. Paramyotonia congenita (PC)
B. Myotonic muscular dystrophy type 1 (DM1)
C. Myotonic muscular dystrophy type 2 (DM2)
D. Myotonia congenita

2892. In which of the following myotonia, muscle weakness is not prominent?
Harrison's 20th Ed. Chapter 441, Page 3242

A. Paramyotonia congenita (PC)
B. Myotonic muscular dystrophy type 1 (DM1)
C. Myotonic muscular dystrophy type 2 (DM2)
D. Myotonia congenita

2893. Which of the following is related to stiff-Person syndrome?
Harrison's 20th Ed. Chapter 441, Page 3242

A. Serum antibodies against PMP22
B. Serum antibodies against ornithine decarboxylase
C. Serum antibodies against dopa decarboxylase
D. Serum antibodies against glutamic acid decarboxylase

Serum antibodies against glutamic acid decarboxylase are present in approximately two-thirds of stiff-Person syndrome cases. This disorder is characterized by progressive muscle rigidity, stiffness & painful spasms mostly of lower extremity, triggered by auditory, sensory, or emotional stimuli. Sometimes, only one extremity is affected (stiff-limb syndrome).

2894. Which of the following antibodies are associated with Stiff-Person syndrome?
Harrison's 20th Ed. Chapter 441, Page 673

A. GAD
B. Amphiphysin
C. GlyR
D. All of the above

The three main targets of autoantibodies in patients with Stiff-Person spectrum disorders are presynaptic proteins GAD and amphiphysin, and postsynaptic glycine receptor (GlyR). Presence of amphiphysin antibodies indicates a paraneoplastic etiology related to SCLC and breast cancer. GAD antibodies are much more frequently present in nonparaneoplastic disorders. GlyR antibodies are also detectable in patients with PERM.

2895. Which of the following is false about Stiff-Person Syndrome?
Harrison's 20th Ed. Chapter 441, Page 673

A. Muscle stiffness & superimposed spasms
B. Involves jaw
C. Associated with cancers
D. Serum antibody against glutamic acid decarboxylase present

Rigidity mainly involves lower trunk & legs, but it can affect the upper extremities & neck. Sometimes, only one extremity is affected when it is called Stiff Limb syndrome.

2896. Acquired neuromyotonia is also called?
Harrison's 20th Ed. Chapter 441, Page 3242

A. Rett syndrome
B. Munchausen's syndrome
C. Isaacs syndrome
D. Andersen-Tawil syndrome

Peripheral nerve hyperexcitability (neuromyotonia, or Isaacs' syndrome) is characterized by spontaneous and continuous muscle fiber activity of peripheral nerve origin.

2897. Which of the following is false about 'Neuromyotonia'?
Harrison's 20th Ed. Chapter 441, Page 3242

A. Muscle stiffness at rest & during sleep
B. Distal limb muscles most severely affected
C. Myokymia
D. None of the above

2898. Which of the following is a feature of Isaacs syndrome?
Harrison's 20th Ed. Chapter 441, Page 674

A. Hypertrophic muscles
B. Paresthesias
C. Hyperhidrosis
D. All of the above

2899. Drugs that cause true myalgia include?
Harrison's 19th Ed. 462e-4 Table 462e-3

A. Cimetidine
B. Labetalol
C. Statins
D. All of the above

Drugs that cause true myalgia include Cimetidine, Cocaine, Cyclosporine, Danazol, Emetine, Gold, Heroin, Labetalol, Methadone, d-Penicillamine, Statins, L-Tryptophan, Zidovudine.

2900. Which of the following is a painful muscle condition?
Harrison's 20th Ed. Chapter 441, Page 3243

A. Paramyotonia congenita
B. Amyotrophic lateral sclerosis
C. Fibromyalgia
D. All of the above

Painful muscle conditions not associated with muscle weakness include fibromyalgia and polymyalgia rheumatica.

2901. Which of the following is associated with polymyalgia rheumatica?
Harrison's 20th Ed. Chapter 13, Page 86

A. Takayasu's arteritis
B. Henoch-Schönlein purpura
C. Temporal arteritis
D. Granulomatosis with polyangiitis (Wegener's)

Giant cell arteritis, also referred to as cranial arteritis or temporal arteritis, is an inflammatory disorder of medium- and large-sized arteries, may accompany polymyalgia rheumatica.

2902. Which of the following enzymes is not found in muscles?
Harrison's 20th Ed. Chapter 441, Page 3243

A. Creatine kinase (CK)
B. Aldolase
C. Lactic dehydrogenase (LDH)
D. Gamma-glutamyl transferase (GGT)

Creatine kinase (CK), aspartate aminotransferase (AST), alanine aminotransferase (ALT), aldolase, and lactic dehydrogenase (LDH) are enzymes sharing an origin in both muscle and liver. Gamma-glutamyl transferase (GGT) has a liver origin and is not found in muscle.

2903. Which of the following enzyme is not found in muscle?
Harrison's 20th Ed. Chapter 441, Page 3243

A. Aspartate aminotransferase (AST)
B. Alanine aminotransferase (ALT)
C. Lactic dehydrogenase (LDH)
D. g-glutamyl transferase (GGT)

Enzymes AST, ALT, aldolase and LDH originate in both muscle & liver. Origin of GGT is liver and is not found in muscle.

2904. Which of the following is helpful in differentiating myopathies from neuropathies & neuromuscular junction diseases?
Harrison's 20th Ed. Chapter 441, Page 3243

A. EMG
B. Repetitive nerve stimulation
C. Nerve conduction studies (NCS)
D. All of the above

2905. Which of the following is the gold standard for diagnosing patients with hereditary myopathies?
Harrison's 20th Ed. Chapter 441, Page 3243

A. Muscle biopsy
B. Genetic testing
C. Electrodiagnostic studies
D. All of the above

Genetic testing is the gold standard for diagnosing patients with hereditary myopathies. Muscle biopsy is extremely helpful in evaluation of acquired myopathies but is performed less frequently in suspected hereditary myopathies as genetic testing has become more widely available.

2906. Which of the following is accompanied by myoglobinuria?
Harrison's 20th Ed. Chapter 441, Page 3243

A. Myasthenia gravis
B. Polymyositis
C. Paramyotonia congenita
D. Myoadenylate deaminase deficiency

The states of metabolic energy deficiencies of glycolysis (myophosphorylase deficiency), fatty acid utilization (carnitine palmitoyltransferase deficiency), cause activity-related muscle breakdown accompanied by myoglobinuria, appearing as light-brown- to dark-brown-colored urine.

2907. Mutations affecting nuclear membrane proteins are responsible for?
Harrison's 20th Ed. Chapter 441, Page 3247 Figure 441-6

A. LGMD
B. Distal myopathies
C. EDMD
D. All of the above

2908. Mutations in genes that encode for sarcomeric and Z-disk proteins cause?
Harrison's 20th Ed. Chapter 441, Page 3247 Figure 441-6

A. Myofibrillar myopathy
B. Hereditary inclusion body myopathy
C. Nemaline rod myopathy
D. All of the above

Mutations in genes that encode for sarcomeric & Z-disk proteins cause forms of LGMD & distal myopathies like myofibrillar myopathy, forms of hereditary inclusion body myopathy, also, nemaline rod myopathy & other congenital myopathies. Mutations affecting nuclear membrane proteins cause most forms of EDMD.

2909. Nationality of Guillaume Benjamin Amand Duchenne de Boulogne was?
Journal of the History of Medicine and Allied Sciences. 2000;55(2):158-178

A. Polish
B. French
C. German
D. Danish

2910. Who discovered dystrophin gene?
Cell. 1987;51(6):919-28

A. Little
B. Gowers
C. Kunkel
D. Meryon

2911. The largest known human gene is?
Harrison's 20th Ed. Chapter 456, Page 3358

A. GNAS1
B. CFTR
C. Dystrophin
D. Emerin

2912. Which of the following is not a cytoskeletal protein?
Harrison's 20th Ed. Chapter 252, Page 1763

A. Desmin
B. Myosin
C. Laminin
D. Vinculin

Cytoskeletal proteins are desmin, cardiac myosin and vinculin while laminin is a nuclear membrane protein.

2913. Dilated cardiomyopathy is associated with?
Harrison's 20th Ed. Chapter 252, Page 1763

A. Duchenne's muscular dystrophy
B. Becker's muscular dystrophy
C. Limb-Girdle muscular dystrophies
D. All of the above

2914. Duchenne muscular dystrophy is present at?
Harrison's 20th Ed. Chapter 441, Page 3244

A. Birth
B. 1–2 years
C. 3–5 years
D. 5–7 years

Duchenne dystrophy is present at birth, but it usually becomes apparent between ages 3 & 5.

2915. Which of the following about Duchenne Muscular Dystrophy is false?
Harrison's 20th Ed. Chapter 441, Page 3244

A. X-linked recessive muscular dystrophy
B. Affects 1 in 3000 male births
C. Caused by mutations in dystrophin gene
D. None of the above

2916. Patients with Duchenne dystrophy are typically in a wheelchair by the age of?
Drug Des Devel Ther. 2017; 11: 533–545

A. 8
B. 10
C. 12
D. 14

Patients with Duchenne dystrophy are typically in wheelchair by age of 12.

2917. Which of the following virus can cleave dystrophin?
Harrison's 20th Ed. Chapter 254, Page 1780

A. Echovirus
B. Epstein-Barr virus
C. Coxsackie virus
D. West Nile virus

Abnormal dystrophin can be acquired when the coxsackie virus cleaves dystrophin during viral myocarditis.

2918. Clinical picture of which of the following resembles that of Duchenne muscular dystrophy?
Harrison's 20th Ed. Chapter 254, Page 1780

A. Tay-Sachs disease
B. Amyotrophic lateral sclerosis (ALS)
C. Pompe's disease
D. Gaucher disease

In the childhood form of α-glucosidase, or acid maltase, deficiency (type II glycogenosis) or Pompe's disease, clinical picture resembles Duchenne muscular dystrophy with delayed motor milestones resulting from proximal limb muscle weakness and involvement of respiratory muscles with calf muscle hypertrophy.

2919. The most important endocrine alteration in DMD/BMD patients is?
doi:10.1155/2012/485376

A. Hypothyroidism
B. Hypogonadism
C. Type II diabetes mellitus
D. Addison's syndrome

The most important endocrine alteration in DMD/BMD patients is hypogonadism. Consequences are delayed puberty, growth failure, osteoporosis, and metabolic abnormalities.

2920. Which of the following diseases can also cause Duchenne muscular dystrophy?
American Journal of Human Genetics. 1987;40(3):212-227

A. Pyruvate kinase deficiency
B. Glycerol kinase deficiency (GKD)
C. Adenosine kinase deficiency
D. Mevalonate kinase deficiency

Glycerol kinase deficiency (GKD) is an X-linked recessive enzyme defect. The responsible gene lies in a region containing genes in which deletions can cause Duchenne muscular dystrophy and adrenal hypoplasia congenita. Combinations of these three genetic defects are addressed as Complex GKD.

2921. 'Gowers' maneuver' is diagnostic of?
Harrison's 20th Ed. Chapter 441, Page 3242 Table 441-4

A. Duchenne muscular dystrophy (DMD)
B. Limb-Girdle muscular dystrophy
C. Emery-Dreifuss muscular dystrophy
D. Facioscapulohumeral muscular dystrophy

2922. Gowers' sign is due to weakness of which group of muscles?
Harrison's 20th Ed. Chapter 441, Page 3242 Table 441-2

A. Knee extensor muscles
B. Hip muscles
C. Anterior compartment of leg muscles
D. Posterior compartment of leg muscles

Gowers' sign refers to the inability to get up from the floor without climbing up the extremities. Weakness is in the hip, thigh, and trunk muscles.

2923. In DMD, which of the following muscle groups are preferentially involved?
DeJong's The Neurologic Examination, 7th Ed. Page 481

A. Distal limb muscles
B. Neck flexors
C. Neck extensors
D. Anterior abdominal muscles

Loss of muscle strength is progressive, with predilection for proximal limb muscles and neck flexors.

2924. Which of the following muscles undergo pseudohypertrophy in DMD?
DeJong's The Neurologic Examination, 7th Ed. Page 481

A. Supraspinatus
B. Infraspinatus
C. Latissimus dorsi
D. Serratus anterior

Pseudohypertrophy is common in Duchenne & Becker dystrophy. Calf muscles & infraspinatus are often strikingly enlarged due to pseudohypertrophy. Wasting of axillary folds is also seen.

2925. Kocher-Debré-Semelaigne (infant Hercules) syndrome is best related to?
DeJong's The Neurologic Examination, 7th Ed. Page 482

A. Hypothyroidism
B. Hyperthyroidism
C. Polymyositis
D. Central core disease

Kocher-Debré-Semelaigne (infant Hercules) syndrome is diffuse muscular hypertrophy due to hypothyroidism, early in life. Hoffman syndrome refers to hypertrophic myopathy due to hypothyroidism in adults.

2926. Muscle enlargement may occur in?
DeJong's The Neurologic Examination, 7th Ed. Page 482

A. Cysticercosis
B. Sarcoidosis
C. Amyloidosis
D. All of the above

Muscle enlargement may occur due to interstitial infiltrates, as in cysticercosis, trichinosis, sarcoidosis & amyloidosis.

2927. Which of the following about DMD is false?
doi:10.1155/2012/485376

A. Due to mutation in dystrophin gene
B. Dystrophin is the largest identified human gene
C. Dystrophin is on X chromosome
D. Mostly due to gene duplication

DMD is caused by a mutation of gene encoding 427-kDa dystrophin protein on the inner surface of sarcolemma. Dystrophin gene is one of the largest identified human genes (>2000 kb) on the short arm of X chromosome (Xp21). Most common gene mutation is a deletion. Less often, Duchenne's dystrophy is caused by a gene duplication or point mutation.

2928. Which of the following is an uncommon cause of death in Duchenne's muscular dystrophy?
doi:10.1155/2012/485376

A. Pulmonary infection
B. Aspiration of food
C. Acute gastric dilation
D. Cardiac cause (cardiomyopathy)

By age 16–18 years, patients of DMD are predisposed to serious, sometimes fatal pulmonary infections. Other causes of death include aspiration of food and acute gastric dilation. Cardiac cause of death is uncommon despite the presence of a cardiomyopathy in almost all patients.

2929. Which of the following statements about serum CK levels in DMD is false?
doi:10.1155/2012/485376

A. Invariably elevated
B. Serum CK levels are abnormal at birth
C. Decline late in the disease
D. None of the above

In DMD, serum CK levels are invariably elevated (20 to 100 times). Levels are abnormal at birth but decline late in the disease because of inactivity & loss of muscle mass.

2930. The most common gene mutation in DMD is?
Harrison's 20th Ed. Chapter 441, Page 3255

A. Deletion
B. Duplication
C. Point mutation
D. Any of the above

The most common gene mutation is a deletion. The size varies but does not correlate with disease severity. Deletions are not uniformly distributed over the gene but rather are most common near the beginning (5' end) and middle of the gene.

2931. Which of the following about dystrophin gene is false?
doi:10.1155/2012/485376

A. > 2000 kb in size
B. Localized to short arm of X chromosome at Xp21
C. Most common gene mutation is a deletion
D. None of the above

2932. Which of the following about dystrophin is false?
doi:10.1155/2012/485376

A. 427-kDa protein
B. Localized to inner surface of sarcolemma of muscle fiber
C. Western blot analysis of muscle biopsy helps in revealing abnormalities of dystrophin protein
D. None of the above

2933. Muscle biopsy of a patient of DMD shows which of the following?
doi:10.1155/2012/485376

A. Muscle fibers of varying size
B. Small groups of necrotic and regenerating fibers
C. Connective tissue & fat replace lost muscle fibers
D. None of the above

2934. Dystrophin binds to which of the following in sarcolemma?
Harrison's 20th Ed. Chapter 441, Page 3247 Figure 441-6

A. Laminin
B. Alpha-dystroglycan
C. F-actin
D. Caveolin-3

Dystrophin is part of a large complex of sarcolemmal proteins and glycoproteins. Dystrophin binds to F-actin at its amino terminus and to beta-dystroglycan at the carboxyl terminus.

2935. In essence, the key defect in DMD due to abnormal dystrophin protein is?
Harrison's 20th Ed. Chapter 441, Page 3247 Figure 441-6

A. Physical weakening of the sarcolemma
B. Disruption of Golgi apparatus
C. Abnormal mitochondria
D. Abnormal extracellular matrix (ECM)

Dystrophin-glycoprotein complex confer stability to the sarcolemma. Disruption of dystrophin-glycoprotein complexes weakens sarcolemma, causing membrane tears and a cascade of events leading to muscle fiber necrosis and eventually muscular dystrophy.

2936. Which of the following significantly slows progression of Duchenne's dystrophy?
Harrison's 20th Ed. Chapter 441, Page 3244

A. Azathioprine
B. Glucocorticoids
C. Cyclosporine
D. IVIg

Glucocorticoids (prednisone 0.75 mg/kg per day), significantly slows progression of Duchenne's dystrophy for up to 3 years.

2937. First and currently only FDA-approved drug for DMD is?
Drug Des Devel Ther. 2017; 11: 533–545

A. Apalutamide
B. Tecovirimat
C. Eteplirsen
D. Stiripentol

Eteplirsen is beneficial for DMD patients with deletions ending at exon 50 and starting at exon 52. It acts to promote dystrophin production by restoring the translational reading frame of DMD through specific skipping of exon 51 in defective gene variants.

2938. Becker's Muscular Dystrophy resembles which of the following muscular dystrophy?
Harrison's 20th Ed. Chapter 441, Page 3239

A. Duchenne's muscular dystrophy
B. Limb-Girdle muscular dystrophy
C. Emery-Dreifuss muscular dystrophy
D. Myotonic dystrophy

Becker's muscular dystrophy is a less severe and 10 times less frequent form of X-linked recessive Duchenne's muscular dystrophy.

2939. Most patients with Becker's muscular dystrophy first experience difficulties at what age?
Harrison's 20th Ed. Chapter 441, Page 3240

A. Birth
B. 1–2 years
C. 3–5 years
D. 5–15 years

Most patients with Becker's dystrophy first experience difficulties between ages 5 and 15 years.

2940. Calpains are Ca^{++} dependent?
N Engl J Med. 2005;352:2413-23

A. Cysteine proteases
B. Arginine proteases
C. Methionine proteases
D. Leucine proteases

2941. Tissue-specific calpains have been implicated in?
N Engl J Med. 2005;352:2413-23

A. Diabetes
B. Multiple sclerosis
C. Limb-girdle muscular dystrophy type 2A (LGMD2A)
D. All of the above

2942. Which of the following statements about Calpain is false?
N Engl J Med. 2005;352:2413-23

A. Calpain activity is regulated by calpastatin
B. Calpains are involved in apoptosis
C. Calpain is a cytoplasmic protease
D. None of the above

2943. Which of the following is a type of adult-onset LGMD?
Harrison's 20th Ed. Chapter 441, Page 3247

A. Calpainopathy
B. Fukutin-related protein (FKRP) deficiency
C. Anoctaminopathy
D. All of the above

The most common types of adult-onset LGMD are calpainopathy (LGMD2A), Fukutin-related protein (FKRP) deficiency (LGMD2I), and anoctaminopathy (LGMD2L).

2944. Which of the following statements is false?
Harrison's 20th Ed. Chapter 441, Page 3244 Table 441-3

A. Abnormal protein associated with LGMD1A is Myotilin
B. Abnormal protein associated with LGMD1B is Lamin A/C
C. Abnormal protein associated with LGMD1C is Caveolin-3
D. Abnormal protein associated with LGMD1D is Desmin

Abnormal protein associated with LGMD1D is DNAJB6 while abnormal protein associated with LGMD1E is Desmin.

2945. Abnormal protein Calpain-3 is associated with?
Harrison's 20th Ed. Chapter 441, Page 3244 Table 441-3

A. LGMD1F
B. LGMD1G
C. LGMD1H
D. LGMD1I

2946. Gower sign, calf hypertrophy & rippling muscles are clinical features of?
Harrison's 20th Ed. Chapter 441, Page 3244 Table 441-3

A. LGMD1A
B. LGMD1B
C. LGMD1C
D. LGMD1D

2947. Which of the following about LGMD2A is false?
Harrison's 20th Ed. Chapter 441, Page 3247

A. Marked scapular winging
B. Calf muscle hypertrophy
C. Lack of cardiac involvement
D. Lack of lung involvement

LGMD2A is associated with marked scapular winging, lack of calf muscle hypertrophy, and lack of cardiac and lung involvement.

2948. LGMD2A is caused by gene mutations in?
Harrison's 20th Ed. Chapter 441, Page 3245 Table 441-4

A. Calpain-1
B. Calpain-2
C. Calpain-3
D. Calpain-4

2949. LGMD2B is due to defect in?
Harrison's 20th Ed. Chapter 441, Page 3245 Table 441-4

A. Dysferlin
B. Emerin
C. Telethonin
D. Titin

2950. Which of the following is a variant of LGMD2B?
Harrison's 20th Ed. Chapter 441, Page 3245 Table 441-4

A. Welander distal myopathy
B. Tibial muscular dystrophy (Udd)
C. Laing distal myopathy
D. Miyoshi myopathy

Miyoshi's myopathy is variant of LGMD2B with calf muscles affected at onset.

2951. In which of the following gastrocnemius muscles are preferentially affected at onset?

Harrison's 20th Ed. Chapter 441, Page 3245, Table 441-4

A. Welander distal myopathy
B. Tibial muscular dystrophy (Udd's)
C. Laing distal myopathy
D. Miyoshi myopathy

In dysferlinopathies (LGMD2B) there is a predilection for early atrophy of gastrocnemius muscles. Miyoshi myopathy is unique in that gastrocnemius muscles are preferentially affected at onset.

2952. Which of the following muscular dystrophy has its onset in infancy?

Harrison's 20th Ed. Chapter 441, Page 3245 Table 441-4

A. Muscle-eye-brain disease
B. Walker-Warburg syndrome
C. Fukuyama congenital muscular dystrophy
D. All of the above

Merosin deficiency, Fukitin-related protein deficiency, Fukuyama congenital muscular dystrophy, Muscle-eye-brain disease, Walker-Warburg syndrome are congenital muscular dystrophies that have an onset at birth. Clinically, Walker-Warburg syndrome is more severe, with death by 1 year.

2953. Which of the following is a lipid myopathy?

DeJong's The Neurologic Examination, 7th Ed. Page 773

A. Carnitine deficiency
B. McArdle's disease
C. Phosphofructokinase deficiency
D. Kearnes-Sayre syndrome

2954. Which of the following statements is false?

Harrison's 20th Ed. Chapter 441, Page 3245 Table 441-4

A. Abnormal protein associated with LGMD2A is Calpain-3
B. Abnormal protein associated with LGMD2B is Dysferlin
C. Abnormal protein associated with LGMD2C is Telethonin
D. None of the above

Abnormal protein associated with LGMD2C is γ sarcoglycan.

2955. Which of the following is clinically similar to Duchenne or Becker dystrophies?

Harrison's 20th Ed. Chapter 441, Page 3245 Table 441-4

A. LGMD2G
B. LGMD2H
C. LGMD2I
D. LGMD2J

LGMD2C, D, E, F and I are clinically similar to Duchenne or Becker dystrophies.

2956. Udd type distal myopathy is due to deficiency of?

Harrison's 20th Ed. Chapter 441, Page 3245 Table 441-4

A. Desmin
B. Titin
C. Plectin 1
D. Fukutin

2957. Which of the following is best related to congenital myasthenic syndrome?

Harrison's 20th Ed. Chapter 441, Page 3245 Table 441-4

A. Dermatitis herpetiformis
B. Cicatricial pemphigoid
C. Epidermolysis bullosa
D. Pemphigus foliaceus

LGMD2Q has onset in infancy to fourth decade. Presentation may includes proximal weakness, ptosis & extraocular weakness with epidermolysis bullosa (a congenital myasthenic syndrome).

2958. Which of the following LGMD has Hutterite descent?

Harrison's 20th Ed. Chapter 441, Page 3245 Table 441-4

A. LGMD2P
B. LGMD2Q
C. LGMD2R
D. LGMD2S

Hutterites, Amish and Mennonites are ethno-religious, isolated groups that have their origins from early 16th century.

2959. Which of the following distal myopathy begins in hands?

Harrison's 20th Ed. Chapter 441, Page 3246 Table 441-5

A. Welander distal myopathy
B. Tibial muscular dystrophy
C. Nonanka distal myopathy
D. Miyoshi myopathy

In autosomal dominant Welander's distal myopathy, onset is in 5th decade, weakness begins in hands and slowly progresses to involve distal lower extremities. Lifespan is normal.

2960. Which of the following distal myopathies begin in lower limbs?

Harrison's 20th Ed. Chapter 441, Page 3246 Table 441-5

A. Tibial muscular dystrophy
B. Nonanka distal myopathy
C. Miyoshi myopathy
D. All of the above

2961. Serum CK is elevated most in which of the following distal myopathies?

Harrison's 20th Ed. Chapter 441, Page 3246 Table 441-5

A. Welander distal myopathy
B. Tibial muscular dystrophy
C. Nonanka distal myopathy
D. Miyoshi myopathy

Serum CK level is is very elevated in Miyoshi myopathy. In other distal myopathies, serum CK is only slightly increased.

2962. Which of the following gene mutation is the most common cause of X-linked EDMD?

Harrison's 20th Ed. Chapter 441, Page 3247

A. FHL1
B. Lamin A/C
C. Nesprin-1
D. Emerin

Emerin mutations are the most common cause of X-linked EDMD.

2963. Which of the following gene mutation is the most common cause of autosomal dominant EDMD?

Harrison's 20th Ed. Chapter 441, Page 3247

A. FHL1
B. Lamin A/C
C. Nesprin-1
D. Emerin

2964. Autosomal dominant EDMD is also known as?

Harrison's 20th Ed. Chapter 441, Page 3247

A. LGMD1A
B. LGMD1B
C. LGMD1C
D. LGMD1D

2965. Autosomal dominant EDMD can occur with mutations in?

Harrison's 20th Ed. Chapter 441, Page 3247

A. Nesprin-1 gene
B. Nesprin-2 gene
C. TMEM43 gene
D. All of the above

2966. In EDMD, which of the following precedes muscle weakness?

Harrison's 20th Ed. Chapter 441, Page 3247

A. Cardiomyopathy
B. Atrial fibrillation
C. Atrioventricular heart block
D. Contractures

2967. In EDMD, prominent contractures are present at?

Harrison's 20th Ed. Chapter 441, Page 3248

A. Elbows
B. Ankles
C. Neck
D. All of the above

2968. In which of the following myopathies, fixed contractures occur early & are a distinctive feature of the disease?

Harrison's 20th Ed. Chapter 441, Page 3242

A. Facioscapulohumeral (FSH) Muscular Dystrophy
B. Bethlem myopathy
C. Nemaline (rod) myopathy
D. Fukuyama congenital muscular dystrophy (FCMD)

in Emery-Dreifuss muscular dystrophy and Bethlem myopathy, fixed contractures occur early and represent distinctive features of the disease.

2969. Which of the following is caused by mutations in LMNA gene?

Harrison's 20th Ed. Chapter 441, Page 3357

A. Lipodystrophies
B. Emery-Dreifuss muscular dystrophy
C. Progeria syndromes
D. All of the above

LMNA gene encodes nuclear lamins A and C. Autosomal dominant and autosomal recessive disorders are caused by mutations in LMNA gene. They include several forms of lipodystrophies, Emery-Dreifuss muscular dystrophy, progeria syndromes, a form of neuronal Charcot-Marie-Tooth disease (type 2B1), and a group of overlapping syndromes.

2970. Proximal myotonic myopathy (PROMM) is best related to?

Harrison's 20th Ed. Chapter 441, Page 3248

A. Myotonic dystrophy type 1 (DM1)
B. Myotonic dystrophy type 2 (DM2)
C. Myotonic dystrophy type 3 (DM3)
D. Myotonic dystrophy type 4 (DM4)

Myotonic dystrophy type 2 (DM2) is also called proximal myotonic myopathy (PROMM).

2971. "Hatchet-faced" appearance is typical of which of the following conditions?

Harrison's 20th Ed. Chapter 441, Page 3248

A. Facioscapulohumeral (FSH) Muscular Dystrophy
B. Myotonic dystrophy
C. Emery-Dreifuss muscular dystrophy
D. Limb-Girdle muscular dystrophy

Patients with myotonic dystrophy have a typical "hatchet-faced" appearance due to temporalis, masseter and facial muscle atrophy and weakness. Frontal baldness is also a characteristic feature.

2972. Footdrop is a feature of?

Harrison's 20th Ed. Chapter 441, Page 3248

A. Facioscapulohumeral (FSH) muscular dystrophy
B. Myotonic dystrophy type 1 (DM1)
C. Type 1 lepra reactions
D. All of the above

Besides the above, also Welander, Udd, and Markesbery-Griggs type distal myopathies cause footdrop.

2973. Hypersomnia is a feature of?

Harrison's 20th Ed. Chapter 441, Page 3248

A. Myotonic dystrophy type 1 (DM1)
B. Paraneoplastic encephalomyelitis and focal encephalitis
C. Acute radiation central nervous system (CNS) toxicity
D. All of the above

2974. In Myotonic dystrophy, involvement of which of the following muscles leads to dysarthria and dysphagia?

Harrison's 20th Ed. Chapter 441, Page 3248

A. Palatal
B. Pharyngeal
C. Tongue
D. All of the above

2975. Trinucleotide expansion is best related to?

Harrison's 20th Ed. Chapter 441, Page 3356

A. Fragile X syndrome
B. Huntington's disease
C. X-linked spinobulbar muscular atrophy
D. All of the above

Trinucleotide expansion is a a cause of the fragile X syndrome, Huntington's disease, X-linked spinobulbar muscular atrophy, and myotonic dystrophy.

2976. Which of the following is due to a CTG repeat expansion?
Harrison's 20th Ed. Chapter 441, Page 3155

- A. SCA6
- B. SCA7
- C. SCA8
- D. SCA17

Spinocerebellar ataxia1, SCA2, SCA3 (Machado-Joseph disease), SCA6, SCA7, and SCA17 are caused by CAG triplet repeat expansions in different genes. SCA8 is due to an untranslated CTG repeat expansion, SCA12 is linked to an untranslated CAG repeat, and SCA10 is caused by an untranslated pentanucleotide repeat. Myotonic dystrophy type 1 (DM1) is transmitted by an intronic mutation consisting of an unstable expansion of a CTG trinucleotide repeat in a serine-threonine protein kinase gene - DMPK.

2977. Which of the following is an "antimyotonia drug"?
Harrison's 20th Ed. Chapter 441, Page 3248

- A. Mexiletine
- B. Amiodarone
- C. Flecainide
- D. Sotalol

Phenytoin & mexiletine are the preferred antimyotonia drugs.

2978. Which of the following is the initial manifestation of FSHD?
Harrison's 20th Ed. Chapter 441, Page 3248

- A. Scapular winging
- B. Footdrop
- C. Facial weakness
- D. Nerve deafness

Facial weakness is the initial manifestation in FSHD appearing as an inability to smile, whistle, or fully close eyes.

2979. Scapular winging becomes apparent with attempts at?
Harrison's 20th Ed. Chapter 441, Page 3248

- A. Abduction and forward movement of arms
- B. Adduction and forward movement of arms
- C. Abduction and backward movement of arms
- D. Adduction and backward movement of arms

Scapular winging becomes apparent with attempts at abduction & forward movement of arms.

2980. Which of the following muscles is relatively spared in Facioscapulohumeral (FSH) muscular dystrophy?
Harrison's 20th Ed. Chapter 441, Page 3248

- A. Facial
- B. Biceps
- C. Triceps
- D. Deltoid

Weakness of shoulder girdles brings patient to the doctor. Scapular winging is common. Biceps, triceps, wrist extensors & muscles weakness of anterior compartment muscles of legs are severely affected, with relative sparing of deltoid muscles.

2981. Coats' disease is a disorder consisting of?
Harrison's 20th Ed. Chapter 441, Page 3248, Indian J Ophthalmol. 2010;58(2):119-124.

- A. Retinal telangiectasia
- B. Intra- and/or subretinal exudation
- C. Retinal detachment
- D. All of the above

The hallmark lesion of Coats' disease is idiopathic retinal telangiectasia which appears as 'light bulb appearance' on fluorescein angiography. Other features include irregular retinal vessel dilatations, retinal vessel tortuosity, areas of capillary non-perfusion, intra- and/or subretinal exudation and retinal detachment.

2982. Which of the following gene is related to FSHD1?
Harrison's 20th Ed. Chapter 441, Page 3249

- A. MYO7A
- B. SIX1
- C. GJB2
- D. DUX4

FSHD1 is associated with deletions of tandem 3.3-kb repeats at 4q35. Within these repeats lies DUX4 gene, which usually is not expressed after early muscle development. In patients with FSHD1 these deletions lead to toxic expression of DUX4 gene. In FSHD2, there is no deletion, but a mutation in SMCHD1, leading to permissive expression of DUX4 gene.

2983. Which of the following is false about oculopharyngeal muscular dystrophy (OPMD)?
Harrison's 20th Ed. Chapter 441, Page 3249

- A. Progressive external ophthalmoplegia
- B. Normal pupillary reactions for light & accommodation
- C. No diplopia
- D. None of the above

2984. Muscle fibers with rimmed vacuoles is a feature of?
Harrison's 20th Ed. Chapter 441, Page 3249

- A. Welander distal myopathy
- B. Oculopharyngeal muscular dystrophy (OPMD)
- C. Tibial muscular dystrophy (Udd)
- D. All of the above

On electron microscopy, a distinctive feature of OPMD is the presence of 8.5 nm tubular filaments in muscle cell nuclei.

2985. Which of the following gene is related to OPMD?
Harrison's 20th Ed. Chapter 441, Page 3249

- A. WFS1
- B. TECTA
- C. COCH
- D. PABP2

The molecular defect in OPMD is an expansion of a polyalanine repeat tract in a poly-RNA-binding protein (PABP2) gene.

2986. Muscle fibers with rimmed vacuoles is a feature of all except?
Harrison's 20th Ed. Chapter 441, Page 3249

- A. Miyoshi myopathy
- B. Inclusion body myositis (IBM)
- C. Markesbery-Griggs distal myopathy
- D. GNE myopathy

2987. Large deposits of myosin heavy chain in muscle fibers is a feature of?
Harrison's 20th Ed. Chapter 441, Page 3249

- A. Laing distal myopathy
- B. Miyoshi myopathy
- C. Williams myopathy
- D. Tibial muscular dystrophy (Udd)

2988. Which of the following is not a late-onset distal myopathy?
Harrison's 20th Ed. Chapter 441, Page 3249

A. Welander distal myopathy
B. Tibial muscular dystrophy (Udd)
C. Markesbery-Griggs distal myopathy
D. Laing distal myopathy

Laing distal myopathy has its onset in childhood or early adult life while rest appear after 40 years of age.

2989. Which of the following has autosomal recessive inheritance?
Harrison's 20th Ed. Chapter 441, Page 3249

A. Welander distal myopathy
B. Miyoshi myopathy
C. Tibial muscular dystrophy (Udd)
D. Markesbery-Griggs distal myopathy

GNE myopathy (Nonaka distal myopathy) and Miyoshi myopathy have autosomal recessive inheritance.

2990. Which of the following produce prominent anterior tibial weakness?
Harrison's 20th Ed. Chapter 441, Page 3249

A. GNE myopathy
B. Williams myopathy
C. Laing distal myopathy
D. All of the above

2991. In which of the following gastrocnemius muscles are preferentially affected at onset?
Harrison's 20th Ed. Chapter 441, Page 3249

A. Welander distal myopathy
B. Tibial muscular dystrophy (Udd's)
C. Laing distal myopathy
D. Miyoshi myopathy

2992. Serum CK levels are markedly elevated in?
Harrison's 20th Ed. Chapter 441, Page 3249

A. Welander distal myopathy
B. Tibial muscular dystrophy (Udd's)
C. Laing distal myopathy
D. Miyoshi myopathy

2993. Which of the following is not a congenital myopathy?
Harrison's 20th Ed. Chapter 441, Page 3240 Table 441-1

A. Central core disease
B. Nemaline (rod) myopathy
C. Miyoshi myopathy
D. Centronuclear (myotubular) myopathy

Miyoshi myopathy is a type of distal myopathy. Minicore myopathy (multi-minicore disease), fingerprint body myopathy, and sarcotubular myopathy are also congenital myopathies.

2994. Patients with which of the following congenital myopathies are susceptibile to malignant hyperthermia?
Harrison's 20th Ed. Chapter 64, Page 433

A. Central core disease
B. Nemaline (rod) myopathy
C. Centronuclear (myotubular) myopathy
D. All of the above

Malignant hyperthermia during anesthesia may occur in central core disease. C-terminal mutations of the RYR1 gene (ryanodine receptor gene on chromosome 19q) predispose to this complication.

2995. Severe brain impairment is seen in which of the following congenital muscular dystrophies?
Harrison's 20th Ed. Chapter 441, Page 3249

A. Fukuyama congenital muscular dystrophy (FCMD)
B. Muscle-eye-brain (MEB) disease
C. Walker-Warburg syndrome (WWS)
D. All of the above

Congenital muscular dystrophy with severe brain impairment are FCMD, MEB disease & WWS. In MEB & WWS, but not in FCMD, vision is impaired. WWS is the most severe congenital muscular dystrophy.

2996. Which of the following is a principal source of energy for skeletal muscles?
Harrison's 20th Ed. Chapter 441, Page 3249

A. Amino acid
B. Fatty acid
C. Lactic acid
D. All of the above

Fatty acids and glucose are the two principal sources of energy for skeletal muscles.

2997. Alpha-glucosidase or acid maltase deficiency is also called?
Harrison's 20th Ed. Chapter 441, Page 3249

A. Leigh's syndrome
B. Kearns-Sayre syndrome (KSS)
C. Pompe's disease
D. McArdle's disease

Alpha-glucosidase or acid maltase deficiency is also called Pompe's Disease. It is caused by mutations of the α-glucosidase gene.

2998. Which out of the following is the most common alpha-glucosidase, or acid maltase deficiency?
Harrison's 20th Ed. Chapter 441, Page 3249

A. Infantile form
B. Childhood form
C. Adult form
D. None of the above

There are three clinical forms of alpha-glucosidase, or acid maltase deficiency (type II glycogenosis). The infantile form is the most common, with onset of symptoms in the first 3 months of life.

2999. Which of the following about Pompe's disease is false?
Harrison's 20th Ed. Chapter 441, Page 3249

A. Autosomal recessive disorder
B. Caused by mutations of the alpha-glucosidase gene
C. Enzyme replacement tt beneficial in infantile-onset type
D. None of the above

Enzyme replacement therapy (ERT) with IV recombinant human alpha-glucosidase is beneficial in infantile-onset type.

3000. De-branching enzyme deficiency is also called?
Harrison's 20th Ed. Chapter 441, Page 3249

A. Type I glycogenosis
B. Type II glycogenosis
C. Type III glycogenosis
D. Type IV glycogenosis

α-glucosidase, or acid maltase, deficiency is called type II glycogenosis. De-branching enzyme deficiency is called type III glycogenosis while branching enzyme deficiency is called type IV glycogenosis.

3001. von Gierke's disease is also called?
Ann Neurol. 2014;76(6):891-898

A. Type I glycogenosis
B. Type II glycogenosis
C. Type III glycogenosis
D. Type IV glycogenosis

Type 0 glycogen storage disease (GSD) is called Lewis' disease. The names of various other GSD's are Type I (von Gierke's disease), Type II (Pompe's disease), Type III (Forbes-Cori disease), Type IV (Andersen's disease), Type V (McArdle's disease), Type VI (Hers' disease), Type VII (Tarui's disease), Type XI (Fanconi-Bickel syndrome).

3002. Which of the following is a disorder of glycolysis causing exercise intolerance?
Harrison's 20th Ed. Chapter 441, Page 3250

A. Myophosphorylase deficiency
B. Phosphofructokinase deficiency
C. Lactate dehydrogenase deficiency
D. All of the above

Disorders of glycolysis causing exercise intolerance include myophosphorylase deficiency (type V glycogenosis), phosphofructokinase deficiency (type VII glycogenosis), phosphoglycerate kinase deficiency (type IX glycogenosis), phosphoglycerate mutase deficiency (type X glycogenosis), lactate dehydrogenase deficiency (glycogenosis type XI), and beta-enolase deficiency. These glycolytic defects are associated with recurrent myoglobinuria.

3003. Which of the following is called McArdle's disease?
Harrison's 20th Ed. Chapter 441, Page 3250

A. Myophosphorylase deficiency
B. Phosphofructokinase deficiency
C. Lactate dehydrogenase deficiency
D. Beta-enolase deficiency

Myophosphorylase deficiency is also called McArdle's disease and is the most common of the glycolytic defects associated with exercise intolerance.

3004. McArdle disease caused by mutations in?
Harrison's 20th Ed. Chapter 441, Page 3250

A. KCNQ4 gene
B. EYA4 gene
C. ACTG1 gene
D. PYGM gene

McArdle disease caused by mutations in the PYGM gene leading to myophosphorylase deficiency.

3005. Seizure disorder with mental retardation is a feature of which of the following?
Harrison's 20th Ed. Chapter 441, Page 3250

A. Myophosphorylase deficiency
B. Phosphofructokinase deficiency
C. Phosphoglycerate kinase deficiency
D. Beta-enolase deficiency

In McArdle's disease, exercise tolerance is enhanced by warm-up or brief periods of rest. Hemolytic anemia accompany deficiencies of phosphofructokinase & phosphoglycerate kinase. Seizure disorder with mental retardation is the usual clinical presentation in phosphoglycerate kinase deficiency.

3006. Which of the following is a X-linked recessive disorder?
Harrison's 20th Ed. Chapter 441, Page 3250

A. Myophosphorylase deficiency
B. Phosphofructokinase deficiency
C. Phosphoglycerate mutase deficiency
D. Phosphoglycerate kinase deficiency

Myophosphorylase deficiency, phosphofructokinase deficiency & phosphoglycerate mutase deficiency are inherited as autosomal recessive disorders. Phosphoglycerate kinase deficiency has X-linked recessive inheritance.

3007. Which of the following statements about lipid as energy source is false?
Harrison's 20th Ed. Chapter 441, Page 3250

A. Fatty acids are derived from circulating VLDL in blood
B. Fatty acids are derived from triglycerides in muscle fibers
C. Oxidation of fatty acids occurs in mitochondria
D. None of the above

3008. To enter mitochondria, a fatty acid must first be converted to?
Harrison's 20th Ed. Chapter 441, Page 3250

A. Enoyl–acyl carrier
B. Acyl-NADH
C. Acyl-CoA
D. Amino-acyl-tRNA

Oxidation of fatty acids occurs in mitochondria. To enter mitochondria, a fatty acid must first be converted to an "activated fatty acid," acyl-CoA.

3009. Acyl-CoA must be linked to which of the following for transport into mitochondria?
Harrison's 20th Ed. Chapter 441, Page 3250

A. Acyl-CoA dehydrogenase
B. Cystinosin
C. Carnitine
D. Carnitine palmitoyltransferase (CPT) I

Acyl-CoA must be linked with carnitine by enzyme carnitine palmitoyltransferase (CPT) I for transport into mitochondria.

3010. Enzyme carnitine palmitoyltransferase (CPT) I is present on?
Harrison's 20th Ed. Chapter 441, Page 3250

A. Outer side of outer mitochondrial membrane
B. Inner side of outer mitochondrial membrane
C. Outer side of inner mitochondrial membrane
D. Inner side of inner mitochondrial membrane

Carnitine palmitoyltransferase (CPT) I is present on inner side of outer mitochondrial membrane.

3011. Enzyme carnitine palmitoyltransferase (CPT) II is present on?
Harrison's 20th Ed. Chapter 441, Page 3250

A. Outer side of outer mitochondrial membrane
B. Inner side of outer mitochondrial membrane
C. Outer side of inner mitochondrial membrane
D. Inner side of inner mitochondrial membrane

Carnitine is removed by CPT II, an enzyme attached to the inside of inner mitochondrial membrane, allowing transport of acyl-CoA into the mitochondrial matrix for beta-oxidation.

3012. Myoglobinuria in CPT2 deficiency is precipitated by?
Harrison's 20th Ed. Chapter 441, Page 3250

A. Prolonged exercise
B. Fasting
C. Infections
D. All of the above

CPT2 deficiency is much more common in men than women (5:1) and is the most common recognizable cause of recurrent myoglobinuria. Muscle pain and myoglobinuria can be precipitated by prolonged exercise, fasting or infections.

3013. Which of the following is false about human mitochondrial DNA (mtDNA)?
Harrison's 20th Ed. Chapter 441, Page 3250

A. Double-stranded circular molecule
B. Codes for transfer & ribosomal RNAs & polypeptides
C. Directly inherited from cytoplasm of oocyte mainly
D. None of the above

Each mitochondrion possesses a DNA genome that is distinct from that of nuclear DNA. Human mitochondrial DNA (mtDNA) consists of a double-strand, circular molecule comprising 16,569 base pairs. It codes for 22 transfer RNAs, 2 ribosomal RNAs, and 13 polypeptides of the respiratory chain enzymes. Genetics of mitochondrial diseases differ from genetics of chromosomal disorders. DNA of mitochondria is directly inherited from the cytoplasm of gametes, mainly oocyte. Sperm contributes very little. Thus, mitochondrial genes are derived almost exclusively from mother.

3014. Which of the following is a mitochondrial myopathy?
Harrison's 20th Ed. Chapter 441, Page 3250

A. Chronic progressive external ophthalmoplegia (CPEO)
B. Skeletal muscle - CNS syndromes
C. Pure myopathy
D. All of the above

Mitochondrial myopathies include chronic progressive external ophthalmoplegia (CPEO), skeletal muscle - CNS syndromes & pure myopathy.

3015. Which of the following about Kearns-Sayre Syndrome (KSS) is false?
Harrison's 20th Ed. Chapter 441, Page 3250

A. Onset before 20 years of age
B. CPEO
C. Pigmentary retinopathy
D. Diplopia

In CPEO, varying degrees of ptosis & weakness of extraocular muscles are seen, usually in the absence of diplopia, a point of distinction from myasthenia gravis. Triad of clinical findings in KSS includes onset before age 20, CPEO, and pigmentary retinopathy, plus one or more of the following features: complete heart block, cerebrospinal fluid protein >100 mg/dL, or cerebellar ataxia.

3016. Which of the following is the most common endocrine abnormality in Kearns-Sayre Syndrome?
Harrison's 20th Ed. Chapter 441, Page 3250

A. Diabetes mellitus
B. Addison's disease
C. Hypoparathyroidism
D. Hyperaldosteronism

Diabetes mellitus occurs in 13% of KSS patients.

3017. Which of the following about KSS is false?
Harrison's 20th Ed. Chapter 441, Page 3250

A. Sporadic disorder
B. Caused by single mtDNA deletions
C. Spontaneous deletion occur in ovum or zygote
D. Spontaneous deletion occur in spermatozoa

KSS is a sporadic disorder. The disease is caused by single mtDNA deletions arising spontaneously in the ovum or zygote. The most common deletion removes 4,977 bp of contiguous mtDNA.

3018. Which of the following is false about progressive external ophthalmoplegia (PEO)?
Harrison's 20th Ed. Chapter 441, Page 3250

A. Due to mtDNA mutations
B. Inherited in a Mendelian fashion
C. Onset is usually after puberty
D. Ragged red fibers seen in muscle biopsy

PEO is caused by nuclear DNA mutations affecting mtDNA copy number & integrity. It is inherited in a Mendelian fashion. Onset is usually after puberty. CSF protein is normal. Ragged red fibers are prominently seen in muscle biopsy.

3019. Which of the following chromosome is affected in autosomal dominant form of CPEO?
Harrison's 20th Ed. Chapter 441, Page 3250

A. 4q35
B. 10q24
C. 15q22–26
D. All of the above

Autosomal dominant form of CPEO is linked to loci on 3 chromosomes - 4q35, 10q24 & 15q22–26.

3020. "Twinkle" is the gene product of?
Harrison's 19th Ed. 462e-16

A. 4q35
B. 10q24
C. 15q22–26
D. All of the above

In chromosome 10q–related CPEO, mutations occur in C10orf2 gene. Its gene product is twinkle, named for its punctate, starlike staining properties. It co-localizes with mtDNA and is critical for lifetime maintenance of mitochondrial integrity.

3021. Enzyme important in mtDNA replication is?
Harrison's 20th Ed. Chapter 441, Page 3251

A. Carnitine palmitoyltransferase (CPT) I
B. Acid maltase
C. Myoadenylate deaminase
D. POLG

In CPEO mapped to chromosome 15q, a mutation affects the gene encoding mtDNA polymerase (POLG), an enzyme important in mtDNA replication.

3022. Characteristic feature of myoclonic epilepsy with ragged red fibers (MERRF) is?
Harrison's 20th Ed. Chapter 441, Page 3251

A. Myoclonic epilepsy
B. Cerebellar ataxia
C. Progressive muscle weakness
D. All of the above

Characteristic features include myoclonic epilepsy, cerebellar ataxia, and progressive muscle weakness in a limb-girdle distribution. Other more variable features include dementia, peripheral neuropathy, optic atrophy, hearing loss, and diabetes mellitus.

3023. To be called ragged red fiber, which of the following is abnormal in a muscle cell?
Harrison's 20th Ed. Chapter 441, Page 3250

A. Golgi apparatus
B. Mitochondria
C. Cell membrane
D. Nucleus

Term ragged red fibers was coined by Olson (1972) to describe muscle fibers with significant numbers of abnormal mitochondria (enlarged, bizarrely shaped with crystalline inclusions) highlighted with modified trichrome stain.

3024. Which of the following is caused by maternally inherited point mutations of mitochondrial tRNA gene?

Harrison's 20th Ed. Chapter 441, Page 3251

- A. Kearns-Sayre syndrome (KSS)
- B. MERRF
- C. Pompe's disease
- D. All of the above

MERRF & MELAS are caused by maternally inherited point mutations of mitochondrial tRNA genes.

3025. Which of the following about Mitochondrial Myopathy, Encephalopathy, Lactic Acidosis, and Stroke like Episodes (MELAS) is false?

Harrison's 20th Ed. Chapter 441, Page 3251

- A. Cerebral lesions conform to a vascular distribution
- B. Partial motor or generalized seizures
- C. Serum lactic acid is elevated
- D. Muscle biopsies show ragged red fibers

In MELAS, the term stroke like is appropriate because cerebral lesions do not conform to a strictly vascular distribution. Like KSS, onset is before age 20. Seizures are partial motor or generalized. Cerebral insults cause hemiparesis, hemianopia, and cortical blindness. Serum lactic acid is typically elevated. CSF protein is increased. Muscle biopsies show ragged red fibers.

3026. Which of the following about Mitochondrial Myopathy, Encephalopathy, Lactic Acidosis, and Stroke like Episodes (MELAS) is false?

Harrison's 20th Ed. Chapter 441, Page 3251

- A. Focal lesions in frontal lobes
- B. Basal ganglia calcification
- C. Vascular territories are not respected
- D. Cerebral angiography essentially normal

IN MELAS, neuroimaging shows basal ganglia calcification. Focal lesions mimiking infarction are seen mainly in occipital & parietal lobes. Strict vascular territories are not respected, and cerebral angiography does not show lesions of the major cerebral blood vessels.

3027. Which of the following is caused by maternally inherited point mutations of mitochondrial tRNA gene?

Harrison's 20th Ed. Chapter 441, Page 3251

- A. Kearns-Sayre syndrome (KSS)
- B. MELAS
- C. Pompe's disease
- D. Mitochondrial DNA depletion syndrome (MDS)

MERRF & MELAS are caused by maternally inherited point mutations of mitochondrial tRNA genes.

3028. Which of the following point mutation is most common in MELAS?

Harrison's 20th Ed. Chapter 441, Page 3251

- A. A3243G point mutation in tRNALeu(UUR)
- B. 3252G point mutation in tRNALeu(UUR)
- C. 3256T point mutation in tRNALeu(UUR)
- D. 3271C point mutation in tRNALeu(UUR)

In MELAS, A3243G point mutation in tRNALeu(UUR) is the most common (80%).

3029. Which of the following is a calcium channelopathy?

Harrison's 20th Ed. Chapter 441, Page 3251

- A. Hypokalemic periodic paralysis
- B. Hyperkalemic periodic paralysis
- C. Paramyotonia congenita
- D. Andersen-Tawil syndrome

3030. Which of the following is a potassium channelopathy?

Harrison's 20th Ed. Chapter 441, Page 3251

- A. Hypokalemic periodic paralysis
- B. Hyperkalemic periodic paralysis
- C. Paramyotonia congenita
- D. Andersen-Tawil Syndrome

3031. Hypokalemic periodic paralysis type 1 is caused by mutation in which of the following gene?

Harrison's 20th Ed. Chapter 441, Page 3251

- A. CALCL1A1
- B. CALCL1A2
- C. CALCL1A3
- D. CALCL1A4

HypoKPP type 1 is inherited as an autosomal dominant disorder with incomplete penetrance. It is due to mutations in voltage-sensitive, skeletal muscle calcium channel gene, CALCL1A3. HypoKPP type 2 is due to mutations in voltage-sensitive sodium channel gene (SCN4A). The muscle cell depolarizes when potassium levels are low.

3032. Onset of hypokalemic periodic paralysis (HypoKPP) is at?

Harrison's 20th Ed. Chapter 441, Page 3251

- A. Childhood
- B. Adolescence
- C. Adulthood
- D. Middle age

Onset of hypokalemic periodic paralysis (Hypokpp) occurs at adolescence. Episodic weakness with onset after age 25 is almost never due to periodic paralyses.

3033. In hypokalemic periodic paralysis, preferred vehicle for administration of IV potassium is?

Harrison's 20th Ed. Chapter 441, Page 3251

- A. Normal saline
- B. GDW
- C. Ringer lactate
- D. Mannitol

Treatment of hypokalemic periodic paralysis is oral KCl (0.2–0.4 mmol/kg), every 30 minutes. Should IV therapy become necessary (swallowing problems or vomiting), Mannitol is the preferred vehicle for administration of IV potassium as glucose solution may further reduce serum potassium levels.

3034. Hyperkalemic periodic paralysis (HyperKPP) is caused by mutation in which of the following gene?

Harrison's 20th Ed. Chapter 441, Page 3252

- A. SCN1A
- B. SCN2A
- C. SCN3A
- D. SCN4A

HyperKPP is an autosomal dominant disorder due to mutations of voltage-gated sodium channel SCN4A gene.

3035. Attacks of muscle weakness are induced by cold in which of the following?
Harrison's 20th Ed. Chapter 441, Page 3252

A. Thomsen's disease
B. Becker's disease
C. Paramyotonia congenita
D. All of the above

In paramyotonia congenita (PC), the attacks of weakness are cold-induced or occur spontaneously. Myotonia in chloride channel disorders - Thomsen's disease and Becker's disease is worsened by cold and improved by activity.

3036. Long QT syndrome is a feature of which of the following?
Harrison's 20th Ed. Chapter 441, Page 3252

A. Thomsen's disease
B. Becker's disease
C. Paramyotonia congenita
D. Andersen-Tawil Syndrome

Autosomal dominant Andersen-Tawil Syndrome is a potassium channel disorder characterized by episodic weakness, cardiac arrhythmias (long QT, ventricular ectopy, bidirectional ventricular arrhythmias), and dysmorphic features (short stature, scoliosis, clinodactyly, hypertelorism, small or prominent low-set ears, micrognathia, and broad forehead). It is caused by mutations of the inwardly rectifying potassium channel (Kir 2.1) gene that heighten muscle cell excitability.

3037. Serum CK level is most conspicuously elevated in which of the following endocrine myopathies?
Harrison's 20th Ed. Chapter 441, Page 3252

A. Hyperthyroidism
B. Hypothyroidism
C. Hyperparathyroidism
D. Diabetes mellitus

In hypothyroidism, serum CK level is elevated (up to 10 times normal), even when there is minimal clinical evidence of muscle disease. EMG is typically normal.

3038. Characteristic prolongation of relaxation phase of muscle stretch reflexes in hypothyroidism is best observed in?
Harrison's 20th Ed. Chapter 441, Page 3252

A. Triceps reflex
B. Biceps reflex
C. Supinator reflex
D. Knee reflex

Relaxation phase of muscle stretch reflexes is characteristically prolonged in hypothyroidism and is best observed at the ankle or biceps brachii reflexes.

3039. Which class of the following lipid-lowering agents cause myopathy?
Harrison's 20th Ed. Chapter 441, Page 3253

A. Fibrates
B. HMG-CoA reductase inhibitors (statins)
C. Niacin (nicotinic acid)
D. All of the above

All classes of lipid-lowering agents have been implicated in muscle toxicity, including fibrates (clofibrate, gemfibrozil), HMG-CoA reductase inhibitors (statins), niacin (nicotinic acid) & ezetimibe.

3040. "Acute quadriplegic" myopathy best relates to?
Harrison's 20th Ed. Chapter 441, Page 3253

A. Glucocorticoid related myopathy
B. Lipid-lowering agent related myopathy
C. Vitamin D related myopathy
D. Vitamin E related myopathy

Glucocorticoid myopathy occurs with chronic treatment or as "acute quadriplegic" myopathy secondary to high-dose IV glucocorticoid use. Acute quadriplegic myopathy can also occur in sepsis.

3041. Which of the following glucocorticoid pose a high risk for myopathy?
Harrison's 20th Ed. Chapter 441, Page 3253

A. Triamcinolone
B. Betamethasone
C. Dexamethasone
D. All of the above

Fluorinated glucocorticoids like triamcinolone, betamethasone and dexamethasone pose a high risk for myopathy.

3042. Which of the following medication can cause mitochondrial myopathy with ragged red fibers?
Harrison's 20th Ed. Chapter 441, Page 3253 Table 441-6

A. Zidovudine
B. D-penicillamine
C. Glucocorticoids
D. Vitamin D

Zidovudine myopathy produces muscle atrophy affecting thigh & calf muscles. Muscle biopsy shows ragged red fibers with minimal inflammation.

3043. Drug-related inflammatory or antibody-mediated myopathy is caused by which of the following medications?
Harrison's 20th Ed. Chapter 441, Page 3253 Table 441-6

A. Zidovudine
B. D-penicillamine
C. Glucocorticoids
D. Vitamin D

Drug-related inflammatory or antibody-mediated myopathy is most consistently caused by D-penicillamine. Myasthenia gravis and polymyositis can also occur with D-penicillamine.

Chronic Fatigue Syndrome

3044. Which of the following is not a characteristic of Chronic fatigue syndrome (CFS)?
Harrison's 20th Ed. Chapter 442, Page 3254

A. Persistent fatigue
B. Unexplained fatigue
C. Fatigue alleviated by rest
D. Severe impairment in daily functioning

Chronic fatigue syndrome (CFS) is a disorder characterized by persistent & unexplained fatigue resulting in severe impairment in daily functioning. CFS is a constellation of symptoms with no pathognomonic features and remains a diagnosis of exclusion.

3045. Institute of Medicine has renamed CFS as?
Harrison's 20th Ed. Chapter 442, Page 3254

A. Fatigue syndrome
B. Exhaustion malady
C. Systemic weariness complex
D. Systemic exercise intolerance disease

The Institute of Medicine has changed the diagnostic criteria & proposed the name of CFS as systemic exercise intolerance disease (SEID).

3046. Which of the following is a characteristic of fatigue in CFS?
Harrison's 20th Ed. Chapter 442, Page 3254 Table 442-1

A. Lasts for at least 6 months
B. Not the result of organic disease or of continuing exertion
C. Not alleviated by rest
D. All of the above

3047. In CFS, which of the following symptoms is concurrently present for 6 months?
Harrison's 20th Ed. Chapter 442, Page 3254 Table 442-1

A. Tender cervical or axillary lymph nodes
B. Impaired memory or concentration
C. Sore throat
D. All of the above

In CFS, four or more of the following symptoms are concurrently present for 6 months: impaired memory or concentration, sore throat, tender cervical or axillary lymph nodes, muscle pain, pain in several joints, new headaches, unrefreshing sleep, or malaise after exertion.

3048. Which of the following is included in the exclusion criteria of CFS?
Harrison's 20th Ed. Chapter 442, Page 3254 Table 442-1

A. Alcohol or substance abuse
B. Severe obesity
C. Schizophrenia
D. All of the above

Exclusion Criteria for defining CFS include medical condition explaining fatigue, major depressive disorder (psychotic features) or bipolar disorder, schizophrenia, dementia, or delusional disorder, anorexia nervosa, bulimia nervosa, alcohol or substance abuse and severe obesity (body mass index >40).

3049. Which of the following about CFS is false?
Harrison's 20th Ed. Chapter 442, Page 3254

A. Prevalence is higher among women
B. Associated with an increase in mortality from suicide
C. Mean age of onset is between 29 & 35 years
D. None of the above

3050. Which of the following infection state acts as a precipitating factor for CFS?
Harrison's 20th Ed. Chapter 442, Page 3254

A. Lyme disease
B. Mononucleosis
C. Q fever
D. All of the above

Mononucleosis, Q fever, Lyme disease act as the trigger of fatigue in CFS.

3051. Excessive production of which of the following induces asthenia?
Harrison's 20th Ed. Chapter 442, Page 3255

A. Interleukin 1
B. Interleukin 4
C. Interleukin 8
D. Interleukin 17

Excessive production of interleukin 1 induces asthenia and other flulike symptoms.

3052. Which of the following is beneficial in CFS?
Harrison's 20th Ed. Chapter 442, Page 3256

A. Cognitive-behavioral therapy (CBT)
B. Community reinforcement approach (CRA)
C. Contingency management (CM)
D. Motivational enhancement therapy (MET)

Cognitive-behavioral therapy (CBT) and graded exercise therapy (GET) are the only beneficial interventions in CFS.

Biology of Psychiatric Disorders

3053. Psychiatric disorder is characterized by disturbance in?
Harrison's 20th Ed. Chapter 443, Page 3256

A. Emotion
B. Cognition
C. Socialization
D. All of the above

Psychiatric disorders are central nervous system diseases characterized by disturbances in emotion, cognition, motivation & socialization. They are highly heritable, with genetic risk comprising 20–90% of disease vulnerability.

3054. Which of the following is a diagnostic scheme for classification of psychiatric illnesses?
Harrison's 20th Ed. Chapter 443, Page 3256

A. Beers criteria
B. Research domain criteria (RDoC)
C. STOPP criteria
D. Wells' criteria

Research Domain Criteria (RDoC) is proposed by National Institute of Mental Health to provide a causal framework for classification of behavioral disturbance.

3055. Which of the following is an intellectual disability syndrome?
Harrison's 20th Ed. Chapter 443, Page 3257

A. Fragile X
B. Rett syndrome
C. Tuberous sclerosis
D. All of the above

Intellectual disability syndromes include fragile X, Rett syndrome and tuberous sclerosis.

3056. Which of the following genes is related to autism spectrum disorders (ASD)?
Harrison's 20th Ed. Chapter 443, Page 3257

A. PTEN
B. TSC1
C. TSC2
D. All of the above

Genes TSC1, TSC2, and PTEN are negative regulators of signaling through the target of rapamycin complex 1 (TORC1), which regulates protein synthesis. Rapamycin is a selective inhibitor of TORC1.

3057. Fragile X syndrome is related to which of the following?
Harrison's 20th Ed. Chapter 443, Page 3257

A. CACNA1C
B. CACNB2
C. FMR1
D. MECP2

Fragile X syndrome is a cause of inherited autism and mental disability. It is due to mutations in FMR1 that result in loss of encoded fragile X mental retardation protein (FMRP). FMRP is a polyribosome-associated mRNA binding protein that represses translation of a subset of all mRNAs, several of which encode proteins that comprise postsynaptic density, including metabotropic glutamate receptor 5 (mGluR5).

3058. Copy number variants (CNVs) best relate to?
Harrison's 20th Ed. Chapter 443, Page 3257

A. Deletions
B. Duplications
C. Deletions and duplications
D. All of the above

There is striking overlap among submicroscopic deletions and duplications, called copy number variants (CNVs). They carry large risks for ASD, schizophrenia, and bipolar disorders, as well as epilepsy and intellectual disability.

3059. CHRNA5-A3-B4 nicotinic acetylcholine receptor gene cluster on chromosome 15 is associated with?
Harrison's 20th Ed. Chapter 443, Page 3257

A. Alcohol addiction
B. Cocaine addiction
C. Marijuana addiction
D. Phencyclidine addiction

CHRNA5-A3-B4 nicotinic acetylcholine receptor gene cluster on chromosome 15 is associated with nicotine and alcohol addiction.

3060. Mutations in which of the following genes can cause obsessive-compulsive & attention-deficit hyperactivity disorders?
Harrison's 20th Ed. Chapter 443, Page 3257

A. MECP2
B. FMR1
C. TSC1
D. NRXN1

Mutations in MECP2 gene can cause obsessive-compulsive & attention-deficit hyperactivity disorders.

3061. Which of the following neurotransmitter is affected in nicotine abuse?
Harrison's 20th Ed. Chapter 443, Page 3259 Table 443-1

A. GABA
B. Glutamate
C. Acetylcholine
D. Serotonin

3062. Which of the following neurotransmitter is affected in ethanol abuse?
Harrison's 20th Ed. Chapter 443, Page 3259 Table 443-1

A. GABA
B. Glutamate
C. Acetylcholine
D. All of the above

3063. Which of the following neurotransmitter is affected in cocaine abuse?
Harrison's 20th Ed. Chapter 443, Page 3259 Table 443-1

A. Endorphin
B. Glutamate
C. Dopamine
D. Serotonin

3064. Which of the following is a noncompetitive antagonist of N-methyl-D-aspartate (NMDA) glutamate receptors?

Harrison's 20th Ed. Chapter 443, Page 3259

A. Imipramine
B. Lithium
C. Tranylcypromine
D. Ketamine

Ketamine is a noncompetitive antagonist of N-methyl-D-aspartate (NMDA) glutamate receptors.

3065. Which of the following is related to morphine use?

Harrison's 20th Ed. Chapter 443, Page 3260

A. Nociceptin/orphanin
B. µ-opioid receptors
C. δ-opioid receptors
D. κ-opioid receptors

Acute activation of µ-opioid receptors by morphine activates Gi/o proteins, leading to inhibition of adenylyl cyclase (AC), resulting in reduced cyclic AMP production, protein kinase A (PKA) activation, and activation of transcription factor CREB. Other known opioid receptors are kappa, delta, and nociceptin/orphanin.

3066. Which of the following is the rate-limiting enzyme in catecholamine biosynthesis?

Harrison's 20th Ed. Chapter 443, Page 3260 Figure 443-2

A. 11β-hydroxylase
B. Tyrosine hydroxylase
C. Lysyl hydroxylase
D. Tryptophan hydroxylase

3067. Which of the following provides dopaminergic input to the limbic structures?

Harrison's 20th Ed. Chapter 443, Page 3261 Figure 443-3

A. Nucleus accumbens (NAc)
B. Ventral tegmental area (VTA)
C. Locus coeruleus (LC)
D. All of the above

Ventral tegmental area (VTA) provides dopaminergic input to all of the limbic structures.

3068. Norepinephrine best relates to which of the following?

Harrison's 20th Ed. Chapter 443, Page 3261 Figure 443-3

A. Locus coeruleus (LC)
B. Dorsal raphe (DR)
C. Arcuate nucleus
D. All of the above

3069. Arcuate nucleus releases which of the following?

Harrison's 20th Ed. Chapter 443, Page 3261 Figure 443-3

A. Norepinephrine
B. β-endorphin
C. Serotonin
D. Orexin

Arcuate nucleus releases β-endorphin and melanocortin.

3070. In schizophrenia, there is reduction of cortical & subcortical gray matter in?

Harrison's 20th Ed. Chapter 443, Page 3260

A. Frontal lobes
B. Temporal lobes
C. Limbic system
D. All of the above

3071. Neuropil includes?

Harrison's 20th Ed. Chapter 443, Page 3260

A. Axons
B. Dendrites
C. Glial cell processes
D. All of the above

The reduction in cortical thickness in schizophrenia is associated with increased cell packing density & reduced neuropil (axons, dendrites & glial cell processes) without an apparent change in neuronal cell number.

3072. The principal inhibitory neurotransmitter in the brain is?

Harrison's 20th Ed. Chapter 443, Page 3260

A. Glutamate
B. γ-aminobutyric acid (GABA)
C. Acetylcholine
D. Dopamine

Enzyme glutamic acid decarboxylase 1 (GAD1) is involved in the synthesis of γ-aminobutyric acid (GABA), GABA is the principal inhibitory neurotransmitter in the brain.

3073. Which of the following is strongly associated with schizophrenia risk?

Harrison's 20th Ed. Chapter 443, Page 3261

A. Complement component 1
B. Complement component 2
C. Complement component 3
D. Complement component 4

3074. Drugs of abuse alter neurotransmission through initial actions at?

Harrison's 20th Ed. Chapter 443, Page 3261

A. Ion channels
B. Neurotransmitter receptors
C. Neurotransmitter transporters
D. All of the above

Psychiatric Disorders

3075. Which of the following provides framework for classification of behavioral disturbance?
Harrison's 20th Ed. Chapter 444, Page 3262

A. DSM-5
B. ICD-10
C. RDoC
D. All of the above

Diagnostic and Statistical Manual of Mental Disorders (DSM-5) of the American Psychiatric Association, tenth revision of the International Classification of Diseases (ICD-10) and Research Domain Criteria (RDOC) proposed by National Institute of Mental Health are used to classify behavioral disturbances.

3076. DSM-IVTR was released in which year?
Harrison's 20th Ed. Chapter 445, Page 3280

A. 2000
B. 2001
C. 2002
D. 2004

Diagnostic and Statistical Manual of Mental Disorders of the American Psychiatric Association, 4th edition, text revision (DSM-IVTR) was released in year 2000.

3077. DSM-V was released in which year?
Harrison's 20th Ed. Chapter 444, Page 3280

A. 2008
B. 2010
C. 2012
D. 2013

3078. General medical condition leading to mental disorders is denoted by which of the following in the multiaxial system of classification?
Harrison's 18th Ed. 3529

A. Axis I
B. Axis II
C. Axis III
D. Axis IV

3079. In DSM-IV-PC, axis III disorders refer to?
Harrison's 18th Ed. 3529

A. Presence or absence of a major mental disorder
B. Any underlying personality disorder
C. General medical condition
D. Psychosocial and environmental problems

The revised fourth edition for use by primary care physicians of the Diagnostic and Statistical Manual (DSM-IV-PC) provides the current multiaxial system of classification. Presence or absence of a major mental disorder (axis I), any underlying personality disorder (axis II), general medical condition (axis III), psychosocial and environmental problems (axis IV), and overall rating of general psychosocial functioning (axis V).

3080. The most prevalent psychiatric illnesses in the general community is?
Harrison's 20th Ed. Chapter 444, Page 3262

A. Anxiety disorders
B. Personality disorders
C. Feeding and eating disorders
D. Somatic symptom disorders

Anxiety disorders are the most prevalent psychiatric illnesses in the general community, present in 15-20% of medical clinic patients.

3081. Subjective sense of unease best relates to?
Harrison's 20th Ed. Chapter 444, Page 3262

A. Anxiety
B. Panic attack
C. Obsessive-compulsive disorder
D. All of the above

Anxiety is defined as a subjective sense of unease, dread, or foreboding.

3082. Which of the following is not an anxiety disorder?
Harrison's 20th Ed. Chapter 444, Page 3262

A. Obsessive-compulsive disorder
B. Phobic disorder
C. Bipolar disorder
D. Stress disorder

3083. Which of the following about panic disorder is false?
Harrison's 20th Ed. Chapter 444, Page 3262

A. Diagnostic criteria require at least 1 month history
B. Sudden onset, usually resolving in an hour
C. First attack is usually outside the home
D. None of the above

3084. Agoraphobia commonly accompanies?
Harrison's 20th Ed. Chapter 444, Page 3263

A. Bipolar disorder
B. Panic disorder
C. Obsessive-compulsive disorder
D. All of the above

Agoraphobia occurs commonly in patients with panic disorder. It is an acquired irrational fear of being in places where one might feel trapped or unable to escape.

3085. Which of the following medical disorders can present as an attack of panic disorder?
Harrison's 20th Ed. Chapter 444, Page 3263

A. Pheochromocytoma
B. Thyrotoxicosis
C. Hypoglycemia
D. All of the above

3086. Which of the following can evoke an attack of panic disorder?
Harrison's 20th Ed. Chapter 444, Page 3263

A. Intravenous infusion of sodium lactate
B. Carbon dioxide inhalation
C. Cholecystokinin tetrapeptide (CCK-4)
D. All of the above

IV sodium lactate, alpha2-adrenergic antagonist yohimbine, cholecystokinin tetrapeptide (CCK-4), and carbon dioxide inhalation evoke a panic attack in panic disorder patients by activating a pathway involving noradrenergic neurons in locus coeruleus and serotonergic neurons in dorsal raphe. Agents that block serotonin reuptake can prevent attacks.

3087. **Which of the following SSRIs has very long half-life?**
Harrison's 20th Ed. Chapter 444, Page 3264 Table 444-1

A. Fluoxetine
B. Citalopram
C. Paroxetine
D. Sertraline

3088. **Which of the following is a serotonin-norepinephrine reuptake inhibitor (SNRI)?**
Harrison's 20th Ed. Chapter 444, Page 3263

A. Fluoxetine
B. Venlafaxine
C. Paroxetine
D. Sertraline

Fluoxetine, paroxetine, sertraline are selective serotonin reuptake inhibitors (SSRIs), and venlafaxine is a serotonin-norepinephrine reuptake inhibitor (SNRI).

3089. **Which of the following is the most noradrenergic of SNRIs?**
Harrison's 20th Ed. Chapter 444, Page 3264 Table 444-1

A. Vortioxetine
B. Levomilnacipran
C. Mirtazapine
D. Duloxetine

3090. **Which of the following tricyclic antidepressants (TCA) is best tolerated, especially by elderly?**
Harrison's 20th Ed. Chapter 444, Page 3264 Table 444-1

A. Amitriptyline
B. Nortriptyline
C. Imipramine
D. Doxepin

3091. **MAOIs should not be used concomitantly with?**
Harrison's 20th Ed. Chapter 444, Page 3263

A. Selective serotonin reuptake inhibitors (SSRIs)
B. Serotonin-norepinephrine reuptake inhibitor (SNRI)
C. Tricyclic antidepressants (TCA)
D. All of the above

MAOIs should not be used concomitantly with SSRIs, because of the risk of serotonin syndrome, or with TCAs, because of possible hyperadrenergic effects.

3092. **Antidepressants typically take how much time to become effective?**
Harrison's 20th Ed. Chapter 444, Page 3263

A. 24–36 hours
B. 5–10 days
C. 1–3 weeks
D. 2–6 weeks

Antidepressants typically take 2–6 weeks to become effective.

3093. **In treatment resistant panic disorder cases, which of the following is efficacious?**
Harrison's 20th Ed. Chapter 444, Page 3263

A. Aripiprazole
B. Divalproex sodium
C. Pindolol
D. All of the above

In treatment resistant panic disorder cases, short-term augmentation with aripiprazole, divalproex sodium or pindolol is efficacious.

3094. **In panic disorders, following recovery, drug treatment should be continued for what length of time?**
Harrison's 20th Ed. Chapter 444, Page 3263

A. 3–6 months
B. 1–2 years
C. 2–5 years
D. Life long

In panic disorders, once patients have achieved a satisfactory response, drug treatment should be maintained for 1–2 years to prevent relapse.

3095. **Which of the following is a mixed norepinephrine/serotonin reuptake inhibitors and receptor blocker?**
Harrison's 20th Ed. Chapter 444, Page 3264 Table 444-1

A. Venlafaxine
B. Duloxetine
C. Mirtazapine
D. All of the above

Venlafaxine, Desvenlafaxine, Duloxetine, Mirtazapine, Vilazodone, Vortioxetine and Levomilnacipran are mixed norepinephrine/serotonin reuptake inhibitors (SNRI) and receptor blockers.

3096. **Which of the following is a monoamine oxidase inhibitor (MAOI)?**
Harrison's 20th Ed. Chapter 444, Page 3264 Table 444-1

A. Amoxapine
B. Bupropion
C. Phenelzine
D. Trazodone

Phenelzine, Tranylcypromine, Isocarboxazid, and selegiline are MAOIs.

3097. **Extrapyramidal symptoms can appear with the use of?**
Harrison's 20th Ed. Chapter 444, Page 3264 Table 444-1

A. Amoxapine
B. Bupropion
C. Phenelzine
D. Trazodone

3098. **Which of the following is to be avoided when monoamine oxidase inhibitors (MAOIs) are used?**
Harrison's 20th Ed. Chapter 444, Page 3263

A. Tobacco
B. Coffee
C. Wine
D. Whisky

Patients taking monoamine oxidase inhibitors (MAOIs) need to maintain a low-tyramine die, i.e. avoidance of cheese and wine.

3099. Which of the following is a weak, reversible monoamine oxidase inhibitor?
Harrison's 20th Ed. Chapter 139, Page 1055

A. Rifamycin
B. Colistin
C. Linezolid
D. Nitrofurantoin

Linezolid is a weak, reversible monoamine oxidase inhibitor and coadministration with sympathomimetics and foods rich in tyramine should be avoided. Linezolid has been associated with serotonin syndrome when coadministered with selective serotonin-reuptake inhibitors.

3100. Which of the following is contraindicated to use along with monoamine oxidase inhibitor?
Harrison's 20th Ed. Chapter 422, Page 3103

A. Tyramine containing foods
B. Decongestants
C. Meperidine
D. All of the above

3101. Which of the following is a monoamine oxidase inhibitor?
Harrison's 20th Ed. Chapter 217, Page 1563

A. Mebendazole
B. Halofantrine
C. Furazolidone
D. Ivermectin

Furazolidone is a monoamine oxidase (MAO) inhibitor. Furazolidone inhibits MAOs gradually over several days, so the risks are small if treatment is limited to a 5-day course.

3102. Anorgasmia/impotence occurring as side effect of antidepressant medication is managed with?
Harrison's 20th Ed. Chapter 444, Page 3265 Table 444-2

A. Cyproheptadine
B. Bupropion
C. Amantadine
D. Any of the above

3103. Diarrhea occurring as side effect of antidepressant medication is managed with?
Harrison's 20th Ed. Chapter 444, Page 3265 Table 444-2

A. Cyproheptadine
B. Bupropion
C. Fluoxetine
D. Famotidine

3104. Which of the following anxiolytic drugs has no active metabolite?
Harrison's 20th Ed. Chapter 444, Page 3266 Table 444-4

A. Oxazepam
B. Temazepam
C. Clonazepam
D. All of the above

Oxazepam, Temazepam, Clonazepam, Lorazepam, and Triazolam have no active metabolites. Diazepam, Alprazolam, Chlordiazepoxide, and Buspirone have active metabolites.

3105. Which of the following benzodiazepines is difficult to withdraw?
Harrison's 20th Ed. Chapter 444, Page 3266 Table 444-4

A. Alprazolam
B. Clonazepam
C. Chlordiazepoxide
D. Oxazepam

3106. Which of the following benzodiazepines is a prodrug?
Harrison's 20th Ed. Chapter 444, Page 3266 Table 444-4

A. Flurazepam
B. Triazolam
C. Lorazepam
D. Temazepam

3107. Many patients with generalized anxiety disorder (GAD) also suffer from?
Harrison's 20th Ed. Chapter 444, Page 3263

A. Major depression
B. Dysthymia
C. Social phobia
D. All of the above

3108. Which of the following complaints are relatively rare in generalized anxiety disorder (GAD)?
Harrison's 20th Ed. Chapter 444, Page 3263

A. Shortness of breath
B. Palpitations
C. Tachycardia
D. All of the above

Unlike panic disorders, complaints of shortness of breath, palpitations, and tachycardia are relatively rare in generalized anxiety disorder (GAD).

3109. Which of the following statements is false?
Harrison's 20th Ed. Chapter 444, Page 3263

A. All anxiogenic agents act on GABA-A receptor/chloride ion channel complex
B. Serotonin (5-HT) has a role in anxiety
C. 3α-reduced neuroactive steroids has a role in anxiety
D. None of the above

All anxiogenic agents act on the γ-aminobutyric acid (GABA)A receptor/chloride ion channel complex.

3110. Which of the following is a GABA-A type II receptor site?
Harrison's 20th Ed. Chapter 444, Page 3263

A. Hippocampus
B. Striatum
C. Neocortex
D. All of the above

Benzodiazepines bind two separate GABA-A receptor sites: type I, has wide neuroanatomic distribution, and type II, which is concentrated in hippocampus, striatum & neocortex.

3111. Sedation & memory impairment of benzodiazepines is related to?
Harrison's 20th Ed. Chapter 444, Page 3263

A. Alpha 1 subunit of GABA-A receptor
B. Alpha 2 subunit of GABA-A receptor
C. Alpha 3 subunit of GABA-A receptor
D. All of the above

Anti-anxiety effects of benzodiazepines are influenced by their relative binding to alpha 2 & 3 subunits of GABA-A receptor, and sedation and memory impairment to the alpha 1 subunit.

3112. Which of the following is a 5-HT1A agonist?
Harrison's 20th Ed. Chapter 444, Page 3263

A. Lorazepam
B. Buspirone
C. Oxazepam
D. Alprazolam

Buspirone and tandospirone are 5-HT1A agonists.

3113. Which of the following is a 5-HT2A & 5-HT2C receptor antagonist?
Harrison's 20th Ed. Chapter 444, Page 3263

A. Mirtazapine
B. Nefazodone
C. Lorcaserin
D. Pimavanserin

Mirtazapine is a 5-HT2A receptor antagonist. Lorcaserin is a selective 5-HT2C receptor agonist. Pimavanserin is an inverse agonist of serotonin 5-HT2A receptor.

3114. Benzodiazepines should not be prescribed for more than how many weeks to avoid risk of abuse and dependence?
Harrison's 20th Ed. Chapter 444, Page 3264

A. 1–2 weeks
B. 2–3 weeks
C. 3–4 weeks
D. 4–6 weeks

Benzodiazepines should not be prescribed for >4–6 weeks because of the development of tolerance and the risk of abuse & dependence.

3115. Which of the following is not a long-acting benzodiazepine?
Harrison's 20th Ed. Chapter 444, Page 3264

A. Diazepam
B. Alprazolam
C. Flurazepam
D. Clonazepam

Longer-acting benzodiazepines are diazepam, chlordiazepoxide, flurazepam, and clonazepam. Shorter-acting benzodiazepines are alprazolam, lorazepam and oxazepam. It is more difficult to taper patients off shorter-acting benzodiazepines.

3116. Which of the following is a non-benzodiazepine anxiolytic agent?
Harrison's 20th Ed. Chapter 444, Page 3265

A. Diazepam
B. Buspirone
C. Flurazepam
D. Clonazepam

Buspirone is a nonbenzodiazepine anxiolytic agent. It is nonsedating, does not produce tolerance or dependence, does not interact with benzodiazepine receptors or alcohol, and has no abuse or disinhibition potential. But, requires several weeks to take effect and thrice-daily dosing.

3117. Which of the following is contraindicated during pregnancy?
Harrison's 20th Ed. Chapter 118, Page 887

A. Live-virus vaccines
B. Clarithromycin
C. Primaquine
D. All of the above

Pregnancy is not a contraindication to administration of inactivated vaccines, but should be avoided.

3118. Which of the following is contraindicated during pregnancy?
Harrison's 20th Ed. Chapter 264, Page 1831

A. Angiotensin converting enzyme (ACE) inhibitors
B. Angiotensin receptor blockers
C. Endothelin-receptor blockers
D. All of the above

3119. Which of the following is contraindicated during pregnancy?
Harrison's 20th Ed. Chapter 264, Page 1831

A. Miltefosine
B. IFN-based therapy
C. Ribavirin
D. All of the above

3120. Which of the following is contraindicated during pregnancy?
Harrison's 20th Ed. Chapter 444, Page 3265

A. Methotrexate
B. Leflunomide
C. Benzodiazepines
D. All of the above

Benzodiazepines are contraindicated during pregnancy and breast-feeding.

3121. Which of the following is contraindicated during breast-feeding?
Harrison's 20th Ed. Chapter 444, Page 3265

A. Treatment for TB
B. Live-virus or other vaccines
C. Warfarin
D. None of the above

Treatment for TB, live-virus or other vaccines & warfarin are not contraindicated in breast-feeding women. Breast-feeding is not contraindicated in women with hepatitis B. Breast-feeding does not increase the risk of HCV infection between an infected mother and her infant.

3122. Which of the following is contraindication for breast-feeding?
Harrison's 20th Ed. Chapter 444, Page 3265

A. HIV
B. Diloxanide furoate
C. Furazolidone
D. All of the above

Pregnancy and breast-feeding are absolute contraindications to radioiodine treatment. Also, use of Atovaquone-proguanil & ivermectin should be avoided.

3123. Which of the following anticonvulsants with GABAergic properties is beneficial in anxiety-related syndromes?
Harrison's 20th Ed. Chapter 444, Page 3265

A. Gabapentin
B. Pregabalin
C. Divalproex
D. All of the above

Anticonvulsants with GABAergic properties like gabapentin, oxcarbazepine, tiagabine, pregabalin, and divalproex are beneficial in anxiety-related syndromes.

3124. Which of the following about phobic disorders is false?
Harrison's 20th Ed. Chapter 444, Page 3265

A. Marked & persistent fear of objects or situations
B. Usually experience anxiety only in specific situations
C. Processing of fear stimulus occurs in lateral nucleus of amygdala
D. None of the above

Processing of fear stimulus occurs through lateral nucleus of the amygdala, extending through central nucleus & projecting to periaqueductal gray region, lateral hypothalamus & paraventricular hypothalamus.

3125. Which of the following is useful in treatment of "performance anxiety"?
Harrison's 20th Ed. Chapter 444, Page 3265

A. Benzodiazepines
B. Propranolol
C. MAOIs
D. All of the above

Beta blockers like propranolol, 20–40 mg orally 2 hours before the event, are effective in the treatment of "performance anxiety".

3126. Which of the following is useful in treatment of social anxiety?
Harrison's 20th Ed. Chapter 444, Page 3265

A. Paroxetine
B. Sertraline
C. Venlafaxine
D. All of the above

3127. Risk factor for the development of Posttraumatic Stress Disorder (PTSD) is?
Harrison's 20th Ed. Chapter 444, Page 3266

A. Past psychiatric history
B. High neuroticism
C. Extroversion
D. All of the above

3128. Which of the following is related to PTSD?
Harrison's 20th Ed. Chapter 444, Page 3266

A. Central tegmental area (VTA)
B. Locus coeruleus
C. Nucleus accumbens (NAc)
D. All of the above

In PTSD, there is excessive release of norepinephrine from locus coeruleus in response to stress & increased noradrenergic activity at projection sites in hippocampus & amygdala.

3129. Which of the following may be beneficial in preventing development of PTSD?
Harrison's 20th Ed. Chapter 444, Page 3267

A. Hydrocortisone
B. Intranasal oxytocin
C. Morphine
D. All of the above

3130. Comorbid alcoholism in PTSD is best treated with?
Harrison's 20th Ed. Chapter 444, Page 3267

A. Nefazadone
B. Topiramate
C. Naltrexone
D. Mirtazepine

Comorbid alcoholism in PTSD is best treated with naltrexone.

3131. In obsessive-compulsive disorder (OCD), obsession pertains to?
Harrison's 20th Ed. Chapter 444, Page 3267

A. Thoughts
B. Actions
C. Behavior
D. All of the above

Obsessive-compulsive disorder (OCD) is characterized by obsessive thoughts and compulsive behaviors that impair everyday functioning.

3132. Which of the following is the most frequent comorbid condition in OCD?
Harrison's 20th Ed. Chapter 444, Page 3267

A. Depression
B. Eating disorders
C. Tics
D. All of the above

In OCD, comorbid conditions are common, the most frequent being depression, other anxiety disorders, eating disorders, and tics.

3133. Obsessive-compulsive disorder (OCD) is related to which of the following clinical conditions?
Harrison's 20th Ed. Chapter 444, Page 3268

A. Wilson's disease
B. Myoclonus
C. Tourette's syndrome
D. Parkinson's disease

Family studies show an aggregation of OCD with Tourette's disorder. Both are more common in males and in first-born children.

3134. Anatomy of obsessive-compulsive behavior includes?
Harrison's 20th Ed. Chapter 444, Page 3268

A. Orbital frontal cortex
B. Caudate nucleus
C. Globus pallidus
D. All of the above

3135. Which of the following part of the brain is responsible for acquisition and maintenance of habit and skill learning?
Harrison's 20th Ed. Chapter 444, Page 3268

A. Hippocampus
B. Amygdala
C. Caudate nucleus
D. Mammillary bodies

Anatomical localization of obsessive-compulsive behavior is to orbital frontal cortex, caudate nucleus, & globus pallidus. Caudate nucleus is involved in acquisition & maintenance of habit & skill learning.

3136. Which of the following is useful in the treatment of obsessive-compulsive disorder (OCD)?

Harrison's 20th Ed. Chapter 444, Page 3268

A. Clomipramine
B. Fluoxetine
C. Fluvoxamine
D. All of the above

3137. In treatment resistant cases of OCD, which of the following is added to treatment?

Harrison's 20th Ed. Chapter 444, Page 3268

A. Buspirone
B. Neuroleptic
C. Benzodiazepine
D. Any of the above

Clomipramine, fluoxetine, fluvoxamine, and sertraline are useful in the treatment of OCD. In treatment-resistant cases, augmentation with buspirone, neuroleptic or benzodiazepine is beneficial and in severe cases deep brain stimulation is effective.

3138. Which of the following about Obsessive-Compulsive Disorder is false?

N Engl J Med. 2014;371:646-53

A. Male:female sex ratio is approximately 1:1
B. Onset after 30 years of age is unusual
C. Hyperactivity in orbitofrontal cortex & caudate
D. None of the above

Studies have consistently shown hyperactivity in the orbitofrontal cortex and caudate in OCD. Other key implicated regions suggesting abnormalities in functional or structural connections include anterior cingulate cortex, thalamus, amygdala, and parietal cortex.

3139. Obsessions are?

N Engl J Med. 2014;371:646-53

A. Recurrent thoughts
B. Recurrent urges
C. Recurrent images
D. All of the above

Obsessions are recurrent thoughts, urges, or images that are experienced, at some time, as intrusive and unwanted. Compulsions are repetitive behaviors (hand washing, ordering, and checking) or mental acts (praying and counting) that the person feels driven to perform in response to an obsession. The diagnosis of OCD requires that a person have obsessions, compulsions, or both.

3140. Persons with OCD may have which of the following?

N Engl J Med. 2014;371:646-53

A. Hallucinations
B. Smell disorder
C. Color blindness
D. Tic disorder

Up to 30% of persons with OCD have a tic disorder. Its presence is associated with a poor response to pharmacotherapy for OCD in children & adolescents. An early age at OCD onset, more severe OCD, coexisting tics, and hoarding symptoms have all been associated with a poor response to clomipramine and SSRIs.

3141. Which of the following is not a selective serotonin-reuptake inhibitor (SSRI)?

N Engl J Med. 2014;371:646-53

A. Paroxetine
B. Fluvoxamine
C. Clomipramine
D. Sertraline

Clomipramine is a tricyclic antidepressant. Paroxetine, fluvoxamine, fluoxetine, citalopram, escitalopram, and sertralineor are selective serotonin-reuptake inhibitor (SSRI) and in OCD are the first-line pharmacologic treatment.

3142. Mood disorders are characterized by a disturbance in the regulation of?

Harrison's 20th Ed. Chapter 444, Page 3268

A. Mood
B. Behavior
C. Affect
D. All of the above

Mood disorders are characterized by a disturbance in the regulation of mood, behavior, and affect.

3143. Which of the following is a mood disorder?

Harrison's 20th Ed. Chapter 444, Page 3268

A. Depressive disorders
B. Bipolar disorders
C. Depression in association with medical illness or alcohol and substance abuse
D. All of the above

3144. Which of the following about major depressive disorder (MDD) is false?

Harrison's 20th Ed. Chapter 444, Page 3268

A. Absence of manic or hypomanic episode in MDD
B. MDD more frequent in families of bipolar individuals
C. Bipolar disorder more frequent in families of MDD individuals
D. None of the above

3145. Depressive symptoms can be triggered by which of the following group of drugs?

Harrison's 20th Ed. Chapter 444, Page 3268

A. Antihypertensive drugs
B. Anticholesterolemic drugs
C. Antiarrhythmic drugs
D. All of the above

3146. Iatrogenic depression can be caused by which of the following group of drugs?

Harrison's 20th Ed. Chapter 444, Page 3268

A. Glucocorticoids
B. Antimicrobials
C. Systemic analgesics
D. All of the above

Iatrogenic depression can be induced by antihypertensives, anticholesterolemics, antiarrhythmics, glucocorticoids, antimicrobials, systemic analgesics, antiparkinsonian medications, and anticonvulsants.

3147. Which of the following occurs in patients with depression?

Harrison's 20th Ed. Chapter 444, Page 3268

A. Reduced parasympathetic nervous system activity
B. Increased platelet aggregation
C. Increased risk of subsequent diagnosis of Alzheimer's disease
D. All of the above

3148. Which of the following can produce hyperglycemia and carbohydrate craving?
Harrison's 20th Ed. Chapter 444, Page 3268

A. MAOI
B. TCAs
C. SSRIs
D. All of the above

MAOIs can induce hypoglycemia and weight gain, while TCAs can produce hyperglycemia and carbohydrate craving. SSRIs, like MAOIs, may reduce fasting plasma glucose.

3149. Major depression is defined as depressed mood on a daily basis for?
Harrison's 20th Ed. Chapter 444, Page 3268

A. A minimum duration of 1 week
B. A minimum duration of 2 weeks
C. A minimum duration of 4 weeks
D. A minimum duration of 6 weeks

Major depression is defined as depressed mood on a daily basis for a minimum duration of 2 weeks.

3150. In patients with depression, mood is worse in?
Harrison's 20th Ed. Chapter 444, Page 3269

A. Morning
B. Afternoon
C. Evening
D. Night

Major depression is defined as depressed mood on a daily basis for a minimum duration of 2 weeks. Patients with depression often notice a diurnal variation in mood, worse in morning hours.

3151. Presence of which of the following significantly increases near-term suicidal risk in depressed patients?
Harrison's 20th Ed. Chapter 444, Page 3269

A. Anxiety
B. Agitation
C. Panic
D. All of the above

Presence of anxiety, panic, or agitation significantly increases near-term suicidal risk in depressed patients. ~4–5% of all depressed patients will commit suicide.

3152. Dysthymic disorder best relates to?
Harrison's 20th Ed. Chapter 444, Page 3269

A. Seasonal affective disorder
B. Persistent depressive disorder
C. Pseudodementia
D. Cyclothymic disorder

Dysthymic disorder refers to a persistent depressive disorder that consists of a pattern of chronic (at least 2 years), ongoing depressive symptoms that are usually less severe and/or less numerous than those found in major depression, but the functional consequences may be equivalent to or even greater. The two conditions can occur together and it is labeled as "double depression".

3153. Which of the following about depression is false?
Harrison's 20th Ed. Chapter 444, Page 3269

A. Men : women ration in depression is ~1 : 2
B. Incidence of depression increases with age in both sexes
C. Major depression of early onset is largely genetic in origin
D. None of the above

3154. Which of the following about unipolar depressive disorders is false?
Harrison's 20th Ed. Chapter 444, Page 3269

A. Usually begin in early adulthood
B. Recur episodically
C. Best predictor of future risk is the number of past episodes
D. None of the above

3155. Seasonal affective disorder best relates to?
Harrison's 20th Ed. Chapter 444, Page 3269

A. Seasonal pattern of depression
B. Depression in seasoned individuals
C. Depression in other members of family
D. Any of the above

A seasonal pattern of depression, which is more common in women, is called seasonal affective disorder. It manifests with onset & remission of episodes at predictable times of the year. The prevalence of depression increases with distance from equator, and improvement may occur by altering light exposure.

3156. Neuro-endocrine abnormality that reflect neuro-vegetative signs & symptoms of depression is?
Harrison's 20th Ed. Chapter 444, Page 3269

A. Increased cortisol & CRH secretion
B. Blunted response of TSH level to infusion of TRH
C. Decreased inhibitory response of glucocorticoids to dexamethasone
D. All of the above

Neuroendocrine abnormalities that reflect the neurovegetative signs & symptoms of depression include increased cortisol and corticotropin-releasing hormone (CRH) secretion, decreased inhibitory response of glucocorticoids to dexamethasone and blunted response of thyroid-stimulating hormone (TSH) level to infusion of thyroid-releasing hormone (TRH). Antidepressant treatment normalizes these abnormalities. Major depression is also associated with an upregulation of proinflammatory cytokines, and neurotrophins, an increase in measures of oxidative stress & cellular aging, telomere shortening & mitochondrial dysfunction.

3157. Sleep abnormality in patients with major depression is?
Harrison's 20th Ed. Chapter 444, Page 3269

A. Decrease in REM sleep
B. Increase in REM density
C. Decrease in stage IV delta slow-wave sleep
D. All of the above

Patients with major depression show a decrease in rapid eye movement (REM) sleep onset (REM latency), an increase in REM density, and, a decrease in stage IV delta slow-wave sleep.

3158. Which of the following is an ideal antidepressant?
Harrison's 20th Ed. Chapter 444, Page 3270

A. SSRI
B. TCA
C. MAOI
D. None of the above

There is no ideal antidepressant. No current compound combines rapid onset of action, moderate half-life, a meaningful relationship between dose & blood level, a low side effect profile, minimal interaction with other drugs, and safety in overdose.

3159. Which tricyclic antidepressant carries the greatest risk in overdose?
Harrison's 20th Ed. Chapter 444, Page 3270

A. Desipramine
B. Imipramine
C. Nortriptyline
D. Amitriptyline

Overdoses of tricyclic agents can be lethal, with desipramine carrying the greatest risk. TCAs are contraindicated in patients with serious cardiovascular risk factors.

3160. Which of the following is false about serotonin syndrome?
Harrison's 20th Ed. Chapter 444, Page 3270

A. Myoclonus
B. Abdominal cramping
C. Hyperpyrexia
D. Hypotension

MAOIs used concomitantly with SSRIs can lead to serotonin syndrome that results from hyperstimulation of brainstem 5HT1A receptors and is characterized by myoclonus, agitation, abdominal cramping, hyperpyrexia, hypertension, and potentially death.

3161. Akathisia refers to?
Harrison's 20th Ed. Chapter 444, Page 3270

A. Phobias for high pitched sounds
B. Inner sense of restlessness and anxiety
C. Obsession for cleanliness
D. Transient blindness

Akathisia refers to an inner sense of restlessness and anxiety.

3162. SSRI induced sexual dysfunction can be ameliorated by?
Harrison's 20th Ed. Chapter 444, Page 3270

A. Amantadine
B. Bethanechol
C. Buspirone
D. All of the above

All SSRIs impair sexual function. Sexual dysfunction can be ameliorated by lowering dose, weekend drug holidays, or by treatment with amantadine, bethanechol, buspirone, or bupropion.

3163. Principal active metabolite of Fluoxetine is?
Harrison's 20th Ed. Chapter 444, Page 3270

A. Isofluoxetine
B. Parfluoxetine
C. Norfluoxetine
D. Metafluoxetine

Principal active metabolite of Fluoxetine is Norfluoxetine.

3164. Which of the following is the most noradrenergic of the SNRI?
Harrison's 20th Ed. Chapter 444, Page 3271

A. Mirtazapine
B. Desvenlafaxine
C. Levomilnacipran
D. Vortioxetine

Levomilnacipran is the most noradrenergic of the SNRIs and theoretically may be appropriate for patients with more severe fatigue and anergia.

3165. Which of the following gene relates to serotonin transporter?
N Engl J Med. 2009;360:957

A. PCDH10
B. SHANK3
C. 5-HTT/SLC6A4
D. OXTR

In CNS, serotonin synthesis is catalyzed by Tph2. It is released at neural synapses, and its reuptake is controlled by 5-HTT. Circulating serotonin does not cross blood–brain barrier, so all its activity in brain is mediated by synthesis, reuptake, and binding to a 5-HT receptor (Htr). Pharmacologic inhibition of 5-HTT by SSRIs enhances serotonin activity.

3166. Which amino acid is the precursor of serotonin?
Harrison's 20th Ed. Chapter 80, Page 604

A. Tryptophan
B. Leucine
C. Isoleucine
D. Arginine

Serotonin (5-HT) is synthesized from tryptophan.

3167. Which of the following is a biologic effect of serotonin?
Harrison's 20th Ed. Chapter 80, Page 604

A. Stimulating intestinal secretion with inhibition of absorption
B. Stimulating increases in intestinal motility
C. Stimulating fibrogenesis
D. All of the above

3168. Which of the following about Mirtazapine is false?
Harrison's 20th Ed. Chapter 9, Page 56, 3271

A. Sedating, antiemetic and anxiolytic
B. Increases noradrenergic & serotonergic neurotransmission
C. Strongly antihistaminic
D. Weight loss

Mirtazapine is an antagonist at the postsynaptic serotonin receptors.

3169. Which of the following is a nonamphetamine psychostimulant with minimal abuse potential?
Harrison's 20th Ed. Chapter 9, Page 56

A. Dextroamphetamine
B. Methylphenidate
C. Modafinil
D. Pemoline

Pemoline is a nonamphetamine psychostimulant with minimal abuse potential.

3170. Which of the following SSRI is preferred in a patient in whom fatigue is a major symptom?
Harrison's 20th Ed. Chapter 9, Page 57

A. Paroxetine
B. Fluoxetine
C. Citalopram
D. Sertraline

For a patient in whom fatigue is a major symptom, a more activating SSRI (fluoxetine) is appropriate. For a patient in whom anxiety & sleeplessness are major symptoms, a sedating SSRI (paroxetine) is appropriate.

3171. Which of the following antidepressants can cause priapism?
Harrison's 20th Ed. Chapter 9, Page 57

A. Paroxetine
B. Trazodone
C. Bupropion
D. Sertraline

Antidepressant Trazodone is sedating, can cause orthostatic hypotension and priapism.

3172. Which of the following SSRI is associated with significant risk of sexual dysfunction?
Harrison's 20th Ed. Chapter 390, Page 2818

A. Escitalopram
B. Bupropion
C. Nefazodone
D. Mirtazapine

Among the SSRIs, paroxetine & escitalopram are associated with the highest risk of sexual dysfunction.

3173. Which of the following is a postsynaptic agonist of serotonin receptor 1A and antagonist of serotonin receptor 2A?
Harrison's 20th Ed. Chapter 390, Page 2818

A. Cyproterone acetate
B. Safinamide
C. Alprostadil
D. Flibanserin

Flibanserin, a postsynaptic agonist of serotonin receptor 1A and antagonist of serotonin receptor 2A, increases sexual desire and reduces resultant stress in women with HypoSexual Desire Disorder (HSDD).

3174. Which of the following SSRIs has no specific inhibitory effects on the P450 system?
Harrison's 20th Ed. Chapter 444, Page 3271

A. Sertraline
B. Escitalopram
C. Fluoxetine
D. Paroxetine

With the exception of citalopram & escitalopram, each of the SSRIs inhibits one or more cytochrome P450 enzymes.

3175. Which of the following is useful in managing treatment-resistant depression?
Harrison's 20th Ed. Chapter 444, Page 3271

A. Repetitive transcranial magnetic stimulation (rTMS)
B. Vagus nerve stimulation (VNS)
C. Deep brain stimulation (DBS)
D. All of the above

Electroconvulsive therapy, Transcranial magnetic stimulation (TMS), Vagus nerve stimulation (VNS) and Deep brain stimulation (DBS) are useful in managing treatment resistant depression.

3176. Response to treatment of depression should be evaluated after how many months?
Harrison's 20th Ed. Chapter 444, Page 3271

A. 1 month
B. 2 months
C. 3 months
D. 6 months

Regardless of the modality of treatment for depression, response should be evaluated after 2 months.

3177. Which of the following distinguish bipolar I mania from bipolar II hypomania?
N Engl J Med. 2011;364:51-9

A. Suicidal tendancy
B. Voluntarily produced physical symptoms of illness
C. Severity of elevated mood
D. Intentionally produced deficit symptoms

The greater severity of elevated mood and associated functional disability distinguish bipolar I mania (which is characterized by psychosis, the need for urgent care or hospitalization, or marked impairment) from bipolar II hypomania.

3178. Montgomery and Åsberg Depression Rating Scale (MADRS) ranges from?
N Engl J Med. 2011;364:51-9

A. 0 to 20
B. 0 to 40
C. 0 to 60
D. 0 to 80

Montgomery and Åsberg Depression Rating Scale [MADRS] ranges from 0 to 60.

3179. Which of the following is a feature of bipolar disorders?
Harrison's 20th Ed. Chapter 444, Page 3271

A. Mania
B. Hypomania
C. Depression
D. All of the above

Bipolar disorder is characterized by unpredictable swings in mood from mania (or hypomania) to depression.

3180. Which of the following is not a feature of mania?
Harrison's 20th Ed. Chapter 444, Page 3271

A. Increased psychomotor activity
B. Excessive social extroversion
C. Increased need for sleep
D. Impulsivity

3181. Mania in its pure form is associated with?
Harrison's 20th Ed. Chapter 444, Page 3271

A. Increased psychomotor activity
B. Impulsivity and impairment in judgment
C. Decreased need for sleep
D. All of the above

Mania in its pure form is associated with increased psychomotor activity, excessive social extroversion, decreased need for sleep, impulsivity and impaired judgment and expansive, grandiose mood.

3182. Which of the following is a feature of cyclothymic disorder?
Harrison's 20th Ed. Chapter 444, Page 3271

A. Many hypomanic periods usually of relatively short duration
B. Clusters of depressive symptoms
C. Manifestations present for at least 2 years
D. All of the above

In cyclothymic disorder, there are many hypomanic periods of short duration, alternating with clusters of depressive symptoms that do not meet the criteria of major depression. Mood fluctuations are chronic and should be present for at least 2 years before the diagnosis is made.

3183. Term rapid cycling is used for patients who have how many episodes of either depression or mania in a given year?
Harrison's 20th Ed. Chapter 444, Page 3271

- A. One or more
- B. Two or more
- C. Three or more
- D. Four or more

Term rapid cycling is used for patients, mostly women, who have four or more episodes of either depression or mania in a given year.

3184. Secondary mania may be induced by?
Harrison's 20th Ed. Chapter 444, Page 3272

- A. Stimulant or sympathomimetic drugs
- B. Hyperthyroidism
- C. Huntington's or Wilson's disease
- D. All of the above

Secondary mania may be induced by stimulant or sympathomimetic drugs, hyperthyroidism, AIDS, Huntington's or Wilson's disease and cerebrovascular accidents.

3185. Risk genes for bipolar disorder include?
Harrison's 20th Ed. Chapter 444, Page 3272

- A. CACNA1C
- B. Teneurin transmembrane protein 4 (ODZ4)
- C. Neurocan (NCAN)
- D. All of the above

Bipolar disorder concordance rate for monozygotic twins is ~80%. Risk genes identified include CACNA1C, teneurin transmembrane protein 4 (ODZ4), ankryn 3 (ANK3), neurocan (NCAN), and tetratricopeptide repeat and ankyrin repeat containing 1 (TRANK1).

3186. Drug for treatment of bipolar disorders include?
Harrison's 20th Ed. Chapter 444, Page 3272

- A. Lithium carbonate
- B. Sodium valproate
- C. Olanzapine
- D. All of the above

3187. Which of the following about lithium therapy is false?
Harrison's 20th Ed. Chapter 444, Page 3272

- A. Side effects include polyuria & weight gain
- B. Lithium exerts an antithyroid effect
- C. No prophylactic effect in prevention of recurrent mania
- D. Excreted mainly by kidneys

3188. Lithium carbonate is of use in which of the following?
Harrison's 20th Ed. Chapter 444, Page 3272

- A. Acute mania
- B. Prophylactically to prevent recurrent mania
- C. Prevention of recurrent depression
- D. All of the above

Lithium carbonate is the mainstay of treatment in bipolar disorder. Lithium also has a prophylactic effect in prevention of recurrent mania and, to a lesser extent, in prevention of recurrent depression.

3189. Which of the following about lithium therapy is false?
Harrison's 20th Ed. Chapter 310, Page 2525, 303, 2157 Table 310-1, 2162

- A. Can induce lupus-like disease
- B. Can cause chronic tubulointerstitial nephritis
- C. Can cause nephrogenic diabetes insipidus
- D. None of the above

3190. Which of the following about lithium therapy is false?
Harrison's 20th Ed. Chapter 56, Page 365

- A. Can cause multifocal myoclonus
- B. Can restore myelopoiesis in patients with neutropenia due to impaired production
- C. Can induce onychomadesis
- D. None of the above

3191. Which of the following about lithium therapy is false?
Harrison's 20th Ed. Chapter 54, Page 341, 342, 364

- A. Can induce acne
- B. Can exacerbate plaque psoriasis
- C. Can cause alopecia
- D. None of the above

3192. Which of the following about lithium therapy is false?
Harrison's 20th Ed. Chapter 240, Page 193, 1728 Table 240-1

- A. Can decrease anionic gap (AG)
- B. Can cause downbeat nystagmus
- C. Can cause bradycardia & atrioventricular block
- D. None of the above

3193. Concomitant administration of which of the following with lithium can result in increased serum levels of lithium?
Harrison's 20th Ed. Chapter 139, Page 1055

- A. Benzodiazapine
- B. Olanzapine
- C. Metronidazole
- D. Valproic acid

Concomitant administration of metronidazole with lithium can result in increased serum levels of lithium and associated toxicity.

3194. What proportion of a given dose of lithium carbonate is excreted unchanged through kidneys within 24 hours?
Harrison's 20th Ed. Chapter 444, Page 3272

- A. 25%
- B. 50%
- C. 75%
- D. 95%

~95% of a given dose of lithium carbonate is excreted unchanged through the kidneys within 24 hours.

3195. Which of the following is not a side effect of lithium therapy?
Harrison's 20th Ed. Chapter 444, Page 3272

- A. Weight loss
- B. Alopecia
- C. Antithyroid effect
- D. Polyuria

Side effects of lithium include gastrointestinal discomfort, nausea, diarrhea, polyuria, weight gain, skin eruptions, alopecia, edema, and antithyroid effect.

3196. In bipolar disorders, which of the following is effective in the depressed phase?
Harrison's 20th Ed. Chapter 444, Page 3272

A. Lithium carbonate
B. Sodium valproate
C. Olanzapine
D. Lamotrigine

Lithium carbonate is the mainstay of treatment in bipolar disorder. Sodium valproate & olanzapine are equally effective in acute mania, as is lamotrigine in the depressed phase.

3197. Therapeutic blood levels of lithium in the treatment of acute mania is?
Harrison's 20th Ed. Chapter 444, Page 3272

A. 0.4–0.8 mEq/L
B. 0.8–1.2 mEq/L
C. 1.4–2.2 mEq/L
D. 2.5–3.2 mEq/L

In the treatment of acute mania, lithium is initiated at 300 mg bid or tid. Dose is titrated every 2–3 days to achieve blood levels of 0.8–1.2 mEq/L.

3198. Therapeutic blood levels of valproic acid is?
Harrison's 20th Ed. Chapter 444, Page 3272 Table 444-9

A. 50–125 µg/mL
B. 100–225 µg/mL
C. 200–350 µg/mL
D. 380–525 µg/mL

3199. Therapeutic blood levels of carbamazepine is?
Harrison's 20th Ed. Chapter 444, Page 3272 Table 444-9

A. 1–4 µg/mL
B. 4–12 µg/mL
C. 12–22 µg/mL
D. 25–42 µg/mL

3200. Stevens-Johnson syndrome can occur with all except?
Harrison's 20th Ed. Chapter 444, Page 3272 Table 444-9

A. Lithium
B. Valproic acid
C. Carbamazepine
D. Lamotrigine

3201. Which of the following drugs is appropriate for patients who experience rapid cycling?
Harrison's 20th Ed. Chapter 444, Page 3272

A. Lithium carbonate
B. Sodium valproate
C. Olanzapine
D. Lamotrigine

Valproic acid is better for patients who experience rapid cycling (> 4 episodes a year) or who present with a mixed or dysphoric mania.

3202. Blood level of lithium is increased by all except?
Harrison's 20th Ed. Chapter 444, Page 3272 Table 444-9

A. Thiazides
B. Verapamil
C. Tetracyclines
D. NSAIDs

Blood level of lithium is increased by thiazides, tetracyclines, and NSAIDs, decreased by bronchodilators, verapamil, and carbonic anhydrase inhibitors.

3203. Which of the following is effective in bipolar disorder?
Harrison's 20th Ed. Chapter 444, Page 3272

A. Social rhythm therapy
B. ECT
C. Light therapy
D. All of the above

3204. In somatization disorder, which of the following is true to fulfill the diagnostic criteria?
Harrison's 20th Ed. Chapter 444, Page 3273

A. 2 pain, 2 GI, 2 sexual, & 2 pseudoneurologic symptom
B. 3 pain, 2 GI, 2 sexual, & 1 pseudoneurologic symptom
C. 3 pain, 2 GI, 1 sexual, & 2 pseudoneurologic symptom
D. 4 pain, 2 GI, 1 sexual, & 1 pseudoneurologic symptom

Formal diagnostic criteria for somatization disorder requires the recording of at least four pain, two gastrointestinal, one sexual, and one pseudoneurologic symptom.

3205. Munchausen's syndrome best relates to?
Harrison's 20th Ed. Chapter 444, Page 3273

A. Factitious disorder
B. Hypochondriasis
C. Conversion disorder
D. Feeding & eating disorder

Munchausen's syndrome is characterized by dramatic, chronic, or severe factitious illness.

3206. In conversion disorder, deficit symptoms involve?
Harrison's 20th Ed. Chapter 444, Page 3273

A. Motor
B. Sensory
C. Psychological
D. All of the above

In conversion disorder, deficit symptoms are not intentionally produced or simulated and involve motor or sensory function & psychological factors that initiate or exacerbate medical presentation.

3207. Which of the following best relates to hypochondriasis?
Harrison's 20th Ed. Chapter 444, Page 3273

A. Voluntarily produced physical symptoms of illness
B. Belief of serious medical illness
C. Intentionally produced deficit symptoms
D. Simulated deficit symptoms

In factitious disorder (malingering), patient consciously & voluntarily produces physical symptoms of illness. Essential feature in hypochondriasis is a belief of serious medical illness that persists despite reassurance & appropriate medical evaluation.

3208. Which of the following is required for the diagnosis of borderline personality disorder?
N Engl J Med. 2011;364:2037-42

A. Interpersonal hypersensitivity
B. Impulsivity
C. Affective dysregulation
D. All of the above

3209. Most distinctive characteristic of patients with BPD is?
N Engl J Med. 2011;364:2037-42

- A. Excessive involvement in pleasurable activities
- B. Decreased need for sleep
- C. Hypersensitivity to rejection
- D. Inflated self-esteem or grandiosity

Most distinctive characteristics of patients with BPD are their hypersensitivity to rejection and their fearful preoccupation with expected abandonment.

3210. Which of the following has the highest mortality among psychiatric conditions?
Harrison's 20th Ed. Chapter 444, Page 3274

- A. Anorexia nervosa
- B. Schizophrenia
- C. Bipolar disorders
- D. Posttraumatic stress disorder

Untreated anorexia nervosa has a mortality of 5.1/1000 which is highest among psychiatric conditions.

3211. Which of the following is false about anorexia nervosa?
Harrison's 20th Ed. Chapter 444, Page 3274

- A. Extreme weight loss
- B. Behavior of dieting/food restriction (self-starvation)
- C. Excessive exercise (obsession with having a thin body)
- D. None of the above

Anorexia nervosa (AN) is a highly distinctive disorder at the brain-body interface. A defining characteristic of anorexia nervosa is that the individual denial of the problem and ambivalence to take treatment.

3212. Which of the following is seen in blood picture of a patient of anorexia nervosa?
Harrison's 20th Ed. Chapter 444, Page 3274

- A. Leukopenia with lymphocytosis
- B. Elevated blood urea nitrogen
- C. Metabolic alkalosis and hypokalemia
- D. All of the above

3213. Endocrine disturbances seen in anorexia nervosa include?
Harrison's 20th Ed. Chapter 444, Page 3274

- A. Hypogonadism
- B. Growth hormone resistance
- C. Hypercortisolemia
- D. All of the above

3214. ARFID refers to?
N Engl J Med. 2017;376:2377-86

- A. Appetite restrictive food intake disorder
- B. Anxiety restrictive food intake disorder
- C. Avoidant restrictive food intake disorder
- D. Acute restrictive food intake disorder

ARFID is defined by the presence of avoidant or restrictive eating that results in persistent failure to meet nutritional needs.

3215. Purging in a patient of anorexia nervosa is suggested by?
N Engl J Med. 2005;353:1481-8

- A. Enlargement of the salivary glands (chubby cheeks)
- B. Eroded dental enamel
- C. Scars on dorsum of hands from repeated, induced vomiting
- D. All of the above

Anorexia nervosa occurs in two types: food restricting, and binge eating and purging.

3216. Which of the following treatment plan has proved to be effective in anorexia nervosa?
Harrison's 20th Ed. Chapter 444, Page 3274

- A. CAT
- B. CBT-E
- C. MANTRA
- D. SSCM

In 2017, the National Institute for Health and Care Excellence (NICE) has recommended Maudsley Anorexia Nervosa Treatment for Adults (MANTRA) as a first line treatment for adults with anorexia nervosa.

3217. Psychiatric conditions that coexist with anorexia nervosa include?
Harrison's 20th Ed. Chapter 444, Page 3274

- A. Major depression or dysthymia
- B. Anxiety disorders
- C. Obsessive - compulsive disorder
- D. All of the above

3218. Transition from bulimia nervosa to anorexia occurs in what percentage of cases?
Harrison's 20th Ed. Chapter 444, Page 3274

- A. 2–5%
- B. 10–15%
- C. 20–30%
- D. 30–50%

3219. Which of the following is not a feature of personality disorders?
Harrison's 20th Ed. Chapter 444, Page 3274

- A. Characteristic patterns of thinking & feeling
- B. Relative flexibility
- C. Significant functional impairment
- D. Subjective distress

Personality disorders are characteristic patterns of thinking, feeling & interpersonal behavior that are relatively inflexible & cause significant functional impairment or subjective distress.

3220. Obsessive-compulsive personality types is grouped in which personality cluster disorder?
Harrison's 20th Ed. Chapter 444, Page 3274

- A. Cluster A
- B. Cluster B
- C. Cluster C
- D. Any of the above

3221. Paranoid personality type is grouped in which personality cluster disorder?
Harrison's 20th Ed. Chapter 444, Page 3274

- A. Cluster A
- B. Cluster B
- C. Cluster C
- D. Any of the above

3222. Antisocial personality type is grouped in which personality cluster disorder?

Harrison's 20th Ed. Chapter 444, Page 3274

A. Cluster A
B. Cluster B
C. Cluster C
D. Any of the above

Personality disorders are grouped into 3 overlapping clusters. Cluster A includes paranoid (unjustified pervasive mistrust & suspiciousness), schizoid, and schizotypal personality disorders. Cluster B disorders include antisocial, borderline, histrionic & narcissistic types (impulsive behavior, excessively emotional, erratic). Cluster C includes avoidant, dependent & obsessive-compulsive personality types.

3223. In Mini Mental Status Examination, scoring is done out of?

Harrison's 20th Ed. Chapter 25, Page 155

A. 20
B. 30
C. 40
D. 50

3224. Depressive episodes that occur in conjunction with manic episodes are called?

N Engl J Med. 2005;353:1819-34

A. Anxiety disorders
B. Schizophrenic disorders
C. Bipolar disorders
D. Major depressive disorders

3225. "Dysthymia" is the term used for?

N Engl J Med. 2005;353:1819-34

A. Persistent, residual depressive symptoms
B. Generalized weakness
C. Absence of sweating
D. Difficulty in swallowing

3226. As regards risk of problems in depressed patients, which of the following statements is true?

N Engl J Med. 2005;353:1819-34

A. Suicide
B. Heart disease
C. Stroke
D. All of the above

3227. Which of the following about depression is false?

N Engl J Med. 2005;353:1819-34

A. Elevated cortisol levels
B. Higher levels of N-acetyl aspartate
C. Deficiencies of serotonin, norepinephrine, dopamine & GABA
D. Overactivity of acetylcholine, corticotropin-releasing factor, and substance P

3228. Disordered neurocircuitry in depression is observed in which of the following structures?

N Engl J Med. 2005;353:1819-34

A. Anterior and posterior cingulate cortex
B. Ventral, medial, and dorsolateral prefrontal cortex
C. Insula
D. All of the above

3229. Disordered neurocircuitry in depression is observed in which of the following structures?

N Engl J Med. 2005;353:1819-34

A. Ventral striatum
B. Hippocampus
C. Medial thalamus
D. All of the above

3230. Tricyclic antidepressants have greater efficacy than SSRIs in?

N Engl J Med. 2005;353:1819-34

A. Severe major depressive disorder
B. Depression with melancholic features
C. Depression in which physical symptoms or pain are prominent
D. All of the above

3231. Which of the following drugs has no direct action on the serotonin system?

N Engl J Med. 2005;353:1819-34

A. Bupropion
B. Venlafaxine
C. Duloxetine
D. Milnacipran

3232. Monoamine oxidase (MAO) is the enzyme involved in?

N Engl J Med. 2005;353:1819-34

A. Norepinephrine breakdown
B. Epinephrine breakdown
C. Dopamine breakdown
D. All of the above

3233. Mirtazapine blocks?

N Engl J Med. 2005;353:1819-34

A. Alpha2-adrenergic autoreceptors
B. Serotonin 5-HT2A and 5-HT3 receptors
C. Histamine H1 receptors
D. All of the above

Mirtazapine is a TCA. It increases noradrenergic & serotonergic neurotransmission through a blockade of central α2-adrenergic receptors and postsynaptic 5HT2 and 5HT3 receptors. It is also strongly antihistaminic and may produce sedation.

3234. Which of the following are classified as mood stabilizers?

N Engl J Med. 2005;353:1819-34

A. Lithium
B. Lamotrigine
C. Divalproex
D. All of the above

Mood Stabilizers include lithium, valproic acid, carbamazepine/oxcarbazepine & lamotrigine.

3235. ECT can be a first-line treatment for patients who have?
N Engl J Med. 2005;353:1819-34

- A. Severe major depressive disorder with psychotic features
- B. Psychomotor retardation
- C. Medication resistance
- D. All of the above

3236. Akinetic mutism can be caused by?
Harrison's 20th Ed. Chapter 300, Page 2069

- A. Damage of the medial thalamic nuclei
- B. Damage of the frontal lobes
- C. Hydrocephalus
- D. All of the above

3237. Milder form of akinetic mutism is called?
Harrison's 20th Ed. Chapter 300, Page 2069

- A. Agnosia
- B. Abulia
- C. Akathesia
- D. None of the above

Abulia describes a milder form of akinetic mutism characterized by mental & physical slowness & diminished ability to initiate activity, usually the result of damage to frontal lobes & its connections.

3238. Hypomobile and mute syndrome associated with a major psychosis is?
Harrison's 20th Ed. Chapter 300, Page 2069

- A. Catatonia
- B. Abulia
- C. Agnosia
- D. Akathesia

Catatonia is a hypomobile & mute syndrome that occurs as part of a major psychosis, usually schizophrenia or major depression.

3239. Beclouded dementia refers to?
Dement Geriatr Cogn Disord. 1999;10:310-314

- A. Acute medical problem, or a poorly tolerated medication supervenes in a mildly demented patient
- B. Transient confusion & drowsiness with febrile infection
- C. Awake but unresponsive state
- D. Awake but cannot produce speech

3240. MASA syndrome includes all except?
European Journal of Human Genetics. 1995;3(5):273-84

- A. Mental retardation
- B. Aphasia
- C. Syncope
- D. Adducted thumbs

MASA syndrome (Mental retardation, Aphasia, Spastic paraplegia, Adducted thumbs) is a historical term used to describe a phenotype now considered to be part of the X-linked L1 clinical spectrum (L1 syndrome), CRASH syndrome or Gareis-Mason syndrome.

3241. Asperger's syndrome best relates to?
Reviews in Neurological Diseases. 2006;3(1):1-7

- A. Autism spectrum disorders (ASD)
- B. Schizophrenia
- C. Mood disorders
- D. Substance use disorders

Individuals with autism-like symptoms (delays or abnormal functioning in social interactions, language as used in social communication, and symbolic or imaginative play, with onset prior to age 3) with relatively preserved cognitive functioning and language skills have Asperger's syndrome.

Schizophrenia

3242. Out of the following, who performed original research in schizophrenia?

A. Maurer D
B. Sachs GS
C. Kraepelin E
D. Kohn R

Dementia praecox, a term used by Emil Kraepelin, was replaced by Eugen Bleuler who called those closely related diseases characterized not by deterioration of intellect but by splitting of cognitive sides of personality from the affective or emotional sides by the name of schizophrenia. Kraepelin and Bleuler were the first to suggest that schizophrenia is an organic brain disease with significant cognitive deficits.

3243. Schizophrenia presents typically in?
Harrison's 20th Ed. Chapter 444, Page 3275

A. Early childhood
B. Late adolescence
C. Middle age
D. Old age

Schizophrenia presents typically in late adolescence and early adulthood as a lifelong phenomenon.

3244. Which of the following is a pathognomonic feature of schizophrenia?
Harrison's 20th Ed. Chapter 444, Page 3275

A. Perturbations of language
B. Perturbations of perception
C. Perturbations of thinking
D. None of the above

There are no pathognomonic features of schizophrenia.

3245. Major symptom cluster seen in schizophrenia is?
Harrison's 20th Ed. Chapter 444, Page 3275

A. Positive
B. Negative
C. Cognitive
D. All of the above

Three major symptom clusters seen in schizophrenia are positive (conceptual disorganization, hallucinations & delusions), negative (loss of function, anhedonia, decreased emotional expression, impaired concentration, and diminished social engagement), and cognitive symptoms (disabling deficits in working memory & cognitive control of behavior). Delusions & hallucinations of schizophrenia are more complex, bizarre, and threatening than those of dementia.

3246. Which of the following is false about the negative symptoms of schizophrenia?
Harrison's 20th Ed. Chapter 444, Page 3275

A. Carry a poor long-term outcome
B. Respond inadequately to drug treatment
C. Predominate in one-third of the schizophrenic population
D. None of the above

Negative symptoms carry a poor long-term outcome and a respond inadequately to drug treatment. Negative symptoms develop prior to positive symptoms.

3247. Patients with symptoms of schizophrenia and independent periods of mood disturbance are called?
Harrison's 20th Ed. Chapter 444, Page 3275

A. Schizoaffective disorder
B. Schizophreniform disorder
C. Schizocognitive disorder
D. Schizopolar disorder

Patients with symptoms of schizophrenia and independent periods of mood disturbance are termed to have schizoaffective disorder. Schizophreniform disorder describes patients who meet the symptom requirements but not the duration requirements for schizophrenia. Schizotypal and schizoid personality disorders refers to individuals who show a lifetime pattern of social & interpersonal deficits (inability to form close interpersonal relationships, eccentric behavior, and mild perceptual distortions).

3248. What percentage of schizophrenic patients commit suicide?
Harrison's 20th Ed. Chapter 444, Page 3275

A. 10%
B. 20%
C. 30%
D. 40%

About 10% of schizophrenic patients commit suicide.

3249. Worldwide lifetime prevalence of schizophrenia is?
Harrison's 20th Ed. Chapter 444, Page 3275

A. 1.5%
B. 3.8%
C. 5.2%
D. 7.6%

Schizophrenia is a sporadic or familial mental disorder of yet unknown etiology. It occurs in all ethnic populations with a worldwide lifetime prevalence of ~1–1.5%. Schizophrenia affects males & females roughly equally.

3250. Which of the following about schizophrenia is false?
Harrison's 20th Ed. Chapter 444, Page 3275, 3114

A. Equal prevalence rates in men & women
B. Peak age of onset is in III decade of life
C. Rate of completed suicide is about 10%
D. None of the above

Schizophrenia & bipolar disorders are equally frequent in both men and women. There may be sex differences in symptoms though. Schizophrenia has an earlier age of onset (II & III decades) and is associated with intact memory.

3251. Which of the following neurologic findings may be seen in untreated patients of schizophrenia?
Harrison's 20th Ed. Chapter 444, Page 3275

A. Motor rigidity
B. Tremor
C. Dyskinesias
D. All of the above

Neurologic examination in patients with schizophrenia is usually normal, but motor rigidity, tremor, and dyskinesias are noted in one-quarter of untreated patients of schizophrenia.

3252. Which out of the following prescription medications is frequently associated with symptoms of schizophrenia?
Harrison's 20th Ed. Chapter 444, Page 3275

A. Clonidine
B. Lorazepam
C. Tizanidine
D. Reserpine

Most common prescription medications associated with symptoms of schizophrenia are clonidine, quinacrine, and procaine derivatives.

3253. Risk factors for schizophrenia include all except?
Harrison's 20th Ed. Chapter 444, Page 3275

A. Summer birth
B. Increasing paternal age
C. Prenatal nutritional deficiency
D. Intrauterine exposure to viral infection.

Risk factors for schizophrenia include urban birth, winter birth, migration, increasing paternal age, fetal hypoxia, maternal-fetal Rhesus blood-group incompatibility, pronatal nutritional deficiency & intrauterine exposure to viral infection.

3254. Among monozygotic twins, the incidence of schizophrenia is?
Harrison's 20th Ed. Chapter 444, Page 3275

A. ~ 25%
B. ~ 50%
C. ~ 75%
D. ~ 100%

Among twins, the incidence of schizophrenia is ~10% in dizygotic twins of affected individuals, and ~50% in monozygotic twins.

3255. If both parents are affected with schizophrenia, the risk for offspring is?
Harrison's 20th Ed. Chapter 444, Page 3275

A. 20%
B. 40%
C. 60%
D. 80%

If both parents are affected with schizophrenia, the risk for offspring is 40%.

3256. Alleles of which of the following genes is associated with both ASDs and schizophrenia?
Harrison's 20th Ed. Chapter 443, Page 3257

A. MeCP2
B. NRXN1
C. TSC 1 & 2
D. FMR1

Mutations in MeCP2, FMR1 and TSC1&2 can cause mental retardation without autism spectrum disorders (ASDs), and alleles of NRXN1 is associated with both ASDs and schizophrenia. Polymorphisms in CACNA1C are strongly associated with both schizophrenia & bipolar disorder.

3257. Which of the following is with both schizophrenia?
Harrison's 20th Ed. Chapter 443, Page 3257

A. Alleles of NRXN1
B. Common polymorphisms in CACNA1C
C. Duplication of chromosome 16p
D. All of the above

3258. In schizophrenia, reduction of cortical & subcortical gray matter is seen in?
Harrison's 20th Ed. Chapter 443, Page 3260

A. Frontal lobe
B. Temporal lobe
C. Limbic system
D. All of the above

In schizophrenia, reduction of cortical & subcortical gray matter is seen in frontal and temporal lobes and in the limbic system.

3259. The best-established neuropathologic finding in schizophrenia is?
Harrison's 20th Ed. Chapter 443, Page 3260

A. Cerebral hemisphere asymmetry
B. Reduced number of gyri & sulci
C. Enlargement of lateral ventricles
D. Increase in cortical thickness

The best-established neuropathologic finding in schizophrenia is enlargement of the lateral ventricles of the cerebral hemispheres accompanied by a reduction in cortical thickness.

3260. Which of the following is a neuropathological finding in brain of schizophrenia patients?
Harrison's 20th Ed. Chapter 443, Page 3260

A. No change in neuronal cell number
B. Increased cell packing density & reduced neuropil
C. Reduction in cortical thickness
D. All of the above

In schizophrenia, reduction in cortical thickness is associated with increased cell packing density & reduced neuropil (axons, dendrites, and glial cell processes) with no reduction in neuronal cell number.

3261. Current antipsychotic drugs are efficacious for which symptom cluster seen in schizophrenia?
Harrison's 20th Ed. Chapter 444, Page 3275

A. Positive
B. Negative
C. Cognitive
D. All of the above

Positive symptoms cluster seen in schizophrenia responds to current antipsychotic drugs that generally lack efficacy for negative and cognitive symptoms.

3262. Which of the following is not a typical feature of schizophrenia?
Harrison's 20th Ed. Chapter 444, Page 3275

A. Bizzare psychosis
B. Frequent mood disturbances
C. Hypervigilance
D. Altered short term memory

Features that preclude the diagnosis of schizophrenia are significant mood symptoms, any relevant medical disease, temporal-lobe epilepsy, evidence of substance abuse and drug reaction. Delusions & hallucinations of schizophrenia are more complex & bizarre than those of dementia.

3263. Anhedonia refers to?
Harrison's 20th Ed. Chapter 65, Page 441

A. Depressed mood
B. Loss of reality
C. Loss of interest in pleasure
D. Loss of self-esteem

Anhedonia refers to loss of interest in pleasure or decreased ability to experience pleasure.

3264. Which of the following diseases can begin with schizophrenia-like features?
Harrison's 20th Ed. Chapter 423, Page 3114

A. Frontotemporal dementia
B. Huntington's disease
C. Alzheimer's disease
D. All of the above

FTD, HD, vascular dementia, Dementia with Lewy bodies (DLB), AD, or leukoencephalopathy can begin with schizophrenia-like features.

3265. Which of the following is not a schizophrenia subtype?
N Engl J Med. 2003;349:1738-49

A. Catatonic
B. Atonic
C. Paranoid
D. Residual

Four subtypes of schizophrenia are catatonic, paranoid, disorganized, and residual.

3266. In which of the following subtypes of schizophrenia, negative symptomatology exists in the absence of delusions, hallucinations, or motor disturbance?
N Engl J Med. 2003;349:1738-49

A. Catatonic
B. Disorganized
C. Paranoid
D. Residual

In residual-type subtype of schizophrenia, negative symptomatology exists in the absence of delusions, hallucinations, or motor disturbance.

3267. Echolalia or echopraxia is a feature of which of the following subtypes of schizophrenia?
N Engl J Med. 2003;349:1738-49

A. Catatonic
B. Disorganized
C. Paranoid
D. Residual

Catatonic subtype patients have profound changes in motor activity, negativism & echolalia or echopraxia.

3268. Which of the following is related to schizophrenia?
N Engl J Med. 2003;349:1738-49

A. Split personality
B. Multiple-personality
C. 'Functional' psychosis
D. None of the above

3269. Which of the following term was used to address schizophrenia in past?
N Engl J Med. 2003;349:1738-49

A. Frontotemporal dementia
B. Dementia with Lewy bodies
C. Dementia praecox
D. Conversion reaction

3270. Mostly, people do not get schizophrenia after the age of?
N Engl J Med. 2003;349:1738-49

A. 15 years
B. 25 years
C. 35 years
D. 45 years

Mostly, people do not get schizophrenia after the age of 45 years.

3271. Area of the brain that are predominantly and consistently affected in schizophrenia is?
N Engl J Med. 2003;349:1738-49

A. Amygdala
B. Anterior & medial nuclei of thalamus
C. Dorsolateral prefrontal cortex (DLPFC)
D. All of the above

3272. Which of the following cortical layers is thinner than normal in schizophrenia?
N Engl J Med. 2003;349:1738-49

A. I
B. II
C. IV
D. V

Cortical layers II and III are thinner than normal in schizophrenia.

3273. Which of the following is not a structural abnormality in brain of schizophrenia individuals?
N Engl J Med. 2003;349:1738-49

A. Ventricular enlargement
B. Absence of glial proliferation
C. Reduction in neuropil
D. Decreased volume of Nucleus accumbens

3274. Which of the following recreational drugs can mimic symptoms of schizophrenia in healthy individuals?
N Engl J Med. 2003;349:1738-49

A. Amphetamine
B. Phencyclidine (PCP)
C. Lysergic acid diethylamide (LSD)
D. All of the above

3275. Which of the following is related to the increased occurrence of schizophrenia?
N Engl J Med. 2003;349:1738-49

A. Tsunami
B. Plague epidemic
C. Nuclear holocaust in Japan
D. Dutch hunger winter

During severe famine, pregnant mothers tend to deliver children who have an increased incidence of schizophrenia later in their life. This observation stems from the experiences of the "Dutch hunger winter" during 1944 – 1945.

3276. The most prevalent excitatory transmitter in brain is?
N Engl J Med. 2003;349:1738-49

A. GABA
B. Glutamate
C. Serotonin
D. Dopamine

Most prevalent transmitter in the human brain is glutamate. It is mostly excitatory at synapses.

3277. Most prevalent inhibitory transmitter in brain is?
N Engl J Med. 2003;349:1738-49

A. GABA
B. Glutamate
C. Serotonin
D. Dopamine

Neurotransmitter is γ-amino-butyric acid (GABA) is mostly inhibitory at the synapses.

3278. Serotonergic neurons in the CNS are found primarily in?
N Engl J Med. 2003;349:1738-49

A. Midline raphe nuclei
B. Locus coeruleus
C. Striatum
D. Thalamus

Serotonergic neurons in the CNS are found primarily in the midline raphe nuclei, located in the brain stem from the midbrain to the medulla.

3279. Principal site for synthesis of norepinephrine in human brain is?
N Engl J Med. 2003;349:1738-49

A. Midline raphe nuclei
B. Locus coeruleus
C. Striatum
D. Thalamus

Locus coeruleus is the principal site for synthesis of norepinephrine (NE) that has an excitatory effect on most of the brain.

3280. Which of the following is a dopamine pathway in the brain?
N Engl J Med. 2003;349:1738-49

A. Mesolimbic
B. Mesocortical
C. Nigrostriatal
D. All of the above

Dopamine pathways in the brain are mesolimbic, mesocortical, nigrostriatal & tuberoinfundibular.

3281. Dopaminergic fibers in brain arise in which of the following?
N Engl J Med. 2003;349:1738-49

A. Amygdala
B. Hippocampus
C. Ventral tegmental area (VTA)
D. Nucleus accumbens

Dopaminergic fibers in brian arise in the ventral tegmental area (VTA).

3282. Which of the following dopamine receptor subtype is excitatory?
N Engl J Med. 2003;349:1738-49

A. D1
B. D2
C. D3
D. D4

Dopamine receptor subtypes D1 and D5 are excitatory while D2, D3 and D4 are inhibitory.

3283. Which of the following dopamine receptor subtype is most abundant in nucleus accumbens?
N Engl J Med. 2003;349:1738-49

A. D1
B. D2
C. D3
D. D4

D3 receptors are mainly present in nucleus accumbens while D4 receptors express themselves in frontal cortex. D1 receptors tend to be distributed in cortical regions, while D2 are subcortical.

3284. Schizophrenia is characterized by?
N Engl J Med. 2003;349:1738-49

A. Hypodopaminergia in mesocortical neurons
B. Hyperdopaminergia in mesocortical neurons
C. Hypodopaminergia in mesolimbic neurons
D. None of the above

Schizophrenia is characterized by hypodopaminergia in mesocortical neurons and hyperdopaminergia in mesolimbic neurons.

3285. Which of the following is an ionotropic glutamate receptor?
N Engl J Med. 2003;349:1738-49

A. AMPA
B. Kainate
C. NMDA
D. All of the above

Ionotropic glutamate receptors (iGluRs) are AMPA (a-amino-3-hydroxy-5-methyl-4-isoxazole propionic acid), kainate, and NMDA.

3286. AMPA-receptor subunits are derived from which of the following genes?
N Engl J Med. 2003;349:1738-49

A. GluR4
B. GluR5
C. GluR6
D. GluR7

AMPA-receptor subunits are derived from GluR1, GluR2, GluR3 and GluR4 genes. Kainate receptors are derived from GluR5, GluR6, GluR7 and KA1, KA2 genes. NMDA receptor subunits are encoded by NR1, NR2A, NR2B, NR2C, NR2D genes.

3287. Glycine co-agonist essential for glutamatergic transmission is?
N Engl J Med. 2003;349:1738-49

A. Tyrosine
B. Serenine
C. Melanin
D. D-serine

3288. Serotonin is produced from?
N Engl J Med. 2003;349:1738-49

A. Arginine
B. L-tryptophan
C. Histidine
D. Leucine

Serotonin is produced by decarboxylation & hydroxylation of L-tryptophan.

3289. Which of the following hallucinogen is a 5-HT agonist?
N Engl J Med. 2003;349:1738-49

A. Amphetamine
B. LSD (lysergic acid diethylamide)
C. Ketamine
D. All of the above

Hallucinogen LSD (lysergic acid diethylamide) is a 5-HT agonist.

3290. GABA is synthesized from?
N Engl J Med. 2003;349:1738-49

A. Glutamic acid
B. Butyric acid
C. Sialic acid
D. Glycine

GABA is synthesized from glutamic acid by removal of alpha-carboxl group from glutamate by the action of glutamic acid decarboxylase (GAD).

3291. Which of the following scales is used for severity of clinical symptoms of schizophrenia?
N Engl J Med. 2003;349:1738-49

A. ESRS
B. BAS
C. PANSS
D. LNS

Positive and Negative Syndrome Scale (PANSS) is used for severity of clinical symptoms of schizophrenia. Brown–Peterson procedure and the Letter-Number Sequencing (LNS) task are measures of verbal working memory. Extrapyramidal Symptom Rating Scale (ESRS) and the Barnes Akathisia Scale (BAS) are used to assess movement disorders that occur with antipsychotic medication of schizophrenia.

3292. Reduction in volume of which of the following correlate with positive symptoms of schizophrenia?
N Engl J Med. 2003;349:1738-49

A. Medial temporal lobes (MTL)
B. Superior temporal gyrus (STG)
C. Hippocampus
D. Amygdala

Reduction in volume of superior temporal gyrus correlate with positive symptoms of schizophrenia while MTL reductions correlate with memory impairment.

3293. Term neuroleptic in Greek means?
N Engl J Med. 2003;349:1738-49

A. To straighten the neuron
B. To clasp the neuron
C. To thin the neuron
D. To energise the neuron

Term neuroleptic in Greek means "to clasp the neuron".

3294. Which of the following is not a typical antipsychotic drug?
Harrison's 20th Ed. Chapter 444, Page 3276 Table 444-10

A. Haloperidol
B. Risperidone
C. Chlorpromazine
D. Thiothixene

3295. Which of the following is not an atypical antipsychotic drug?
Harrison's 20th Ed. Chapter 444, Page 3276 Table 444-10

A. Ziprasidone
B. Perphenazine
C. Asenapine
D. Aripiprazole

First-generation or "typical" antipsychotic agents include Chlorpromazine, Perphenazine, Trifluoperazine, Thiothixene and Haloperidol. Second-generation or "atypical" antipsychotic agents are Clozapine, Risperidone, Olanzapine, Quetiapine, Ziprasidone, Aripiprazole and Amisulpride. Intramuscular depot preparations available are Fluphenazine decanoate, Haloperidol decanoate, Flupentixol decanoate and Risperidone microspheres.

3296. Agranulocytosis is a side effect of which of the following antipsychotic drug?
Harrison's 20th Ed. Chapter 444, Page 3276 Table 444-10

A. Olanzapine
B. Clozapine
C. Quetiapine
D. Chlorpromazine

3297. In UK, Clozaril Patient Monitoring Services (CPMS) monitors patient's?
N Engl J Med. 2003;349:1738-49

A. Hematological profile
B. Weight gain
C. Lenticular opacities
D. Myocarditis

In UK, it is mandatory for all patients receiving Clozapine to register with Clozaril Patient Monitoring Services (CPMS) that monitors patient's hematological profile.

3298. Which of the following antipsychotic drug is unlikely to increase prolactin levels?
Harrison's 20th Ed. Chapter 444, Page 3276

A. Aripiprazole
B. Clozapine
C. Ziprasidone
D. None of the above

3299. In schizophrenia, if antipsychotic medications are completely discontinued, the relapse rate is?
Harrison's 20th Ed. Chapter 444, Page 3276

A. 1% per month
B. 5% per month
C. 10% per month
D. 20% per month

If antipsychotic medications are completely discontinued in schizophrenia, the relapse rate is 60% within 6 months or 10% per month, until eventually almost all patients undergo relapse.

3300. Use of which of the following is least likely to cause hyperglycemia, weight gain, and hypertriglyceridemia?
Harrison's 20th Ed. Chapter 444, Page 3276

A. Clozapine
B. Ziprasidone
C. Olanzapine
D. Quetiapine

Clozapine, olanzapine & quetiapine cause hyperglycemia, weight gain & hypertriglyceridemia more than Ziprasidone.

3301. Which of the following may reduce tardive dyskinesia with the use of antipsychotic agents if given early in the syndrome?
Harrison's 20th Ed. Chapter 444, Page 3276

A. Vitamin E
B. Vitamin B12
C. Zinc
D. Calcium

Vitamin E may reduce abnormal involuntary movements with the use of antipsychotic agents, if given early in the syndrome.

3302. Which of the following is most commonly involved in tardive dyskinesia (TD)?
Harrison's 20th Ed. Chapter 444, Page 3276

A. Tongue
B. Trunk
C. Limbs
D. Respiratory muscles

TD comprises of choreiform movements involving mouth, lips & tongue. In severe cases trunk, limbs & respiratory muscles may be affected.

3303. Sleep disturbance in chronic schizophrenia includes?
Harrison's 20th Ed. Chapter 444, Page 3276

A. Day-night reversal
B. Sleep fragmentation
C. Insomnia
D. All of the above

3304. Which of the following anti-malarials should not be prescribed to patients of schizophrenia?
Harrison's 20th Ed. Chapter 444, Page 3276

A. Quinine
B. Lumefantrine
C. Mefloquine
D. Primaquine

Mefloquine should not be prescribed to patients with depression, generalized anxiety disorder, psychosis, schizophrenia, and seizure disorder.

3305. Dysthymia best relates to?
Harrison's 20th Ed. Chapter 444, Page 3276

A. Depressive disorder
B. Bipolar disorder
C. Seizure disorder
D. Schizophrenia

Mood disorders can be either depressive or bipolar disorders. Depressive disorders include the major & minor depressive disorders and dysthymia

3306. Neurovegetative symptoms best relate to?
Harrison's 20th Ed. Chapter 444, Page 3260

A. Depressive disorder
B. Bipolar disorder
C. Posttraumatic stress disorder (PTSD)
D. Schizophrenia

Symptoms of depression are referred to as neurovegetative symptoms.

3307. Deep brain stimulation (DBS) of which of the following elevates mood in normal and depressed individuals?
Harrison's 20th Ed. Chapter 444, Page 3260

A. Subgenual area 23
B. Subgenual area 24
C. Subgenual area 25
D. Subgenual area 26

Deep brain stimulation (DBS) of either nucleus accumbens or subgenual area 25 elevates mood in normal and depressed individuals.

3308. Which of the following is a broad group of psychoses?
N Engl J Med. 2018;379:270-80

A. Idiopathic psychoses
B. Psychoses due to medical conditions
C. Toxic psychoses
D. All of the above

3309. Psychosis due to SLE begins at what age?
N Engl J Med. 2018;379:270-80

A. Late second or third decade
B. Middle age
C. Senescence
D. Any age

Schizophrenia, bipolar disorder & depression with psychotic symptoms, begin in late II or III decade of life. Delusional disorders more often develop in middle age. Psychoses due to neurodegenerative diseases begin during senescence. Psychotic symptoms caused by drug abuse or prescribed medications & symptoms caused by medical disorders like SLE, seizures, or fevers can occur at any age.

3310. Diagnosis of secondary psychosis is favoured by which of the following?
N Engl J Med. 2018;379:270-80

A. Absence of a family history of psychotic disorders
B. A history of headaches, seizures, or hallucinations
C. An abrupt onset of symptoms without clear precipitants
D. All of the above

Features that suggest a secondary psychosis (toxic psychosis or psychosis due to medical conditions) rather than idiopathic type include a rapid decline in functional capacity from premorbid levels, an abrupt onset of symptoms without clear precipitants, a history of headaches, seizures, or hallucinations (visual, olfactory, or tactile) and an absence of a family history of psychotic disorders. Idiopathic psychotic disorders (schizophrenia & schizoaffective disorder, usually evolve through premorbid, prodromal, syndromal, progressive, and chronic stages.

3311. Persons with psychotic disorders are at risk for?
N Engl J Med. 2018;379:270-80

A. Suicide
B. Substance abuse
C. Committing acts of violence
D. All of the above

Persons with psychotic disorders are at risk for complications & derivative effects of psychosis like suicide attempts (lifetime prevalence, 34.5%), substance abuse (lifetime prevalence, 74%), homelessness (annual prevalence, 5%), victimization by others (prevalence over a 3-year period, 38%), and committing acts of violence.

3312. The most common genetic abnormality associated with a psychotic disorder is?
N Engl J Med. 2018;379:270-80

A. Chromosome 19q11.2 microdeletion
B. Chromosome 20q11.2 microdeletion
C. Chromosome 21q11.2 microdeletion
D. Chromosome 22q11.2 microdeletion

Chromosome 22q11.2 deletion syndrome (velocardiofacial syndrome or the DiGeorge syndrome) occurs in ~1 in 4000 live births. It is associated with cardiac, facial & limb abnormalities, and ~25% of affected patients have symptoms of schizophrenia or schizophrenia-like features that are indistinguishable from idiopathic schizophrenia.

Primary and Metastatic Tumors of the Nervous System

3313. Which is the most common primary CNS tumor?
Harrison's 20th Ed. Chapter 86, Page 643

A. Glial tumors
B. Meningiomas
C. Schwannomas
D. Pituitary adenoma

Glial tumors account for 30% of all primary brain tumors, meningiomas for 35%, vestibular schwannomas for 10%, & central nervous system (CNS) lymphomas ~2%.

3314. Brain tumors usually present with?
Harrison's 20th Ed. Chapter 86, Page 643

A. Progressive focal neurologic deficits
B. Seizure
C. Non-focal neurologic disorder
D. Any of the above

Brain tumors may present with subacute progression of a focal neurologic deficit, seizure, or nonfocal neurologic disorder like headache, dementia, personality change or gait disorder. All seizures that arise from a brain tumor will have a focal onset.

3315. Features of headache due to increased ICP include all except?
Harrison's 20th Ed. Chapter 86, Page 643

A. Frontal
B. Episodic
C. Frequency more than once a day
D. Develop rapidly, subside quickly

Headaches due to increased ICP are usually holocephalic.

3316. Which of the following is a MRI feature of malignant brain tumors?
Harrison's 20th Ed. Chapter 86, Page 643

A. Enhance with gadolinium
B. May have central areas of necrosis
C. Surrounded by edema of neighboring white matter
D. All of the above

Malignant brain tumors (primary or metastatic) typically enhance with gadolinium and may have central areas of necrosis. They are characteristically surrounded by edema of the neighboring white matter.

3317. Fluid-attenuated inversion recovery (FLAIR) MRI best appreciates which of the following?
Harrison's 20th Ed. Chapter 86, Page 643

A. Low-grade gliomas
B. Meningiomas
C. Metastatic brain tumors
D. Dural lymphoma

Low-grade gliomas usually do not enhance with gadolinium and are best appreciated on fluid-attenuated inversion recovery (FLAIR) MRIs.

3318. Which of the following is useful to diagnose a brain tumor?
Harrison's 20th Ed. Chapter 86, Page 643

A. Cerebral angiogram
B. Electroencephalogram (EEG)
C. Lumbar puncture
D. None of the above

3319. Which of the following helps in distinguishing brain tumor progression from necrotic tissue?
Harrison's 20th Ed. Chapter 86, Page 643

A. Fluid-attenuated inversion recovery (FLAIR) MRI
B. Positron emission tomography (PET)
C. MR perfusion and spectroscopy
D. All of the above

MR perfusion & spectroscopy provides information on blood flow or tissue composition. It also helps in distinguishing tumor progression from necrotic tissue as a consequence of treatment with radiation & chemotherapy.

3320. Headache as a presenting symptom is least common in?
Harrison's 20th Ed. Chapter 86, Page 644 Table 86-1

A. High-grade glioma
B. Low-grade glioma
C. Meningioma
D. Metastases

3321. Hemiparesis as a presenting symptom is most common in?
Harrison's 20th Ed. Chapter 86, Page 644 Table 86-1

A. High-grade glioma
B. Low-grade glioma
C. Meningioma
D. Metastases

3322. Impaired cognitive function as a presenting symptom is most common in?
Harrison's 20th Ed. Chapter 86, Page 644 Table 86-1

A. High-grade glioma
B. Low-grade glioma
C. Meningioma
D. Metastases

3323. Seizures as a presenting symptom is most common in?
Harrison's 20th Ed. Chapter 86, Page 644 Table 86-1

A. High-grade glioma
B. Low-grade glioma
C. Meningioma
D. Metastases

3324. Antiepileptic drug that does not induce hepatic microsomal enzyme system is?
Harrison's 20th Ed. Chapter 86, Page 644

A. Levetiracetam
B. Topiramate
C. Lacosamide
D. All of the above

Antiepileptic drugs that do not induce hepatic microsomal enzyme system include levetiracetam, topiramate, lamotrigine, valproic acid and lacosamide.

3325. Exposure to ionizing radiation is a risk factor for?
Harrison's 20th Ed. Chapter 86, Page 644

- A. Meningiomas
- B. Gliomas
- C. Schwannomas
- D. All of the above

The only established risk factor for meningiomas, gliomas and schwannomas is exposure to ionizing radiation.

3326. The established risk factor for primary CNS lymphoma is?
Harrison's 20th Ed. Chapter 86, Page 644

- A. Foods containing N-nitroso compounds
- B. Immunosuppression
- C. Exposure to electromagnetic fields (cellular telephones)
- D. Positive family history

3327. Well-documented environmental risk factor for the development of gliomas is?
Harrison's 20th Ed. Chapter 86, Page 644

- A. Benzene
- B. Cadmium
- C. Ionizing radiation
- D. Ozone

For majority of primary brain tumors, the only established risk factors are exposure to ionizing radiation (meningiomas, gliomas, and schwannomas) and immunosuppression (primary CNS lymphoma).

3328. Which of the following is associated with increased risk for deep vein thrombosis & pulmonary embolism?
Harrison's 20th Ed. Chapter 86, Page 644

- A. Leptomeningeal metastases
- B. Brain metastases
- C. Medulloblastoma
- D. All of the above

High-grade gliomas & brain metastases are associated with increased risk for DVT & PE because these tumors secrete procoagulant factors.

3329. Hereditary syndromes associated with an increased risk of brain tumors includes all except?
Harrison's 20th Ed. Chapter 86, Page 645 Table 86-2

- A. Li-Fraumeni syndrome
- B. Turcot syndrome
- C. Werner syndrome
- D. Pearson syndrome

Pearson syndrome is a mitochondrial disease consisting of pancreatic insufficiency, pancytopenia and lactic acidosis.

3330. Pheochromocytoma is associated with which of the following hereditary syndrome?
Harrison's 20th Ed. Chapter 86, Page 645 Table 86-2

- A. Li-Fraumeni syndrome
- B. Turcot syndrome
- C. Werner syndrome
- D. von Hippel-Lindau syndrome

3331. Lhermitte-Duclos disease is best related to?
Harrison's 20th Ed. Chapter 86, Page 645 Table 86-2

- A. Gardner's syndrome
- B. Gorlin syndrome
- C. Cowden's syndrome
- D. Werner's syndrome

3332. Which of the following about Foster Kennedy syndrome is false?
DeJong's The Neurologic Examination, 7th Ed. Page 141

- A. Anosmia
- B. Unilateral ipsilateral optic atrophy
- C. Contralateral papilledema
- D. None of the above

Foster Kennedy syndrome consists of anosmia accompanied by unilateral ipsilateral optic atrophy & contralateral papilledema, classically due to a large tumor involving orbitofrontal region (olfactory groove meningioma). It was first described by Sir William Gowers, later and more thoroughly by R. Foster Kennedy.

3333. Which of the following is absent in pseudo - Foster Kennedy syndrome?
DeJong's The Neurologic Examination, 7th Ed. Page 141

- A. Anosmia
- B. Unilateral ipsilateral optic atrophy
- C. Contralateral papilledema
- D. Anterior ischemic optic neuropathy

Ophthalmologic picture similar to Foster Kennedy syndrome, without anosmia, is more often due to anterior ischemic optic neuropathy, involving first one eye, leading to atrophy, then the other, leading to disc edema is termed as the pseudo - Foster Kennedy syndrome.

3334. Which of the following is false about Cogan's rule?
DeJong's The Neurologic Examination, 7th Ed. Page 210

- A. Asymmetric optokinetic nystagmus (OKN)
- B. Etiology in parietal lobe
- C. More likely to be a tumor
- D. None of the above

With asymmetric optokinetic nystagmus (OKN), the lesion is more likely to reside in the parietal lobe, and more likely to be nonvascular, that is, a tumor (Cogan's rule).

3335. Which of the following is a tumor-suppressor gene?
Harrison's 20th Ed. Chapter 86, Page 644

- A. Epidermal growth factor receptor (EGFR)
- B. Platelet-derived growth factor receptors (PDGFR)
- C. Phosphatase and tensin homolog (PTEN)
- D. All of the above

Tumor-suppressor genes include p53, cyclin-dependent kinase inhibitor 2A and 2B (CDKN2A/B) and phosphatase and tensin homolog on chromosome 10 [PTEN]). Proto-oncogenes include epidermal growth factor receptor (EGFR) and platelet-derived growth factor receptors (PDGFR).

3336. Molecular alterations in gliomas include?
Harrison's 20th Ed. Chapter 86, Page 644

- A. Isocitrate dehydrogenase (IDH) mutations & 1p/19q codeletion
- B. ATRX
- C. p53
- D. All of the above

3337. Which of the following is not a low-grade astrocytoma?
Harrison's 20th Ed. Chapter 86, Page 644

A. Astrocytoma
B. Pilocytic astrocytoma
C. Subependymal giant cell astrocytoma
D. Anaplastic astrocytoma

3338. Anaplastic astrocytoma belongs to which WHO prognostic grade of astrocytomas?
Harrison's 20th Ed. Chapter 86, Page 644

A. Grade I
B. Grade II
C. Grade III
D. Grade IV

3339. Out of the following, most common childhood brain tumor is?
Harrison's 20th Ed. Chapter 86, Page 644

A. Pilocytic astrocytoma
B. Subependymal giant cell astrocytoma
C. Pleomorphic xanthoastrocytoma
D. Glioblastoma multiforme

Pilocytic astrocytoma (spindle-shaped cells) is the most common childhood brain tumor and is typically benign. They occur typically in the cerebellum.

3340. Nervous system neoplasm seen in tuberous sclerosis is?
Harrison's 20th Ed. Chapter 86, Page 644

A. Astrocytoma
B. Schwannoma
C. Medulloblastoma
D. Hemangioblastoma

Subependymal giant cell astrocytoma mostly occurs in tuberous sclerosis.

3341. Which of the following is the preferred drug for high-grade astrocytomas?
Harrison's 20th Ed. Chapter 86, Page 645

A. Temozolomide
B. Carmustine (BCNU)
C. Lomustine (CCNU)
D. Vincristine

3342. Resistance to temozolomide best relates to?
Harrison's 20th Ed. Chapter 86, Page 645

A. Histone deacetylases (HDAC)
B. Ataxia telangiectasia mutated (ATM) gene
C. O6-methylguanine-DNA methyltransferase (MGMT)
D. Cyclic AMP response element binding (CREB) protein

Patients whose tumor contains DNA repair enzyme O6-methylguanine-DNA methyltransferase (MGMT) are relatively resistant to temozolomide and have a worse prognosis compared to those whose tumors contain low levels of MGMT as a result of silencing of the MGMT gene by promoter hypermethylation.

3343. Most important adverse prognostic factor in patients with glioblastoma is?
Harrison's 20th Ed. Chapter 86, Page 646

A. Older age
B. Absence of IDH mutations
C. Unresectable tumor
D. All of the above

Most important adverse prognostic factors in patients with glioblastomas are older age, absence of IDH mutations, unmethylated MGMT promoter, poor Karnofsky performance status, and unresectable tumor.

3344. Fried-egg appearance best relates to?
Harrison's 20th Ed. Chapter 86, Page 646

A. Ependymoma
B. Glioblastoma
C. Oligodendroglioma
D. Gliomatosis cerebri

3345. Oligodendrogliomas with deletions of which chromosome always respond to chemotherapy?
Harrison's 20th Ed. Chapter 86, Page 646

A. 1 p
B. 2 p
C. 3 p
D. 4 p

Oligodendrogliomas with deletions of chromosome 1p always respond to chemotherapy.

3346. Systemic combination chemotherapy (PCV) for oligodendrogliomas includes all except?
Harrison's 20th Ed. Chapter 86, Page 646

A. Procarbazine
B. Lomustine
C. Temozolomide
D. Vincristine

Oligodendrogliomas respond well to systemic combination chemotherapy with procarbazine, lomustine, and vincristine (PCV), or to temozolomide.

3347. In adults, ependymomas of spinal canal are mostly located in?
Harrison's 20th Ed. Chapter 86, Page 646

A. Cervical region
B. Thoracic region
C. Lumbosacral region
D. All of the above

In adults, myxopapillary histologic type is the most frequent ependymoma, which typically arises from the filum terminale of the spinal cord and appears in the lumbosacral region.

3348. Which of the following is associated with medulloblastoma?
Harrison's 20th Ed. Chapter 86, Page 645 Table 86-2

A. Gorlin syndrome
B. Turcot syndrome
C. Li-Fraumeni syndrome
D. All of the above

3349. Homer-Wright rosettes are best related to?
Harrison's 20th Ed. Chapter 86, Page 647

A. Meningioma
B. Primary central nervous system lymphoma (PCNSL)
C. Acoustic neuroma
D. Medulloblastoma

Histologically, medulloblastomas are highly cellular tumors with abundant dark staining, round nuclei, and rosette formation called Homer-Wright rosettes.

3350. Which of the following molecular subgroup of medulloblastoma has the worst outcome?
Harrison's 20th Ed. Chapter 86, Page 647

A. WNT-activated
B. SHH-activated
C. Non-WNT/non-SHH, group 3
D. Non-WNT/non-SHH, group 4

3351. Patients of medulloblastoma present with?
Harrison's 20th Ed. Chapter 86, Page 647

A. Headache
B. Ataxia
C. Signs of brainstem involvement
D. All of the above

Regardless of subtype, patients of medulloblastoma present with headache, ataxia, and signs of brainstem involvement.

3352. Meningiomas are more common in?
Harrison's 20th Ed. Chapter 86, Page 648

A. Women
B. In patients with neurofibromatosis type 2 (NF2)
C. In patients with a past history of cranial irradiation
D. All of the above

Meningiomas are the most common primary brain tumor. They are more common in women, in patients with neurofibromatosis type 2 (NF2) and in patients with a past history of cranial irradiation.

3353. Which of the following is the main in differential diagnosis of meningioma?
Harrison's 20th Ed. Chapter 86, Page 648

A. Hemangiopericytoma
B. Solitary fibrous tumors
C. Dural metastasis
D. Schwannoma

The main differential diagnosis of meningioma is a dural metastasis. Hemangiopericytomas and solitary fibrous tumors resemble meningiomas.

3354. On MRI, dural tail is seen in?
Harrison's 20th Ed. Chapter 86, Page 648

A. Meningioma
B. Dural metastases
C. Dural lymphoma
D. All of the above

3355. Neurofibromatosis type 1 (NF1) is associated with an increased incidence of schwannomas of?
Harrison's 20th Ed. Chapter 86, Page 648

A. Trigeminal nerve
B. Facial nerve
C. Eighth cranial nerve
D. Spinal nerve roots

Neurofibromatosis type 1 is associated with an increased incidence of schwannomas of spinal nerve roots.

3356. Schwannoma most frequently involves which cranial nerve?
Harrison's 20th Ed. Chapter 86, Page 648

A. II
B. III
C. V
D. VIII

3357. Cranial nerve where Schwannoma never occur is?
Harrison's 20th Ed. Chapter 86, Page 648

A. II
B. III
C. VIII
D. XI

Schwannomas are most frequent in the vestibular division of VIII cranial nerve, fifth cranial nerve is the second most frequent site. Schwannomas are not found in optic & olfactory nerves as they are myelinated by oligodendroglia rather than by Schwann cells.

3358. Radiographically, which of the following resemble lipomas?
Harrison's 20th Ed. Chapter 86, Page 649

A. Dysembryoplastic neuroepithelial tumors (DNTs)
B. Colloid cyst
C. Dermoid cyst
D. Epidermoid cyst

3359. Which of the following occurs in cerebellopontine angle?
Harrison's 20th Ed. Chapter 86, Page 649

A. Dysembryoplastic neuroepithelial tumors (DNTs)
B. Colloid cyst
C. Dermoid cyst
D. Epidermoid cyst

3360. Bruns' nystagmus best relates to?
DeJong's The Neurologic Examination, 7th Ed. Page 622

A. Occipital lobe
B. Temporal lobe
C. Cerebellopontine angle
D. Medulla oblongata

When a tumor of the cerebellopontine angle is present, nystagmus is coarse on looking toward the side of lesion and fine & rapid on gaze to the opposite side (Bruns' nystagmus).

3361. High-dose methotrexate is used in the treatment of?
Harrison's 20th Ed. Chapter 86, Page 649

A. Craniopharyngioma
B. Schwannoma
C. Primary central nervous system lymphoma
D. Oligodendroglioma

3362. NF1 gene is on chromosome?
Harrison's 20th Ed. Chapter 86, Page 649

A. 1
B. 4
C. 9
D. 17

Tumor-suppressor NF1 gene on chromosome 17. Its mutation causes von Recklinghausen's disease. It encodes protein neurofibromin. NF2 gene is on chromosome 22q, & encodes neurofibromin 2, schwannomin, or merlin (moesin, ezrin, radixin-like protein).

3363. Mutations of NF1 result in?
Harrison's 20th Ed. Chapter 86, Page 649

A. Optic nerve gliomas
B. Astrocytomas
C. Meningiomas
D. All of the above

Mutations of NF1 result in neurofibromas, plexiform neurofibromas, optic nerve gliomas, astrocytomas and meningiomas.

3364. Manifestation of NF1 (von Recklinhausen's disease) is?
Harrison's 20th Ed. Chapter 86, Page 649

A. Cafe-au-lait spots
B. Axillary freckling
C. Lisch nodules
D. All of the above

In addition to neurofibromas, which appear as multiple, soft, rubbery cutaneous tumors, other cutaneous manifestations of NF1 include cafe-au-lait spots and axillary freckling. NF1 is also associated with hamartomas of the iris termed Lisch nodules, pheochromocytomas, pseudoarthrosis of the tibia, scoliosis, epilepsy and mental retardation.

3365. Lisch nodules relate best to?
Harrison's 20th Ed. Chapter 86, Page 649

A. Ocular lens
B. Iris
C. Retina
D. Conjunctiva

Hamartomas of the iris are called Lisch nodules.

3366. NF2 is characterized by all except?
Harrison's 20th Ed. Chapter 86, Page 649

A. Bilateral vestibular schwannomas
B. Multiple meningiomas
C. Periungual fibromas
D. Astrocytomas

NF2 is characterized by bilateral vestibular schwannomas in over 90% of patients, multiple meningiomas and spinal ependymomas and astrocytomas.

3367. Bourneville's disease is also called?
Harrison's 20th Ed. Chapter 86, Page 649

A. Meningioma
B. Tuberous sclerosis
C. Ependymoma
D. Primary CNS lymphoma

Tuberous sclerosis is also called Bourneville's disease.

3368. TSC stands for?
Harrison's 20th Ed. Chapter 86, Page 649

A. Tuberous sclerosis complex
B. Tuberous sclerosis candidate
C. Tuberous sclerosis compound
D. Tuberous sclerosis combination

Tuberous sclerosis is caused by mutations in either TSC1 gene (9q34) and encodes hamartin, or TSC2 gene (16p13.3) and encodes the protein tuberin.

3369. Shagreen patches are best related to?
Harrison's 20th Ed. Chapter 86, Page 649

A. Secondary syphilis
B. Neurofibromatosis Type 1
C. Tuberous sclerosis
D. Von Hippel–Lindau syndrome

Shagreen patches are yellowish thickenings of skin over lumbosacral region of the back, seen in tuberous sclerosis.

3370. Tuberous sclerosis is characterized by all except?
Harrison's 20th Ed. Chapter 86, Page 649

A. Cutaneous lesions
B. Seizures
C. Deafness
D. Mental retardation

Tuberous sclerosis is characterized by cutaneous lesions, seizures, and mental retardation.

3371. Cutaneous lesions in tuberous sclerosis include all except?
Harrison's 20th Ed. Chapter 86, Page 345

A. Adenoma sebaceum
B. Ash leaf - shaped hypopigmented macules
C. Lentigo
D. Shagreen patches

In tuberous sclerosis, earliest cutaneous sign is an ash leaf spot. Other manifestations include adenoma sebaceum (facial angiofibromas), shagreen patch, hypomelanotic macules, periungual fibromas, renal angiomyolipomas, and cardiac rhabdomyomas. These patients have an increased incidence of subependymal nodules, cortical tubers, and subependymal giant-cell astrocytomas (SEGAs).

3372. Most effective therapy for subependymal giant-cell astrocytomas (SEGAs) is?
Harrison's 20th Ed. Chapter 86, Page 649

A. Alemtuzumab
B. Antithymocyte globulin
C. Sirolimus
D. Mycophenolate mofetil

3373. Hemangioblastomas in Von Hippel-Lindau syndrome are seen in?
Harrison's 20th Ed. Chapter 86, Page 666

A. Retina
B. Cerebellum
C. Spinal cord
D. All of the above

VHL syndrome consists of retinal, cerebellar, and spinal hemangioblastomas, which are slowly growing cystic tumors.

3374. Hemangioblastomas in Von Hippel-Lindau syndrome produce which hormone?
Harrison's 20th Ed. Chapter 86, Page 666

A. Parathyroid hormone (PTH)
B. Calcitonin
C. Erythropoietin
D. Antidiuretic hormone

Erythropoietin produced by hemangioblastomas results in polycythemia.

3375. Which of the following is the most common origin of brain metastases?
Harrison's 20th Ed. Chapter 86, Page 649

A. Ca. lung
B. Ca. ovary
C. Ca. thyroid
D. Ca. prostate

Lung cancers (primary & metastatic) are the most common origin of brain metastases.

3376. Breast cancer has a propensity to metastasize to?
Harrison's 20th Ed. Chapter 86, Page 649

A. Leptomeninges
B. Dura
C. Spinal cord
D. All of the above

3377. Breast cancer has a propensity to metastasize to?
Harrison's 20th Ed. Chapter 86, Page 649

A. Anterior pituitary gland
B. Posterior pituitary gland
C. Hypothalamus
D. Hippocampus

Breast cancer (esp. ductal carcinoma) has a propensity to metastasize to the cerebellum and the posterior pituitary gland.

3378. Which of the following cancers rarely metastasize to brain?
Harrison's 20th Ed. Chapter 86, Page 649

A. Prostate cancer
B. Ovarian cancer
C. Hodgkin's disease
D. All of the above

Prostate & ovarian cancer & Hodgkin's disease rarely metastasize to brain.

3379. Breast cancer that metastasizes to which of the following tends not to metastasize to brain?
Harrison's 20th Ed. Chapter 86, Page 649

A. Pleura
B. Bone
C. Lung
D. Liver

3380. Which of the following cancer has the greatest propensity to intracranial metastases with hemorrhage?
Harrison's 20th Ed. Chapter 86, Page 649

A. Melanoma
B. Thyroid cancer
C. Kidney cancer
D. All of the above

Melanoma, thyroid and kidney cancer have the greatest propensity to intracranial metastases hemorrhage.

3381. Ommaya reservoir best relates to?
Harrison's 20th Ed. Chapter 86, Page 651

A. Bone marrow transplantation
B. Ventriculoperitoneal shunt
C. Intraventricular cannula
D. Spinal cord compression

Ommaya reservoir is an intraventricular cannula to deliver chemotherapy intrathecally.

3382. Brain tumor metastases that spread to spinal cord via CSF pathways are termed?
Surg Neurol 1991;35:377-80

A. Pin metastases
B. Hanging metastases
C. Drop metastases
D. Confluent metastases

Intradural extramedullary spinal metastases that arise from intracranial lesions are called drop metastases.

3383. Which of the following is a cellular marker for proliferation?
Harrison's 20th Ed. Chapter 75, Page 560

A. Ki-66
B. Ki-67
C. Ki-68
D. Ki-69

Ki-67 protein (also known as MKI67) is a cellular marker for proliferation. Proliferation index (mitotic activity) can be determined with monoclonal antibody Ki-67 which recognizes a histone protein expressed in proliferating but not quiescent cells.

3384. Which of the following is a germ cell tumor?
Harrison's 20th Ed. Chapter 86, Page 640

A. Teratoma
B. Yolk sac tumor
C. Choriocarcinoma
D. All of the above

Malignant germ cell tumors include dysgerminomas, yolk sac tumors, immature teratomas, embryonal & choriocarcinomas.

3385. What level of 'Karnofsky performance status' have a poor prognosis in patients with brain tumor?
Harrison's 20th Ed. Chapter 65, Page 438 Table 65-4

A. < 70
B. < 80
C. < 90
D. < 100

Karnofsky performance scale and Eastern Cooperative Oncology Group (ECOG) performance scale are meant to assess patients with brain tumors. A Karnofsky score ≥ 70 indicates that patient is ambulatory & independent in self-care activities.

3386. Differential diagnosis of ring-enhancement lesions include?
Harrison's 20th Ed. Chapter 135, Page 1014

A. Glioblastoma
B. Brain abscess stage 3
C. L. monocytogenes meningoencephalitis
D. All of the above

3387. Differential diagnosis of ring-enhancement lesions include?
Harrison's 20th Ed. Chapter 197, Page 1450, 1445

A. Actinomycosis
B. CNS lymphomas
C. Toxoplasmosis
D. All of the above

3388. In vegetative state which of the following persists?
Harrison's 20th Ed. Chapter 300, Page 2068

A. Yawning
B. Coughing
C. Swallowing
D. All of the above

Encephalitis

3389. Sporadic cases of encephalitis in immunocompetent adults are mostly caused by?
Harrison's 20th Ed. Chapter 132, Page 992

- A. HSV
- B. West Nile virus (WNV)
- C. St. Louis encephalitis virus
- D. La Crosse virus

Most important viruses causing sporadic cases of encephalitis in immunocompetent adults are HSV, VZV and EBV. Epidemics of encephalitis are caused by arboviruses.

3390. Which of the following is a member of Flaviviruses?
Harrison's 20th Ed. Chapter 132, Page 992

- A. Eastern equine encephalitis virus
- B. Western equine encephalitis virus
- C. West Nile virus (WNV)
- D. California encephalitis virus

Epidemics of encephalitis are caused by arboviruses of which there are several groups like Alphaviruses (Eastern equine encephalitis virus, Western equine encephalitis virus), Flaviviruses (WNV, St. Louis encephalitis virus, Powassan virus), and Bunyaviruses (California encephalitis virus serogroup, La Crosse virus).

3391. Which of the following is a togavirus?
Harrison's 20th Ed. Chapter 132, Page 992

- A. Toscana
- B. Nipah
- C. Chikungunya
- D. Human parechovirus 3 (HPeV3)

3392. Viral "hemorrhagic" encephalitis can be seen in?
Harrison's 20th Ed. Chapter 132, Page 992

- A. HSV
- B. Colorado tick fever virus
- C. California encephalitis virus
- D. All of the above

~20% of patients with encephalitis have RBC's (>500/µL) in CSF tap (hemorrhagic encephalitis) which is also seen with HSV, Colorado tick fever virus and California encephalitis virus.

3393. Which of the following seizure type occurs in a case of severe viral encephalitis?
Harrison's 20th Ed. Chapter 132, Page 992

- A. Absence (petit mal)
- B. Tonic-clonic (grand mal)
- C. Myoclonic
- D. Any of the above

Virtually every possible type of focal neurologic disturbance can occur in viral encephalitis.

3394. Which of the following focal neurological findings is commonly encountered in viral encephalitis?
Harrison's 20th Ed. Chapter 132, Page 992

- A. Aphasia
- B. Ataxia
- C. Involuntary movements
- D. All of the above

Most common focal findings in viral encephalitis are aphasia, ataxia, hemiparesis, involuntary movements & cranial nerve deficits.

3395. "Atypical lymphocytes" in CSF of viral encephalitis are commonly seen in?
Harrison's 20th Ed. Chapter 132, Page 992

- A. EBV
- B. CMV
- C. HSV
- D. Enteroviruses

Atypical lymphocytes in CSF may be seen in EBV infection and less commonly with other viruses like CMV, HSV and enteroviruses.

3396. CSF PCR is most sensitive for which of the following viruses causing viral encephalitis?
Harrison's 20th Ed. Chapter 132, Page 993

- A. WNV
- B. HSV
- C. Enterovirus
- D. VZV

Sensitivity is ~98% & specificity is ~94% of CSF HSV PCR.

3397. Presence in CSF of which class of antibody against WNV indicates WNV encephalitis?
Harrison's 20th Ed. Chapter 132, Page 993

- A. IgA
- B. IgG
- C. IgM
- D. IgE

Demonstration of WNV intrathecally synthesized IgM antibodies is diagnostic of WNV encephalitis. They do not cross blood-brain barrier.

3398. Which of the following about HSV-1 encephalitis is false?
Harrison's 20th Ed. Chapter 132, Page 993

- A. Focal findings in MRI
- B. Invariably negative CSF cultures
- C. Most sensitive CSF HSV PCR
- D. None of the above

Focal findings in encephalitis raises the possibility of HSV encephalitis. Cultures are invariably negative in cases of HSV-1 encephalitis. CSF HSV PCR has a sensitivity of ~98%.

3399. In MRI, which cortical lobe of brain is most affected in HSV encephalitis?
Harrison's 20th Ed. Chapter 132, Page 993

- A. Frontal
- B. Temporal
- C. Parietal
- D. Occipital

~10% of patients with PCR-documented HSV encephalitis have normal MRI, although ~90% will have abnormalities in the temporal lobe.

3400. In MRI of viral encephalitis, abnormalities involving deep brain structures like thalamus, basal ganglia, and brainstem rather than cortex indicate infection with which of the following viruses?

Harrison's 20th Ed. Chapter 132, Page 993

A. HSV
B. VZV
C. WNV
D. All of the above

MRI abnormalities of patients with WNV encephalitis involve deep brain structures like thalamus, basal ganglia & brainstem rather than cortex. Presentation is therefore with prominent movement disorders (tremor, myoclonus) or Parkinsonism. Patients with WNV infection can also present with acute poliomyelitis-like areflexic paralysis.

3401. In MRI of viral encephalitis, areas of hemorrhagic infarction reflect infection with which of the following viruses?

Harrison's 20th Ed. Chapter 132, Page 993

A. HSV
B. VZV
C. WNV
D. All of the above

Patients with VZV encephalitis show areas of hemorrhagic infarction pointing towards a CNS vasculopathy rather than a true encephalitis.

3402. Which of the following bacterial infection can mimic viral encephalitis?

Harrison's 20th Ed. Chapter 132, Page 993

A. Listeria
B. Bartonella
C. Mycoplasma
D. All of the above

Bartonella infection is the most common bacterial infection mimicking viral encephalitis.

3403. In viral encephalitis, infection with which of the following can present as acute ascending paralysis resembling Guillain-Barre' syndrome?

Harrison's 20th Ed. Chapter 132, Page 993

A. HIV infection
B. Rabies
C. WNV
D. All of the above

Acute ascending paralysis resembling Guillain-Barre' syndrome but associated with CSF pleocytosis can occur with HIV infection, rabies, and WNV infection.

3404. Abnormalities in MRI are found in which of the following regions of the brain in viral encephalitis caused by rabies?

Harrison's 20th Ed. Chapter 132, Page 993

A. Brainstem
B. Hippocampus
C. Hypothalamus
D. All of the above

In rabies, CSF lymphocytic pleocytosis with areas of increased T2 signal abnormality in brainstem, hippocampus & hypothalamus are seen.

3405. PCR amplification of viral nucleic acid for diagnosis of viral encephalitis caused by rabies can be done from?

Harrison's 20th Ed. Chapter 132, Page 994

A. CSF
B. Saliva
C. Tears
D. All of the above

PCR amplification of viral nucleic acid from CSF and saliva or tears may also enable diagnosis.

3406. Enzyme in HSV, VZV, and EBV that phosphorylates acyclovir to produce acyclovir-5` monophosphate is?

Harrison's 20th Ed. Chapter 132, Page 995

A. 2`deoxyguanosine
B. 3`deoxyguanosine
C. Deoxypyrimidine kinase
D. Pyrimidine kinase

HSV, VZV, & EBV encode enzyme, deoxypyrimidine (thymidine) kinase, that phosphorylates acyclovir to produce acyclovir-5`-monophosphate.

3407. Which of the following metabolite of acyclovir acts as an antiviral agent by inhibiting viral DNA polymerase?

Harrison's 20th Ed. Chapter 132, Page 995

A. Monophosphate
B. Biphosphate
C. Triphosphate
D. Any of the above

Infected host cell enzymes phosphorylate acyclovir-5`-monophosphate to form a triphosphate derivative which acts as an antiviral agent by inhibiting viral DNA polymerase & by causing premature termination of nascent viral DNA chains.

3408. In adults suffering from HSV encephalitis, duration of intravenous acyclovir therapy should be for a minimum period of?

Harrison's 20th Ed. Chapter 132, Page 995

A. 3 days
B. 7 days
C. 10 days
D. 14 days

3409. In neonates suffering from HSV encephalitis, duration of intravenous acyclovir therapy should be for a minimum period of?

Harrison's 20th Ed. Chapter 132, Page 995

A. 5 days
B. 10 days
C. 14 days
D. 21 days

Adults should receive a dose of 10 mg/kg of acyclovir IV 8 hourly (30 mg/kg/day) for at least 14 days. Neonates with HSV encephalitis receive 20 mg/kg of acyclovir 8 hourly (60 mg/kg/day) for at least 21 days.

3410. Which of the following is not a side effect of IV acyclovir?

Harrison's 20th Ed. Chapter 132, Page 995

A. Hemolysis
B. Elevations in BUN & creatinine
C. Thrombocytopenia
D. Neurotoxicity

Complications of acyclovir therapy are elevations in BUN & creatinine levels (5%), thrombocytopenia (6%), GI toxicity (7%) & neurotoxicity (lethargy, obtundation, disorientation, confusion, agitation, hallucinations, tremors, seizures) (1%). Hemolysis, with resulting anemia, is a major side effect of IV ribavarin therapy.

3411. Which of the following drug is effective in CMV-related CNS infections?
Harrison's 20th Ed. Chapter 132, Page 995

A. Ganciclovir
B. Foscarnet
C. Cidofovir
D. All of the above

Ganciclovir & foscarnet (often used in combination) are effective in CMV-related CNS infections. Cidofovir may provide an alternative in patients who fail to respond to ganciclovir and foscarnet.

3412. Which of the following drugs is useful for treatment of WNV encephalitis?
Harrison's 20th Ed. Chapter 132, Page 995

A. Ganciclovir
B. Foscarnet
C. Cidofovir
D. None of the above

3413. Incidence & severity of sequelae in patients surviving viral encephalitis is more in infections with?
Harrison's 20th Ed. Chapter 132, Page 995

A. Eastern equine encephalitis virus
B. EBV
C. California encephalitis virus
D. Venezuelan equine encephalitis virus

In Eastern equine encephalitis virus infection, ~80% of survivors have severe neurologic sequelae. Severe sequelae are unusual in EBV, California & Venezuelan equine encephalitis.

3414. Incidence & severity of sequelae of viral encephalitis depends on which of the following?
Harrison's 20th Ed. Chapter 132, Page 996

A. Age of patient
B. Level of consciousness at time of initiation of therapy
C. Amount of HSV DNA in CSF at time of presentation
D. All of the above

Incidence & severity of sequelae are directly related to age of patient & level of consciousness at initiation of therapy. Clinical outcome following treatment correlates with amount of HSV DNA in CSF at presentation.

3415. Most common pathogen causing fungal meningitis is?
Harrison's 20th Ed. Chapter 132, Page 995

A. Coccidioides immitis
B. Histoplasma capsulatum
C. Cryptococcus neoformans
D. Candida

The most common pathogen causing fungal meningitis is C. neoformans.

3416. Which of the following cranial nerve is most frequently involved in T. pallidum invasion of CNS?
Harrison's 20th Ed. Chapter 132, Page 996

A. II
B. III
C. VII
D. XII

Cranial nerves VII and VIII are most frequently involved in syphilis.

3417. Negative result of which of the following does not rule out neurosyphilis?
Harrison's 20th Ed. Chapter 132, Page 996

A. CSF VDRL
B. CSF FTA-ABS
C. MHA-TP
D. All of the above

A negative CSF VDRL does not rule out neurosyphilis. A negative CSF FTA-ABS or MHA-TP rules out neurosyphilis.

3418. In tuberculous meningitis, which sample of CSF is best for detecting acid-fast bacilli (AFB)?
Harrison's 20th Ed. Chapter 132, Page 996

A. First tube
B. Middle tube
C. Last tube
D. Any of the above

In TBM, last tube of CSF collected at LP is the best tube to send for a smear for AFB. If there is a pellicle in CSF or a cobweb-like clot on surface of fluid, AFB is demonstrated in smear of clot / pellicle.

3419. Eosinophils in the CSF are found in meningitis due to?
Harrison's 20th Ed. Chapter 132, Page 996

A. L. monocytogenes
B. T. pallidum
C. C. immitis
D. La Crosse virus

Eosinophils in the CSF are found in C. immitis meningitis.

3420. The most common complication of fungal meningitis is?
Harrison's 20th Ed. Chapter 132, Page 996

A. Seizure
B. Amnesia
C. Hydrocephalus
D. Hearing loss

The most common complication of fungal meningitis is hydrocephalus.

3421. In progressive multifocal leukoencephalopathy, which of the following is not involved?
Harrison's 20th Ed. Chapter 132, Page 997

A. Frontal cortex
B. Cerebellum
C. Midbrain
D. Spinal cord

In PML, multifocal areas of demyelination distributed throughout the brain but sparing spinal cord and optic nerves are seen.

3422. Which of the following is false about progressive multifocal leukoencephalopathy?
Harrison's 20th Ed. Chapter 132, Page 997

A. Occurs in immunosuppressed population
B. Only known manifestation of JC virus infection
C. Late manifestation of AIDS
D. None of the above

3423. Which of the following is useful for the diagnosis of progressive multifocal leukoencephalopathy?

Harrison's 20th Ed. Chapter 132, Page 997

- A. EEG
- B. CT scan of brain
- C. Positive CSF PCR for JCV DNA
- D. Serologic studies for JC virus

Positive CSF PCR for JCV DNA with typical MRI lesions in appropriate clinical setting is diagnostic of PML.

3424. Typical visual deficit seen in progressive multifocal leukoencephalopathy is?

Harrison's 20th Ed. Chapter 132, Page 997

- A. Achromatopia
- B. Homonymous hemianopia
- C. Cortical blindness
- D. Amaurosis fugax

Patients of progressive multifocal leukoencephalopathy present with visual deficits, typically homonymous hemianopia.

3425. Subacute sclerosing panencephalitis occurs after a latent interval of how many years after measles infection?

Harrison's 20th Ed. Chapter 132, Page 997

- A. 1–2 years
- B. 2–4 years
- C. 4–6 years
- D. 6–8 years

SSPE occurs after a latent interval of 6–8 years after measles infection.

3426. Which of the following is not a manifestation of subacute sclerosing panencephalitis?

Harrison's 20th Ed. Chapter 132, Page 997

- A. Fever and headache
- B. Progressive intellectual deterioration
- C. Focal and/or generalized seizures
- D. Ataxia

Signs of a CNS viral infection - fever & headache do not occur in SSPE.

3427. Which of the following diagnostic modalities are useful in SSPE?

Harrison's 20th Ed. Chapter 132, Page 997

- A. EEG
- B. CSF
- C. MRI
- D. All of the above

3428. CSF finding in SSPE is?

Harrison's 20th Ed. Chapter 132, Page 997

- A. Acellular
- B. Elevated gamma globulin level
- C. Elevated CSF antimeasles antibody level
- D. All of the above

In SSPE, CSF is acellular with markedly elevated gamma globulin level (>20% of total CSF protein). CSF antimeasles antibody levels are invariably elevated & oligoclonal antimeasles antibodies are present.

3429. Which of the following drugs is used in the treatment of SSPE?

Harrison's 20th Ed. Chapter 132, Page 997

- A. Acyclovir
- B. Isoprinosine
- C. Cytarabine
- D. Foscarnet

Isoprinosine (100 mg/kg/day), alone or in combination with intrathecal or intraventricular α-interferon prolongs survival with clinical improvement.

Acute Meningitis: Bacterial Meningitis

3430. In meningoencephalitis, which of the following is involved in the inflammatory reaction?
Harrison's 20th Ed. Chapter 133, Page 998

A. Meninges
B. Subarachnoid space (SAS)
C. Brain parenchyma
D. All of the above

3431. In adults, organism most commonly responsible for community-acquired bacterial meningitis is?
Harrison's 20th Ed. Chapter 133, Page 998

A. N. meningitidis
B. Streptococcus pneumoniae
C. Group B streptococci
D. H. influenzae

Organisms responsible for community-acquired bacterial meningitis are S. pneumoniae (~50%), N. meningitidis (~25%), group B streptococci (~15%), Listeria monocytogenes (~10%) & H. influenzae Type B (<10%).

3432. Most important predisposing condition that increase risk of pneumococcal meningitis is?
Harrison's 20th Ed. Chapter 133, Page 998

A. Acute or chronic pneumococcal sinusitis
B. Alcoholism
C. Pneumococcal pneumonia
D. Splenectomy

The most important predisposing condition that increase the risk of pneumococcal meningitis is pneumococcal pneumonia. Other risk factors include coexisting acute or chronic pneumococcal sinusitis or otitis media, alcoholism, diabetes, splenectomy, hypogammaglobulinemia, complement deficiency & head trauma with basilar skull fracture and CSF rhinorrhea.

3433. The mortality rate in pneumococcal meningitis is?
Harrison's 20th Ed. Chapter 133, Page 998

A. ~2%
B. ~5%
C. ~10%
D. ~20%

The mortality rate in pneumococcal meningitis remains ~20% despite antibiotic therapy.

3434. Quadrivalent meningococcal glycoconjugate vaccine does not contain which serogroup?
Harrison's 20th Ed. Chapter 133, Page 998

A. Serogroup A
B. Serogroup B
C. Serogroup C
D. Serogroup Y

Quadrivalent (serogroups A, C, W-135 and Y) meningococcal glycoconjugate vaccine does not contain serogroup B which is responsible for one-third of cases of meningococcal disease.

3435. Individuals with deficiencies of which of the following are highly susceptible to meningococcal infections?
Harrison's 20th Ed. Chapter 133, Page 998

A. Galectin-1
B. Properdin
C. Pentraxin
D. Cathelin

Complement components are important for bactericidal activity of serum. Individuals with deficiencies of any of the complement components, chiefly of the terminal complement components (C5-9), properdin or factor D are highly susceptible to meningococcal infections. Such a deficiency increases the risk of disease by up to 600-fold and may result in recurrent attacks.

3436. Infection acquired by ingesting "ready-to-eat" foods is due to?
Harrison's 20th Ed. Chapter 133, Page 998

A. Actinobacillus actinomycetemcomitans
B. Kingella kingae
C. Listeria monocytogenes
D. Streptococcus bovis

3437. Which of the following is present in relatively small amounts in normal CSF?
Harrison's 20th Ed. Chapter 133, Page 999

A. White blood cells (WBCs)
B. Complement proteins
C. Immunoglobulins
D. All of the above

Normal CSF contains few WBCs, relatively small amounts of complement proteins & immunoglobulins.

3438. Which of the following is a bacterial cell-wall component?
Harrison's 20th Ed. Chapter 133, Page 999

A. Lipopolysaccharide (LPS)
B. Teichoic acid
C. Peptidoglycan
D. All of the above

3439. Following intracisternal inoculation of LPS, which of the following cytokine is first to appear?
Harrison's 20th Ed. Chapter 133, Page 999

A. Interleukin 1α
B. Interleukin 1β
C. Interleukin 1γ
D. Interleukin 1δ

In meningitis, cytokines like tumor necrosis factor alpha (TNFα) and interleukin 1b (IL-1β) are present in CSF within 1–2 hours of intracisternal inoculation of LPS.

3440. Raised intracranial pressure in bacterial meningitis is due to?
Harrison's 20th Ed. Chapter 133, Page 999

A. Interstitial edema
B. Vasogenic edema
C. Cytotoxic edema
D. All of the above

The combination of interstitial, vasogenic, and cytotoxic edema leads to raised ICP and coma.

3441. Which of the following is not a feature of classic clinical triad of meningitis?
Harrison's 20th Ed. Chapter 133, Page 999

A. Fever
B. Headache
C. Vomiting
D. Nuchal rigidity

The classic clinical triad of meningitis is fever, headache & nuchal rigidity. Decreased level of consciousness occurs in >75% of patients. Nausea, vomiting & photophobia are also common complaints.

3442. Which of the following is the pathognomonic sign of meningeal irritation?
Harrison's 20th Ed. Chapter 133, Page 999

A. Fever
B. Headache
C. Photophobia
D. Nuchal rigidity

Nuchal rigidity ("stiff neck") is the pathognomonic sign of meningeal irritation.

3443. While eliciting Brudzinski's sign, which part of body is moved passively?
Harrison's 20th Ed. Chapter 133, Page 1000

A. Hip joint
B. Knee joint
C. Neck
D. Ankle joint

Brudzinski's sign is positive when passive flexion of neck results in spontaneous flexion of hips & knees.

3444. Kernig and Brudzinski's signs may be absent or reduced in?
Harrison's 20th Ed. Chapter 133, Page 1000

A. Very young patients
B. Elderly patients
C. Immunocompromised individuals
D. All of the above

Kernig and Brudzinski's signs may be absent or reduced in very young or elderly patients, immunocompromised individuals or patients with a severely depressed mental status.

3445. Which of the following sign is positive in meningitis?
DeJong's The Neurologic Examination, 7th Ed. Page 764

A. Kernig sign
B. Brudzinski's neck sign
C. Lasègue's sign
D. All of the above

The Kernig sign, Brudzinski's neck sign and Lasègue's sign (straight leg raising) are positive in meningitis. To avoid spinal flexion, patient with meningitis may sit in bed with hands placed far behind, head thrown back, hips & knees flexed, and the back arched (Amoss's, Hoyne's, or tripod sign).

3446. Which of the following is a sign for meningeal inflammation?
DeJong's The Neurologic Examination, 7th Ed. Page 765

A. Brudzinski's contralateral leg sign
B. Brudzinski's cheek sign
C. Brudzinski's symphysis sign
D. All of the above

In Brudzinski's cheek sign, pressure is applied against the cheeks on or just below the zygoma, which results in flexion at elbows with an upward jerking of the arms. In Brudzinski's symphysis sign, pressure is applied on symphysis pubis that causes flexion of both lower extremities.

3447. Resistance to elbow extension due to meningeal inflammation is?
DeJong's The Neurologic Examination, 7th Ed. Page 765

A. Guilland's sign
B. Bikele sign
C. Lomadtse sign
D. Schrijver-Bernhard reflex

In Bikele sign, with elbow flexed, shoulder abducted, elevated, and externally rotated, examiner attempts to passively extend the elbow. If meningeal inflammation is present or there is brachial plexitis, resistance is observed to elbow extension.

3448. Generalized seizure and status epilepticus in bacterial meningitis may be due to?
Harrison's 20th Ed. Chapter 133, Page 1000

A. Hyponatremia
B. Cerebral anoxia
C. Toxic effects of antimicrobial agents
D. All of the above

Generalized seizure activity & status epilepticus in bacterial meningitis may be due to hyponatremia, cerebral anoxia or less commonly, toxic effects of antimicrobial agents (high-dose penicillin).

3449. Over 90% of patients of bacterial meningitis have a CSF opening pressure of?
Harrison's 20th Ed. Chapter 133, Page 1000

A. > 100 mm H_2O
B. > 120 mm H_2O
C. > 160 mm H_2O
D. > 180 mm H_2O

More than 90% of patients will have a CSF opening pressure >180 mm H_2O.

3450. Signs of increased intracranial pressure (ICP) include?
Harrison's 20th Ed. Chapter 133, Page 1000

A. Deteriorating or reduced level of consciousness
B. Dilated poorly reactive pupils
C. Cushing reflex
D. All of the above

Signs of increased ICP include a deteriorating or reduced level of consciousness, papilledema, dilated poorly reactive pupils, sixth nerve palsies, decerebrate posturing, and the Cushing reflex.

3451. Cushing reflex in raised ICP relates to?
Harrison's 20th Ed. Chapter 133, Page 1000

A. Bradycardia
B. Hypertension
C. Irregular respirations
D. All of the above

Cushing reflex includes bradycardia, hypertension & irregular respirations.

3452. Petechiae due to meningococcemia are found on?
Harrison's 20th Ed. Chapter 133, Page 1000

A. Trunk and lower extremities
B. Mucous membranes and conjunctiva
C. Palms and soles
D. All of the above

Petechiae due to meningococcemia are found on trunk & lower extremities, in mucous membranes & conjunctiva, and occasionally on palms & soles.

3453. In bacterial meningitis, CSF/serum glucose ratio is?
Harrison's 20th Ed. Chapter 133, Page 1000

A. < 0.4
B. < 0.5
C. < 0.6
D. < 0.8

CSF/serum glucose ratio in bacterial meningitis is <0.4 in ~60% of patients.

3454. CSF glucose concentration is low when CSF/serum glucose ratio is?
Harrison's 20th Ed. Chapter 133, Page 1000

A. < 0.4
B. < 0.5
C. < 0.6
D. < 0.8

CSF glucose concentration is low when CSF/serum glucose ratio is <0.6.

3455. CSF/serum glucose ratio of <0.4 is seen in?
Harrison's 20th Ed. Chapter 133, Page 1000

A. Fungal meningitis
B. Tuberculous meningitis
C. Carcinomatous meningitis
D. All of the above

Besides bacterial meningitis, CSF/serum glucose ratio <0.4 is also seen in fungal, tuberculous, and carcinomatous meningitis.

3456. Limulus amebocyte lysate assay in CSF is diagnostic of?
Harrison's 20th Ed. Chapter 133, Page 1001

A. Gram-negative bacterial meningitis
B. Fungal meningitis
C. Tuberculous meningitis
D. Carcinomatous meningitis

Limulus amebocyte lysate assay detects gram-negative endotoxin in CSF & is diagnostic of gram-negative bacterial meningitis. (Specificity 85–100%; sensitivity 100%).

3457. In Rocky Mountain spotted fever (RMSF), skin rash typically begins in?
Harrison's 20th Ed. Chapter 133, Page 1001

A. Face and scalp
B. Wrists and ankles
C. Chest and abdomen
D. Neck

Skin rash in RMSF typically begins in wrist & ankles. It spreads distally & proximally rapidly to involve palms & soles.

3458. Noninfectious CNS disorder that can mimic bacterial meningitis is?
Harrison's 20th Ed. Chapter 133, Page 1001

A. Subarachnoid hemorrhage
B. Behçet's syndrome
C. Pituitary apoplexy
D. All of the above

Noninfectious CNS disorders that can mimic bacterial meningitis are subarachnoid hemorrhage, medication-induced hypersensitivity meningitis, chemical meningitis due to rupture of tumor contents into the CSF, carcinomatous or lymphomatous meningitis, meningitis associated with inflammatory disorders like sarcoid, systemic lupus erythematosus (SLE), and Behçet's syndrome, pituitary apoplexy and Vogt-Koyanagi-Harada syndrome.

3459. Vogt-Koyanagi-Harada syndrome refers to?
Harrison's 20th Ed. Chapter 133, Page 1001

A. Drug-induced hypersensitivity meningitis
B. Carcinomatous meningitis
C. Meningitis associated with sarcoid
D. Uveomeningitic syndromes

Vogt-Koyanagi-Harada syndrome refers to uveomeningitic syndromes.

3460. Which of the following causes a subacutely evolving meningitis?
Harrison's 20th Ed. Chapter 133, Page 1001

A. Mycobacterium tuberculosis
B. Cryptococcus neoformans
C. Treponema pallidum
D. All of the above

Subacutely evolving meningitis is caused by Mycobacterium tuberculosis, Cryptococcus neoformans, Histoplasma capsulatum, Coccidioides immitis and Treponema pallidum.

3461. Which of the following viral infections can mimic the clinical presentation of bacterial meningitis?
Harrison's 20th Ed. Chapter 133, Page 1001

A. Varicella-zoster virus
B. Herpes simplex virus
C. Cytomegalovirus
D. Enterovirus

3462. In bacterial meningitis, the goal is to begin antibiotic therapy within what time of patient's arrival?
Harrison's 20th Ed. Chapter 133, Page 1001

A. 1 hour
B. 3 hours
C. 6 hours
D. 12 hours

In bacterial meningitis, the goal is to begin antibiotic therapy within 60 minutes of patient's arrival in the emergency room.

3463. Which of the following cephalosporin is preferred in CNS infection with P. aeruginosa?
Harrison's 20th Ed. Chapter 133, Page 1002 Table 133-3

A. Ceftriaxone
B. Cefotaxime
C. Ceftazidime
D. None of the above

Meningitis due to P. aeruginosa should be treated with ceftazidime, cefepime, or meropenem.

3464. Close contacts of a patient of meningococcal meningitis should receive chemoprophylaxis with?
Harrison's 20th Ed. Chapter 133, Page 1002

A. Rifampin
B. Ciprofloxacin
C. Azithromycin
D. Any of the above

Close contacts of meningococcal meningitis patient should receive chemoprophylaxis with rifampin, ciprofloxacin, azithromycin or ceftriaxone.

3465. In meningococcal meningitis chemoprophylaxis, adult dose of rifampin is?
Harrison's 20th Ed. Chapter 133, Page 1002

A. 450 mg once a day for 1 day
B. 450 mg twice a day for 2 days
C. 600 mg once a day for 1 day
D. 600 mg twice a day for 2 days

In meningococcal meningitis chemoprophylaxis, rifampin is given as a 2-day regimen of 600 mg every 12 hour for 2 days in adults.

3466. Which antibiotic should be added to the empirical regimen in acute meningitis for coverage of L. monocytogenes?
Harrison's 20th Ed. Chapter 133, Page 1002

A. Ampicillin
B. Nafcillin
C. Penicillin G
D. Metronidazole

Ampicillin should be added to the empirical regimen for coverage of L. monocytogenes.

3467. Which of the following is false about vancomycin therapy in S. pneumoniae meningitis?
Harrison's 20th Ed. Chapter 133, Page 1002

A. Antibiotic of choice if cephalosporin MIC is >1 µg/mL
B. Rifampin produces synergistic effect to vancomycin
C. Vancomycin can be given by intraventricular route
D. None of the above

3468. Which of the following statements about duration of antimicrobial therapy in meningitis is false?
Harrison's 20th Ed. Chapter 133, Page 1002

A. 1 week course of IV penicillin is recommended for meningococcal meningitis
B. 2 week course of IV antimicrobial therapy is recommended for pneumococcal meningitis
C. 3 week course of ampicillin is recommended for L. monocytogenes meningitis
D. 4 week course of IV antibiotic is recommended for gram-negative bacilli meningitis

A 3-week course of IV antibiotic therapy is recommended for meningitis due to gram-negative bacilli.

3469. Dexamethasone exerts its beneficial effect by?
Harrison's 20th Ed. Chapter 133, Page 1002

A. Inhibiting the synthesis of IL-1β & TNF-α at mRNA level
B. Decreasing CSF outflow resistance
C. Stabilizing the blood-brain barrier
D. All of the above

Dexamethasone exerts its beneficial effect by inhibiting the synthesis of IL-1β and TNF-α at the mRNA level, decreasing CSF outflow resistance and stabilizing the blood-brain barrier.

3470. When should dexamethasone be given in acute bacterial meningitis?
Harrison's 20th Ed. Chapter 133, Page 1002

A. Before antibiotic therapy
B. Along with antibiotic therapy
C. After antibiotic therapy
D. Any of the above

Rationale for giving dexamethasone 20 minutes before antibiotic therapy is that it inhibits production of TNF by macrophages & microglia only if it is administered before these cells are activated by endotoxin.

3471. Benefit of dexamethasone therapy is not significant if started how many hours after antimicrobial therapy?
Harrison's 20th Ed. Chapter 133, Page 1003

A. > 1 hour
B. > 3 hours
C. > 6 hours
D. > 12 hours

Dexamethasone therapy is unlikely to be of significant benefit if started > 6 hours after antimicrobial therapy has been initiated.

3472. Benefits of dexamethasone therapy are most striking in patients with?
Harrison's 20th Ed. Chapter 133, Page 1003

A. Gram-negative bacterial meningitis
B. Pneumococcal meningitis
C. Meningococcal meningitis
D. Staphylococcal meningitis

3473. Mortality is higher in meningitis due to?
Harrison's 20th Ed. Chapter 133, Page 1003

A. H. influenzae
B. N. meningitidis
C. L. monocytogenes
D. S. pneumoniae

Mortality is 3–7% for meningitis caused by H. influenzae, N. meningitidis or group B streptococci. 15% for that due to L. monocytogenes and 20% for S. pneumoniae.

3474. Predictors of increased mortality in bacterial meningitis include?
Harrison's 20th Ed. Chapter 133, Page 1003

A. Onset of seizures within 24 hours of admission
B. CSF glucose concentration of < 40 mg/dL
C. CSF protein concentration of > 300 mg/dL
D. All of the above

Risk of death from bacterial meningitis increases with decreased level of consciousness on admission, onset of seizures within 24 hours of admission, signs of increased ICP, young age (infancy) & age >50, presence of shock and/or need for mechanical ventilation, delay in initiation of treatment, CSF glucose concentration <40 mg/dL and CSF protein >300 mg/dL.

3475. Common sequelae of bacterial meningitis include all except?
Harrison's 20th Ed. Chapter 133, Page 1003

A. Decreased intellectual function
B. Seizures
C. Visual loss
D. Hearing loss

Common sequelae of bacterial meningitis include decreased intellectual function, memory impairment, seizures, hearing loss & dizziness & gait disturbances.

Viral Meningitis

3476. Which of the following viruses has a nonseasonal prevalence in causing viral meningitis?
Harrison's 20th Ed. Chapter 133, Page 1003

- A. Arboviruses
- B. LCMV
- C. Mumps
- D. HSV

HSV & HIV viral meningitis have no seasonal predominance. Arboviruses & enteroviruses are frequent during summer/early fall. LCMV & mumps viruses cause viral meningitis during winter months.

3477. Which of the following is uncommon in viral meningitis?
Harrison's 20th Ed. Chapter 133, Page 1003

- A. Fever
- B. Headache
- C. Meningeal irritation
- D. Marked confusion

Viral meningitis presents as fever, headache, meningeal irritation and an inflammatory CSF profile. Fever may be accompanied by malaise, myalgia, anorexia, nausea and vomiting, abdominal pain, and/or diarrhea. Mild degree of lethargy or drowsiness may occur but more profound alterations in consciousness like stupor, coma, or marked confusion, should prompt consideration of alternative diagnoses.

3478. Which of the following is common in viral meningitis?
Harrison's 20th Ed. Chapter 133, Page 1003

- A. Kernig's and Brudzinski's signs
- B. Headache - frontal or retroorbital
- C. Focal neurological deficits
- D. Seizures

Headache in viral meningitis is usually frontal or retro-orbital with photophobia, pain on moving eyes & mild terminal nuchal rigidity. Evidence of severe meningeal irritation, such as Kernig's and Brudzinski's signs, is generally absent. Seizures or other focal neurologic signs or symptoms suggest involvement of the brain parenchyma and do not occur in uncomplicated viral meningitis.

3479. Which of the following viruses is a less common cause of viral meningitis?
Harrison's 20th Ed. Chapter 133, Page 1003

- A. Enteroviruses
- B. Arboviruses
- C. Adenoviruses
- D. HSV-2

Enteroviruses account for > 85% of aseptic meningitis cases. Viruses belonging to the Enterovirus genus are members of the family Picornaviridae and include the coxsackieviruses, echoviruses, polioviruses, and human enteroviruses 68 to 71. Adenoviruses rarely cause viral meningitis.

3480. Typical CSF profile in viral meningitis includes all except?
Harrison's 20th Ed. Chapter 133, Page 1003

- A. Lymphocytic pleocytosis - 25 to 500 cells/μL
- B. Normal or slightly elevated protein - 20 to 80 mg/dL
- C. Reduced glucose concentration
- D. Normal or mildly elevated pressure (100–350 mm H_2O)

Examination of CSF is the most important laboratory test in the diagnosis of viral meningitis. The typical profile is a lymphocytic pleocytosis (25 to 500 cells/μL), a normal or slightly elevated protein concentration (20 to 80 mg/dL), a normal glucose concentration, and a normal or mildly elevated opening pressure (100 to 350 mm H_2O).

3481. PMNs may predominate in CSF of viral meningitis in the first 48 hours of illness in which of the following infections?
Harrison's 20th Ed. Chapter 133, Page 1003

- A. Echovirus 9
- B. West Nile virus
- C. Mumps
- D. All of the above

PMNs may predominate in the first 48 hours of illness, especially in patients with infections due to echovirus 9, West Nile virus or Eastern equine encephalitis (EEE) virus, or mumps.

3482. Cell counts of several thousand per microliter are seen in viral meningitis due to which of the following?
Harrison's 20th Ed. Chapter 133, Page 1003

- A. Echovirus 9
- B. West Nile virus
- C. Mumps
- D. Arboviruses

3483. Cell counts of several thousand per microliter are seen in viral meningitis due to which of the following?
Harrison's 20th Ed. Chapter 133, Page 1003

- A. Echovirus 9
- B. West Nile virus
- C. Lymphocytic choriomeningitis virus (LCMV)
- D. Arboviruses

Total CSF cell count in viral meningitis is typically 25 to 500/μL, although cell counts of several thousand per microliter are occasionally seen, especially with infections due to lymphocytic choriomeningitis virus (LCMV) and mumps virus.

3484. Low CSF glucose concentration is seen in viral meningitis due to which of the following?
Harrison's 20th Ed. Chapter 133, Page 1003

- A. Echovirus 9
- B. West Nile virus
- C. Lymphocytic choriomeningitis virus (LCMV)
- D. Arboviruses

3485. Low CSF glucose concentration is seen in viral meningitis due to which of the following?
Harrison's 20th Ed. Chapter 133, Page 1003

- A. CMV
- B. West Nile virus
- C. Mumps
- D. EBV

The CSF glucose concentration is typically normal in viral infections, although it may be decreased in 10 to 30% of cases due to mumps as well as in cases due to LCMV.

3486. In CSF, lymphocytic pleocytosis with low glucose concentration should suggest which of the following?
Harrison's 20th Ed. Chapter 133, Page 1003

- A. Fungal meningitis
- B. Listerial meningitis
- C. Tuberculous meningitis
- D. All of the above

3487. In CSF, lymphocytic pleocytosis with low glucose concentration should suggest which of the following?

Harrison's 20th Ed. Chapter 133, Page 1003

A. Sarcoid
B. Neoplastic meningitis
C. Tuberculous meningitis
D. All of the above

As a rule, a lymphocytic pleocytosis with a low glucose concentration should suggest fungal, listerial, or tuberculous meningitis or noninfectious disorders (e.g., sarcoid, neoplastic meningitis).

3488. Which of the following is the most important method for diagnosing CNS viral infections?

Harrison's 20th Ed. Chapter 133, Page 1003

A. Neopterin
B. β2-microglobulin
C. LDH
D. PCR amplification of viral nucleic acid

Amplification of viral-specific DNA or RNA from CSF using PCR amplification is the single most important method for diagnosing CNS viral infections.

3489. At what temperature should CSF be stored for culture for diagnosis of viral infection (> 24 hours)?

Harrison's 20th Ed. Chapter 133, Page 1004

A. – 20 °C
B. – 40 °C
C. – 50 °C
D. – 70 °C

Beyond 24 hours, CSF specimens for viral isolation are stored in a (–)70°C freezer.

3490. Enteroviruses may be found in all except?

Harrison's 20th Ed. Chapter 133, Page 1004

A. Feces
B. Blood
C. Urine
D. Throat washings

Enteroviruses & adenoviruses may be found in feces, arboviruses & LCMV in blood, mumps & CMV, in urine and enteroviruses, mumps, and adenoviruses in throat washings.

3491. Serologic studies are a crucial diagnostic tool for which of the following viruses?

Harrison's 20th Ed. Chapter 133, Page 1004

A. West Nile virus (WNV)
B. HSV
C. VZV
D. CMV

For West Nile virus (WNV), serologic studies are a crucial diagnostic tool.

3492. Oligoclonal bands in CSF is not found in which of the following conditions?

Harrison's 20th Ed. Chapter 133, Page 1004

A. HIV infection
B. HSV infections
C. Subacute sclerosing panencephalitis (SSPE)
D. Progressive rubella panencephalitis

Oligoclonal bands in CSF are not seen with arbovirus, enterovirus, or HSV infections. But, seen in infections with HIV, HTLV type I, VZV, mumps, SSPE & progressive rubella panencephalitis.

3493. Oligoclonal bands are found in which of the following?

Harrison's 20th Ed. Chapter 133, Page 1004

A. Multiple sclerosis
B. Neurosyphilis
C. Lyme neuroborreliosis
D. All of the above

Oligoclonal bands are encountered in multiple sclerosis, neurosyphilis & Lyme neuroborreliosis.

3494. Which of the following viruses is the most common cause of viral meningitis?

Harrison's 20th Ed. Chapter 133, Page 1004

A. Enteroviruses
B. Arboviruses
C. Adenoviruses
D. HSV-2

3495. A case of viral meningitis with exanthemata, hand-foot-mouth disease, herpangina, pleurodynia, myopericarditis, and hemorrhagic conjunctivitis suggest the diagnosis of which infection?

Harrison's 20th Ed. Chapter 133, Page 1004

A. HSV-2 infection
B. EBV infection
C. LCMV infection
D. Enterovirus infection

Enteroviruses are the most common cause of viral meningitis. Occur in summer months, especially in children. Physical findings may include exanthemata, hand-foot-mouth disease, herpangina, pleurodynia, myopericarditis, and hemorrhagic conjunctivitis.

3496. A case of viral meningitis occuring in clusters during summer should prompt for infection with?

Harrison's 20th Ed. Chapter 133, Page 1004

A. HSV-2 infection
B. Arbovirus infection
C. LCMV infection
D. Enterovirus infection

Arbovirus infections typically occur in summer months and early fall, in both endemic & epidemic form, reflecting transmission through infected insect vectors. Arboviral meningitis should be considered when clusters of meningitis cases occur in a restricted geographic region during the summer or early fall.

3497. Which of the following arboviruses can cause meningitis & encephalitis?

Harrison's 20th Ed. Chapter 133, Page 1004

A. WNV
B. St. Louis encephalitis virus
C. California encephalitis group of viruses
D. All of the above

Most important causes of arboviral meningitis and encephalitis are WNV, St. Louis encephalitis virus and California encephalitis group of viruses.

3498. In WNV epidemics, which of the following may serve as sentinel infections for subsequent human disease?

Harrison's 20th Ed. Chapter 133, Page 1004

A. Avian deaths
B. Cattle deaths
C. Rodent deaths
D. All of the above

In WNV epidemics, avian deaths may serve as sentinel infections for subsequent human disease.

3499. 'Mollaret's meningitis' is due to?
Harrison's 20th Ed. Chapter 133, Page 1005

A. HIV
B. HSV
C. EBV
D. CMV

'Mollaret's meningitis' appear to be due to HSV.

3500. Which of the following viral infections commonly produces cranial nerve palsies?
Harrison's 20th Ed. Chapter 133, Page 1005

A. HIV
B. HSV
C. EBV
D. CMV

Cranial nerve palsies, most commonly involving cranial nerves V, VII or VIII are more common in HIV meningitis than in other viral infections.

3501. A case of viral meningitis along with orchitis, oophoritis, parotitis, pancreatitis should prompt for infection with?
Harrison's 20th Ed. Chapter 133, Page 1005

A. HSV-2 infection
B. Arbovirus infection
C. LCMV infection
D. Mumps infection

Mumps meningitis occurs in late winter or early spring, especially in males. The presence of orchitis, oophoritis, parotitis, pancreatitis, or elevations in serum lipase and amylase are suggestive of the diagnosis. Clinical meningitis occurs in 5% of patients with parotitis, but only 50% of patients with meningitis have associated parotitis. Mumps infection confers lifelong immunity, so a documented history of previous infection excludes this diagnosis.

3502. Aseptic meningitis occurring in winter, with a history of exposure to house mice excreta, leukopenia, thrombocytopenia and CSF pleocytosis suggest the diagnosis of which infection?
Harrison's 20th Ed. Chapter 133, Page 1005

A. HSV-2 infection
B. EBV infection
C. LCMV infection
D. Mumps

LCMV infection should be considered when aseptic meningitis occurs in late fall or winter, and in individuals with a history of exposure to house mice (Mus musculus) excreta, rash, pulmonary infiltrates, alopecia, parotitis, orchitis, or myopericarditis. Laboratory clues to the diagnosis of LCMV include leukopenia, thrombocytopenia, abnormal LFT, marked CSF pleocytosis (>1000 cells/µL) and hypoglycorrachia (<30%).

3503. A case of viral meningitis complicated by acute cerebellar ataxia should prompt for infection with?
Harrison's 20th Ed. Chapter 133, Page 1005

A. HSV-2 infection
B. Arbovirus infection
C. LCMV infection
D. VZV CNS infection

VZV meningitis should be suspected in the presence of concurrent chickenpox or shingles though up to 40% of VZV meningitis occur in the absence of rash. VZV can produce acute cerebellar ataxia. The syndrome of acute cerebellar ataxia and meningeal inflammation generally appears ~21 days after onset of the rash and rarely develops in the pre-eruptive phase.

3504. Acyclovir therapy is of benefit in patients with meningitis caused by?
Harrison's 20th Ed. Chapter 133, Page 1005

A. HSV-1 or -2
B. Severe EBV infection
C. Severe VZV infection
D. All of the above

Oral or intravenous acyclovir may be of benefit in patients with meningitis caused by HSV-1 or -2 and in cases of severe EBV or VZV infection.

Chronic and Recurrent Meningitis

3505. Chronic meningitis is diagnosed when?
Harrison's 20th Ed. Chapter 134, Page 1007
- A. > 4 weeks duration
- B. Persistent CSF WBC count > 5/μL
- C. Chronic & persistent or recurrent & discrete headache
- D. All of the above

3506. Which of the following can cause chronic meningitis?
Harrison's 20th Ed. Chapter 134, Page 1007
- A. Autoimmune inflammatory disorders
- B. Chemical meningitis
- C. Parameningeal infections
- D. All of the above

Five categories of disease cause most cases of chronic meningitis: meningeal infections, malignancy, autoimmune inflammatory disorders, chemical meningitis, and parameningeal infections.

3507. Which of the following is not a cardinal feature of chronic meningitis?
Harrison's 20th Ed. Chapter 134, Page 1007
- A. Hydrocephalus
- B. Radiculopathies
- C. Cognitive or personality changes
- D. All of the above

Persistent headache, hydrocephalus, cranial neuropathies, radiculopathies, and cognitive or personality changes are the cardinal features of chronic meningitis.

3508. Which of the following is best related to resorbption of CSF?
Harrison's 20th Ed. Chapter 134, Page 1007
- A. Choroid plexus
- B. Arachnoid villi
- C. Virchow-Robin spaces
- D. All of the above

CSF is produced by choroid plexus of cerebral ventricles, exits through narrow foramina into subarachnoid space surrounding brain & spinal cord, circulates around the base of brain and over cerebral hemispheres, and is resorbed by arachnoid villi projecting into superior sagittal sinus. Spread of infectious and other infiltrative processes from subarachnoid space into brain parenchyma may occur via the arachnoid cuffs that surround blood vessels that penetrate brain tissue (Virchow-Robin spaces).

3509. Recurrent meningitis is a feature of all except?
Harrison's 20th Ed. Chapter 134, Page 1008
- A. Vogt-Koyanagi-Harada syndrome
- B. Behçet's syndrome
- C. Wegener's granulomatosis
- D. Mollaret's meningitis

3510. Recurrent meningitis is a feature of?
Harrison's 20th Ed. Chapter 134, Page 1008
- A. Neurocysticercosis
- B. Drug hypersensitivity
- C. Syphilis
- D. Mumps

Exposure to ibuprofen, sulfonamides, isoniazid, tolmetin, ciprofloxacin, phenazopyridine lead to recurrent episodes with recurrent exposure. Improvement occurs after discontinuation of drug.

3511. Uveitis is a feature of?
Harrison's 20th Ed. Chapter 134, Page 1008
- A. Vogt-Koyanagi-Harada syndrome
- B. Sarcoid
- C. CNS lymphoma
- D. All of the above

Uveitis is a feature of Vogt-Koyanagi-Harada syndrome, sarcoid or CNS lymphoma.

3512. Iridocyclitis is a feature of?
Harrison's 20th Ed. Chapter 134, Page 1008
- A. Systemic lupus erythematosus
- B. CNS sarcoidosis
- C. Wegener's granulomatosis
- D. Behçet's syndrome

Iridocyclitis is a feature of Behçet's syndrome.

3513. Which of the following is a feature of Behçet's syndrome?
Harrison's 20th Ed. Chapter 134, Page 1008
- A. Aphthous oral lesions
- B. Genital ulcers
- C. Hypopyon
- D. All of the above

Aphthous oral lesions, genital ulcers and hypopyon suggest Behçet's syndrome.

3514. Fatal levels of raised ICP can occur without enlarged ventricles in?
Harrison's 20th Ed. Chapter 134, Page 1011
- A. Lyme disease
- B. CNS sarcoidosis
- C. Cryptococcal meningitis
- D. Chronic benign lymphocytic meningitis

In cryptococcal meningitis, fatal levels of raised ICP can occur without enlarged ventricles.

3515. Anti-Ro/SSA positivity is associated with?
Harrison's 20th Ed. Chapter 348, Page 2514
- A. Sensorineural hearing loss
- B. Raynaud's phenomenon
- C. Congenital heart block
- D. All of the above

Congenital heart block in newborn due to damage to developing conducting system of heart results from transfer of anti-Ro antibody from mother to child.

3516. Most useful empirical therapy for chronic meningitis is?
Harrison's 20th Ed. Chapter 134, Page 1013
- A. Antituberculous therapy
- B. Antifungal medication
- C. Glucocorticoids
- D. Ventricular-peritoneal shunt

Most useful empirical therapy for chronic meningitis is administration of glucocorticoids rather than antituberculous therapy.

Brain Abscess and Empyema

3517. Cerebritis is best related to?
Harrison's 20th Ed. Chapter 135, Page 1013

A. Encephalitis
B. Meningitis
C. Abscess
D. Thrombophlebitis

Focal bacterial, fungal or parasitic infections involving brain tissue are classified as either cerebritis or abscess, depending on the presence or absence of a capsule. When brain tissue is directly injured by a viral infection the disease is referred to as encephalitis.

3518. Which of the following is true for the capsule of a brain abscess?
Harrison's 20th Ed. Chapter 135, Page 1013

A. Fibrous
B. Vascularized
C. No capsule
D. All of the above

Brain abscess is a focal, suppurative infection within brain parenchyma, typically surrounded by a vascularized capsule. Term cerebritis refers to describe a nonencapsulated brain abscess.

3519. Predisposing conditions for brain abscess include?
Harrison's 20th Ed. Chapter 135, Page 1013

A. Paranasal sinusitis
B. Otitis media/mastoiditis
C. Dental infections
D. All of the above

Predisposing conditions for brain abscess include otitis media/mastoiditis, paranasal sinusitis, dental infections (direct contiguous spread); pyogenic infections (hematogenous spread); penetrating head trauma or neurosurgical procedures.

3520. In immunocompetent individuals the most common pathogen that causes brain abscess is?
Harrison's 20th Ed. Chapter 135, Page 1013

A. Streptococcus
B. Klebsiella
C. Staphylococcus
D. E. coli

3521. In immunocompromised hosts the most common pathogen that causes brain abscess is?
Harrison's 20th Ed. Chapter 135, Page 1013

A. Taenia solium
B. Mycobacterium tuberculosis
C. Nocardia
D. E. coli

In immunocompetent individuals the most important pathogens are Streptococcus spp., Enterobacteriaceae (Proteus spp., E. coli sp., Klebsiella spp.), anaerobes (Bacteroides spp., Fusobacterium spp.) and staphylococci. In immunocompromised hosts most brain abscesses are caused by Nocardia spp., Toxoplasma gondii, Aspergillus spp., Candida spp. and C. neoformans. In Latin America & in immigrants from Latin America, the most common cause of brain abscess is Taenia solium (neurocysticercosis). In India & East Asia, mycobacterial infection (tuberculoma) remains a major cause of focal CNS mass lesions.

3522. Otogenic abscesses occur predominantly in?
Harrison's 20th Ed. Chapter 135, Page 1013

A. Frontal lobe
B. Occipital lobe
C. Cerebellum
D. Pons

Otogenic abscesses occur predominantly in the temporal lobe (55–75%) and cerebellum (20 - 30%).

3523. Abscesses that develop as a result of dental infections are usually located in?
Harrison's 20th Ed. Chapter 135, Page 1013

A. Frontal lobe
B. Occipital lobe
C. Cerebellum
D. Pons

Abscesses that develop as a result of direct spread of infection from frontal, ethmoidal, or sphenoidal sinuses and those that occur due to dental infections are usually located in the frontal lobes.

3524. Which of the following is false about hematogenous brain abscesses?
Harrison's 20th Ed. Chapter 135, Page 1013

A. At the junction of gray & white matter
B. Predilection for MCA territory
C. Multiple
D. Encapsulated

Hematogenous abscesses account for ~25% of brain abscesses. Hematogenous abscesses are multiple, and multiple abscesses (50%) have a hematogenous origin. Hematogenous abscesses are poorly encapsulated.

3525. Late cerebritis stage is seen during?
Harrison's 20th Ed. Chapter 135, Page 1014

A. Days 1–3
B. Days 4–9
C. Days 10–13
D. Day 14 and beyond

3526. Which of the following is not a part of the classic clinical triad of brain abscess?
Harrison's 20th Ed. Chapter 135, Page 1014

A. Headache
B. Fever
C. Nuchal rigidity
D. Focal neurologic deficit

The classic clinical triad of brain abscess consists of headache, fever, and a focal neurologic deficit. Others include new onset of focal or generalized seizure activity, and focal neurologic deficits (hemiparesis, aphasia, or visual field defects). Presence of nuchal rigidity is unusual with brain abscess.

3527. Most common symptom of brain abscess is?
Harrison's 20th Ed. Chapter 135, Page 1014

A. Headache
B. Fever
C. Seizure
D. Focal neurologic deficit

Most common symptom in patients with a brain abscess is headache, occurring in >75% of patients.

3528. The clinical presentation of a brain abscess depends on?
Harrison's 20th Ed. Chapter 135, Page 1014

A. Its location
B. Nature of the primary infection, if present
C. Level of intracranial pressure (ICP)
D. All of the above

Clinical presentation of a brain abscess depends on its location, nature of the primary infection, if present, and the level of ICP.

3529. A temporal lobe abscess may present with?
Harrison's 20th Ed. Chapter 135, Page 1014

A. Hemiparesis
B. Upper homonymous quadrantanopia
C. Nystagmus
D. Ataxia

Hemiparesis is the most common localizing sign of a frontal lobe abscess. A temporal lobe abscess may present with a disturbance of language (dysphasia) or an upper homonymous quadrantanopia. Nystagmus & ataxia are signs of a cerebellar abscess. Signs of raised ICP (papilledema, nausea & vomiting, drowsiness or confusion) can be the dominant presentation of abscesses in cerebellum. Meningismus is not present unless abscess has ruptured into ventricle or infection has spread to subarachnoid space.

3530. When should a lumbar puncture performed in patients suspected of brain abscess?
Harrison's 20th Ed. Chapter 135, Page 1014

A. As early as possible
B. On day 3
C. On day 10
D. Should not be performed

LP should not be performed in those with known or suspected focal intracranial infections (abscess / empyema) as CSF analysis contributes nothing to diagnosis or therapy, & LP increases the risk of herniation.

3531. Conditions that can cause headache, fever, focal neurologic signs, and seizure activity include?
Harrison's 20th Ed. Chapter 135, Page 1014

A. Bacterial meningitis
B. Superior sagittal sinus thrombosis
C. Acute disseminated encephalomyelitis
D. All of the above

Conditions that can cause headache, fever, focal neurologic signs & seizures are brain abscess, subdural empyema, bacterial meningitis, viral meningoencephalitis, superior sagittal sinus thrombosis & acute disseminated encephalomyelitis.

3532. Medical therapy for treatment of brain abscess is for which of the following patients?
Harrison's 20th Ed. Chapter 135, Page 1015

A. Whose abscesses are neurosurgically inaccessible
B. Patients with small (<2–3 cm) abscesses
C. Patients with nonencapsulated abscesses (cerebritis)
D. All of the above

3533. All patients of brain abscess should receive parenteral antibiotic therapy for?
Harrison's 20th Ed. Chapter 135, Page 1015

A. A minimum of 2–4 weeks
B. A minimum of 4–6 weeks
C. A minimum of 6–8 weeks
D. A minimum of 8–12 weeks

All patients of brain abscess should receive a minimum of 6 - 8 weeks of parenteral antibiotic therapy.

3534. Anticonvulsant therapy is continued for at least how many months after resolution of brain abscess?
Harrison's 20th Ed. Chapter 135, Page 1015

A. 3
B. 6
C. 9
D. 12

Anticonvulsant therapy is continued for at least 3 months after resolution of the brain abscess.

3535. The mortality rate in patients of brain abscess is?
Harrison's 20th Ed. Chapter 348, Page 2514

A. <5%
B. <10%
C. <15%
D. <20%

The mortality rate in patients of brain abscess is <15%. Significant sequelae, including seizures, persisting weakness, aphasia, or mental impairment, occur in ≥20% of survivors.

3536. Most common parasitic disease of the CNS worldwide is?
Harrison's 20th Ed. Chapter 135, Page 1015

A. Neurocysticercosis
B. Toxoplasmosis
C. Schistosomiasis
D. Amebiasis

Neurocysticercosis is the most common parasitic disease of the CNS worldwide.

3537. Most common manifestation of neurocysticercosis is?
Harrison's 20th Ed. Chapter 135, Page 1015

A. New-onset partial seizures
B. New-onset generalized seizures
C. Focal neurologic deficit
D. Headache

Most common manifestation of neurocysticercosis is new-onset partial seizures with or without secondary generalization.

3538. Spinal cysticerci can mimic the presentation of?
Harrison's 20th Ed. Chapter 135, Page 1015

A. Chronic arachnoiditis
B. Cauda equina syndrome
C. Conus medullaris syndrome
D. Intraspinal tumors

Spinal cysticerci can mimic the presentation of intraspinal tumors.

3539. In MRI, lesions of neurocysticercosis with viable parasites appear as?
Harrison's 20th Ed. Chapter 135, Page 1015

A. Multiple lesions in the deep white matter
B. Nodular lesion surrounded by edema
C. Cystic lesions
D. Parenchymal brain calcifications

The lesions of neurocysticercosis with viable parasites appear as cystic lesions.

3540. In neurocysticercosis, a very early sign of cyst death is?
Harrison's 20th Ed. Chapter 135, Page 1015

A. Multiple lesions in the deep white matter
B. Hypointensity of vesicular fluid (T2) as compared to CSF
C. Nodular lesion surrounded by edema
D. Parenchymal brain calcifications

In neurocysticercosis, a very early sign of cyst death is hypointensity of the vesicular fluid on T2-weighted images when compared with CSF. Parenchymal brain calcifications are the most common finding and evidence that the parasite is no longer viable.

3541. Which of the following findings on neuroimaging calls for treatment with anticysticidal drugs?
Harrison's 20th Ed. Chapter 135, Page 1015

A. Cysticerci appearing as cystic lesions in brain
B. Cysticerci appearing as enhancing lesions in brain
C. Cysticerci appearing as enhancing lesions in subarachnoid space
D. All of the above

Cysticerci appearing as cystic lesions or as enhancing lesions in the brain parenchyma or in the subarachnoid space at the convexity of the cerebral hemispheres should be treated with anticysticidal therapy.

3542. Which of the following drug is used in the treatment of neurocysticercosis?
Harrison's 20th Ed. Chapter 135, Page 1015

A. Pentamidine isethionate
B. Pyrantel pamoate
C. Suramin
D. Praziquantel

Albendazole and praziquantel are used in the treatment of neurocysticercosis.

3543. The superior sagittal sinus drains into?
Harrison's 20th Ed. Chapter 135, Page 1018

A. Transverse sinus
B. Sigmoid sinus
C. Internal jugular vein
D. Cavernous sinus

Superior sagittal sinus drains into the transverse sinuses which becomes sigmoid sinus before draining into internal jugular vein.

3544. Which of the following communicates with the meningeal veins?
Harrison's 20th Ed. Chapter 135, Page 1018

A. Frontal superior cerebral veins
B. Parietal superior cerebral veins
C. Occipital superior cerebral veins
D. Diploic veins

Diploic veins, which drain into superior sagittal sinus, provide a route for the spread of infection from the meninges as they communicate with the meningeal veins.

3545. Which of the following can spread infection to the superior sagittal sinus?
Harrison's 20th Ed. Chapter 135, Page 1018

A. Bacterial meningitis
B. Subdural empyema (SDE)
C. Epidural abscess
D. All of the above

3546. Which of the following receive venous drainage from the middle ear and mastoid cells?
Harrison's 20th Ed. Chapter 135, Page 1018

A. Transverse sinus
B. Sigmoid sinus
C. Internal jugular vein
D. Cavernous sinus

3547. Which of the following sinuses is the most common site of primary infection resulting in septic cavernous sinus thrombosis?
Harrison's 20th Ed. Chapter 135, Page 1018

A. Frontal sinus
B. Maxillary sinus
C. Sphenoid sinus
D. All of the above

Sphenoid & ethmoid sinuses are the most common sites of primary infection resulting in septic cavernous sinus thrombosis.

3548. Which of the following does not pass through the cavernous sinus?
Harrison's 20th Ed. Chapter 135, Page 1018

A. III, IV & VI cranial nerves
B. Ophthalmic & maxillary branches of trigeminal nerve
C. Middle cerebral artery
D. Internal carotid artery

III, IV & VI and ophthalmic & maxillary branches of V cranial nerve, along with internal carotid artery pass through the cavernous sinus.

3549. Headache & earache are the most frequent symptoms of?
Harrison's 20th Ed. Chapter 135, Page 1018

A. Transverse sinus thrombosis
B. Internal jugular vein thrombosis
C. Superior sagittal sinus thrombosis
D. Cavernous sinus thrombosis

Headache and earache are the most frequent symptoms of transverse sinus thrombosis.

3550. Gradinego's syndrome is due to thrombosis in which of the following intracranial sinuses?
Harrison's 20th Ed. Chapter 135, Page 1018

A. Transverse sinus
B. Sigmoid sinus
C. Internal jugular vein
D. Cavernous sinus

Transverse sinus thrombosis may present with otitis media, sixth nerve palsy & retro-orbital or facial pain (Gradinego's syndrome).

3551. **Retro-orbital pain is a feature of?**

Harrison's 20th Ed. Chapter 135, Page 1018

- A. Viral meningitis
- B. Transverse sinus thrombosis
- C. Cavernous sinus thrombosis
- D. All of the above

Headache of viral meningitis is usually frontal or retroorbital and is often associated with photophobia & pain on eye movement. Retroorbital pain is also a feature of cluster headache, paroxysmal hemicrania, dengue, leptospirosis.

3552. **Pott's puffy tumor best relates to?**

Harrison's 20th Ed. Chapter 31, Page 210

- A. Frontal sinusitis
- B. Maxillary sinusitis
- C. Sphenoid sinusitis
- D. Ethmoid sinusitis

Patients with advanced frontal sinusitis can present with Pott's puffy tumor, with soft-tissue swelling & pitting edema over frontal bone from a communicating subperiosteal abscess.

Alcohol and Alcohol Use Disorders

3553. One typical alcohol drink produces blood levels of?
Harrison's 20th Ed. Chapter 445, Page 3278

A. ~ 10 mg/dL
B. ~ 20 mg/dL
C. ~ 30 mg/dL
D. ~ 40 mg/dL

Blood values of ~20 mg/dL result from ingestion of one typical drink.

3554. Which of the following is a congener in beverages?
Harrison's 20th Ed. Chapter 445, Page 3278

A. Methanol
B. Butanol
C. Acetaldehyde
D. All of the above

3555. Which of the following is a congener in beverages?
Harrison's 20th Ed. Chapter 445, Page 3278

A. Histamine
B. Iron
C. Lead
D. All of the above

Beverages have additional components called congeners that affect the drink's taste and might contribute to adverse effects on the body. Congeners include methanol, butanol, acetaldehyde, histamine, tannins, iron and lead.

3556. The major site of absorption of alcohol is?
Harrison's 20th Ed. Chapter 445, Page 3278

A. Mouth and esophagus
B. Stomach
C. Proximal small intestine
D. Large bowel

Alcohol is absorbed from mucous membranes of mouth & esophagus in small amounts, from stomach & large bowel in modest amounts. The major site of absorption is the proximal portion of small intestine.

3557. Alcohol is excreted directly through which of the following?
Harrison's 20th Ed. Chapter 445, Page 3278

A. Lungs
B. Urine
C. Sweat
D. All of the above

Between 2% and 10% of ethanol is excreted directly through lungs, urine, or sweat. Greater part is metabolized to acetaldehyde in liver.

3558. In liver, which of the following is responsible for metabolism of alcohol?
Harrison's 20th Ed. Chapter 445, Page 3278 Figure 445-1

A. Alcohol dehydrogenase (ADH)
B. Aldehyde dehydrogenase (ALDH)
C. Microsomal ethanol-oxidizing system (MEOS)
D. All of the above

Two pathways operate to metabolise alcohol in body. First pathway (~80%) occurs in cell cytosol where alcohol dehydrogenase (ADH) produces acetaldehyde, which is then rapidly destroyed by aldehyde dehydrogenase (ALDH) in cytosol and mitochondria to either Acetyl CoA or Acetate. Second pathway (~20%) is microsomal ethanol-oxidizing system or MEOS in smooth endoplasmic reticulum.

3559. Alcohol is devoid of which of the following?
Harrison's 20th Ed. Chapter 445, Page 3278

A. Minerals
B. Proteins
C. Vitamins
D. All of the above

Alcohol is devoid of nutrients such as minerals, proteins and vitamins.

3560. Alcohol affects levels of which of the following vitamins?
Harrison's 20th Ed. Chapter 445, Page 3278

A. Folate (folacin or folic acid)
B. Pyridoxine (B6)
C. Nicotinic acid (niacin, B3)
D. All of the above

Alcohol produces modest effects on folate (folacin or folic acid), pyridoxine (B6), thiamine (B1), nicotinic acid (niacin, B3) and vitamin A levels.

3561. Which of the following is false about alcohol ketoacidosis?
Harrison's 20th Ed. Chapter 445, Page 3278

A. Large anion gap
B. Increase in serum lactate
C. Increase in β-hydroxybutyrate/lactate ratio
D. None of the above

Alcohol ketoacidosis patients show an increase in serum ketones with mild increase in glucose but a large anion gap, a mild - moderate increase in serum lactate & increased β-hydroxybutyrate/lactate ratio of between 2:1 and 9:1 (normal 1:1).

3562. Intoxicating effect of alcohol is due to its action on?
Harrison's 20th Ed. Chapter 445, Page 3278

A. Neurotransmitters
B. Receptors
C. Transporters
D. All of the above

Intoxicating effect of alcohol is due to its action on several neurotransmitters, receptors & transporters.

3563. Alcohol affects which of the following neurochemical systems in the brain?
N Engl J Med. 2008;359:715-21

A. γ-aminobutyric acid (GABA)
B. Glutamate
C. Dopamine
D. All of the above

Neurochemical systems in brain influenced by alcohol are γ-aminobutyric acid (GABA), glutamate, dopamine, and opiate systems. GABA and glutamate are involved with alcohol stimulation, sedation, intoxication & many symptoms of alcohol withdrawal. Dopamine & opiate systems are involved with reinforcement, reward, some aspects of craving, sustained use of alcohol and potential relapse after prolonged abstinence in dependent person.

3564. Mutations in which of the following predisposes to the development of alcoholic liver disease?
Harrison's 20th Ed. Chapter 445, Page Table 335-1, N Engl J Med. 2018;378:270-80

A. Chromatin modifying protein 2B
B. Receptor expression enhancing protein 2
C. Patatin-like phospholipase domain-containing 3 (PNLAP3)
D. Patatin-like phospholipase domain-containing protein 6

Genetic mutations in patatin-like phospholipase domain-containing 3 (PNLAP3) & transmembrane 6 superfamily, member 2 (TM6SF2) predispose to the development of alcoholic liver disease/alcoholic cirrhosis.

3565. Which of the following is related to alcohol-use disorders?
N Engl J Med. 2008;359:715-21

A. Nucleus basalis of Meynert
B. Nucleus accumbens
C. Caudate nucleus
D. All of the above

Ethanol inhibits inhibitory neurons in midbrain ventral tegmental area (VTA) leading to increased dopamine release in nucleus accumbens. Blockade of dopamine in nucleus accumbens can terminate rewarding effects of addictive drugs.

3566. Which of the following is false about actions of alcohol?
Harrison's 20th Ed. Chapter 445, Page 3278

A. Alcohol inhibits GABA-A receptors
B. Alcohol inhibits NMDA receptors
C. Inhibition of uptake of adenosine
D. Increases synaptic serotonin levels

Alcohol acutely enhances actions at γ-aminobutyric acid A (GABA-A) receptors and inhibits N-methyl-D-aspartate (NMDA) excitatory glutamate receptors.

3567. Which of the following is false about actions of alcohol?
Harrison's 20th Ed. Chapter 445, Page 3278

A. Increases dopamine levels in ventral tegmentum
B. Increase in cortisol & adrenocorticotropic hormone (ACTH)
C. Release of beta endorphins
D. None of the above

3568. Which of the following is false about actions of alcohol?
Harrison's 20th Ed. Chapter 445, Page 3278

A. Increase in nicotinic acetylcholine system
B. Release of dopamine, GABA and glutamate in brain
C. Upregulation of serotonin receptors
D. None of the above

3569. A standard drink contains how many grams of ethanol?
N Engl J Med. 2013;368:365-73

A. 10 grams
B. 12 grams
C. 14 grams
D. 16 grams

A standard drink (12 oz of beer, 5 oz of wine, or 1.5 oz of 80-proof liquor) contains 14 grams of ethanol.

3570. "Legal intoxication" in USA requires a blood alcohol concentration of at least?
Harrison's 20th Ed. Chapter 445, Page 3279

A. 40 mg/dL
B. 80 mg/dL
C. 120 mg/dL
D. 160 mg/dL

"Legal intoxication" in USA requires a blood alcohol concentration of at least 80–100 mg/dL.

3571. Compensatory mechanism in alcohol tolerance is?
Harrison's 20th Ed. Chapter 445, Page 3279

A. Metabolic or pharmacokinetic tolerance
B. Cellular or pharmacodynamic tolerance
C. Learned or behavioral tolerance
D. All of the above

Alcohol tolerance involves compensatory mechanisms like metabolic or pharmacokinetic tolerance, cellular or pharmacodynamic tolerance and learned or behavioral tolerance.

3572. At low doses, alcohol can have which of the following beneficial effects?
Harrison's 20th Ed. Chapter 445, Page 3279

A. Decreased rates of myocardial infarction
B. Decreased rates of stroke
C. Decreased rates of gallstones
D. All of the above

Beneficial effects of low doses of alcohol are decreased rates of myocardial infarction, stroke, gallstones and vascular & Alzheimer's dementias.

3573. Health-promoting quality at low doses of red wine is due to?
Harrison's 20th Ed. Chapter 445, Page 3279

A. Flavinols
B. Dronabinol
C. Flavonoids
D. Aescin

3574. Which of the following occurs in chronic alcoholism?
Harrison's 20th Ed. Chapter 445, Page 3279

A. Episode of temporary anterograde amnesia
B. Deficiency in REM sleep
C. Exacerbation of sleep apnea
D. All of the above

Alcoholics may experience episodes of temporary anterograde amnesia (blackout), reduced rapid eye movement (REM) and deep sleep, exacerbated sleep apnea & prominent and disturbing dreams.

3575. Hangover syndrome consists of all except?
Harrison's 20th Ed. Chapter 445, Page 3279

A. Abdominal pain
B. Headache
C. Thirst
D. Fatigue

After heavy drinking, on the following day, hangover syndrome consists of headache, thirst, nausea, vomiting, and fatigue.

3576. Which of the following is a feature of Wernicke's syndrome?
Harrison's 20th Ed. Chapter 445, Page 3279

   A. Ophthalmoparesis
   B. Ataxia
   C. Encephalopathy
   D. All of the above

3577. Korsakoff's syndrome in alcoholics is due to the deficiency of?
Harrison's 20th Ed. Chapter 445, Page 3279

   A. Methionine
   B. Thiamine
   C. Tryptophan
   D. All of the above

3578. Korsakoff's syndrome in alcoholics is predisposed by the deficiency of?
Harrison's 20th Ed. Chapter 445, Page 3279

   A. Acetylketolase deficiency
   B. Paraketolase deficiency
   C. Transketolase deficiency
   D. Semiketolase deficiency

Wernicke's syndrome refers to ophthalmoparesis, ataxia & encephalopathy. Korsakoff's syndrome includes retrograde & anterograde amnesia. Both are due to thiamine deficiency, especially in those with transketolase deficiency.

3579. Alcohol-induced intense sadness is a component of?
Harrison's 20th Ed. Chapter 445, Page 3279

   A. Alcohol-induced mood disorder
   B. Alcohol-induced anxiety disorder
   C. Alcohol-induced psychotic disorder
   D. All of the above

3580. Alcohol can cause all except which of the following?
Harrison's 20th Ed. Chapter 445, Page 3280

   A. Impairs gluconeogenesis in liver
   B. Increases lactate production
   C. Increases oxidation of fatty acids
   D. Increases fat accumulation in liver cells

Alcohol impairs gluconeogenesis in liver, increases lactate production and decreases oxidation of fatty acids leading to increased fat accumulation in liver cells. Repeated exposure to ethanol leads to alcohol-induced hepatitis, perivenular sclerosis and cirrhosis.

3581. Alcohol increases the risk of which of the following cancer?
Harrison's 20th Ed. Chapter 445, Page 3280

   A. Breast cancer in women
   B. Oral and esophageal cancer
   C. Rectal cancer
   D. All of the above

Alcohol consumption increases risk of breast cancer (in women), oral, esophageal and rectal cancers.

3582. Alcohol is associated with increased risks of?
N Engl J Med. 2013;368:365-73

   A. Oropharyngeal carcinoma
   B. Esophageal carcinoma
   C. Breast carcinoma
   D. All of the above

Beverage alcohol is a carcinogen, and even light drinking is associated with increased risks of oropharyngeal, esophageal, and breast carcinomas.

3583. "Holiday heart" refers to?
Harrison's 20th Ed. Chapter 445, Page 3280

   A. Dilation of all heart chambers in chronic alcoholics
   B. Paroxysmal tachycardia after a drinking binge in individuals without heart disease
   C. Finding of >25% decrease in heart rarte at times of leisure
   D. Finding of >10% decrease in SBP at times of leisure

Atrial or ventricular arrhythmias, especially paroxysmal tachycardia, can occur after a drinking binge in individuals with no other evidence of heart disease (holiday heart syndrome").

3584. Features of 'Fetal alcohol syndrome' include all except?
Harrison's 20th Ed. Chapter 445, Page 3280

   A. Epicanthal eye folds
   B. Poorly formed concha
   C. Small teeth with faulty enamel
   D. Microglossia

3585. Features of 'Fetal alcohol syndrome' include all except?
Harrison's 20th Ed. Chapter 445, Page 3280

   A. Atrial or ventricular septal defect
   B. Aberrant palmar crease
   C. Polydactyly
   D. Microcephaly with mental retardation

Fetal alcohol syndrome (FAS) can include facial changes with epicanthal eye folds, poorly formed ear concha, small teeth with faulty enamel, cardiac atrial or ventricular septal defects, aberrant palmar crease & limitation in joint movement, and microcephaly with mental retardation.

3586. Polydactyly is a feature of?
Harrison's 20th Ed. Chapter 309, Page 2151

   A. Meckel-Gruber syndrome
   B. Bardet Biedl syndrome (BBS)
   C. Laurence-Moon syndrome
   D. All of the above

Other syndromes with a feature of polydactyly are Meckel-Gruber syndrome, Sensenbrenner's syndrome, Carpenter's syndrome, Bardet-Biedl syndrome (BBS), Laurence-Moon syndrome.

3587. Which of the following is a feature of fetal alcohol spectrum disorder (FASD)?
Harrison's 20th Ed. Chapter 445, Page 3280

   A. Low birth weight
   B. Lower IQ
   C. Hyperactive behavior
   D. All of the above

Features of fetal alcohol spectrum disorder (FASD) include low birth weight, a lower IQ, hyperactive behavior, and some modest cognitive deficits.

3588. Hormonal changes during heavy drinking include?
Harrison's 20th Ed. Chapter 445, Page 3280

   A. Increase in cortisol levels
   B. Inhibition of vasopressin secretion
   C. Decrease in serum triiodothyronine (T3)
   D. All of the above

Hormonal changes during heavy drinking include an increase in cortisol levels, inhibition of vasopressin secretion at rising blood alcohol concentrations & enhanced secretion at falling blood alcohol concentrations, reversible decrease in serum T4 and T3.

3589. How many life areas are included in defining alcohol use disorder (AUD)?

Harrison's 20th Ed. Chapter 445, Page 3280

A. 8
B. 9
C. 10
D. 11

Alcohol use disorder (AUD) is defined as repeated alcohol-related dificulties in at least 2 of 11 life areas that cluster together in the same 12 month period.

3590. What percentage of patients have an alcohol use disorder?

Harrison's 20th Ed. Chapter 445, Page 3281

A. 5%
B. 10%
C. 15%
D. 20%

3591. Blood tests useful in identifying individuals consuming six or more standard drinks per day include?

Harrison's 20th Ed. Chapter 445, Page 3281

A. γ-glutamyl transferase (GGT)
B. Carbohydrate-deficient transferrin (CDT)
C. Serum uric acid (>7 mg/dL)
D. All of the above

Laboratory tests that are likely to be abnormal in persons with regular alcohol consumption of 6 to 8 or more drinks per day are γ-glutamyl transferase (GGT) (>35 U), carbohydrate-deficient transferrin (CDT) (>20 U/L), high-normal MCVs (≥91 μm³) and serum uric acid (>7 mg/dL).

3592. Alcohol withdrawal symptoms peak in intensity on day?

Harrison's 20th Ed. Chapter 445, Page 3282

A. 1–2
B. 2–3
C. 3–4
D. 4–5

Alcohol withdrawal symptoms begin within 5–10 hours of decreasing ethanol intake, peak in intensity on day 2 or 3, and improve by day 4 or 5.

3593. Delirium in delirium tremens includes all except?

Harrison's 20th Ed. Chapter 445, Page 3282

A. Mental confusion
B. Agitation
C. Hallucinations
D. Fluctuating levels of consciousness

Delirium tremens (DTs) is a state of intense acute alcohol withdrawal. It includes delirium (mental confusion, agitation, and fluctuating levels of consciousness) associated with a tremor & autonomic overactivity (tachycardia, hypertension, and tachypnea).

3594. Medication helpful in alcoholic rehabilitation include?

Harrison's 20th Ed. Chapter 445, Page 3283

A. Naltrexone
B. Acamprosate
C. Disulfiram
D. All of the above

Naltrexone is a mu opioid receptor antagonist given in doses of 50–150 mg/day. It decreases activity in dopamine-rich ventral tegmental reward system. Acamprosate in doses of 2 gm/day inhibits the actions of NMDA receptors. Disulfiram (250 mg/day) is an ALDH inhibitor. It produces an unpleasant reaction in presence of alcohol due to rapidly rising blood levels of acetaldehyde. Other drugs under investigation are selective 5-HT3 receptor antagonist ondansetron, anticonvulsant topiramate, nalmefene (opioid receptor antagonist) and cannabinol receptor antagonist ramonibant.

3595. Which of the following drugs is an opioid antagonist?

Harrison's 20th Ed. Chapter 445, Page 3283

A. Varenicline
B. Baclofen
C. Nalmefene
D. Topiramate

Additional drugs under investigation for the alcohol rehabilitation treatment phase include opioid antagonist nalmefene, nicotinic receptor agonist varenicline, serotonin antagonist ondansetron, α-adrenergic agonist prazosin, GABA-B receptor agonist baclofen, anticonvulsant topiramate, and cannabinol receptor antagonists.

3596. Which of the following is a toxic alcohol?

N Engl J Med. 2018;378:270-80

A. Methanol
B. Isopropanol
C. Propylene glycol
D. All of the above

Toxic alcohols include methanol, ethylene glycol, isopropanol, diethylene glycol, and propylene glycol. Isopropanol is directly toxic while others exert toxic effects from their metabolites.

3597. Which of the following statements is false?

N Engl J Med. 2018;378:270-80

A. Methanol is metabolized to formic acid
B. Ethylene glycol is metabolized to oxalic and glycolic acid
C. Propylene glycol is metabolized to D-lactic and L-lactic acid
D. None of the above

Methanol is metabolized to formic acid,3 ethylene glycol to oxalic and glycolic acid,3 diethylene glycol to 2-hydroxyethoxyacetic acid and glycolic acid,4 and propylene glycol to D-lactic and L-lactic acid.

3598. Which of the following about alcohol dehydrogenase is false?

N Engl J Med. 2018;378:270-80

A. It catalyzes the first oxidation of toxic alcohols
B. Fomepizole is a strong inhibitor of alcohol dehydrogenase
C. Fomepizole has an affinity for alcohol dehydrogenase 8000 times that of ethanol
D. None of the above

3599. Poisoning with which of the following leads to formation of oxalate crystals?

N Engl J Med. 2018;378:270-80

A. Methanol
B. Isopropanol
C. Propylene glycol
D. Ethylene glycol

3600. Which of the following leads to elevation of osmolal or anion gap?

N Engl J Med. 2018;378:270-80

A. Ketoacidosis
B. Chronic kidney disease
C. Sick cell syndrome
D. All of the above

An elevated osmolal or anion gap does not always indicate toxic alcohol poisoning. Lactic acidosis, ketoacidosis, chronic kidney disease, and the sick cell syndrome all may increase both gaps.

ANSWERS

1. D	45. D	89. A	133. D	177. D	221. B
2. D	46. D	90. D	134. D	178. D	222. D
3. D	47. D	91. C	135. A	179. C	223. A
4. D	48. D	92. D	136. C	180. B	224. B
5. B	49. D	93. A	137. D	181. D	225. B
6. D	50. D	94. D	138. C	182. A	226. B
7. D	51. D	95. D	139. B	183. C	227. B
8. D	52. A	96. D	140. D	184. C	228. A
9. D	53. A	97. D	141. D	185. A	229. D
10. D	54. B	98. D	142. D	186. D	230. C
11. D	55. A	99. D	143. A	187. D	231. A
12. D	56. C	100. D	144. A	188. C	232. A
13. A	57. D	101. B	145. C	189. D	233. B
14. D	58. A	102. C	146. D	190. D	234. D
15. D	59. D	103. C	147. A	191. A	235. D
16. C	60. B	104. D	148. D	192. C	236. A
17. D	61. D	105. C	149. D	193. B	237. B
18. A	62. D	106. D	150. A	194. A	238. C
19. C	63. C	107. C	151. C	195. A	239. A
20. C	64. D	108. D	152. D	196. B	240. B
21. C	65. D	109. A	153. D	197. A	241. B
22. C	66. D	110. C	154. C	198. D	242. D
23. C	67. B	111. D	155. D	199. A	243. D
24. C	68. C	112. D	156. D	200. A	244. D
25. B	69. A	113. D	157. C	201. D	245. D
26. D	70. D	114. D	158. A	202. C	246. C
27. D	71. B	115. D	159. C	203. A	247. B
28. D	72. C	116. D	160. D	204. B	248. D
29. B	73. B	117. A	161. D	205. D	249. D
30. D	74. D	118. B	162. D	206. A	250. D
31. D	75. B	119. D	163. D	207. B	251. D
32. D	76. C	120. D	164. B	208. B	252. D
33. D	77. D	121. D	165. D	209. C	253. C
34. A	78. B	122. D	166. D	210. D	254. A
35. A	79. C	123. D	167. D	211. B	255. A
36. A	80. D	124. B	168. D	212. D	256. A
37. D	81. A	125. B	169. D	213. D	257. C
38. A	82. A	126. D	170. D	214. D	258. D
39. C	83. D	127. D	171. D	215. C	259. D
40. C	84. D	128. A	172. D	216. C	260. C
41. D	85. B	129. D	173. B	217. B	261. D
42. D	86. D	130. D	174. D	218. D	262. D
43. D	87. B	131. D	175. D	219. D	263. D
44. D	88. C	132. D	176. D	220. C	264. C

ANSWERS

265. C	309. A	353. D	397. B	441. D	485. A
266. A	310. C	354. A	398. B	442. A	486. D
267. A	311. C	355. D	399. A	443. B	487. D
268. A	312. A	356. B	400. D	444. D	488. D
269. C	313. D	357. D	401. C	445. D	489. D
270. A	314. B	358. D	402. D	446. C	490. C
271. C	315. B	359. D	403. B	447. B	491. C
272. A	316. C	360. B	404. D	448. A	492. D
273. D	317. C	361. C	405. D	449. D	493. D
274. D	318. C	362. A	406. A	450. D	494. A
275. D	319. D	363. D	407. D	451. D	495. A
276. C	320. D	364. D	408. B	452. D	496. C
277. C	321. D	365. D	409. A	453. C	497. D
278. D	322. A	366. D	410. B	454. C	498. D
279. D	323. C	367. D	411. C	455. D	499. C
280. A	324. D	368. D	412. D	456. D	500. B
281. D	325. D	369. D	413. D	457. C	501. A
282. D	326. D	370. D	414. C	458. D	502. D
283. D	327. B	371. D	415. D	459. D	503. B
284. C	328. C	372. A	416. D	460. D	504. C
285. C	329. B	373. D	417. D	461. D	505. D
286. D	330. C	374. D	418. C	462. C	506. A
287. A	331. B	375. D	419. A	463. A	507. B
288. A	332. D	376. A	420. D	464. D	508. D
289. A	333. D	377. D	421. A	465. C	509. D
290. D	334. D	378. D	422. D	466. D	510. D
291. B	335. D	379. D	423. B	467. D	511. B
292. A	336. C	380. B	424. D	468. C	512. C
293. B	337. C	381. C	425. B	469. A	513. C
294. C	338. C	382. A	426. D	470. D	514. D
295. A	339. D	383. D	427. D	471. A	515. D
296. D	340. D	384. A	428. D	472. D	516. C
297. C	341. C	385. A	429. D	473. D	517. D
298. C	342. D	386. C	430. C	474. A	518. D
299. A	343. C	387. D	431. B	475. D	519. B
300. B	344. D	388. B	432. D	476. B	520. B
301. A	345. D	389. D	433. D	477. D	521. C
302. C	346. A	390. A	434. D	478. A	522. D
303. D	347. B	391. D	435. D	479. C	523. D
304. B	348. C	392. A	436. D	480. D	524. B
305. C	349. D	393. B	437. D	481. D	525. B
306. D	350. B	394. A	438. B	482. D	526. A
307. D	351. C	395. C	439. C	483. C	527. B
308. D	352. D	396. D	440. D	484. A	528. D

ANSWERS

529. A	573. D	617. A	661. D	705. D	749. C
530. B	574. B	618. C	662. B	706. D	750. D
531. D	575. B	619. D	663. C	707. D	751. B
532. D	576. C	620. D	664. A	708. D	752. C
533. C	577. D	621. A	665. A	709. D	753. B
534. D	578. B	622. A	666. B	710. D	754. D
535. A	579. C	623. B	667. D	711. D	755. D
536. D	580. D	624. C	668. D	712. D	756. C
537. C	581. D	625. B	669. D	713. D	757. D
538. D	582. C	626. D	670. D	714. B	758. C
539. D	583. C	627. D	671. D	715. A	759. D
540. C	584. B	628. D	672. B	716. D	760. C
541. B	585. C	629. B	673. D	717. D	761. B
542. B	586. C	630. B	674. C	718. D	762. D
543. B	587. C	631. A	675. C	719. D	763. D
544. C	588. D	632. B	676. D	720. D	764. C
545. B	589. C	633. A	677. D	721. B	765. A
546. B	590. C	634. B	678. D	722. B	766. A
547. D	591. B	635. A	679. D	723. D	767. D
548. B	592. B	636. B	680. D	724. B	768. C
549. D	593. C	637. D	681. A	725. D	769. D
550. D	594. C	638. D	682. D	726. C	770. D
551. D	595. A	639. A	683. C	727. C	771. D
552. D	596. C	640. C	684. D	728. C	772. C
553. B	597. C	641. D	685. C	729. A	773. D
554. B	598. D	642. C	686. C	730. D	774. C
555. C	599. A	643. B	687. D	731. D	775. B
556. B	600. A	644. B	688. D	732. B	776. D
557. C	601. D	645. D	689. C	733. D	777. A
558. A	602. C	646. D	690. C	734. D	778. A
559. D	603. D	647. C	691. D	735. B	779. A
560. D	604. D	648. A	692. C	736. D	780. C
561. D	605. D	649. B	693. A	737. C	781. B
562. D	606. C	650. A	694. C	738. D	782. C
563. D	607. D	651. B	695. C	739. A	783. D
564. C	608. D	652. C	696. D	740. A	784. D
565. C	609. D	653. D	697. C	741. B	785. D
566. C	610. A	654. D	698. D	742. B	786. C
567. C	611. D	655. A	699. D	743. B	787. B
568. D	612. B	656. D	700. D	744. D	788. B
569. D	613. D	657. D	701. D	745. D	789. D
570. D	614. D	658. A	702. D	746. D	790. A
571. B	615. A	659. B	703. D	747. D	791. A
572. D	616. B	660. C	704. D	748. D	792. A

ANSWERS

793. C	837. D	881. C	925. D	969. D	1013. C
794. B	838. D	882. D	926. A	970. A	1014. D
795. D	839. D	883. B	927. B	971. D	1015. D
796. A	840. A	884. A	928. B	972. B	1016. D
797. D	841. C	885. D	929. D	973. C	1017. D
798. D	842. B	886. A	930. C	974. B	1018. D
799. D	843. B	887. D	931. B	975. C	1019. C
800. B	844. D	888. C	932. D	976. D	1020. D
801. C	845. A	889. C	933. A	977. D	1021. B
802. C	846. D	890. D	934. A	978. B	1022. B
803. C	847. A	891. D	935. D	979. D	1023. D
804. D	848. D	892. C	936. B	980. D	1024. A
805. D	849. C	893. D	937. D	981. D	1025. D
806. A	850. A	894. B	938. D	982. C	1026. A
807. D	851. B	895. D	939. D	983. C	1027. C
808. B	852. D	896. D	940. B	984. C	1028. C
809. B	853. A	897. D	941. C	985. C	1029. D
810. B	854. A	898. A	942. D	986. B	1030. A
811. A	855. C	899. A	943. A	987. D	1031. D
812. A	856. D	900. D	944. D	988. B	1032. D
813. D	857. A	901. D	945. D	989. A	1033. C
814. C	858. A	902. B	946. D	990. B	1034. B
815. D	859. D	903. A	947. C	991. B	1035. D
816. D	860. A	904. A	948. C	992. D	1036. C
817. D	861. C	905. B	949. D	993. D	1037. A
818. A	862. B	906. A	950. D	994. D	1038. D
819. B	863. D	907. A	951. D	995. C	1039. C
820. C	864. D	908. A	952. A	996. C	1040. D
821. D	865. D	909. D	953. C	997. A	1041. B
822. B	866. B	910. D	954. D	998. D	1042. A
823. D	867. C	911. C	955. C	999. D	1043. D
824. D	868. D	912. D	956. A	1000. D	1044. A
825. C	869. D	913. D	957. A	1001. B	1045. D
826. D	870. B	914. D	958. D	1002. D	1046. B
827. D	871. A	915. A	959. D	1003. C	1047. D
828. B	872. D	916. D	960. D	1004. C	1048. C
829. B	873. D	917. D	961. B	1005. D	1049. D
830. D	874. A	918. B	962. C	1006. D	1050. D
831. C	875. C	919. A	963. A	1007. B	1051. D
832. D	876. C	920. A	964. A	1008. D	1052. D
833. D	877. D	921. A	965. B	1009. D	1053. B
834. A	878. D	922. D	966. C	1010. C	1054. D
835. D	879. D	923. A	967. B	1011. C	1055. D
836. A	880. C	924. D	968. C	1012. C	1056. D

ANSWERS

1057. B	1101. D	1145. C	1189. A	1233. D	1277. D
1058. C	1102. B	1146. D	1190. D	1234. A	1278. B
1059. C	1103. B	1147. C	1191. B	1235. C	1279. A
1060. A	1104. A	1148. D	1192. B	1236. D	1280. D
1061. B	1105. D	1149. D	1193. C	1237. C	1281. D
1062. B	1106. D	1150. D	1194. C	1238. D	1282. C
1063. C	1107. A	1151. D	1195. A	1239. A	1283. D
1064. A	1108. A	1152. D	1196. B	1240. D	1284. A
1065. B	1109. B	1153. D	1197. D	1241. D	1285. C
1066. A	1110. B	1154. D	1198. D	1242. D	1286. D
1067. A	1111. B	1155. D	1199. D	1243. D	1287. C
1068. D	1112. D	1156. C	1200. C	1244. D	1288. C
1069. B	1113. D	1157. A	1201. D	1245. D	1289. C
1070. B	1114. B	1158. B	1202. C	1246. A	1290. D
1071. A	1115. D	1159. D	1203. C	1247. C	1291. D
1072. D	1116. B	1160. B	1204. D	1248. D	1292. D
1073. A	1117. B	1161. D	1205. A	1249. D	1293. D
1074. B	1118. C	1162. B	1206. D	1250. A	1294. D
1075. D	1119. C	1163. B	1207. D	1251. B	1295. A
1076. B	1120. A	1164. D	1208. D	1252. D	1296. A
1077. A	1121. D	1165. A	1209. A	1253. B	1297. C
1078. D	1122. C	1166. A	1210. C	1254. B	1298. D
1079. D	1123. C	1167. D	1211. B	1255. D	1299. D
1080. B	1124. D	1168. C	1212. D	1256. C	1300. D
1081. C	1125. B	1169. C	1213. D	1257. B	1301. C
1082. C	1126. C	1170. A	1214. D	1258. C	1302. D
1083. B	1127. B	1171. D	1215. D	1259. C	1303. D
1084. D	1128. C	1172. C	1216. D	1260. A	1304. B
1085. A	1129. D	1173. B	1217. D	1261. D	1305. D
1086. D	1130. B	1174. D	1218. A	1262. C	1306. C
1087. D	1131. C	1175. C	1219. D	1263. D	1307. C
1088. C	1132. B	1176. B	1220. D	1264. C	1308. B
1089. B	1133. A	1177. A	1221. A	1265. B	1309. D
1090. C	1134. A	1178. D	1222. D	1266. D	1310. B
1091. C	1135. A	1179. A	1223. C	1267. D	1311. D
1092. D	1136. A	1180. A	1224. A	1268. D	1312. A
1093. D	1137. B	1181. D	1225. D	1269. D	1313. D
1094. D	1138. B	1182. D	1226. B	1270. A	1314. D
1095. A	1139. A	1183. C	1227. C	1271. B	1315. C
1096. A	1140. B	1184. D	1228. A	1272. D	1316. D
1097. D	1141. D	1185. C	1229. B	1273. C	1317. D
1098. A	1142. B	1186. A	1230. B	1274. D	1318. D
1099. A	1143. D	1187. C	1231. B	1275. D	1319. A
1100. C	1144. B	1188. D	1232. D	1276. A	1320. A

ANSWERS

1321. D	1365. A	1409. C	1453. D	1497. C	1541. B
1322. C	1366. C	1410. D	1454. B	1498. D	1542. D
1323. D	1367. D	1411. C	1455. A	1499. D	1543. D
1324. D	1368. D	1412. C	1456. D	1500. D	1544. C
1325. D	1369. C	1413. D	1457. D	1501. A	1545. B
1326. D	1370. C	1414. D	1458. D	1502. D	1546. D
1327. A	1371. D	1415. D	1459. C	1503. D	1547. C
1328. D	1372. D	1416. A	1460. D	1504. D	1548. C
1329. A	1373. C	1417. D	1461. D	1505. B	1549. A
1330. B	1374. D	1418. B	1462. D	1506. D	1550. B
1331. D	1375. C	1419. A	1463. C	1507. D	1551. D
1332. D	1376. D	1420. B	1464. B	1508. C	1552. D
1333. D	1377. A	1421. B	1465. B	1509. D	1553. C
1334. D	1378. D	1422. A	1466. B	1510. B	1554. D
1335. D	1379. A	1423. C	1467. A	1511. D	1555. D
1336. D	1380. D	1424. C	1468. A	1512. D	1556. D
1337. D	1381. D	1425. B	1469. B	1513. C	1557. B
1338. D	1382. D	1426. D	1470. C	1514. A	1558. D
1339. D	1383. D	1427. D	1471. C	1515. D	1559. D
1340. D	1384. B	1428. C	1472. D	1516. C	1560. B
1341. D	1385. A	1429. B	1473. B	1517. C	1561. A
1342. A	1386. C	1430. D	1474. D	1518. C	1562. D
1343. A	1387. B	1431. A	1475. D	1519. D	1563. D
1344. D	1388. D	1432. D	1476. B	1520. B	1564. B
1345. D	1389. D	1433. D	1477. A	1521. D	1565. C
1346. D	1390. D	1434. B	1478. D	1522. D	1566. A
1347. D	1391. C	1435. C	1479. C	1523. D	1567. D
1348. C	1392. D	1436. A	1480. D	1524. B	1568. D
1349. D	1393. B	1437. C	1481. A	1525. D	1569. D
1350. A	1394. B	1438. B	1482. D	1526. D	1570. C
1351. D	1395. C	1439. D	1483. B	1527. D	1571. C
1352. C	1396. D	1440. B	1484. D	1528. C	1572. A
1353. C	1397. C	1441. D	1485. D	1529. D	1573. A
1354. A	1398. D	1442. D	1486. D	1530. D	1574. B
1355. D	1399. A	1443. C	1487. C	1531. D	1575. C
1356. B	1400. D	1444. D	1488. D	1532. D	1576. D
1357. C	1401. D	1445. A	1489. B	1533. A	1577. C
1358. D	1402. C	1446. D	1490. A	1534. C	1578. C
1359. D	1403. D	1447. D	1491. D	1535. B	1579. B
1360. C	1404. C	1448. D	1492. B	1536. C	1580. C
1361. A	1405. B	1449. B	1493. D	1537. D	1581. B
1362. C	1406. D	1450. D	1494. B	1538. C	1582. D
1363. A	1407. D	1451. D	1495. D	1539. D	1583. D
1364. D	1408. A	1452. D	1496. D	1540. A	1584. B

ANSWERS

1585. B	1629. D	1673. C	1717. D	1761. D	1805. C
1586. D	1630. B	1674. D	1718. D	1762. D	1806. D
1587. D	1631. D	1675. D	1719. B	1763. D	1807. D
1588. B	1632. C	1676. D	1720. C	1764. C	1808. C
1589. C	1633. D	1677. D	1721. D	1765. D	1809. A
1590. D	1634. C	1678. D	1722. D	1766. D	1810. D
1591. B	1635. C	1679. D	1723. B	1767. B	1811. D
1592. C	1636. D	1680. B	1724. D	1768. A	1812. A
1593. B	1637. B	1681. D	1725. D	1769. B	1813. A
1594. C	1638. D	1682. D	1726. D	1770. D	1814. D
1595. A	1639. B	1683. D	1727. B	1771. D	1815. C
1596. D	1640. D	1684. C	1728. D	1772. C	1816. B
1597. A	1641. C	1685. D	1729. C	1773. D	1817. C
1598. D	1642. B	1686. D	1730. B	1774. A	1818. D
1599. D	1643. B	1687. A	1731. D	1775. D	1819. D
1600. A	1644. D	1688. D	1732. C	1776. D	1820. B
1601. D	1645. D	1689. D	1733. C	1777. A	1821. C
1602. A	1646. C	1690. D	1734. A	1778. C	1822. D
1603. B	1647. B	1691. D	1735. C	1779. A	1823. D
1604. C	1648. B	1692. D	1736. A	1780. A	1824. C
1605. A	1649. B	1693. A	1737. A	1781. D	1825. C
1606. C	1650. B	1694. D	1738. A	1782. B	1826. B
1607. B	1651. A	1695. D	1739. D	1783. D	1827. D
1608. D	1652. A	1696. A	1740. D	1784. D	1828. D
1609. D	1653. D	1697. C	1741. D	1785. D	1829. D
1610. C	1654. C	1698. D	1742. D	1786. A	1830. D
1611. D	1655. D	1699. D	1743. D	1787. D	1831. D
1612. A	1656. D	1700. D	1744. D	1788. B	1832. D
1613. D	1657. A	1701. D	1745. D	1789. B	1833. D
1614. C	1658. B	1702. C	1746. C	1790. D	1834. A
1615. C	1659. B	1703. D	1747. C	1791. D	1835. A
1616. B	1660. C	1704. D	1748. D	1792. D	1836. D
1617. D	1661. C	1705. D	1749. B	1793. C	1837. D
1618. B	1662. D	1706. D	1750. D	1794. A	1838. A
1619. D	1663. D	1707. D	1751. B	1795. D	1839. C
1620. D	1664. C	1708. D	1752. C	1796. C	1840. D
1621. D	1665. C	1709. D	1753. C	1797. D	1841. C
1622. C	1666. D	1710. A	1754. D	1798. B	1842. D
1623. D	1667. D	1711. B	1755. D	1799. A	1843. D
1624. B	1668. D	1712. C	1756. A	1800. D	1844. C
1625. B	1669. D	1713. A	1757. A	1801. D	1845. C
1626. D	1670. B	1714. D	1758. D	1802. A	1846. D
1627. D	1671. A	1715. C	1759. B	1803. D	1847. D
1628. D	1672. D	1716. C	1760. B	1804. D	1848. D

ANSWERS

1849. D	1893. C	1937. D	1981. D	2025. D	2069. C
1850. A	1894. D	1938. D	1982. A	2026. D	2070. D
1851. C	1895. D	1939. C	1983. D	2027. C	2071. B
1852. D	1896. D	1940. B	1984. D	2028. D	2072. D
1853. D	1897. B	1941. D	1985. C	2029. D	2073. D
1854. C	1898. D	1942. A	1986. D	2030. B	2074. D
1855. C	1899. B	1943. D	1987. C	2031. B	2075. D
1856. B	1900. A	1944. D	1988. A	2032. D	2076. D
1857. D	1901. D	1945. D	1989. D	2033. C	2077. B
1858. D	1902. D	1946. D	1990. A	2034. C	2078. D
1859. D	1903. D	1947. C	1991. C	2035. C	2079. D
1860. B	1904. A	1948. B	1992. B	2036. D	2080. C
1861. D	1905. D	1949. D	1993. D	2037. D	2081. D
1862. A	1906. C	1950. B	1994. D	2038. D	2082. D
1863. B	1907. B	1951. A	1995. D	2039. C	2083. D
1864. C	1908. C	1952. A	1996. D	2040. A	2084. D
1865. A	1909. D	1953. D	1997. C	2041. D	2085. D
1866. B	1910. A	1954. B	1998. D	2042. C	2086. D
1867. C	1911. A	1955. B	1999. D	2043. D	2087. B
1868. B	1912. A	1956. D	2000. D	2044. D	2088. D
1869. D	1913. D	1957. D	2001. C	2045. A	2089. D
1870. D	1914. B	1958. B	2002. D	2046. A	2090. D
1871. A	1915. D	1959. B	2003. C	2047. B	2091. A
1872. D	1916. B	1960. A	2004. B	2048. D	2092. B
1873. D	1917. D	1961. D	2005. B	2049. D	2093. C
1874. C	1918. D	1962. D	2006. D	2050. B	2094. D
1875. B	1919. A	1963. C	2007. A	2051. A	2095. D
1876. D	1920. A	1964. D	2008. B	2052. D	2096. D
1877. D	1921. D	1965. D	2009. C	2053. C	2097. A
1878. B	1922. D	1966. B	2010. C	2054. D	2098. A
1879. B	1923. C	1967. B	2011. A	2055. D	2099. A
1880. C	1924. D	1968. C	2012. D	2056. C	2100. B
1881. B	1925. D	1969. D	2013. C	2057. D	2101. B
1882. C	1926. D	1970. A	2014. B	2058. B	2102. D
1883. D	1927. B	1971. D	2015. B	2059. A	2103. A
1884. D	1928. B	1972. B	2016. D	2060. D	2104. D
1885. B	1929. B	1973. D	2017. D	2061. C	2105. D
1886. C	1930. B	1974. D	2018. D	2062. B	2106. D
1887. C	1931. D	1975. A	2019. A	2063. C	2107. D
1888. D	1932. D	1976. D	2020. D	2064. D	2108. D
1889. C	1933. D	1977. D	2021. B	2065. D	2109. C
1890. B	1934. A	1978. C	2022. D	2066. C	2110. C
1891. D	1935. D	1979. A	2023. A	2067. C	2111. B
1892. C	1936. D	1980. A	2024. D	2068. C	2112. B

ANSWERS

2113. C	2157. C	2201. D	2245. B	2289. B	2333. A
2114. D	2158. B	2202. D	2246. C	2290. B	2334. A
2115. D	2159. C	2203. D	2247. D	2291. A	2335. A
2116. A	2160. B	2204. D	2248. A	2292. D	2336. A
2117. C	2161. D	2205. D	2249. B	2293. D	2337. D
2118. A	2162. D	2206. A	2250. C	2294. C	2338. C
2119. B	2163. D	2207. B	2251. D	2295. D	2339. C
2120. A	2164. D	2208. D	2252. A	2296. D	2340. B
2121. B	2165. D	2209. A	2253. B	2297. D	2341. B
2122. A	2166. A	2210. D	2254. C	2298. D	2342. C
2123. D	2167. A	2211. D	2255. A	2299. C	2343. B
2124. D	2168. D	2212. D	2256. B	2300. D	2344. B
2125. D	2169. D	2213. D	2257. C	2301. C	2345. B
2126. D	2170. D	2214. D	2258. D	2302. D	2346. A
2127. D	2171. B	2215. D	2259. A	2303. D	2347. D
2128. B	2172. B	2216. C	2260. A	2304. C	2348. D
2129. D	2173. D	2217. D	2261. D	2305. A	2349. D
2130. D	2174. C	2218. D	2262. D	2306. A	2350. B
2131. B	2175. C	2219. D	2263. C	2307. D	2351. D
2132. B	2176. C	2220. D	2264. A	2308. D	2352. B
2133. A	2177. D	2221. A	2265. A	2309. A	2353. A
2134. C	2178. C	2222. A	2266. D	2310. D	2354. C
2135. D	2179. C	2223. D	2267. C	2311. B	2355. D
2136. A	2180. D	2224. D	2268. B	2312. D	2356. D
2137. C	2181. B	2225. C	2269. D	2313. B	2357. B
2138. D	2182. D	2226. B	2270. D	2314. B	2358. C
2139. D	2183. B	2227. D	2271. D	2315. A	2359. C
2140. B	2184. D	2228. D	2272. D	2316. B	2360. B
2141. A	2185. D	2229. D	2273. D	2317. D	2361. A
2142. C	2186. C	2230. D	2274. B	2318. C	2362. A
2143. D	2187. C	2231. D	2275. D	2319. D	2363. D
2144. D	2188. C	2232. D	2276. D	2320. C	2364. D
2145. B	2189. C	2233. C	2277. B	2321. D	2365. D
2146. A	2190. B	2234. D	2278. D	2322. A	2366. D
2147. B	2191. B	2235. D	2279. D	2323. D	2367. D
2148. D	2192. D	2236. D	2280. D	2324. A	2368. C
2149. C	2193. D	2237. D	2281. C	2325. A	2369. D
2150. C	2194. A	2238. B	2282. D	2326. B	2370. D
2151. C	2195. D	2239. D	2283. D	2327. A	2371. D
2152. A	2196. D	2240. B	2284. D	2328. A	2372. A
2153. C	2197. B	2241. C	2285. A	2329. C	2373. A
2154. C	2198. D	2242. D	2286. A	2330. B	2374. A
2155. B	2199. D	2243. B	2287. B	2331. B	2375. B
2156. C	2200. D	2244. A	2288. A	2332. D	2376. A

ANSWERS

2377. C	2421. A	2465. B	2509. C	2553. B	2597. B
2378. D	2422. A	2466. D	2510. C	2554. D	2598. B
2379. D	2423. D	2467. C	2511. B	2555. D	2599. D
2380. A	2424. A	2468. D	2512. B	2556. D	2600. D
2381. D	2425. D	2469. D	2513. D	2557. D	2601. D
2382. D	2426. A	2470. A	2514. C	2558. D	2602. A
2383. D	2427. D	2471. A	2515. D	2559. D	2603. A
2384. D	2428. D	2472. B	2516. D	2560. C	2604. B
2385. C	2429. D	2473. C	2517. D	2561. D	2605. D
2386. D	2430. C	2474. D	2518. D	2562. A	2606. D
2387. B	2431. D	2475. D	2519. B	2563. A	2607. A
2388. A	2432. B	2476. D	2520. A	2564. A	2608. A
2389. D	2433. D	2477. D	2521. B	2565. D	2609. D
2390. B	2434. C	2478. C	2522. C	2566. D	2610. D
2391. A	2435. B	2479. C	2523. A	2567. C	2611. C
2392. D	2436. B	2480. B	2524. D	2568. C	2612. D
2393. B	2437. A	2481. D	2525. D	2569. D	2613. D
2394. B	2438. D	2482. A	2526. A	2570. C	2614. D
2395. B	2439. D	2483. A	2527. C	2571. D	2615. D
2396. D	2440. D	2484. B	2528. D	2572. D	2616. C
2397. D	2441. C	2485. D	2529. D	2573. D	2617. D
2398. C	2442. B	2486. C	2530. D	2574. D	2618. D
2399. D	2443. D	2487. C	2531. D	2575. D	2619. D
2400. D	2444. D	2488. D	2532. D	2576. C	2620. C
2401. D	2445. B	2489. D	2533. B	2577. D	2621. B
2402. D	2446. A	2490. C	2534. C	2578. D	2622. B
2403. D	2447. C	2491. B	2535. D	2579. D	2623. A
2404. B	2448. D	2492. D	2536. B	2580. D	2624. D
2405. D	2449. D	2493. D	2537. A	2581. D	2625. B
2406. D	2450. D	2494. D	2538. D	2582. D	2626. B
2407. D	2451. D	2495. D	2539. C	2583. D	2627. A
2408. D	2452. C	2496. D	2540. D	2584. D	2628. A
2409. A	2453. D	2497. D	2541. D	2585. B	2629. D
2410. B	2454. C	2498. B	2542. D	2586. D	2630. D
2411. D	2455. A	2499. A	2543. D	2587. C	2631. C
2412. D	2456. D	2500. D	2544. A	2588. B	2632. B
2413. D	2457. A	2501. D	2545. B	2589. B	2633. D
2414. B	2458. D	2502. D	2546. A	2590. D	2634. B
2415. A	2459. A	2503. A	2547. D	2591. B	2635. D
2416. B	2460. D	2504. D	2548. D	2592. D	2636. D
2417. D	2461. D	2505. A	2549. A	2593. D	2637. C
2418. B	2462. D	2506. B	2550. D	2594. A	2638. D
2419. B	2463. B	2507. B	2551. C	2595. D	2639. A
2420. D	2464. A	2508. A	2552. D	2596. D	2640. D

ANSWERS

2641. D	2685. B	2729. C	2773. C	2817. A	2861. B
2642. C	2686. C	2730. D	2774. B	2818. A	2862. B
2643. D	2687. A	2731. D	2775. D	2819. D	2863. B
2644. D	2688. A	2732. A	2776. D	2820. B	2864. D
2645. D	2689. C	2733. D	2777. D	2821. A	2865. B
2646. B	2690. D	2734. D	2778. D	2822. D	2866. B
2647. D	2691. D	2735. D	2779. C	2823. B	2867. D
2648. A	2692. D	2736. D	2780. B	2824. D	2868. C
2649. B	2693. D	2737. D	2781. C	2825. D	2869. D
2650. A	2694. B	2738. D	2782. C	2826. D	2870. C
2651. B	2695. D	2739. A	2783. B	2827. A	2871. D
2652. D	2696. C	2740. D	2784. D	2828. B	2872. D
2653. A	2697. D	2741. D	2785. B	2829. A	2873. D
2654. A	2698. A	2742. D	2786. B	2830. B	2874. C
2655. A	2699. C	2743. D	2787. D	2831. D	2875. D
2656. B	2700. D	2744. D	2788. D	2832. D	2876. D
2657. B	2701. A	2745. B	2789. C	2833. D	2877. C
2658. C	2702. C	2746. A	2790. D	2834. D	2878. D
2659. D	2703. D	2747. D	2791. D	2835. D	2879. A
2660. D	2704. D	2748. D	2792. B	2836. D	2880. B
2661. C	2705. D	2749. A	2793. D	2837. D	2881. D
2662. D	2706. C	2750. C	2794. D	2838. D	2882. D
2663. C	2707. D	2751. C	2795. D	2839. C	2883. D
2664. D	2708. B	2752. D	2796. C	2840. C	2884. D
2665. D	2709. B	2753. A	2797. B	2841. D	2885. D
2666. D	2710. A	2754. A	2798. B	2842. D	2886. D
2667. C	2711. D	2755. D	2799. D	2843. D	2887. D
2668. D	2712. D	2756. C	2800. D	2844. D	2888. D
2669. D	2713. D	2757. D	2801. B	2845. D	2889. D
2670. D	2714. D	2758. A	2802. D	2846. A	2890. C
2671. D	2715. A	2759. A	2803. D	2847. D	2891. D
2672. D	2716. D	2760. D	2804. B	2848. A	2892. D
2673. D	2717. D	2761. D	2805. D	2849. D	2893. D
2674. B	2718. D	2762. D	2806. D	2850. D	2894. D
2675. D	2719. D	2763. B	2807. D	2851. C	2895. B
2676. B	2720. B	2764. D	2808. A	2852. C	2896. C
2677. C	2721. B	2765. A	2809. B	2853. D	2897. D
2678. C	2722. C	2766. C	2810. A	2854. A	2898. D
2679. B	2723. D	2767. C	2811. C	2855. D	2899. D
2680. C	2724. A	2768. B	2812. B	2856. D	2900. C
2681. B	2725. C	2769. D	2813. B	2857. D	2901. C
2682. D	2726. D	2770. C	2814. A	2858. D	2902. D
2683. D	2727. D	2771. D	2815. A	2859. A	2903. D
2684. D	2728. C	2772. B	2816. D	2860. C	2904. D

ANSWERS

2905. B	2949. A	2993. C	3037. B	3081. A	3125. B
2906. D	2950. D	2994. A	3038. B	3082. C	3126. D
2907. C	2951. D	2995. D	3039. D	3083. D	3127. D
2908. D	2952. D	2996. B	3040. A	3084. B	3128. B
2909. B	2953. A	2997. C	3041. D	3085. D	3129. D
2910. C	2954. C	2998. A	3042. A	3086. D	3130. C
2911. C	2955. C	2999. D	3043. B	3087. A	3131. A
2912. C	2956. B	3000. C	3044. C	3088. B	3132. A
2913. D	2957. C	3001. A	3045. D	3089. B	3133. C
2914. A	2958. D	3002. D	3046. D	3090. B	3134. D
2915. D	2959. A	3003. A	3047. D	3091. D	3135. C
2916. C	2960. D	3004. D	3048. D	3092. D	3136. D
2917. C	2961. D	3005. C	3049. D	3093. D	3137. D
2918. C	2962. D	3006. D	3050. D	3094. B	3138. D
2919. B	2963. B	3007. D	3051. A	3095. D	3139. D
2920. B	2964. B	3008. C	3052. A	3096. C	3140. D
2921. A	2965. D	3009. C	3053. D	3097. A	3141. C
2922. B	2966. D	3010. B	3054. B	3098. C	3142. D
2923. B	2967. D	3011. D	3055. D	3099. C	3143. D
2924. B	2968. B	3012. D	3056. D	3100. D	3144. C
2925. A	2969. D	3013. D	3057. C	3101. C	3145. D
2926. D	2970. B	3014. D	3058. C	3102. D	3146. D
2927. D	2971. B	3015. D	3059. A	3103. D	3147. D
2928. D	2972. D	3016. A	3060. A	3104. D	3148. B
2929. D	2973. D	3017. D	3061. C	3105. A	3149. B
2930. A	2974. D	3018. A	3062. D	3106. A	3150. A
2931. D	2975. D	3019. D	3063. C	3107. D	3151. D
2932. D	2976. C	3020. B	3064. D	3108. D	3152. B
2933. D	2977. A	3021. D	3065. B	3109. D	3153. D
2934. C	2978. C	3022. D	3066. B	3110. D	3154. D
2935. A	2979. A	3023. B	3067. B	3111. A	3155. A
2936. B	2980. D	3024. B	3068. A	3112. B	3156. D
2937. C	2981. D	3025. A	3069. B	3113. B	3157. D
2938. A	2982. D	3026. A	3070. D	3114. D	3158. D
2939. D	2983. D	3027. B	3071. D	3115. B	3159. A
2940. A	2984. D	3028. A	3072. B	3116. B	3160. D
2941. D	2985. D	3029. A	3073. D	3117. D	3161. B
2942. D	2986. A	3030. D	3074. D	3118. D	3162. D
2943. D	2987. A	3031. C	3075. D	3119. D	3163. C
2944. D	2988. D	3032. B	3076. A	3120. D	3164. C
2945. D	2989. B	3033. D	3077. D	3121. D	3165. C
2946. C	2990. D	3034. D	3078. C	3122. D	3166. A
2947. B	2991. D	3035. D	3079. C	3123. D	3167. D
2948. C	2992. D	3036. D	3080. A	3124. D	3168. D

ANSWERS

3169. D	3213. D	3257. D	3301. A	3345. A	3389. A
3170. B	3214. C	3258. D	3302. A	3346. C	3390. C
3171. B	3215. D	3259. C	3303. D	3347. C	3391. C
3172. A	3216. C	3260. D	3304. C	3348. D	3392. D
3173. D	3217. D	3261. A	3305. A	3349. D	3393. D
3174. B	3218. B	3262. B	3306. A	3350. C	3394. D
3175. D	3219. B	3263. C	3307. C	3351. D	3395. A
3176. B	3220. C	3264. D	3308. D	3352. D	3396. B
3177. C	3221. A	3265. B	3309. D	3353. C	3397. C
3178. C	3222. B	3266. D	3310. D	3354. D	3398. D
3179. D	3223. B	3267. A	3311. D	3355. D	3399. B
3180. C	3224. C	3268. D	3312. D	3356. D	3400. C
3181. D	3225. A	3269. C	3313. B	3357. A	3401. B
3182. D	3226. D	3270. D	3314. D	3358. C	3402. D
3183. D	3227. B	3271. D	3315. A	3359. D	3403. D
3184. D	3228. D	3272. B	3316. D	3360. C	3404. D
3185. D	3229. D	3273. D	3317. A	3361. C	3405. D
3186. D	3230. D	3274. D	3318. D	3362. D	3406. C
3187. C	3231. A	3275. D	3319. C	3363. D	3407. C
3188. D	3232. A	3276. B	3320. C	3364. D	3408. D
3189. D	3233. D	3277. A	3321. D	3365. B	3409. D
3190. D	3234. D	3278. A	3322. D	3366. C	3410. A
3191. D	3235. D	3279. B	3323. B	3367. B	3411. D
3192. D	3236. D	3280. D	3324. D	3368. A	3412. D
3193. C	3237. B	3281. C	3325. D	3369. C	3413. A
3194. D	3238. A	3282. A	3326. B	3370. C	3414. D
3195. A	3239. A	3283. C	3327. C	3371. C	3415. C
3196. D	3240. C	3284. A	3328. B	3372. C	3416. C
3197. B	3241. A	3285. D	3329. D	3373. D	3417. A
3198. A	3242. C	3286. A	3330. D	3374. C	3418. C
3199. B	3243. B	3287. D	3331. C	3375. A	3419. C
3200. A	3244. D	3288. B	3332. D	3376. D	3420. C
3201. B	3245. D	3289. B	3333. A	3377. B	3421. D
3202. B	3246. D	3290. A	3334. D	3378. D	3422. D
3203. D	3247. A	3291. C	3335. C	3379. B	3423. C
3204. D	3248. A	3292. B	3336. D	3380. D	3424. B
3205. A	3249. A	3293. B	3337. D	3381. C	3425. D
3206. D	3250. D	3294. B	3338. C	3382. C	3426. A
3207. B	3251. D	3295. B	3339. A	3383. B	3427. D
3208. D	3252. A	3296. B	3340. A	3384. D	3428. D
3209. C	3253. A	3297. A	3341. A	3385. A	3429. B
3210. A	3254. B	3298. D	3342. C	3386. D	3430. D
3211. D	3255. B	3299. C	3343. D	3387. D	3431. B
3212. D	3256. B	3300. B	3344. C	3388. D	3432. C

ANSWERS

3433. D	3461. B	3489. D	3517. C	3545. D	3573. A
3434. B	3462. A	3490. C	3518. B	3546. A	3574. D
3435. B	3463. C	3491. A	3519. D	3547. C	3575. A
3436. C	3464. D	3492. B	3520. A	3548. C	3576. D
3437. D	3465. D	3493. D	3521. C	3549. A	3577. B
3438. D	3466. A	3494. A	3522. C	3550. A	3578. C
3439. B	3467. D	3495. D	3523. A	3551. D	3579. A
3440. D	3468. D	3496. B	3524. D	3552. A	3580. C
3441. C	3469. D	3497. D	3525. B	3553. B	3581. D
3442. D	3470. A	3498. A	3526. C	3554. D	3582. D
3443. C	3471. C	3499. B	3527. A	3555. D	3583. B
3444. D	3472. B	3500. A	3528. D	3556. C	3584. D
3445. D	3473. D	3501. D	3529. B	3557. D	3585. C
3446. D	3474. D	3502. C	3530. D	3558. D	3586. D
3447. B	3475. C	3503. D	3531. D	3559. D	3587. D
3448. D	3476. D	3504. D	3532. D	3560. D	3588. D
3449. D	3477. D	3505. D	3533. C	3561. D	3589. D
3450. D	3478. B	3506. D	3534. A	3562. D	3590. D
3451. D	3479. C	3507. D	3535. C	3563. D	3591. D
3452. D	3480. C	3508. B	3536. A	3564. C	3592. B
3453. A	3481. D	3509. C	3537. A	3565. B	3593. C
3454. C	3482. C	3510. B	3538. D	3566. A	3594. D
3455. D	3483. C	3511. D	3539. C	3567. D	3595. C
3456. A	3484. C	3512. D	3540. B	3568. D	3596. D
3457. B	3485. C	3513. D	3541. D	3569. C	3597. D
3458. D	3486. D	3514. C	3542. D	3570. B	3598. D
3459. D	3487. D	3515. C	3543. A	3571. D	3599. D
3460. D	3488. D	3516. C	3544. D	3572. D	3600. D